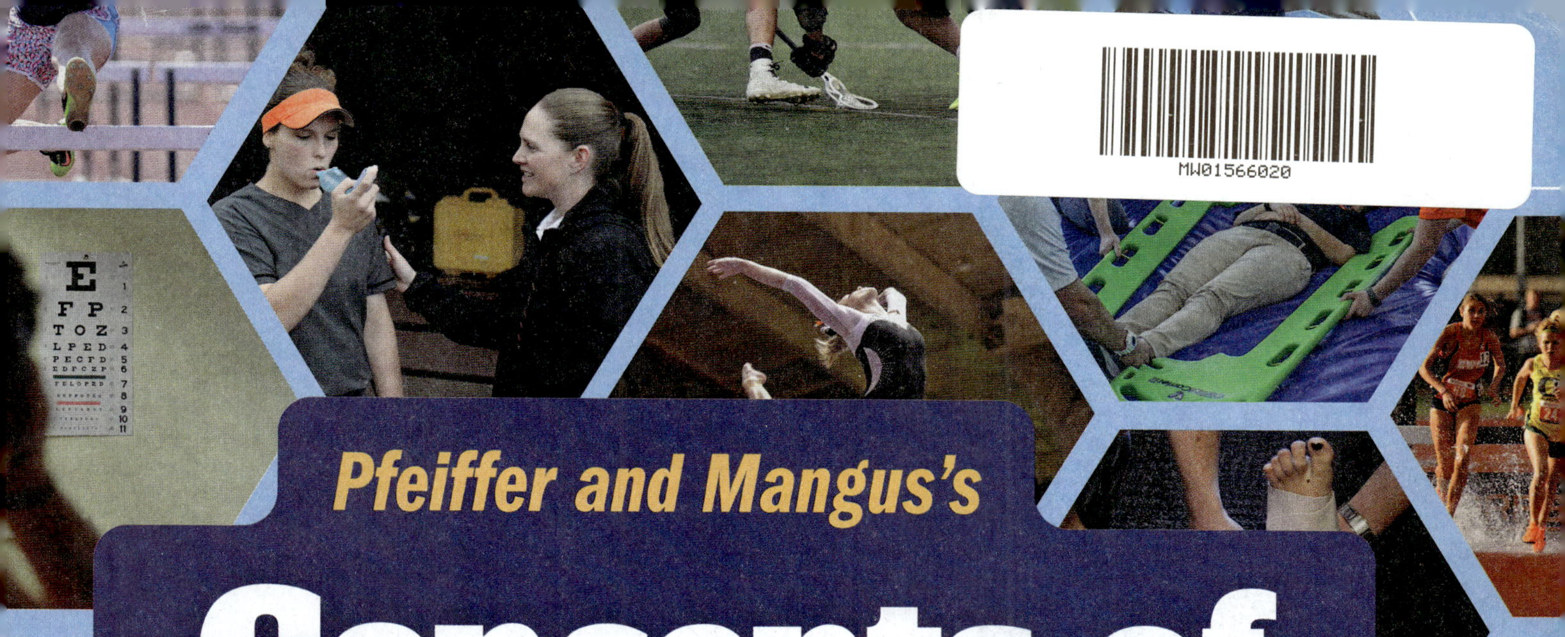

Pfeiffer and Mangus's
Concepts of Athletic Training

EIGHTH EDITION

Cynthia A. Trowbridge, PhD, LAT, ATC, CSCS
Associate Professor, Department of Kinesiology
University of Texas at Arlington
Arlington, Texas

Cheryl M. Ferris, PhD, LAT, ATC, LMT
Lucia Health, LLC
Certified Bowenwork® Practitioner
Tensegrity Medicine™ Practitioner
Pittsburgh, Pennsylvania

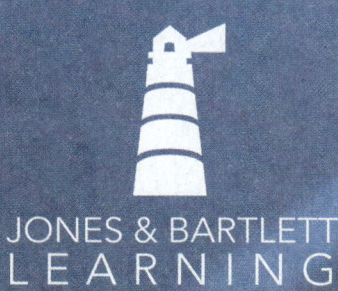

JONES & BARTLETT
LEARNING

World Headquarters
Jones & Bartlett Learning
25 Mall Road
Burlington, MA 01803
978-443-5000
info@jblearning.com
www.jblearning.com

Jones & Bartlett Learning books and products are available through most bookstores and online booksellers. To contact Jones & Bartlett Learning directly, call 800-832-0034, fax 978-443-8000, or visit our website, www.jblearning.com.

Substantial discounts on bulk quantities of Jones & Bartlett Learning publications are available to corporations, professional associations, and other qualified organizations. For details and specific discount information, contact the special sales department at Jones & Bartlett Learning via the above contact information or send an email to specialsales@jblearning.com.

Copyright © 2023 by Jones & Bartlett Learning, LLC, an Ascend Learning Company

All rights reserved. No part of the material protected by this copyright may be reproduced or utilized in any form, electronic or mechanical, including photocopying, recording, or by any information storage and retrieval system, without written permission from the copyright owner.

The content, statements, views, and opinions herein are the sole expression of the respective authors and not that of Jones & Bartlett Learning, LLC. Reference herein to any specific commercial product, process, or service by trade name, trademark, manufacturer, or otherwise does not constitute or imply its endorsement or recommendation by Jones & Bartlett Learning, LLC and such reference shall not be used for advertising or product endorsement purposes. All trademarks displayed are the trademarks of the parties noted herein. *Pfeiffer and Mangus's Concepts of Athletic Training, Eighth Edition* is an independent publication and has not been authorized, sponsored, or otherwise approved by the owners of the trademarks or service marks referenced in this product.

There may be images in this book that feature models; these models do not necessarily endorse, represent, or participate in the activities represented in the images. Any screenshots in this product are for educational and instructive purposes only. Any individuals and scenarios featured in the case studies throughout this product may be real or fictitious but are used for instructional purposes only.

This publication is designed to provide accurate and authoritative information in regard to the Subject Matter covered. It is sold with the understanding that the publisher is not engaged in rendering legal, accounting, or other professional service. If legal advice or other expert assistance is required, the service of a competent professional person should be sought.

12752-2

Production Credits
Vice President, Product Management: Marisa R. Urbano
Vice President, Product Operations: Christine Emerton
Director, Product Management: Matthew Kane
Product Manager: Whitney Fekete
Director, Content Management: Donna Gridley
Manager, Content Strategy: Carolyn Pershouse
Content Strategist: Carol Brewer Guerrero
Content Coordinator: Samantha Gillespie
Director, Project Management and Content Services: Karen Scott
Manager, Project Management: Jackie Reynen
Project Manager: Kelly Mahoney
Senior Digital Project Specialist: Angela Dooley
Director, Marketing: Andrea DeFronzo
Content Services Manager: Colleen Lamy
VP, Manufacturing and Inventory Control: Therese Connell
Composition: Exela Technologies
Cover Design: Kristin E. Parker
Senior Media Development Editor: Troy Liston
Rights & Permissions Manager: John Rusk
Rights Specialist: Maria Leon Maimone
Cover Image (Title Page, Section Opener): © Kameleon007/iStock/Getty Images Plus/Getty Images; Courtesy of Mark Hoffman.
Printing and Binding: LSC Communications

Library of Congress Cataloging-in-Publication Data
Names: Trowbridge, Cynthia A., author. | Ferris, Cheryl M., author. | Pfeiffer, Ronald P. Concepts of athletic training.
Title: Pfeiffer's concepts of athletic training / Cynthia Trowbridge, Cheryl M. Ferris.
Other titles: Concepts of athletic training
Description: Eighth edition. | Burlington, MA: Jones & Bartlett Learning, [2021] | Preceded by: Concepts of athletic training / Ronald Pfeiffer. Seventh edition. [2015] | Includes bibliographical references and index. | Summary: "Pfeiffer's Concepts of Athletic Training focuses on the care and management of sport- and activity-related injuries while presenting key concepts in a comprehensive, logically sequential manner that will assist future professionals in making the correct decisions when confronted with an activity-related injury or illness in their scope of practice. The eighth edition of Pfeiffer's Concepts of Athletic Training features new, full-color presentation as well as deeper and updated coverage on topics"– Provided by publisher.
Identifiers: LCCN 2021053238 | ISBN 9781284127300 (paperback)
Subjects: MESH: Athletic Injuries–therapy | Sports Medicine–methods | BISAC: SPORTS & RECREATION / Coaching / General
Classification: LCC RD97 | NLM QT 261 | DDC 617.1/027–dc23/eng/20211124
LC record available at https://lccn.loc.gov/2021053238

6048

Printed in the United States of America
26 25 24 23 22   10 9 8 7 6 5 4 3 2 1

Brief Contents

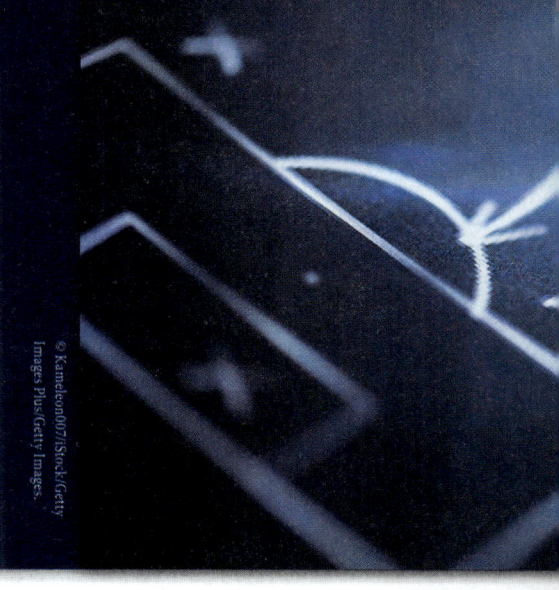

Preface	xvii
How to Use This Book	xxi
Acknowledgments	xxv
Reviewers	xxvii
Chapter 1 The Concept of Sports Injury	1
Chapter 2 The Athletic Healthcare Team	37
Chapter 3 The Law of Sports Injury	51
Chapter 4 Sports-Injury Prevention	65
Chapter 5 The Psychology of Athletes and Sports Injury	89
Chapter 6 Nutritional Considerations	109
Chapter 7 Emergency Plan and Initial Injury Evaluation	151
Chapter 8 The Injury and Healing Processes	169

Chapter 9	Injuries to the Head, Neck, and Face	191
Chapter 10	Injuries to the Thoracic Through Coccygeal Spine	247
Chapter 11	Injuries to the Shoulder Region	261
Chapter 12	Injuries to the Wrist, Arm, and Hand	285
Chapter 13	Injuries to the Thorax and Abdomen	321
Chapter 14	Injuries to the Hip and Pelvis	339
Chapter 15	Injuries to the Thigh, Leg, and Knee	353
Chapter 16	Injuries to the Lower Leg, Ankle, and Foot	379
Chapter 17	Skin Conditions in Sports	409
Chapter 18	Environmental Injuries and Athletics	431
Chapter 19	General Medical Concerns for Athletes	461
Chapter 20	Special Medical Concerns for the Adolescent Athlete	487
Glossary of Terms		507
Index		523

Contents

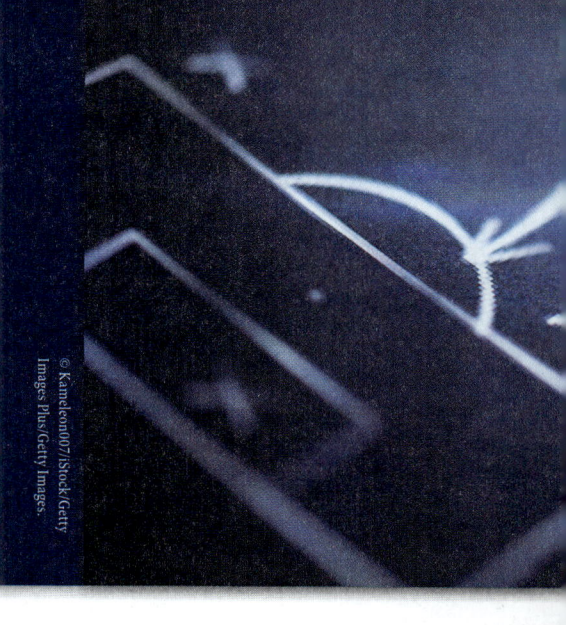

Preface		xvii
How to Use This Book		xxi
Acknowledgments		xxv
Reviewers		xxvii
Chapter 1	**The Concept of Sports Injury**	**1**
	Youth Sports and Fitness Participation	1
	Definition of Sports Injury	4
	Injury Classifications	8
	Sprains	9
	Strains	9
	Contusions	10
	Fractures	10
	Dislocations	13
	Injury Recognition	14
	Epidemiology of Sports Injury	14
	Classification of Sports	15
	Extent of the Injury Problem: Epidemiology Reports	18
	Tackle Football	18
	Basketball	20
	Baseball and Softball	21
	Wrestling	23
	Volleyball	24

	Soccer	25
	Gymnastics	27
	Cheerleading	27
	Recurrent Injuries	28
Youth Sport Specialization		29
Review Questions		31
References		32

Chapter 2 The Athletic Healthcare Team — 37

Sports Medicine		38
Key Members of the Team		39
	Coaches	39
	Team Physician	39
	BOC-Certified Athletic Trainer	40
Settings of Employment for the Practice of Athletic Training		43
	Colleges and Universities	44
	Secondary Schools	45
	Clinics and Hospitals	46
	AT Salaries	46
Importance of Athletic Training Services for Youth Athletes		46
AHCT at the Secondary School Level		47
Review Questions		49
References		50

Chapter 3 The Law of Sports Injury — 51

Ethics of Sports-Injury Care	52
The Concept of Tort	54
What Is the Physical Educator's or Coach's Liability?	56
Are Coaches and Physical Educators Protected?	58
How to Reduce the Chances of Going to Court	59
What Coaches or Physical Educators Can Do If They Are Sued	61
Role of the AT	62
Review Questions	63
Recommended Reading	63
References	63

| Chapter 4 | Sports-Injury Prevention | 65 |

- Causative Factors in Injury — 66
- Intervention Strategies — 67
  - Extrinsic Factors — 67
  - Intrinsic Factors — 69
- Sport-Specific Injury Prevention Considerations — 82
  - Overuse Injuries — 82
- Review Questions — 85
- References — 85

| Chapter 5 | The Psychology of Athletes and Sports Injury | 89 |

- Psychology of Competition — 89
  - Competitive Stress and the Athlete — 89
  - Personality Variables and Competition — 91
- Psychology of Injury — 91
  - Personality Traits and Injury — 91
  - Psychosocial Variables and Injury — 92
  - Psychological Stress and Injury — 92
- Psychology of the Injured Athlete — 93
  - Recommendations — 95
- Mental Health Concerns — 95
  - Mood Disorders — 95
  - Anxiety Disorders — 98
  - Behavioral Disorders — 98
  - Anorexia Nervosa and Bulimia Nervosa — 100
  - Research of Eating Habits — 101
  - Sport Specificity and Eating Disorders — 101
  - Prevention — 102
  - Treatment — 103
  - Neurodevelopmental Disorders — 103
- Plan to Manage Mental Health Concerns and Role of Care Provider — 104
- Review Questions — 105
- References — 106

Chapter 6 Nutritional Considerations — 109

Nutrients: An Overview — 110
- Energy Expenditure — 110
- Weight Loss — 111
- Energy Systems — 113
- Carbohydrate — 113
- Protein — 116
- Fat — 118
- Vitamins — 121
- Minerals — 123
- Water — 126

Special Considerations — 129
- Female Athletes — 129
- Endurance Athletes — 129
- Strength/Power Athletes — 130
- Team Sport Athletes — 131
- Wrestling — 132
- Conclusions — 134

Nutritional Knowledge of Athletes and Coaches: What the Research Shows — 135
- Educating Athletes: What Can the Coach Do? — 135

General Dietary Guidelines for Athletes — 136
- Daily Diet: Nutritional Maintenance — 136
- Precompetition Diets — 138
- Nutrition During Competition — 138
- Postexercise Nutrition — 138
- Nutrition and Injury Recovery — 139
- Managing Body Weight — 140

Ergogenic Aids — 142
- Nutritional Ergogenic Aids — 145
- Pharmacological Ergogenic Aids: Stimulants and Anabolic-Androgenic Substances — 146

Review Questions — 148
References — 149

Chapter 7 Emergency Plan and Initial Injury Evaluation — 151

Emergency Team — 153
Best Practices for Emergency Planning for Athletics — 154
- Institution-Based Athletics — 154
- Youth Sports–Based Athletics — 154

Emergency Care Training	**155**
Injury Evaluation Procedures	156
Initial Responders' Limitations	157
Assessment of the Injured Athlete: Scene Safety	**158**
Assessment of the Injured Athlete: Initial Check and Physical Exam	**158**
Initial Check (Primary Assessment)	159
Physical Exam (Secondary Assessment)	162
Return to Play	**165**
Review Questions	**166**
References	**167**

Chapter 8 The Injury and Healing Processes — 169

The Physics of Sports Injury	**169**
The Physiology of Sports Injury	**171**
Inflammatory Response Phase	172
Fibroblastic Repair Phase	176
Maturation and Remodeling Phase	178
Pain and Acute Injury	**178**
Intervention Procedures	**180**
Cryotherapy and Thermotherapy	181
Pharmacological Agents	184
Role of Exercise Rehabilitation	**186**
Review Questions	**187**
References	**188**

Chapter 9 Injuries to the Head, Neck, and Face — 191

Anatomy Review	**192**
Skull	192
The Meninges	192
Central Nervous System	194
Peripheral Nervous System	**194**
Face	195
Neck (Cervical Spine)	195
Head Injuries in Sports	**195**
Background Information	195
Mechanism of Injury and Type	197
Concussion	198
Postconcussive Syndrome	200

Second Impact Syndrome	200
Intracranial Injury	201
Cranial Injury	203

Initial Treatment of a Suspected Head Injury, Including Sports-Related Concussion: Guidelines — 203

Consensus Statements Regarding Concussion Management	204
Baseline Concussion Screening	205
Initial Assessment for Head Injury	208
Physical Examination	209

Cervical Spine Injuries — 218

Background Information	218
Mechanisms of Injury	219
Brachial Plexus Injuries	221
Sprains	222
Strains	222
Fractures and Dislocations	222

Initial Management of a Suspected Cervical Spine Injury: Guidelines — 224

Prehospital Care for the Treatment of Head and Neck Injuries in Football — 226

Injuries to the Maxillofacial Region — 231

Dental Injuries	232
Eye Injuries	234
Nose Injuries	237
Fractures of the Face (Non-Nasal)	239
Wounds of the Facial Region	239

Review Questions — 240
References — 241

Chapter 10 Injuries to the Thoracic Through Coccygeal Spine 247

Anatomy Review of the Thoracic Spine — 247
Common Sports Injuries for the Thoracic Spine and Thoracic Cage — 248

Skeletal Injuries	249
Sprains	251
Strains	251
Thoracic Outlet Syndrome	251
Intervertebral Disk Injuries in Thoracic Vertebrae	253

Anatomy Review of the Lumbar, Sacral, and Coccygeal
Regions of the Spine — 253
Common Sports Injuries — 254
- Sprains and Strains — 255
- Lumbar Disk Injuries — 256
- Spondylolysis and Spondylolisthesis — 257
- Traumatic Fractures — 257
- Sacral and Coccyx Injuries — 258

Review Questions — 258
References — 259

Chapter 11 Injuries to the Shoulder Region — 261

Anatomy Review — 261
Common Sports Injuries — 267
- Skeletal Injuries — 267
- Soft-Tissue Injuries — 269

Review Questions — 282
References — 283

Chapter 12 Injuries to the Wrist, Arm, and Hand — 285

Anatomy Review — 285
Soft-Tissue Injuries to the Upper Arm — 286
- Myositis Ossificans Traumatica — 288
- Biceps Brachii Injuries — 289
- Triceps Brachii Injuries — 291

Fractures of the Upper Arm/Humerus — 291
Elbow Injuries — 293
- Elbow Sprains and Dislocations — 294
- Elbow Fractures — 295
- Epicondylitis of the Elbow — 296
- Osteochondritis Dissecans of the Elbow — 299
- Contusions of the Elbow — 300

Wrist and Forearm Injuries — 300
- Wrist Fractures — 302
- Wrist Sprains and Dislocations — 303
- Nerve Injuries to the Wrist — 304
- Unique Tendon Problems of the Wrist — 306

	Hand Injuries	**307**
	Hand Fractures	308
	Sprains, Dislocations, and Muscle Avulsions of the Hand	310
	Wrist and Thumb Taping	**314**
	Review Questions	**317**
	References	**318**
Chapter 13	**Injuries to the Thorax and Abdomen**	**321**
	Anatomy Review	**321**
	Internal Organs	**322**
	Common Sports Injuries	**323**
	External Injuries	325
	Internal Injuries	327
	Review Questions	**336**
	References	**336**
Chapter 14	**Injuries to the Hip and Pelvis**	**339**
	Anatomy Review	**339**
	Common Sports Injuries	**343**
	Skeletal Injuries	343
	Soft-Tissue Injuries	346
	Prevention	**350**
	Review Questions	**351**
	References	**351**
Chapter 15	**Injuries to the Thigh, Leg, and Knee**	**353**
	Anatomy Review	**353**
	Common Sports Injuries	**357**
	Skeletal Injuries	357
	Soft-Tissue Injuries to the Thigh	358
	Patellofemoral Joint Injuries	362
	Patellofemoral Conditions	366
	Menisci Injuries	366
	Knee Ligament Injuries	367
	Prevention	**373**
	Knee Bracing	374

	Review Questions	376
	References	376

Chapter 16 Injuries to the Lower Leg, Ankle, and Foot — 379

Anatomy Review — 379
Common Sports Injuries — 383
- Skeletal Injuries — 383
- Soft-Tissue Injuries — 384
- Foot Disorders — 394

Preventive Ankle Taping — 400
Review Questions — 405
References — 405

Chapter 17 Skin Conditions in Sports — 409

Traumatic Skin Conditions — 410
- Wounds — 410
- Friction Blisters — 413
- Calluses and Corns — 413
- Talon or Tâche Noir — 414

Skin Inflammatory Conditions — 414
- Contact Dermatitis — 414
- Poison (Plants) Allergy — 414
- Latex Allergy — 415
- Ultraviolet Light–Related Skin Problems — 415

Exacerbation Skin Conditions — 416
- Acne Mechanica — 416
- Urticaria — 416

Skin Infections — 416
- Fungus — 417
- Bacterial Infections — 418
- Viral Infections — 422
- Parasites — 424
- Wrestling and Skin Infections — 426

Role of the Care Provider — 426
Review Questions — 428
References — 428

Chapter 18   Environmental Injuries and Athletics — 431

Heat-Related Conditions — 431
- Exertional Heat Illnesses — 434
- Prevention of Exertional Heat Illnesses — 440
- Heat Illness Prevention — 441

Cold-Related Conditions — 449
- Hypothermia — 451
- Frostbite and Frostnip — 452
- Chilblain and Immersion (Trench) Foot — 453
- Cold Urticaria — 454

Altitude-Related Conditions — 454
- Altitude Sickness or Acute Mountain Sickness — 455
- High Altitude Pulmonary Edema — 455
- High Altitude Cerebral Edema — 455
- Treatment and Prevention of Altitude Illnesses — 456

Lightning — 456
- Lightning Safety — 457
- Lightning Treatment — 457

Review Questions — 457
References — 458

Chapter 19   General Medical Concerns for Athletes — 461

Exercise and the Immune Response — 461
- Respiratory Infections — 462
- Gastrointestinal Infections — 464
- Other Infectious Diseases — 465

Allergies — 469
Asthma — 469
- Exercise-Induced Asthma — 470
- Exercise-Induced Bronchospasm — 472

The Athlete With Sickle Cell Trait — 472
Exertional Rhabdomyolysis — 473
Athletes With Diabetes — 475
- Blood Sugar 101 — 477
- Blood Sugar and Exercise — 478
- Pregame or Exercise Plan — 479
- During Game or Exercise Plan — 480

Postgame or Exercise Plan	480
Blood Sugar and the Environment	480
Miscellaneous Issues	481
Epilepsy and Sports Participation	481
Review Questions	484
References	484

Chapter 20 Special Medical Concerns for the Adolescent Athlete — 487

Youth Sports in America	488
Factors in Youth Sports Participation	488
Epidemic of Youth Sports Injury	489
The Growing Athlete	490
Prepubescence	490
Puberty	491
Injury Mechanisms	492
Ligament Injuries	492
Tendon and Bone Injuries	492
Growth Plate Injuries	494
Growth Cartilage	494
Contributors to Injury	495
Intrinsic Factors	496
Extrinsic Factors	496
Injury Imitators	498
Oncological Considerations	499
Rheumatological Considerations	499
Infectious Considerations	499
Neurovascular Considerations	499
Psychological Considerations	500
Strength Training	500
Safety	501
Lat Pulldown	502
Bench Press	502
Military Press	502
Squats	502
Prevention of Injury	503
Preparticipation Physical Examination	503
Treatment and Rehabilitation of Injuries	503

	Stretching Programs	503
	Coaching Techniques	503
	Female Athletes	504
	Prescription Stimulant Medications	504
Review Questions		504
References		505

Glossary of Terms 507

Index 523

Preface

Over 60 million youth (ages 6–17 years) participate in some form of organized sports in the United States and over 28 million participate in a team sport (McKay, Cumming, & Blake, 2019). There are many benefits to sports participation, including improved physical health, better behavior, higher self-esteem, stronger peer and familial relationships, and improved attendance and academic performance. However, injury is a natural concern because sport injuries are the second leading cause of emergency department visits for children and adolescents. Therefore, governing bodies of school and youth recreational sports need to focus on the prevention, care, and management of injuries related to physical activity, and this requires a team approach with a variety of professionals. This team includes medical providers as well as coaches, administrators, personal trainers, and parents. Medical providers may not always be present at all practices and competitions, so coaches and others need to be trained and informed regarding initial injury care because they may be the first responders to a sport injury. There are many qualified medical providers who can serve within the medical portion of the team; however, Board of Certification (BOC)–certified athletic trainers (ATs) play a vital role because they are most often present for the continuum of a sport injury, including prevention, recognition, immediate care, management, treatment, and rehabilitation. Collaboration from team members is the key for success, and it begins with education and understanding.

The target audience for *Pfeiffer and Mangus's Concepts of Athletic Training* includes anyone planning a career as a coach, physical educator, or personal trainer as well as current or future parents of young athletes. The primary goal of this book is the prevention, care, and management of sport- and physical activity–related injuries because treatment and rehabilitation are mostly performed by qualified medical providers. To make correct decisions, these personnel must be properly trained not only in basic first aid but also in more advanced knowledge to properly manage injuries that are complicated by sports equipment and personal protective equipment, such as helmets, face masks, and mouth guards. This eighth edition is also excellent for high school or undergraduate college students who are interested in a career as an AT. The general field of sports medicine continues to be a rapidly evolving field of study, and the content will form a solid foundation for more advanced studies in this exciting and constantly evolving allied health field.

New to This Edition

The authors have made every effort to update critical material throughout the text with best practice evidence to make the content as current as possible. This latest edition includes considerable updates in sports injury epidemiology and careers in athletic training (Chapter 1, *The Concept of Sports Injury*, and Chapter 2, *The Athletic Healthcare Team*); proper prevention strategies, including emergency planning (Chapter 7, *Emergency Plan and Initial Injury Evaluation*); legal issues (Chapter 3, *The Law of Sports Injury*); and preparticipation physical exams and strength training and periodization techniques (Chapter 4, *Sports-Injury Prevention*); in addition to updated information on the importance of nutrition in injury prevention (Chapter 6, *Nutritional Considerations*). Response to injury, including the coach's or physical educator's initial decisions and subsequent actions, is critical in determining the outcome of an injury. Therefore, significant updates have been added to chapters that focus on the nature of injury and healing (Chapter 8, *The Injury and Healing Processes*); injuries to the head, neck, face, and mouth (Chapter 9, *Injuries to the Head, Neck, and Face*); upper and lower extremities (Chapter 11, *Injuries to the Shoulder Region*; Chapter 12, *Injuries to the Arm, Wrist, and Hand*; Chapter 14, *Injuries to the Hip and Pelvis*; Chapter 15, *Injuries to the Thigh, Leg, and Knee*; and Chapter 16, *Injuries to the Lower Leg, Ankle, and Foot*); skin (Chapter 17, *Skin Conditions in Sports*); and the low back, thorax, and abdomen (Chapter 10, *Injuries to the Thoracic Through Coccygeal Spine*, and Chapter 13, *Injuries to the Thorax and Abdomen*). Because the majority of sport- and activity-related injuries involve the musculoskeletal system, much of this text's content is devoted to the recognition, immediate care, and management of injuries such as sprains, strains, dislocations, and fractures in the extremities. To help coaches and physical educators provide proper advice for the home management of musculoskeletal injuries, Chapter 8, *The Injury and Healing Processes*, includes the latest information regarding the treatment of inflammation and controversies about using ice or heat for injury treatment. Fortunately, only a small percentage of sports- and activity-related injuries are life threatening or result in permanent disability. However, deaths and permanent disability tragically continue to be an outcome in a small percentage of cases. Most of these injuries are related to trauma to the head or neck or are heat related. Detailed information on head and neck injuries, as well as prevention of heat disorders, is provided in Chapter 9, *Injuries to the Head, Neck, and Face*, and Chapter 18, *Environmental Injuries and Athletics*. These chapters have been updated based on recent publications on the recognition, treatment, and disposition of concussions, neck injuries, and heat illness. New information on cardiac concerns, diabetes, exercise-induced asthma, epilepsy, and sickle cell crisis is also included in Chapter 19, *General Medical Concerns for Athletes*, because coaches and physical educators may be the first to respond to these incidents and proper recognition and activation of an emergency action plan is essential. This newest edition also includes vital information related to the psychology of sports participation and injury (Chapter 5, *The Psychology of Athletes and Sport Injury*). Advice on recognizing symptoms of overspecialization and directions for referral of youth who may be experiencing psychological issues related to sports participation, sports injury, or undue pressure from caregivers is included.

Because coaches and physical educators are often responsible for adolescent athletes, this latest edition continues to feature a chapter devoted to the adolescent athlete (Chapter 20, *Special Medical Concerns for the Adolescent Athlete*). The rationale for this is simple: The vast majority of school-aged athletes (grades 7–12) are, in fact, adolescents or even preadolescents. As such, they represent an anatomically and physiologically distinct population when compared to adult athletes. These differences must be recognized and considered by coaching personnel and parents when making decisions regarding not only injury management but also when designing and implementing injury prevention programs.

What Is Not Included and Why

Our text does not include detailed information on more advanced techniques associated with athletic training, including muscle assessments, rehabilitation techniques, and complex taping and wrapping skills. These procedures clearly fall outside the scope of practice for a coach, physical education teacher, or personal trainer. Because we have targeted this text to these populations, we feel it would be irresponsible to introduce students to clinical skills they should not attempt to execute in the field. Besides, students who complete a Commission on Accreditation of Athletic Training Education (CAATE)–accredited athletic training program will receive extensive training in many advanced skills within a professional degree program and through mentoring from clinical instructors.

Conclusion

This book is a vital resource for personnel who might be involved in providing first aid or emergency care for sports injuries, such as physical education teachers, coaches, and athletic training student aides. The content of this text will provide instructors and students with a wealth of information on topics related to the recognition, care, and prevention of sports injuries. The goal, of course, is to give coaching and teaching personnel the necessary knowledge and critical thinking skills to recognize and differentiate minor from more serious sports injuries. Once decisions are made regarding the nature of the injury, appropriate first aid care and medical referral can be instituted.

Reference

McKay, C. D., Cumming S. P., & Blake, T. (2019). Youth sport: Friend or foe? *Best Practice & Research Clinical Rheumatology, 33,* 141–157.

How to Use This Book

Major Concepts sections provide an introduction that sets the stage for each chapter and an overview of what is to come.

What If? features are real-world scenarios that encourage students to work on critical decision-making skills. These sections provide information typically available to coaching personnel when confronted with an injury-related problem. Applications range from simple decision-making practice sessions to role-playing exercises in the classroom.

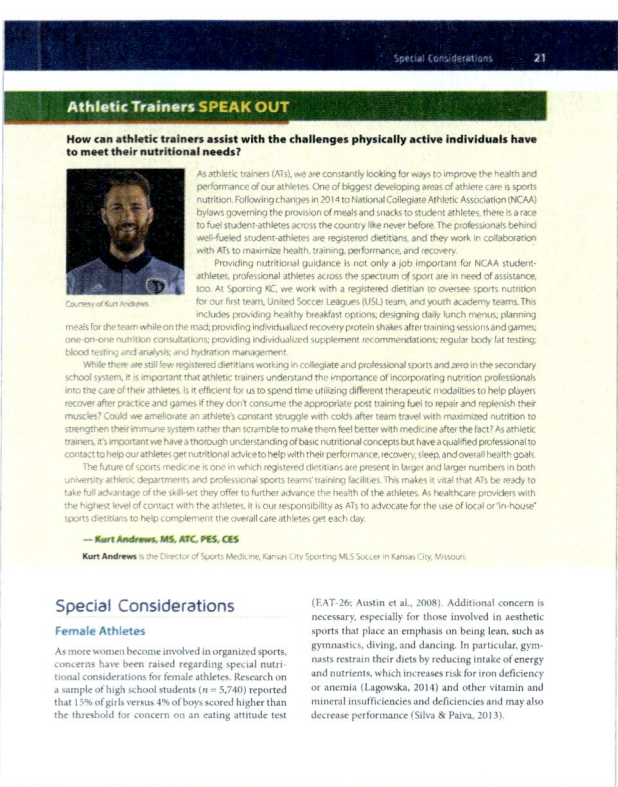

Athletic Trainers Speak Out boxes feature a different athletic trainer in every chapter who discusses an element of athlete care and injury prevention.

Time Out boxes provide additional information related to the text, such as National Athletic Trainers' Association (NATA) Athletic Helmet Removal Guidelines, guidelines for working with an injured athlete, how to recognize the signs of concussion, and much more.

How to Use This Book   xxiii

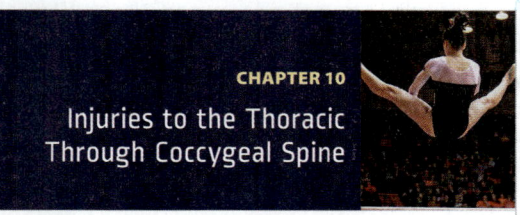

All relevant chapters begin with an **Anatomy Review** to introduce body parts to students unfamiliar with human anatomy and provide a refresher for others who may have taken past anatomy courses.

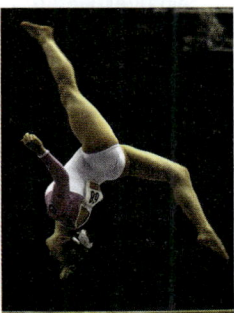

Key terms are bolded within the text and defined in boxes to help students quickly identify and understand new terms.

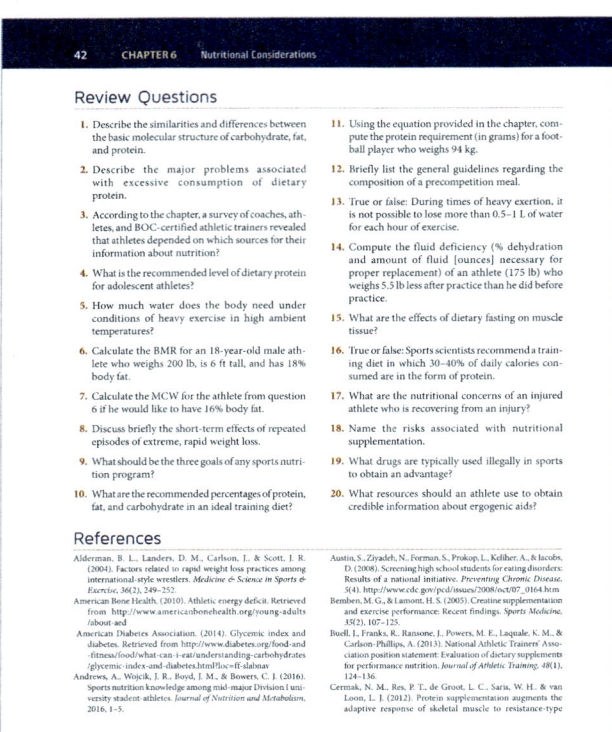

Each chapter closes with **Review Questions**, which continue to engage students in a thoughtful review of important chapter material.

Integrated Teaching and Learning Package

Each new purchase of this textbook includes an access code to Navigate Advantage, which includes the following resources.

For Instructors

- Slides in PowerPoint format
- Instructor Manual
- Lecture Outlines
- Test Bank in LMS-compatible formats
- Answer Key to practice quizzes
- Answer Key to crossword puzzles
- Image Bank

For Students

- Interactive eBook with knowledge check questions and chapter quizzes
- Anatomy and physiology review module
- Anatomical review slides
- Practice quizzes
- Open educational resources
- Online appendices
- Crossword puzzles
- Terminology flashcards

Acknowledgments

The mantle has been passed from two legends in athletic training. Ron Pfeiffer and Brent Mangus have retired and are enjoying life with family and friends. I was fortunate to have met Brent Mangus while serving on the athletic training written exam development committee for the BOC over 20 years ago. He mentored me and gave me opportunities to grow in the area of athletic training scholarship and publishing, and I will forever be thankful for his mentorship and friendship. I was honored when both Ron and Brent included me as a chapter writer and ancillary author and then as a coauthor in the seventh edition, but I was humbled when they passed the textbook on to me for this eighth edition of *Concepts of Athletic Training*. This textbook has guided many teachers and students as they took coursework to establish a future serving physically active participants of all ages. It is my pleasure to introduce you to Dr. Cheryl Ferris, my coauthor and longtime friend. She is an athletic trainer, Bowenwork® Practitioner, and Tensegrity Medicine™ practitioner with over 25 years of experience as an educator, clinician, and scholar. She is a fabulous colleague and is continually discovering new pathways to enhance her education and serve patients. Her dedication to adolescent athletes and their protection is highlighted in her contributions to this textbook. I also want to recognize my family for their continued support and all my former and current colleagues and students. All of you have provided me with opportunities, encouragement, and support over many years, and my life is richer for it. I cannot list all your names, but my specific thanks go to all of you who crossed my path through my involvement with the BOC, NATA and district organizations, NATA Foundation, and United States Olympic Committee Sports Medicine as well as at the University of Colorado Boulder, Indiana State University, Ithaca College, and University of Texas at Arlington. Thank you to all. As Helen Keller said, "*Alone we can do so little, together we can do so much.*"

—Cynthia (Cindy) Trowbridge
Arlington, Texas

As Dr. Trowbridge mentioned, we have had the pleasure and honor of working with Brent Mangus while serving on the athletic training written exam development committee for the BOC over 20 years ago.

I could not have been more excited and amazed when Dr. Trowbridge asked me to be involved with the eighth edition of this book and continue Brent's (and Ron's) legacy; she could have chosen a coauthor from many, many incredible professionals like herself. This process has enriched our long-term friendship, and I am grateful to Dr. Trowbridge for being patient with the new kid on the block. I am delighted for this book to be in the hands of many who seek this information but most importantly, to assist in the safety of physically active individuals. I would like to thank my family for their support and to recognize my numerous teachers and mentors during my lifelong education, colleagues from all my work and volunteer experiences over the years, classmates, and former students for always providing a valuable lesson for me to learn. And last but not least, thank you to those who not only allowed me to assist with their healing journey but also helped me grow, develop, and evolve.

—Cheryl Ferris
Pittsburgh, Pennsylvania

Reviewers

Stefanie Basso
University of Hawaii at Hilo
San Diego, California

Mike Carroll, MEd, ATC
Graham ISD
Graham, Texas

Paul R. Geisler, EdD, ATC
Associate Dean, Health Sciences
Professor, Health Professions
  Education
College of Natural, Behavioral
  and Health Sciences
Simmons University
Boston, Massachusetts

Marsha Grant-Ford, PhD, ATC
Assistant Professor, Clinical Education
  Coordinator
Montclair State University
Clifton, New Jersey

Ky Kugler, EdD, ATC
Chapman University
Orange, California

John Eric Leonard, MS, ATC
Winslow High School
Winslow, Arizona

Christopher Nightingale, EdD, ATC
Associate Professor of Physical
  Education and Athletic Training
University of Maine
Orono, Maine

Hal Strough, PhD, LAT, ATC
Associate Dean/Department Chair
Nova Southeastern University
Fort Lauderdale, Florida

Sherrie Weeks
University of Maine
Orono, Maine

CHAPTER 1
The Concept of Sports Injury

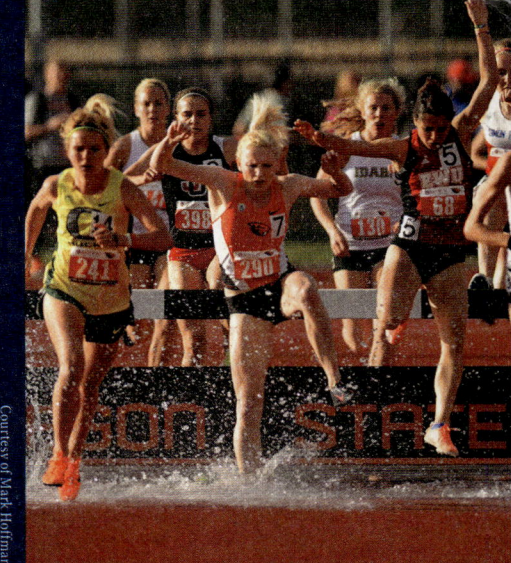

Courtesy of Mark Hoffman.

MAJOR CONCEPTS

After reading and studying this chapter, the reader will be familiar with the scope and breadth of the topic of sports injury. This chapter discusses the most popular definitions of sports injury currently in use, along with a variety of the most commonly used medical terms related to the type and severity of injury. These terms are used throughout the remainder of the text and can prove useful to individuals when communicating with members of the medical community about sports injuries. The last sections of the chapter introduce the concept of epidemiology as it applies to the study of sports injury. A straightforward sports classification system is introduced that is based on the relative amount of physical contact that typically occurs during the activity. This chapter concludes with specific participation and injury data from the most popular interscholastic and collegiate sports in the United States.

Youth Sports and Fitness Participation

Organized competitive youth and interscholastic high school sports continue to be extremely popular among U.S. children because 75% of families have at least one child who participates in organized sports (Merkel, 2013). Recent research indicates that approximately 7.9 million public school children are involved in these activities annually (National Federation of State High School Associations [NFSH], 2020). Youth sports and fitness participation has grown significantly over the years; estimations are that over 28 million youth (ages 6–17 years) participate in a team sport (Endres et al., 2019) and over 60 million, in some form of organized sports in the United States (McKay et al., 2019). Forty-five percent of kids ages 6–12 played in 2008, but as of 2018 only 38% were playing on a regular basis, indicating a decline in the number of adolescent and pediatric-aged children playing sports outside of or in addition to school-sponsored programs (Aspen Institute, 2019). By the time children are 15 years old (transitional year of adolescence), about 70–80% are no longer engaged in regular sport participation (Merkel, 2013).

Youth sports participation is associated with both positive and negative aspects (McKay et al., 2019). Some of the positive aspects include physical, physiological, psychological, and social development (Felfe et al., 2016; Merkel, 2013). Obesity and other disease rates, teen pregnancy, smoking, drug use, depression, and suicide decrease with increasing physical activity and sports participation (Merkel, 2013; McKay et al., 2019). The negative aspects include risk of injury; untrained coaches; overspecialization; time commitment; pressure to perform/win and achieve success; and the expenses associated with elite teams, travel teams, or individual sports that require personal coaches and lessons (Aspen Institute, 2019; McKay et al., 2019; Merkel, 2013). Also of interest is the economic divide that exists as evidenced in the participation rate of children (6–12 years old) from households with incomes <$25,000 (22%) and those from households with incomes ≥$100,000 (43%; Aspen Institute, 2019).

With the implementation of Title IX of the Education Amendments of 1972, growth in the participation of female athletes in the United States occurred exponentially. In 1972–1973, 3,770,621 boys and 817,073 girls participated in youth sports, but by 1975–1976, 4,109,021 boys and 1,645,039 girls were participating, indicating a twofold growth for girls (NFHS, 2020). In the latest available report (2018–2019), still more boys than girls were participating (4,534,758), but the total number of girls (3,402,733) had increased dramatically (NFHS, 2020). Although initially persistent stereotypes in both the lay and coaching communities indicated that girls were not tough enough to play sports, female athletes have dispelled this myth, and young girls can find many role models in collegiate, semiprofessional, Olympic, and professional sports (Figure 1.1).

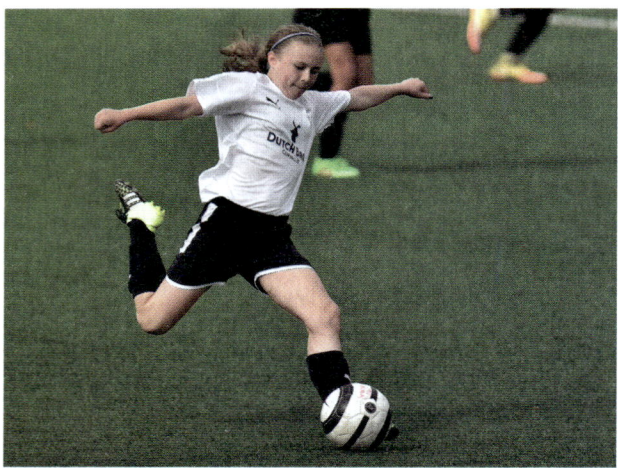

Figure 1.1 Historically, females were discouraged from sport participation based on unfounded fears of gender-based vulnerability to injury.
Courtesy of Mark Hoffman.

The vast majority of sports-related musculoskeletal injuries in children and adolescents are caused by repetitive overuse as opposed to acute macrotrauma, which is seen less frequently in young athletes (Patel, Yamasaki, et al., 2017). Even so, the American Academy of Pediatrics reports that 3.5 million children aged 14 years and younger experience a sports-related injury each year and around 775,000 are treated in hospital emergency departments (EDs) (Stanford Children's Health, n.d.). Of these injuries, falls, collisions, being struck by an object, and overexertion during unorganized or informal sports activities account for most of these visits (Stanford Children's Health, n.d.). Research indicates that EDs are often a likely choice for even low-urgency-related health problems for reasons including, but not limited to, a patient's or parent's perceived urgency and the convenience of the ED location; however, limited access to a primary care physician and views of family and/or friends were also cited as playing a significant role (Coster et al., 2017). Unfortunately, traumatic brain injuries sustained in contact sports accounted for approximately 45% of all the sports- and recreation-related head trauma ED visits by 10- to 17-year-olds (Sarmiento et al., 2019). Rui, Ashman, and Akinseye (2019) reported that for patients aged 5–9 years the most frequent activities causing ED visits for sports injuries were playground (23.1%), pedal cycling (13.8%), gymnastics or cheerleading (9.3%), running or jogging (8.4%); for patients aged 10–14, football (19.9%), basketball (13.0%), pedal cycling (10.1%), soccer (7.4%), and baseball or softball (6.2%); and for patients aged 15–19, basketball (16.6%), football (16.2%), soccer (9.3%), pedal cycling (7.3%), ice or roller skating or skateboarding (5.9%), and baseball or softball (5.9%). From 2007 to 2015, 45 deaths were reported in youth sports with both direct and indirect physiological causes and more incidents occurring during practices than competitions (Endres et al., 2019). The highest percentage of indirect deaths were attributed to cardiac issues, with males experiencing the most sudden deaths and basketball having the highest incidence (Endres et al., 2019).

Available evidence suggests that the injury rates for girls and boys vary based on the sport. High school data, for example, indicate that, in sports in which both sexes compete, such as soccer and basketball, differences exist in injury rates based on sex. Gender differences in the number of injuries that resulted in time loss greater than 1 day were reported in the U.S. National High School Sports-Related Injury Surveillance Study (HS RIO™), which is an analysis of data from 100 representative nationwide high schools, for the 2018–2019 school year (Comstock & Pierpoint, 2020). From reported strata data, boys' soccer resulted in 184,656 and girls' soccer in 227,951 injuries, in both competition and practice, whereas boys' basketball resulted in 87,521 and girls' basketball in 82,383 injuries, in both competition and practice (Comstock & Pierpoint, 2020). Regardless of gender, head/face, ankle, and knee injuries were the top three injuries reported in both competition and practice (Comstock & Pierpoint, 2020). Girls' soccer had an injury rate that was 1.48 times that of boys' soccer for both competition and practice but a greater injury proportion rate for head/face, ankle, and knee than boys' soccer, which had higher injury proportion rates for hip/thigh/upper leg, trunk, and shoulder than girls' soccer (Comstock & Pierpoint, 2020). Although girls' basketball had fewer total injuries than boys' basketball, girls' basketball had an injury rate ratio of 1.21 times that of boys' basketball for both competition and practice, and the injury proportion rate was greater for girls' basketball for head/face, knee, and hip/thigh/upper leg, whereas boys' basketball had higher injury proportion rates for ankle (Comstock & Pierpoint, 2020). Other data suggest that high school girls were twice as likely to sustain knee injuries requiring surgery and to incur noncontact major knee injuries as were high school boys (Ingram et al., 2008; Figure 1.2).

Despite the best efforts of parents, coaches, and officials, sports injury continues to be an unavoidable reality for a significant number of participants. In a recent survey, youth coaches reported that at least one player on their team had suffered an injury. Of those coaches working with children between the ages of 8 and 14 years, the most common types of injuries reported involved either wounds or bruises. Those coaches working with older players (up to 18 years of age) reported higher percentages of injuries such as fractures and concussions/head injuries. Parents reported that football produced the highest number of injuries, whereas swimming, softball,

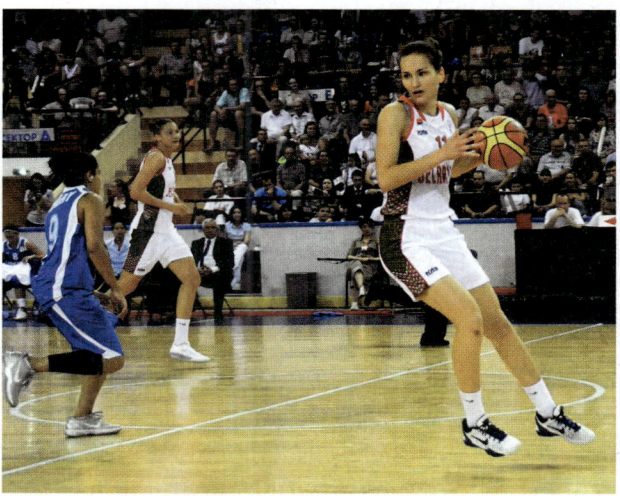

Figure 1.2 Although data show that in some sports females have a higher risk for some injuries compared to their male counterparts, data also show that in other sports rates for males are higher.
© Tumar/Shutterstock.

track, and cheerleading had the lowest. Data were also reported on the kinds of injuries that resulted in players' being forced to miss a game or practice (time loss) and concluded that sprained ankles accounted for 18% of time-loss injuries (Mickalide & Hansen, 2012). Unfortunately, around 50% of players and coaches had seen players put under pressure to play when injured likely because of the desire to win and not let the team down or a lack of knowledge about the type of injury (Whatman et al., 2018).

Although sports injuries are complex and both modifiable and unmodifiable risk factors exist for injury in youth sports, an increased risk seems to exist for injury during periods of rapid growth and in those with a previous injury history (Caine et al., 2008). Poor dynamic balance and ineffective implementation of quality prevention programs have also been linked with an increased risk for injury (DiStefano et al., 2017). Evidence is available, though, supporting the use of injury prevention strategies in children and adolescents (e.g., preseason conditioning, functional training, education, and strength and balance programs) that are continued throughout the playing season (Caine et al., 2008) and are adaptable to the very dynamic settings in which youth sports exist (Tee et al., 2020).

Definition of Sports Injury

The most current definitions of sports injury include direct (i.e., traumatic injury) and indirect (i.e., exertional, or systemic, failure) classifications as well as fatal and nonfatal (i.e., catastrophic or serious) classifications of injuries that result from participation in organized practices or competitions. Traumatic, or direct, injuries result directly from participation in the fundamental skills of the sport, whereas exertional/systemic, or indirect, injuries are caused by systemic failure (usually cardiac or respiratory) as a result of exertion while participating in an activity. Nonfatal injuries are classified as catastrophic when permanent disability results or serious when full recovery happens (Kucera & Cantu, 2019). Given these definitions, a **catastrophic injury** can occur as either a direct result of participation (e.g., sustaining a neck fracture during a tackle in football) or an indirect result (e.g., suffering a systemic heatstroke during a cross-country run).

As early as 1965, football-related fatalities were recorded and reported, but in 1982 the National Center for Catastrophic Sport Injury Research (NCCSIR) was established to track catastrophic injuries and illnesses related to participation in organized sports in the United States at the collegiate, high school, and youth levels of play. Also in 1982, the National Collegiate Athletic Association (NCAA) established the Injury Surveillance Program (ISP), which institutes a common set of injury and risk definitions for use in tracking collegiate sports injuries across Division I, II, and III NCAA institutions (Kerr, Comstock, et al., 2018). In 2005, the HS RIO program was introduced to capture injury data within secondary school sports across the nation (Kerr, Comstock, et al., 2018). Now, all systems for injury tracking data are web based, and the University of North Carolina partners with the NCCSIR (https://nccsir.unc.edu/), the Datalys Center (https://www.datalyscenter.org/index.php) partners with the NCAA for the management and publication of the ISP data, and Colorado School of Public Health (https://coloradosph.cuanschutz.edu/) partners with the HS RIO program to manage its data and publish reports. Because the ISP and the HS RIO focus on nonfatal injuries, they both use the following criteria to define a sports injury (Kerr, Comstock, et al., 2018):

1. Occurs as a result of participation in an organized intercollegiate practice or game
2. Requires medical attention by a team athletic trainer or physician
3. Results in restriction of the student athlete's participation or performance for 1 or more days beyond the day of injury

However, the HS RIO also includes fractures, concussions, and dental injuries that result in less than 1 day of time loss. The ISP, HS RIO, and NCCSIR provide evidence-based knowledge about the associations between sport participation and illness/injury, which can enhance risk-management decisions, injury prevention techniques, and athletic healthcare delivery (Kerr, Comstock, et al., 2018).

Catastrophic sports injuries account for a small portion of all sports-related injuries, but increased awareness by members of the sports medicine community is the only way to prevent these very serious if not fatal injuries. The most recent data available from the NCCSIR (1982–2018) indicate that, during this 36-year period, there were 2,686 catastrophic sports-related injuries/illnesses at the high school and college levels (Kucera & Cantu, 2019). During the 2017–2018 academic year, 85 catastrophic injuries/illnesses occurred among high school and college organized sports participants, and most of them were at the high school level (78%; Kucera & Cantu, 2019). Overall, 24.7% of cases were fatal, 9.4% were nonfatal, 60.0% were serious with recovery, and 5.9% were unknown. Forty-six percent were from direct (i.e., traumatic injury) causes, and over half occurred in competition. For high school sports, football had the highest number of traumatic injuries, followed by female cheerleading, wrestling, baseball, and male track and field; for college sports, football had the highest number of traumatic injuries, followed by female cheerleading, baseball, and male track and field. However, the number of traumatic injuries in the 2017–2018 academic year were not statistically different from those during the 2016–2017 academic year and were actually 26% less than those during the 2015–2016 academic year because of fewer catastrophic head

---

Catastrophic injury Injury involving damage to the brain and/or spinal cord that presents a potentially life-threatening situation or the possibility of permanent disability.

and neck injuries. For both high school and college sports, football also had the highest number of exertional/systemic (i.e., indirect) catastrophic events, followed by male basketball. Cardiac/sudden cardiac arrest accounted for 71%, and heat-related illnesses accounted for 15% of the indirect catastrophic events (Kucera & Cantu, 2019).

Even though time lost is a convenient method for identifying an injury, reporting systems for sports injury often lack a common conceptual basis and definition of sports injury (Timpka, Jacobsson, et al., 2014). The definition of time loss does not lend itself to an accurate reflection of the severity of the injury. Severity of injury determinations may be made by a variety of people, including the coach, physicians or other sports medicine personnel, parents, or perhaps even the athlete (Timpka, Jacobsson, et al., 2014). A related problem is that no standard is currently in use by all organizations monitoring sports injuries for the amount of time (i.e., hours, days, weeks, or months) that must be lost to qualify as a specific level of injury severity. Terms including *sports injury* (defined by clinician), *sports trauma* (defined by self-evaluation), *sports incapacity*, *sports illness*, and *sports sickness* (i.e., relative to time loss), and *sports disease* (i.e., overuse or overexertion syndrome) have been proposed as ways to qualify injury that results in health problems associated with participation in sports (Timpka, Jacobsson, et al., 2014). From a scientific standpoint, using the amount of time lost as the only definition of sports **injury** is subject to some error as previously described, depending on the method of data collection and injury definitions employed. Therefore, once an injury is identified, several qualifiers, such as the type of tissue(s) involved, injury location, the limitation of activity level and participation, and the time frame of the injury (i.e., either acute or chronic), are available to enable sports medicine personnel to better describe the precise characteristics of the injury.

A commonly used medical classification system for injuries uses two major categories: acute and chronic. **Acute injuries** have been defined as those that result from a traumatic event and have a rapid onset (Timpka, Alonso, et al., 2014). Acute injuries are usually associated with a pattern of signs and symptoms, such as pain, swelling, and loss of function (Figure 1.3). In the case of an acute injury, a **critical force** has been defined as the force at which the tissue's ability to withstand stress and strain is exceeded, potentially resulting in complete failure of the tissue (Prentice, 2017). The potential for critical force and subsequent acute injury is clearly seen in tackle football and other contact or collision sports. **Chronic injuries** have been defined as those characterized by a slow, insidious onset, implying a gradual development of structural damage (Prentice, 2017). In contrast to acute injuries, chronic sports injuries are not associated with a single traumatic episode; rather, they develop progressively over time. In many cases, they occur in athletes who are involved in activities that require repeated, continuous movements, such as those in running or dancing (Figure 1.4). Unfortunately, the current literature varies greatly in defining the terms *acute* and *chronic* in common sports injuries (Flint et al., 2014; Timpka, Alonso, et al., 2014). Therefore, several research groups have proposed redefining how sports injuries are classified to better identify causes, so mitigation and risk reduction are easier. One group associated with track and field developed a consensus statement to categorize

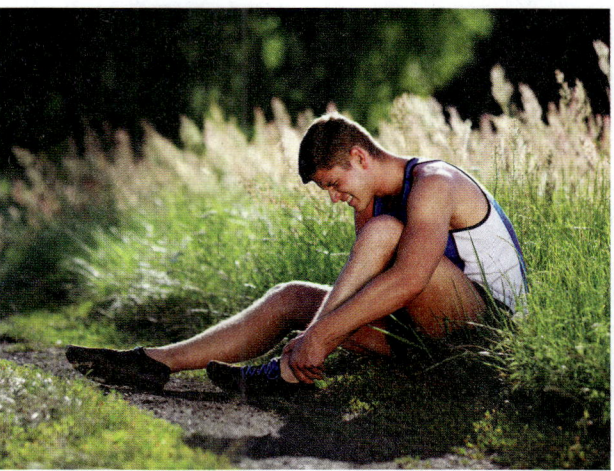

Figure 1.3 Acute injury in an athlete.
© baranq/Shutterstock.

Injury Physical harm or damage to the body.

Acute injury Injury characterized by rapid onset, resulting from a traumatic event.

Critical force The force at which the tissue's ability to withstand stress and strain is exceeded.

Chronic injury Injury characterized by a slow, insidious onset, implying a gradual development of structural damage.

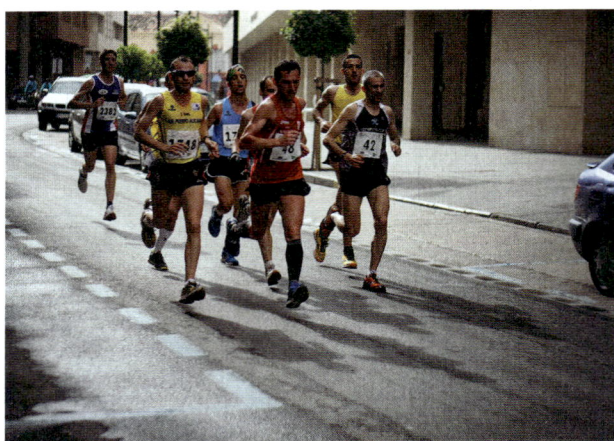

Figure 1.4 Chronic injuries are common in high-impact sports, such as running.
© Porcy/Shutterstock.

injury incidents according to the onset in contrast to the traditional diagnostic classification of acute versus chronic progress (Timpka, Alonso, et al., 2014). They proposed the use of **sudden onset injury** and **gradual onset injury**. A condition resulting from a specific identifiable episode resulting in a rapid onset of experienced distress or disability is classified as a sudden onset injury, whereas a condition that manifests itself over a period of time where there is no single identifiable event and the distress or disability progressively increases is classified as a gradual onset injury (Timpka, Alonso, et al., 2014). Sudden onset injuries are further divided into traumatic and overuse injuries. Traumatic injuries occur from a single external transfer of energy and include contact and noncontact injuries. Contact injuries can be caused by a collision with another athlete, a moveable object, or an immobile object, whereas noncontact injuries occur when a force exceeds the tissue's capacity to adapt. Examples of traumatic sudden onset injuries might include a bone fracture caused by a fall or a ligament tear caused by a twisting force applied to a joint during a sport movement. Overuse injuries occur with no single identifiable external transfer of energy and instead are a result of multiple accumulative bouts of energy transfer over time, which progressively weaken tissue (Timpka, Alonso, et al., 2014).

Overuse injuries in tendons occur when the workload from exercise exceeds the ability of musculotendinous tissues to recover; such injuries are ultimately biomechanical events resulting from the mechanical fatigue of biological tissue (Aicale et al., 2018; Edwards, 2018). Thus, the activity itself serves to cause a progressive breakdown of the tissue, which eventually leads to failure. Common sites for overuse injuries are the Achilles tendon, the patellar tendon, and the rotator cuff tendon in the shoulder (Flint et al., 2014). Edwards (2018) categorized factors contributing to overuse injuries as either intrinsic (e.g., immature/growth cartilage, lack of flexibility, lack of proper conditioning, and psychological factors) or extrinsic (e.g., excessive training or lack of adequate recovery, incorrect technique, and playing on uneven or too hard surfaces).

The Achilles tendon is subjected to tremendous stress during running and jumping (Figure 1.5). Research indicates that these forces may exceed the physiological limits of the tendon, thereby resulting in damage (Lorimer & Hume, 2014). Likewise, the patellar tendon must absorb repeated episodes of stress during sports. For instance, jumping and landing, as well as kicking a soccer ball (Figure 1.6), generate forces in this tendon that are many times greater than those produced during normal gait (Reinking, 2016). The rotator cuff tendons, specifically the supraspinatus tendon, are also vulnerable to injury from

Sudden onset injury A condition resulting from a specific identifiable episode resulting in a rapid onset of experienced distress or disability.

Gradual onset injury A condition that manifests itself over time where there is no single identifiable event and the distress or disability progressively increases.

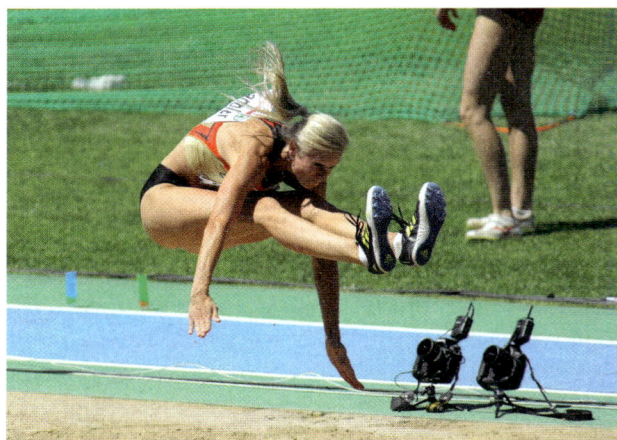

Figure 1.5 Injuries to the Achilles tendon are common in track and field events.
© Maxisport/Shutterstock.

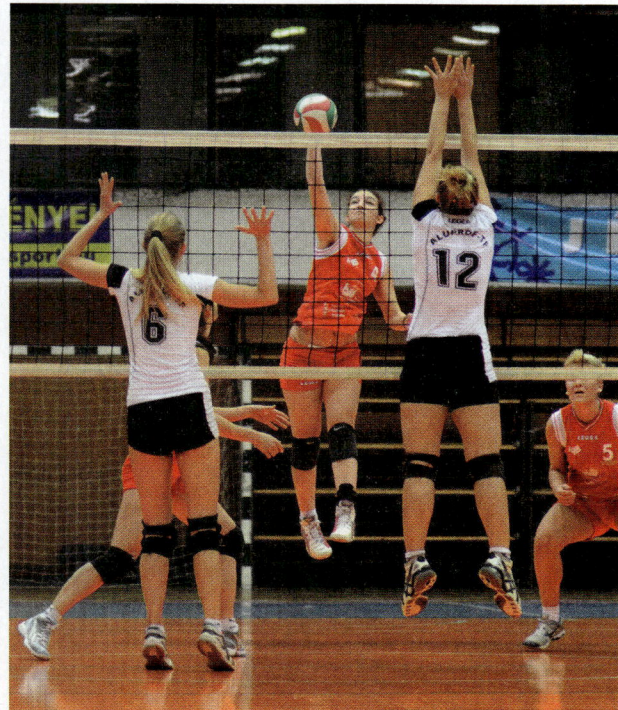

Figure 1.6 Jumping and landing subject the patellar tendon to stress.
© muzsy/Shutterstock.

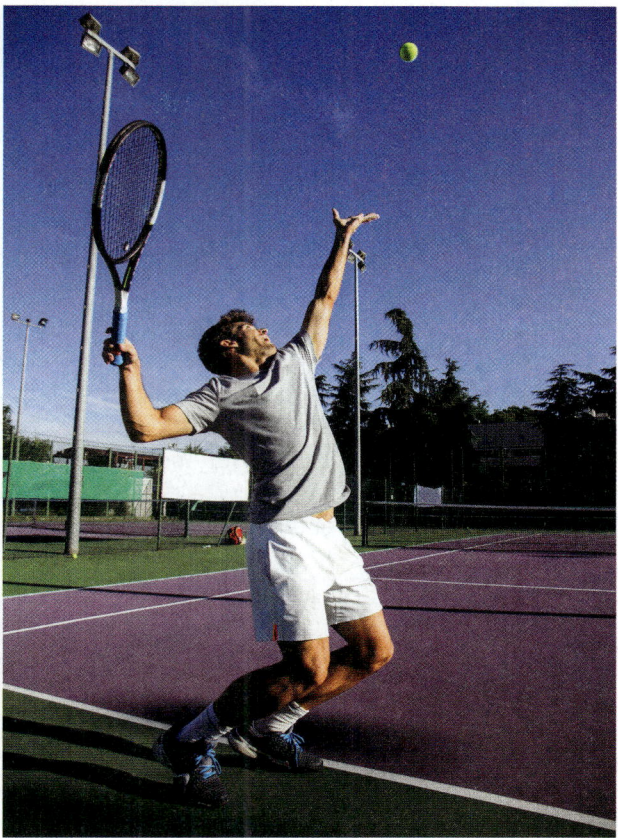

Figure 1.7 Tennis places significant stress on the rotator cuff.
© PabloBenii/Shutterstock.

overuse. Any activity requiring repeated overhead movements of the arm, such as overhead strokes in tennis (Figure 1.7), places significant stress on this tendon (Lewis, 2009). Overuse stress on any tendon is caused by both tensile (i.e., stretching) and compressive loads over time and has not been linked to one type of loading but rather seems to be related to the amount of load, the loading rate, and the loading duration, which when combined may result in a fatigue failure process of the tendon tissue (Edwards, 2018). Eccentric exercises that involve lengthening of the musculotendinous unit while a load is applied to it have proven to be very effective in treating and preventing tendinopathy because they condition the tendon with force fluctuations of loading and unloading, which may be an important stimulus for tendon remodeling (Murtaugh & Ihm, 2013).

Probably the most commonly used terms for differentiating tissues involved in a given injury are soft tissue and skeletal tissue. As a category, soft tissue includes muscles, fascia, tendons, joint capsules, ligaments, blood vessels, and nerves. Most soft-tissue injuries involve contusions (i.e., bruises), sprains (ligaments/capsules), and strains (muscles/tendons). On the contrary, skeletal tissue includes any bony structure in the body. Therefore, under this system, a common ankle sprain would qualify as a soft-tissue injury, and a fractured wrist would be deemed a skeletal injury.

> **Eccentric exercises** Exercises that concentrate or focus on the eccentric contraction of the movement (the muscle lengthens while it contracts); sometimes referred to as the negative muscle contraction.
>
> **Soft tissue** Includes muscles, fascia, tendons, joint capsules, ligaments, blood vessels, and nerves.
>
> **Fascia** Connective tissue that covers, supports, and connects, yet separates muscles, organs, vessels, nerves, and other structures.
>
> **Joint capsule** Saclike structure that encloses the ends of bones in a diarthrodial joint.

Athletic Trainers SPEAK OUT

How does the study of sports injury epidemiology and the continued collection of data assist coaches, parents, and athletic trainers?

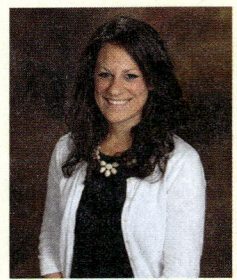

Courtesy of Sara Quetant, MEd, LAT, ATC.

Documentation is a vital part of the athletic training profession. Documenting what would be recorded as part of daily clinical practice, with the addition of a couple research-specific questions about exposures and injuries, contributes to the overall goal of making athletes safer. The continued collection of data is necessary to look at trends over time. Just as with personal goals, measuring changes and improvements takes time and tracking. Participation in sports injury epidemiology allows athletic trainers (ATs) to compare what is happening at their institutions to what is happening within their conference or the overall average of participating institutions. Another major aspect of the AT profession is prevention. Reviewing your injury rates and comparing to either your own previous years or other institutions rates at the end of a season or school year allows you to highlight problem areas and plan for the future. Why was there an increase in anterior cruciate ligament (ACL) tears? What have we implemented since last year that has helped decrease the number of concussions? Although 100% of sports injuries will never be eradicated, improvement is always possible.

The study of sports injury epidemiology can also assist coaches. Coaches want their players fit and performing at their best for competitions, a goal that starts with avoiding injuries. Working closely with ATs may influence coaches to routinely include time at practice for injury prevention to decrease injuries and improve athletes' weaknesses/predispositions to certain injuries. Over the course of my college soccer career, the AT staff had an increasingly involved role each year in communicating with the coaching staff on a daily basis. Anecdotally, we saw a decrease in the number of injured players as the two separate staffs collaborated more.

Furthermore, a child's health is important to parents. All involved parties should be on the same page to maximize safety and success. Having parents educated and included in discussions provides a successful environment for athletes to excel and remain healthy. By participating in the study of sports injury epidemiology, ATs can ensure they are doing the most to provide the best care for their athletes and keep coaches and parents informed.

—**Sara Quetant, MEd, LAT, ATC**

Sara Quetant is a research specialist and project coordinator for High School NATION at the Datalys Center for Sports Injury Research and Prevention in Indianapolis, Indiana.

Injury Classifications

Regardless of the specific force involved in producing an injury, all personnel involved in supervision of sports and physical activities, particularly coaches, must be familiar with and fluent in the use of the basic terminology of soft-tissue injury. Personnel must be able to recognize any injury and whenever possible correctly identify it as quickly as they can after its occurrence. Then, they need to clearly describe it when communicating with other members of the sports medicine team (e.g., the team physician or AT). Also vital is for sports personnel to master a vocabulary of standardized terms universal to all members of the sports medicine team. In 1968, the Committee on the Medical Aspects of Sports, a branch of the American Medical Association, published the Standard Nomenclature of Athletic Injuries (SNAI). Although this text is no longer in print, it provided clearly defined, standardized terms that are still in use today and should be used by those providing care for sports injuries.

Because the vast majority of sports injuries involve damage to soft tissue, the terms that apply to these common conditions are listed hereafter. Obviously, a certain degree of variability is unavoidable in any clinical definition, and newer definitions have recently been developed for tendinopathy (Scott et al., 2020) and muscle injuries (Mueller-Wohlfahrt et al., 2013). However, when used properly, the following terms can greatly reduce the confusion that so often exists regarding specific injuries.

Sprains

Sprains are injuries to ligaments, which surround all synovial joints in the body. The severity of sprains is highly variable depending on the forces involved. The SNAI describes three categories of sprains, based on the level of severity.

First-Degree Sprains

According to the SNAI, first-degree sprains are the mildest form of sprain; only mild pain and disability occur. These sprains demonstrate little or no swelling and are associated with minor ligament damage.

Second-Degree Sprains

Second-degree sprains are more severe than first-degree sprains; they imply more actual damage to the ligament(s) involved, with an increase in the amount of pain and dysfunction. Swelling is more pronounced, and abnormal motion is present. Such injuries tend to recur.

Third-Degree Sprains

Third-degree sprains are the most severe form of sprain of the three categories and imply a complete tear of the ligament(s) involved. Given the extensive damage, pain, swelling, and hemorrhage are significant and are associated with considerable loss of joint stability.

Strains

Strains are injuries to muscles, tendons, or the junction between the two, commonly known as the musculotendinous junction (MTJ). The most common location of a strain is the MTJ, for which the exact reason is unknown. As is the case with sprains, tremendous variability exists in the severity of strains incurred in sports. The SNAI presents three categories of strains.

First-Degree Strains

The SNAI describes first-degree strains as the mildest form, with little associated damage to muscle and tendon structures. Pain is most noticeable during use, and mild swelling and muscle spasm may be present.

Second-Degree Strains

Compared to first-degree strains, second-degree strains imply more extensive damage to the soft-tissue structures involved. Pain, swelling, and muscle spasm are more pronounced, and functional loss is moderate. These types of injuries are associated with excessive, forced stretching or a failure in the synergistic action in a muscle group.

Third-Degree Strains

Third-degree strains are the most severe form of strain of the three categories and imply a complete rupture of the soft-tissue structures involved. Damage may occur at a variety of locations, including the bony attachment of the tendon (i.e., avulsion fracture), the tissues between the tendon and muscle (i.e., MTJ), or in the muscle itself. A defect may be apparent through the skin and will be associated with significant swelling. Obviously, this type of injury involves significant loss of function.

Other Terminology Associated with Muscular Injury

According to a European-developed consensus statement (Mueller-Wohlfahrt et al., 2013), muscle injuries in sports fall into two major classifications: indirect disorder/injury and direct muscle injury. Direct muscle injuries are further classified as being related to lacerations or contusions, whereas indirect muscle disorders/injuries are considered functional muscle disorders or structural muscle injuries. Functional muscle disorders include two types: overexertion-related muscle disorders (type 1) and neuromuscular muscle disorders (type 2). Type 1 muscle disorders

---

Sprain Injury to a joint and the surrounding structures, primarily ligaments and/or joint capsules.

Hemorrhage A profuse escape of blood from a ruptured blood vessel.

Strain Injury involving muscles and tendons or the junction between the two, commonly known as the musculotendinous junction.

Avulsions Forcible tearing away or separation.

fall into two categories: fatigue-induced muscle disorders (type IA) and delayed onset muscle soreness (DOMS; type 1B). Type 2 muscle disorders fall into two categories: spine-related neuromuscular disorders (type 2A) and muscle-related neuromuscular muscle disorders (type 2B). Finally, the typical structural muscle injuries (i.e., first, second, and third degree) are labeled as type 3A (i.e., minor partial muscle tear), type 3B (i.e., moderate partial muscle tear), or type 4 (i.e., total tear or avulsion).

Other Terminology Associated with Tendon Injury

Tendon injuries have also often been classified as first-, second-, and third-degree injuries, based on the amount of tissue damage, and mild tendon injuries were often subclassified as tendinitis (i.e., active inflammation, including redness and heat) and as tendinosis (i.e., no active inflammation, including redness and heat; Prentice, 2017). However, a consensus group (Scott et al., 2020) recently agreed that the term *tendinopathy* is the overall preferred term. Tendinopathy is defined as persistent tendon pain and loss of function related to mechanical loading that causes a loss of tendon microstructure. The group also refers to a tendon tear (partial or complete) as when a load-bearing tendon has a macroscopic discontinuity (Scott et al., 2020).

Contusions

In all probability, common bruises or contusions are the most frequent sports injury, regardless of activity. **Contusions** result from direct blows to the body surface that cause a compression of the underlying tissue(s) as well as the skin (Trojian, 2013). They can occur in almost any activity; however, collision and contact sports, such as tackle football, basketball, and baseball, are more to blame in this regard. Curiously, many athletes and coaches view contusions as routine, minor injuries, but they can be serious or even life-threatening injuries when the tissues involve vital organs, such as the kidneys or the brain.

Contusions are typically characterized as being associated with pain, stiffness, swelling, **ecchymosis** (i.e., discoloration), and **hematoma** (i.e., pooling of blood). If not treated properly, subsequent contusions to the same area of muscles can result in a condition known as **myositis ossificans**, which involves the development of bonelike formations in the muscle tissue.

Fractures

Fractures and dislocations represent two categories of injuries involving either bones or joints of the body. Though such injuries can occur in any activity, they are more common in collision sports in which large forces come into play. **Fractures** have been defined as "a break of a bone" (Venes & Taber, 2009, p. 901). If the fracture does not result in a skin wound it is called a simple or a closed fracture; however, if the bone penetrates the skin, it is called a compound or open fracture (Venes & Taber, 2009, p. 903). Compound fractures are potentially more serious than simple fractures because of the risk of infection related to the open wound. Furthermore, control of bleeding may be necessary depending on the severity and location of the wound.

Acute fractures are relatively uncommon sports injuries. When they occur, however, appropriate first aid is essential to prevent complications, such as shock, excessive blood loss, or permanent damage. Fortunately, with modern diagnostic procedures, identifying traumatic fractures is relatively easy. The National Safety Council (1991) provides the following descriptions of signs and symptoms:

Contusion Bruise or injury to soft tissue that does not break the skin.

Ecchymosis Black-and-blue discoloration of the skin caused by hemorrhage.

Hematoma A localized collection of extravasated blood, usually clotted, that is confined within an organ, tissue, or space.

Myositis ossificans The abnormal calcification or ossification of bone within muscle tissue after an injury.

Fracture A break or crack in a bone.

- **Swelling.** Caused by bleeding, it occurs rapidly after a fracture.
- **Deformity.** This is not always obvious. Compare the injured with the uninjured opposite body part when checking for deformity.
- **Pain and tenderness.** Commonly found only at the injury site. The athlete usually can point to the

site of pain. A useful procedure for detecting fractures is to feel gently along the bones; complaints about pain or tenderness serve as a reliable sign of a fracture.
- **Loss of use.** Inability to use the injured part. Guarded motion occurs because movement produces pain, and the athlete will refuse to use the injured limb. However, sometimes the athlete is able to move the limb with little or no pain.
- **Grating sensation.** Do not move the injured limb to see whether a grating sensation, called crepitation, can be felt (and sometimes even heard) when broken bone ends rub together.
- **History of the injury.** Suspect a fracture whenever severe forces are involved, especially in high-risk sports, such as tackle football, alpine skiing, and ice hockey. The athlete may have heard or felt the bone snap.

Fractures may also be described in terms of the specific nature of the break in the bone. The major types of traumatic fractures are shown in Figure 1.8 and Figure 1.9.

Stress Fracture

A stress fracture is typically linked to sports or active-duty service members because it develops over a relatively long time, as opposed to other fractures caused

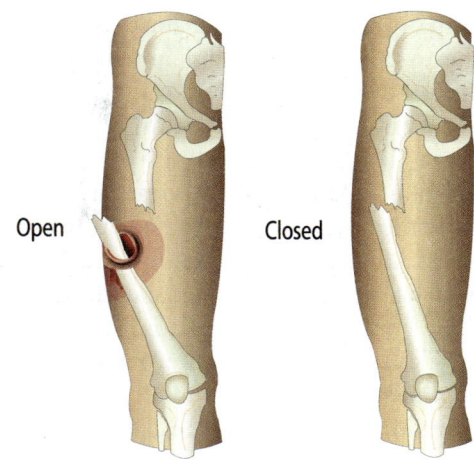

Figure 1.8 Open and closed fracture of the femur bone.
© Songtum Prakobtieng/Shutterstock.

by a single trauma. Stress fractures occur when a bone is subjected to repeated episodes of overloading (stress) that exceeds its rate of recovery (Knapik et al., 2017). In effect, the bone starts to break down

> **Crepitation** Crackling, grating, or grinding sound heard during the movement of a broken bone or joint.
>
> **Stress fracture** Small crack or break in a bone related to excessive, repeated overloads; also known as overuse fracture or march fracture.

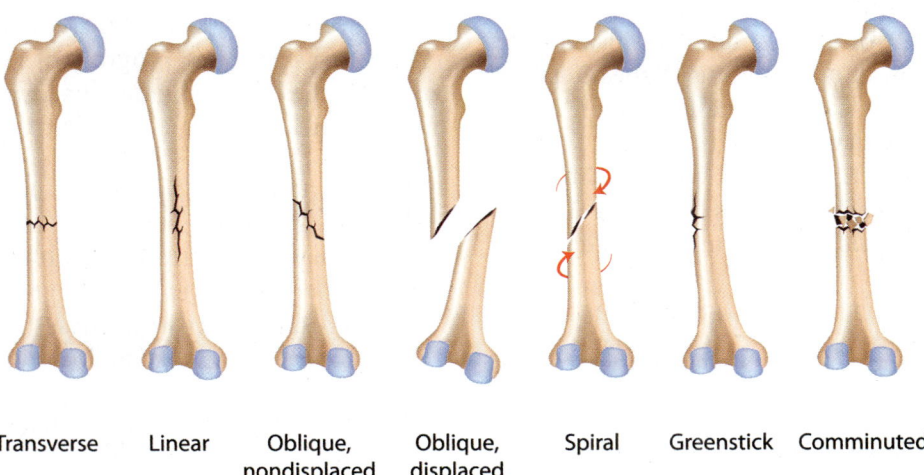

Figure 1.9 Types of fractures.
© Alila Medical Media/Shutterstock.

and eventually begins to fail. Because stress fractures take time to develop, the signs and symptoms are easily confused with other, less serious sports-related problems. This is especially true for stress fractures of the lower leg bones, which are often confused with shin splints. Although stress fractures can occur throughout the body, the majority occur in the lower extremities. Athletes at high risk for stress fractures are those who are in poor physical condition or are overweight. However, even well-conditioned participants may develop such a fracture, particularly when they have made a recent and sudden increase in the intensity or duration of their training program. Stress fractures may even be related to a lack of key nutrients within a diet.

The symptoms of a stress fracture are nebulous at best; nevertheless, certain factors are usually present when one is developing:

- **Pain/tenderness.** Athlete complains of pain and/or tenderness. A constant ache is not relieved with rest.
- **Absence of trauma.** Suspect such a fracture when there is no history of traumatic event, yet the symptoms persist.
- **Repetitive activity.** The athlete is involved in an activity that subjects the suspect area to repeated stressful episodes.
- **Duration.** Symptoms have slowly developed over a period of days, weeks, or even months.

Stress fractures are often difficult to diagnose because, during the initial phases, X-ray examinations may not show the fracture. In fact, the fracture may not be visible on X-ray until several weeks or longer after the onset of symptoms (Venes & Taber, 2009, p. 905). What can eventually be seen on an X-ray that signals that a fracture has occurred is called a callus, which is formed from hyaline cartilage during the healing process (Figure 1.10). As a result, the diagnosis must be made based on the

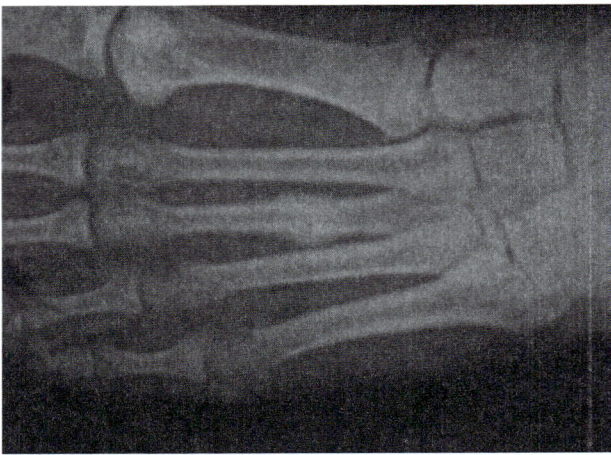

Figure 1.10 Stress fracture of the third metatarsal (approximately midshaft) in the left foot. Note callus formation around the site of the fracture.
Courtesy of Kevin G. Shea, MD, Intermountain Orthopaedics, Boise, Idaho.

factors previously listed. The best approach is to treat athletes as if they have a stress fracture and repeat the X-ray evaluation weekly or biweekly until a callus is seen. In difficult cases, a bone scan or magnetic resonance imaging (MRI) may be used to obtain a positive diagnosis.

Treatment of stress fractures involves rest and splinting or casting, when necessary, followed by a slow, gradual return to participation. Athletes are often encouraged to maintain their fitness levels during recovery by cross-training (e.g., riding a stationary bike, jogging in shallow water, or swimming). All these activities provide good stimulation for aerobic fitness while reducing stress on the skeletal system. Any program of recovery must be structured on an individual basis by the coach, AT, and physician.

Salter-Harris Fractures

A category of fractures unique to the adolescent athlete involves the epiphyseal growth plate known as **Salter-Harris fractures**. These fractures are classified based on the specific location of the fracture line(s) across the epiphyseal region of the bone. Five types (I, II, III, IV, and V) have been identified (Figure 1.11):

- Type I involves a complete separation of the **epiphysis** from the **metaphysis**.

Salter-Harris fracture A category of fractures that involves the growth plate.

Epiphysis Cartilaginous growth region of a bone.

Metaphysis The portion of growing bone located between the shaft and the epiphysis.

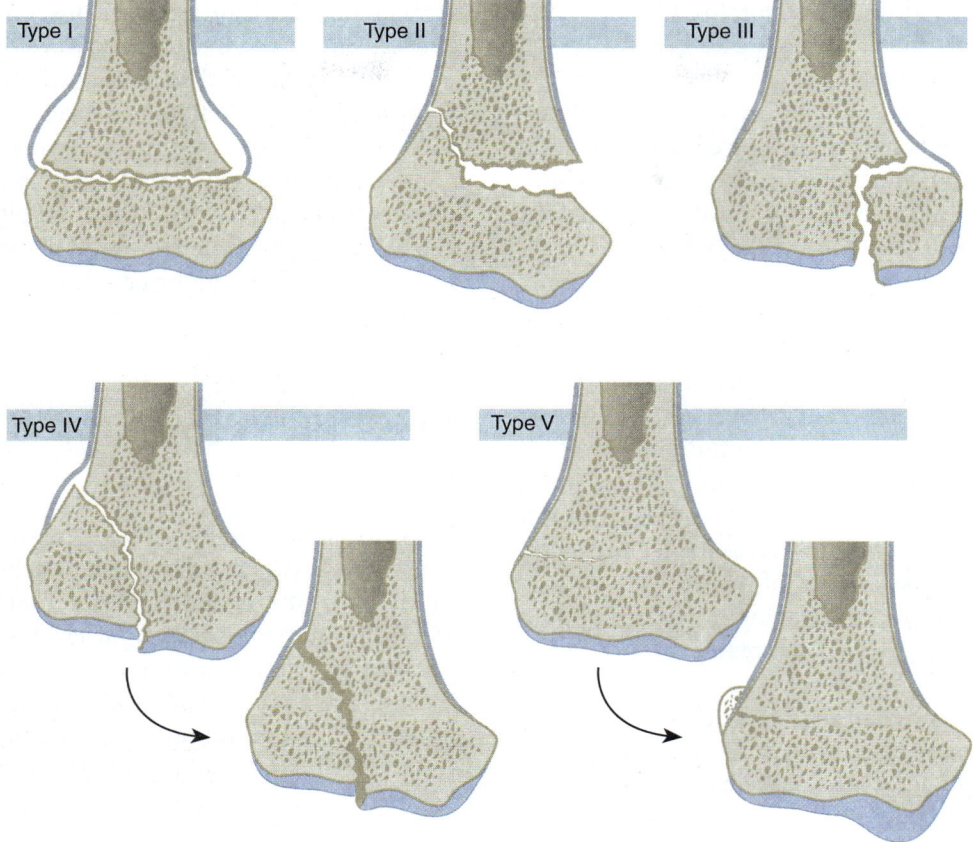

Figure 1.11 Salter-Harris epiphyseal fractures.

- Type II involves a separation of the epiphysis from the metaphysis as well as a fracture through a small part of the metaphysis.
- Type III involves a fracture of the epiphysis.
- Type IV involves fracture of both the epiphysis and metaphysis.
- Type V involves a crushing injury of the epiphysis without displacement.

Salter-Harris fractures can result in long-term complications for bone growth if they are not cared for properly. These complications include premature closure of the growth plate or abnormal joint alignment, both of which can result in different leg lengths when growth ceases. These injuries must be evaluated by a physician to determine the best method of management. A fracture associated with displacement of the fragments requires reduction, which can be accomplished either with or without surgical intervention, depending on the specifics of the pathology as determined by the physician.

Dislocations

Dislocations have been defined as "the temporary displacement of a bone from its normal position in the joint" (Venes & Taber, 2009, p.671). Two types of dislocations can occur, based on the severity of the injury. A **subluxation** occurs when the bones of a joint are only partially displaced, whereas a **luxation** occurs when the bones of a joint are totally displaced. In a sense, both types of dislocation should be viewed as severe sprains. Recall that sprains involve damage to the tissues surrounding joints (i.e., capsules and ligaments). Therefore, dislocations present many of the same signs

Dislocation The displacement of contiguous surfaces of bones comprising a joint.

Subluxation Partial or incomplete dislocation of an articulation.

Luxation Complete dislocation of a joint.

and symptoms as those seen in sprains. First aid treatment for dislocations combines care given for both sprains and fractures.

Dislocations can occur in any articulation; however, specific joints seem to be more vulnerable than others. Two joints in the shoulder complex, the glenohumeral and acromioclavicular joints, are injured frequently in sports such as tackle football and wrestling, and the small joints in the fingers are commonly dislocated in baseball and softball. Fortunately, such dislocations are relatively easy to evaluate because their most definitive sign is deformity of the joint. Deformity is typically easily identified because the joint can be quickly compared to the same joint on the opposite side of the body or an adjacent joint, such as in a finger or toe. Symptoms of dislocation include joint dysfunction as well as the feeling of the joint having been forced out of its normal position. Often, the athlete reports having heard a snapping or popping sound as well. If treated properly, full recovery typically occurs. Note that at no time should the coach or fellow teammate attempt to reduce (put back in place) any dislocation, no matter how minor it may appear to be. All dislocations should be diagnosed and reduced by a physician or other qualified medical personnel (QMP) after a complete medical evaluation.

Injury Recognition

Regardless of the classification system used, coaches or physical educators must learn to recognize injuries and their severity because they are most often the first to arrive at the scene of an injury; thus, the athlete's health and safety are greatly determined by their decisions and subsequent actions. In addition, the dramatic increase in sports-injury litigation should serve as a further incentive for coaching and physical education personnel to be prepared for emergencies. The premise that most injuries are best treated with the "run-it-off" approach is dangerous, to say the least. Today's coach or physical educator should treat all possible injuries as serious until proven otherwise. Sport personnel must develop the knowledge and skills to discriminate between injuries that require immediate medical referral versus those that do not. Decisions regarding nonemergency medical follow-up and/or treatment are best left to QMPs, such as ATs certified by the Board of Certification (BOC). Every effort should be made to have such a QMP employed, either permanently or part-time, by the school or agency sponsoring the sports program.

Epidemiology of Sports Injury

Scientific sports-injury research began over 60 years ago when the American Football Coaches Association funded a study related to football fatalities. Before 1982, the study of sports injuries was in its infancy because early studies were based on collections of case reports (Walter et al., 1985). Although this type of data collection did provide valuable information, it had significant problems because many injuries were not seen as serious, and thus were not tracked, and the actual cause of the specific injury was often not listed.

Therefore, a better approach to sports-injury research involves the application of the principles of **epidemiology**. The science of epidemiology involves the "study of the distribution of diseases, injuries, or other health states in human populations for the purpose of identifying and implementing measures to prevent their development and spread" (Caine et al., 1996, p. 2). The sports epidemiologist collects information to identify **risk factors** that may have contributed to particular injuries. Hypotheses are then developed and tested to confirm statistical relationships typically expressed as injury rate or injury risk. Injury rate is often expressed as the number of injuries per athlete exposures (AEs; i.e., total practices and games), whereas injury risk is the average probability of injury per athlete. The rate of injury is often expressed relative to 1,000 AEs, whereas injury risk is relative to the number of athletes exposed on the team (Comstock & Pierpoint, 2020). Other statistical relationships often reported include rate ratios (use injury rate) and injury proportion ratios (use injury risk) because these ratios allow a comparison

Epidemiology The study of the distribution of disease or injury within a population and its environment.

Risk factor Causative agent in a sports injury.

between genders within the same sport or to compare sports (Comstock & Pierpoint, 2020). Results of epidemiological studies can be used to identify risk factors, such as collisions, equipment, weather, sports techniques, or time period of a season or game/practice. For example, collisions are inherent in tackle football or ice hockey but may be more prevalent in younger participants or later in games or practices. Weather conditions may increase the risk of injury; for example, performing conditioning drills after a full football practice in pads may put athletes at risk for systemic failure if the weather is too hot. The athlete may also possess risk factors, for example, muscle imbalances, obesity, low skill level, or any of a variety of congenital conditions, all of which can be linked to an increased risk or rate of injury. As covered earlier in the chapter, several organizations are dedicated to the collection of epidemiological sports-injury data, including NCAA, Datalys Center, NCCSIR, and HS Rio. The primary goal of all organizations involved in sports-injury research is to identify risk factors for injury and, whenever possible, develop and implement strategies to eliminate or reduce them. The hope is that the information collected by these organizations will lead to continued reductions in both the frequency and severity of sports injuries.

For example, exertional heat illnesses (EHIs), such as heat cramps, heat exhaustion, and, most serious, heatstroke, can affect thousands of athletes each year. However, through the use of geographic temperature ranges (Grundstein et al., 2015) and the identification of statistical relationships between suspected risk factors and EHI occurrence, sports regulatory organizations were able to recommend strategies designed to reduce or eliminate heatstroke, which is the most serious EHI and can result in death. After the Georgia High School Association revised its policy to mandate a 5-day acclimatization period with no practices exceeding 2 hours and the use of wet bulb globe temperature–based activity-modification categories, heat syncope incidences decreased by 35%, and heat exhaustion incidences decreased by 100% (Cooper et al., 2020). The new heat policy also resulted in no heat-related deaths among Georgia high school athletes from 2012 to 2018 (Cooper et al., 2020).

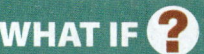

WHAT IF

Student-athletes ask you to explain the difference between a subluxation and a luxation of a joint. What do you tell them?

Classification of Sports

Injuries are often defined and described using a variety of medical and scientific terms, and sports can also be classified based on their comparative risk of injury, which depends on certain criteria, such as the amount of physical contact between participants (Rice, 2008) or the relative intensity of the activities (Levine et al., 2015). Table 1.1 presents the latest sports classifications related to the amount of contact and the classifications based on physiological load.

The American Academy of Pediatrics (AAP) classifies many popular sports into three categories (i.e., contact, limited contact, and noncontact) based on the likelihood of collisions with participants or inanimate objects and relative risk of an acute injury (Rice, 2008). Contact/collision sports involve intentional contact between participants or the potential for contact with equipment or other implements, limited-contact sports involve typically infrequent or inadvertent contact between participants or with inanimate objects, and noncontact sports typically do not involve contact between participants (Rice, 2008). As such, the potential for impact-related injuries is lower in limited-contact and noncontact sports than in contact/collision sports (Table 1.1). Note that this classification system does not imply that sports classified as something other than contact/collision are completely safe. To the contrary, not all injuries are related to the amount of physical contact between participants. For example, temperature-related injuries, such as heat exhaustion and heatstroke, can occur in virtually any sport, especially in aerobically intensive or high-load sports where proper preventive measures are often neglected. The American College of Cardiology and the American Heart Association (AHA) use the relative intensity of sports to classify them (Table 1.1). The sports are classified based on the peak static and dynamic components achieved during competition;

Table 1.1
Classification of Sports by Contact and Physiological Load

	Category of Sport*	Static Component†	Dynamic Component‡
Basketball	Contact/collision	Moderate	High
Cheerleading	Contact/collision	Moderate	Low
Diving	Contact/collision	Moderate	Low
Field hockey	Contact/collision	Moderate	Moderate
Football, tackle	Contact/collision	Moderate	Moderate
Gymnastics	Contact/collision	High	Low
Judo	Contact/collision	High	Low
Ice hockey	Contact/collision	Moderate	High
Lacrosse	Contact/collision	Moderate	Moderate
Rodeo	Contact/collision	High	Moderate
Rugby	Contact/collision	Moderate	Moderate
Skiing (downhill)	Contact/collision	High	Moderate
Snowboarding	Contact/collision	High	Moderate
Soccer	Contact/collision	Moderate	High
Wrestling	Contact/collision	High	Moderate
Baseball	Limited contact	Moderate	Moderate
Canoeing/kayaking (white water)	Limited contact	High	High
Cycling (road, mountain)	Limited contact	High	High
Field events (high jump/pole vault)	Limited contact	Moderate	Moderate
Skateboarding	Limited contact	High	Moderate
Skiing (cross-country)	Limited contact	Moderate	High
Softball	Limited contact	Low	Moderate
Speed skating	Limited contact	High	High
Volleyball	Limited contact	Moderate	Moderate
Weight lifting	Limited contact	High	Low
Badminton	Noncontact	Moderate	High

Bodybuilding	Noncontact	High	Moderate
Bowling	Noncontact	Low	Low
Canoeing/kayaking (flat water)	Noncontact	High	Moderate
Crew/rowing	Noncontact	High	High
Field events (throwing)	Noncontact	High	Low
Golf	Noncontact	Low	Low
Running (distance)	Noncontact	Low	High
Running (middle distance)	Noncontact	Moderate	High
Running (sprints)	Noncontact	Moderate	Moderate
Swimming	Noncontact	Moderate	Moderate
Tennis	Noncontact	Moderate	High

*Category of sport:
- Contact/collision sports involve intentional contact between participants or the potential for contact with equipment or other implements.
- Limited-contact sports involve typically infrequent or inadvertent contact between participants or with inanimate objects.
- Noncontact sports typically do not involve contact between participants.

†Static component of sport—related to the percentage of a maximal voluntary muscular contraction or effort.
- Low (<10%);
- Moderate (10–20%);
- High (>30%)

‡Dynamic component of sport—related to the estimated percentage of maximal oxygen uptake (VO_2 max) achieved.
- Low (<50%);
- Moderate (50–75%);
- High (>75%)

Data from Levine et al. (2015). Eligibility and disqualification recommendations for competitive athletes with cardiovascular abnormalities: Task force 1: Classification of sports: Dynamic, static, and impact: A scientific statement from the American Heart Association and American College of Cardiology. *Journal of American College of Cardiology, 66*(21), 2350–2355; and Rice, S. G. (2008). Medical conditions affecting sports participation. *Pediatrics, 121*(4), 841–848.

however, higher values may be reached during training. The static component is related to the percentage of a maximal voluntary muscular contraction and, in essence, the blood pressure load, whereas the dynamic component is defined in terms of the estimated percentage of maximal oxygen uptake (VO_2 max) achieved and the cardiac output demands (Levine et al., 2015).

Sports medicine personnel, coaches, administrators, and parents can use this information when athletes are found to have specific health-related problems during their preparticipation physical evaluations (PPEs). For example, a child with a history of head injury, such as a concussion, would be identified and required to receive a full neurological evaluation and subsequent physician's recommendation regarding continuing with competitive sports, particularly contact/collision sports. However, contrary to popular belief, noncontact sports can represent a risk to athletes as well. For example, a child with an identified, clinically significant congenital heart disorder might be advised to avoid aerobic activities, such as track, swimming, and aerobic dance.

WHAT IF

Student-athletes ask you the classification of their three favorite sports: softball, golf, and soccer. What are their classifications according to the two different classification schemes?

Extent of the Injury Problem: Epidemiology Reports

This section presents current statistical information on injuries in eight popular interscholastic sports.

Tackle Football

In the United States, tackle football (Figure 1.12) continues to be popular, with an estimated 839,000 children ages 6–12 participating on a regular basis (Aspen Institute, 2019) and 1,040,000 high school students participating in 2018–2019 (NFHS, 2020). There are around 100,000 post–high school tackle football players, including approximately 74,000 NCAA players (NCAA, 2020) and athletes aligned with the National Association of Intercollegiate Athletics (NAIA), National Junior College Athletic Association (NJCAA), National Football League (NFL), and other professional and semiprofessional leagues (Kucera et al., 2019). In addition, USA Football (the national governing body of American football at the youth and amateur levels) estimates there are 2.5 million youth players throughout the United States.

The HS RIO system for the football seasons 2005–2006 to 2013–2014 indicated 18,189 time-loss injuries during 4,539,636 AEs, or an injury rate of 4.01/1,000 AEs (Kerr, Wilkerson, et al., 2018), and for the 2018–2019 academic year an overall injury rate for boys' football at 3.85/1,000 student AEs, with competition having a much higher rate at 12.1/1,000 student AEs versus 2/1,000 in practice (Comstock & Pierpoint, 2020). For both competitions and practices, sprains and strains were most frequent, followed by concussions, contusions, and fractures. Most injuries over the 9-year period (2005–2014) affected the head/face, lower extremity, and shoulder/clavicle, and most extremity injuries were diagnosed as ligament sprains and muscle/tendon strains (Kerr, Wilkerson, et al., 2018). Within the 2018–2019 season, time losses were typically less than 7 days; however, more competition injuries resulted in longer time loss (Comstock & Pierpoint, 2020).

The most recently available multiyear data for NCAA football is from the seasons 2004–2005 to 2013–2014 (Kerr, Wilkerson, et al., 2018). The highest injury rate was found in regular season competitions (32.49/1,000 AEs), followed by competition scrimmages (29.98/1,000 AEs), postseason competitions (21.18/1,000 AEs), preseason practices (8.74/1,000 AEs), and regular practices (2.82/1,000 AEs). Most injuries occurred at the lower extremity (>50%) and consisted of sprains and strains, followed by contusions (Kerr, Wilkerson, et al., 2018). Across competitions, scrimmages, and practices, the top three areas of sprains and strains were the hip/thigh, knee, ankle, and shoulder, with lateral ankle sprains and medial collateral ligament sprains being the most common. The injury rate for concussions was greater in competitions than practices but less than ligament, muscle, and contusion injuries. Overall, most of the practice (about 40%) and competition (about 70%) injuries were related to contact with another player, and the second most common reason was noncontact (around 30% for competition; 14% for practice), whereas in football only a small portion of injuries came from overuse (<4%; Kerr, Wilkerson, et al., 2018).

The most recently available multiyear data for EHI events within NCAA football is from the seasons 2009–2010 to 2014–2015 (Yeargin et al., 2019). Football comprised 75% of all EHI events and had the highest rate (1.55/10,000 AEs) compared to other sports. The EHI rate was higher in preseason football practices with a 5.8 injury rate ratio compared to all other practices and competitions. Overall, nine football athletes required emergency transportation related to heat illness presentation. Most of these

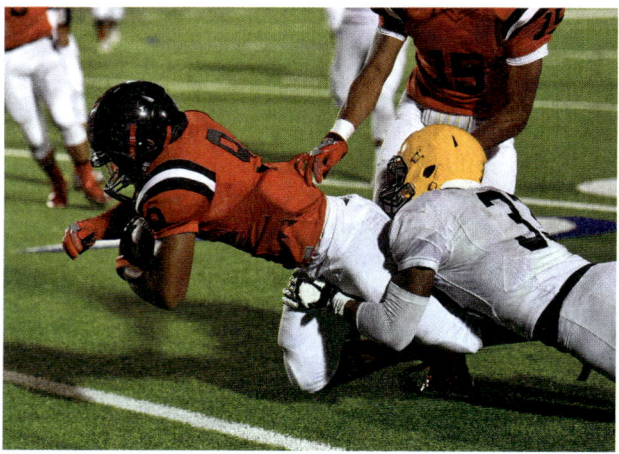

Figure 1.12 Over 40% of participants in interscholastic tackle football can expect to be injured in practice or competition.
© JoeSAPhotos/Shutterstock.

cases were from states with warmer climates, but the data indicate that enhancing preseason EHI prevention policies for football is warranted (Yeargin et al., 2019).

Understandably, an ongoing area of concern in tackle football is the incidence of catastrophic injuries involving the brain or spinal cord and exertional deaths attributed to heatstroke, sickling, or cardiovascular conditions. Kucera and colleagues (2019) found that, although football-related fatalities and nonfatal catastrophic injuries have been significantly reduced since 1976, data for 2018 indicated 16 fatalities among football players at all levels of play (five college, nine high school, one middle school, and one professional/semiprofessional). Nine deaths (56%) were either directly ($n = 2$) or indirectly ($n = 7$) related to football participation, and the other seven deaths (44%) were nonexertional and occurred outside of football-related activities (Kucera et al., 2019). The two direct fatalities occurred at the high school level during competition, and one was attributed to cervical spine and the other to a brain injury. The indirect fatalities occurred in both high school (four cardiac related) and college/university (one heatstroke and two cardiovascular/cardiac related) and in competitions, practices, and conditioning sessions (Kucera et al., 2019). Quantification of the seven deaths that occurred outside of football-related activity (at home or in a public park) determined that two were at the college level, four at the high school and middle school levels, and one at the professional/semiprofessional level; the causes were suspected to be cardiac related ($n = 5$), heatstroke ($n = 1$), and cardiovascular disorder ($n = 1$). Within these data from 2018, there were two noted trends that are likely related to better education and rules established regarding acclimatization, participation in hot weather, and screening for sickle cell traits. First, no deaths were attributed to exertional sickling again this year (last death was 2016), and, second, the number of heatstroke deaths decreased from three to two (one football and one nonfootball activity). Overall, during the most recent 5-year period from 2014–2018, there was an average of 2.2 heatstroke deaths per year compared to 3.2 per year during the previous 5-year period from 2009–2013 (Kucera et al., 2019). Therefore, education and rules do work and should continue to be updated and enforced.

Given the inherently violent nature of the sport, eliminating head and neck injuries from football completely may be impossible. The trends in the data suggest we have made progress, but more work needs to be done to implement effective strategies to reduce the incidence of serious injuries associated with football. Further study of the NCCSIR report reveals that cervical spine injuries have increased and decreased over the years of data collection, with two deaths (1995–2004), five deaths (2005–2014), and three deaths (2015–2018); however, brain injury deaths have steadily declined from 45 (1995–2004), to 32 (2005–2014), to 10 (2015–2018; Kucera et al., 2019). These improvements and overall variations are attributed to football helmet manufacturer and reconditioning rules; updates to spearing rules, including stiff penalties for "targeting" when tackling; and an increased emphasis on the importance of teaching proper tackling techniques; however, football is a contact sport, and aggressive play is often praised and rewarded (Kucera et al., 2019).

Fatalities related to football are also related to concerns regarding repeated head contacts and the occurrence of chronic traumatic encephalopathy (CTE); however, these data are not included in the NCCSIR reports because the deaths tend to happen years after competition ceases. CTE is a neurodegenerative disease associated with head trauma. However, the literature on neurobehavioral sequelae and long-term consequences of exposure to recurrent head trauma is inconsistent (McCrory et al., 2017), and the information remains unknown because of the lack of large, longitudinal studies (Maroon et al., 2015). A cause-and-effect relationship has not yet been demonstrated between CTE and sports-related concussions or exposure to contact sports; therefore, widespread speculation exists that reaches far beyond any conclusions that can be drawn from the current CTE research (McCrory et al., 2017; Maroon et al., 2015). Ultimately, the decision to play football and the age at which a child might start playing football is primarily up to the parents; however, philosophical arguments are made against playing tackle football because of the risks of injury (Findler, 2015) and arguments are made for continued play because the

Spearing A practice in tackle football whereby a player performs either a tackle or a block using the head as the initial point of contact.

benefits of physical activity far outweigh the concerns associated with injuries (MacDonald & Myer, 2017). MacDonald and Myer (2017) emphasized that a sedentary lifestyle is much riskier for youth because physical activity has significant social, psychological, and medical benefits, including better self-esteem; higher academic and career achievement; and decreased susceptibility to obesity, heart disease, mental illness, and diabetes. Medical advances and improved medical care as well as safety rules and prevention strategies are allowing for the more effective prevention and treatment of head injuries so youth can enjoy the various benefits of sports participation (MacDonald & Myer, 2017).

Basketball

Basketball is a very popular sport, with an estimated 4.2 million children ages 6–12 participating on a regular basis (Aspen Institute, 2019). Slightly fewer than 1 million high school students, boys and girls, participated in basketball programs in the United States during the 2018–2019 school year (NFHS, 2020) and about 35,000 participated in NCAA basketball (NCAA, 2020).

For girls' basketball, the HS RIO system (2005–2014) documented 2,930 time-loss injuries during 1,609,733 AEs, and for women's basketball the NCAA ISP (2004–2014) documented 3,887 time-loss injuries during 783,600 AEs. For females, the injury rate was higher in college (4.96/1,000 AEs) than in high school (1.82/1,000 AEs), and the injury rate was higher in competitions than in practices for both groups of players (Clifton, Hertel, et al., 2018). The top three types of injuries with the highest rates in girls' basketball were ankle sprains (0.98/1,000 AEs), concussions (0.94/1,000 AEs), and knee sprains (0.66/1,000 AEs), respectively, whereas the top three areas with the highest rates in women's basketball were knee sprains (1.78/1,000 AEs), ankle sprains (1.71/1,000 AEs), and concussion (1.55/1,000 AEs), respectively. Regardless of level and location, most injuries were caused by contact with another player although a noncontact mechanism was more common than overuse (Clifton, Hertel, et al., 2018).

For boys' basketball, the HS RIO system documented 3,056 time-loss injuries during 1,977,480 AEs, and for men's basketball the NCAA ISP documented 4,607 time-loss injuries during 868,631 AEs.

For males, the injury rate was higher in college (5.3/1,000 AEs) than in high school (1.55/1,000 AEs), and the injury rate was higher in competitions than in practices for both groups of players (Clifton, Onate, et al., 2018). The top three types of injuries with the highest rates in boys' basketball were ankle sprains (0.85/1,000 AEs), concussions or face injuries (0.56/1,000 AEs), and knee sprains (0.33/1,000 AEs), respectively, whereas the top three areas with the highest rates in men's basketball were ankle sprains (2.15/1,000 AEs), knee sprains (1.64/1,000 AEs), and concussion or face injuries (1.27/1,000 AEs), respectively. Similar to females, most injuries were caused by contact with another player (HS RIO: 1.32/1,000 AEs; NCAA: 4.63/1,000 AEs) although a noncontact mechanism (HS RIO: 0.43/1,000 AEs; NCAA: 2.02/1,000 AEs) was overall more common than an overuse mechanism (Clifton, Onate, et al., 2018).

Unfortunately, male basketball players suffer far more catastrophic exertional/systemic injuries than male players in many other sports, including tackle football, ice hockey, and soccer. From 1982–1983 to 2017–2018, the injury rate of all catastrophic exertional/systemic injuries for boys' basketball was 0.84/10,000 AEs compared to 0.78 (football), 0.74 (ice hockey), and 0.34 (soccer), and for men's collegiate basketball was 9.52/10,000 AEs compared to 3.75 (football), 2.84 (ice hockey), and 1.2 (soccer; Kucera & Cantu, 2019). These catastrophic injuries are often linked to sudden cardiac death or other cardiovascular disorders; therefore, having complete preparticipation physical examinations and QMPs on-site is even more important for boys' and men's basketball than for other sports.

Note that the incidence of knee injuries in basketball is consistently higher for females than for males (Figure 1.13). Young female athletes participating in sports involving jumping, landing, running, and pivoting are at increased risk of ACL injury (Leppänen et al., 2017). Knee valgus (knocked knees) plays a critical role in the mechanism of ACL injury, but stiff landings, with less knee flexion and greater landing forces, are particularly associated with ACL injuries in young female basketball players. A recent systematic review of 58 studies determined that, across a variety of sports, females' injury rate was 1.7 times higher than males' and the injury proportion was 1.5 times higher across a season (Montalvo et al., 2019). Unfortunately, 62% of patients with an isolated

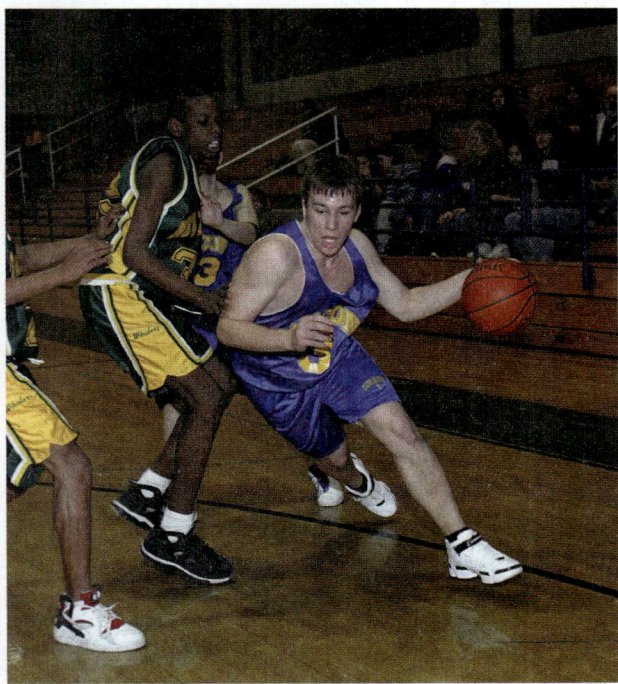

Figure 1.13 Basketball places players' lower extremities at particular risk.
© Larry St. Pierre/Shutterstock.

ACL injury and 80% of patients with combined ACL and cartilage injuries develop osteoarthritis within 10–15 years (Cheung et al., 2020).

Baseball and Softball

Baseball continues to be the most popular sport among young children, with an estimated 4.2 million children ages 6–12 participating on a regular basis, and softball is increasing in popularity, with 359,000 children ages 6–12 participating on a regular basis (Aspen Institute, 2019). The NFHS reports that 484,024 high school students participated in baseball during the 2018–2019 academic year (boys, 482,740; girls, 1,284; NFHS, 2020) and 364,221 high school students participated in fast pitch softball during the 2018–2019 academic year (boys, 2,183; girls 362,038; NFHS, 2020). About 36,011 student athletes participated in NCAA baseball and 20,419 participated in NCAA softball (NCAA, 2020).

For boys' baseball, the HS RIO system (2005–2014) documented 1,537 time-loss injuries during 1,573,257 AEs, and for girls' softball the HS RIO system documented 1,357 time-loss injuries during 1,173,722 AEs. The NCAA ISP (2004–2014) documented 2,574 time-loss injuries during 804,737 AEs for men's baseball and 1,848 time-loss injuries during 579,553 AEs for women's softball. For baseball, the injury rate was higher in college (3.2/1,000 AEs) than in high school (0.98/1,000 AEs), and the injury rate was higher in competitions than in practices for both groups of players (Wasserman, Sauers, et al., 2019). The top three types of injuries with the highest rates in boys' baseball were concussion or face injuries (0.29/1,000 AEs) and hand/wrist (0.24/1,000 AEs), and shoulder, arm, hip, and ankle sprains were all about 0.18/1,000 AEs, respectively, whereas the top three types of injuries with the highest rates in men's baseball were shoulder, arm/elbow, hand/wrist, hip/thigh sprains/strains (around 0.8/1,000 AEs); concussion or face injuries (0.53/1,000 AEs), and ankle sprains (0.38/1,000 AEs), respectively. In both groups of players, baseball demonstrated more injuries in the noncontact and overuse categories than contact with another player or batted ball, with noncontact injuries being greater than overuse injuries (Wasserman, Sauers, et al., 2019). For softball, the injury rate was higher in college (3.19/1,000 AEs) than in high school (1.16/1,000 AEs), and the injury rate was higher in competitions than in practices for both groups of players (Wasserman, Register-Mihalik, et al., 2019). The top three types of injuries with the highest rates in girls' softball were concussion or face injuries (0.35/1,000 AEs), hand/wrist (0.29/1,000 AEs), and ankle sprains (0.3/1,000 AEs), respectively, whereas the top three types of injuries with the highest rates in women's softball were concussion or face injuries (0.73/1,000 AEs), hand/wrist (0.64/1,000 AEs), and knee sprains (0.51/1,000 AEs), respectively. Softball demonstrated different mechanisms of injury based on competition level. Contact with another person was the highest for high school and college, but in high school overuse injuries were next most common, whereas in college noncontact injuries and contact with a batted ball or pitch were the next most common (Wasserman, Register-Mihalik, et al., 2019). In light of the findings that concussion and face injuries have a higher rate and contact with a batted ball or pitch is fairly common, eye injuries are a major concern in baseball. One-third of these injuries result from being struck by a pitched ball. Therefore, the recommendation is for pitchers, infielders, and batters to wear helmets with face shields or wear mouth guards and eye protection. The AAP has made several recommendations designed to reduce the risk of such injuries, including the use of batting helmets and face protectors, both at bat and when on base; outfitting catchers with a helmet, face mask, and chest and neck protector; eliminating the on-deck circle; and adding protective screening around dugouts and player benches (Rice & Congeni, 2012).

Baseball remains a popular favorite for children ages 6–12, with over 4 million playing baseball in 2018, which was a 3.3% increase from 2015 (Aspen Institute, 2019). Baseball is the second most popular sport for children in that age group, after basketball (Aspen Institute, 2019). Unfortunately, statistics from 2009 indicated that around 110,000 children ages 5–14 were treated in hospital EDs for baseball-related injuries and baseball had the highest fatality rate among sports for that age group, with three or four children dying from baseball injuries each year (Stanford Children's Health, n.d.). **Commotio cordis** is a common cause of death in youth athletes, especially baseball players. It occurs when a batted or thrown ball strikes the chest over the heart during its heart rate cycle, which can cause ventricular fibrillation and sudden death. Often, these blows do not seem serious, and individuals will initially get up only to collapse in minutes without a heartbeat (Maron & Estes, 2010). From 1995–2010, 224 cases of commotio cordis in sport were reported, with most of them occurring in children under 15 years of age. Sadly, approximately 100 cases occurred in baseball and softball alone (Maron & Estes, 2010). Education and effective chest protection are the best ways to prevent commotio cordis; however, the presence of an automated external defibrillator and parents or coaches trained in CPR are also key elements in survival if an incidence does occur (Maron & Estes, 2010).

Another persistent area of concern for decades has been the risk of injury to the shoulder or elbow in adolescent pitchers and fielders. This fear was apparently based on the fact that many young pitchers complained of shoulder and elbow pain and subsequently during medical evaluations evidence was sometimes found of overuse injuries in these children. These injuries were thought to be related to throwing excessive numbers of curve balls and/or breaking pitches. Specifically, the area of concern is the proximal humerus or the distal humerus (medial humeral epicondyle) where the muscles and tendons attach to bony outgrowths, or **apophyses**. In the adolescent shoulder or elbow, these attachments represent a growth plate; therefore, they are vulnerable to the repeated stresses that pitching and other throwing can generate (Rice & Congeni, 2012). Elbow injuries have been dubbed **Little League elbow**, and shoulder injuries have been dubbed **Little League shoulder** (Smucny et al., 2016). Fleisig and Andrews (2012) concluded that four factors are responsible for the increased risk of elbow injury in youth players: (1) number of pitches thrown, (2) pitching mechanics, (3) pitch type, and (4) physical condition of the player. Other factors may include using maximum-effort throws (Figure 1.14) and not resting enough

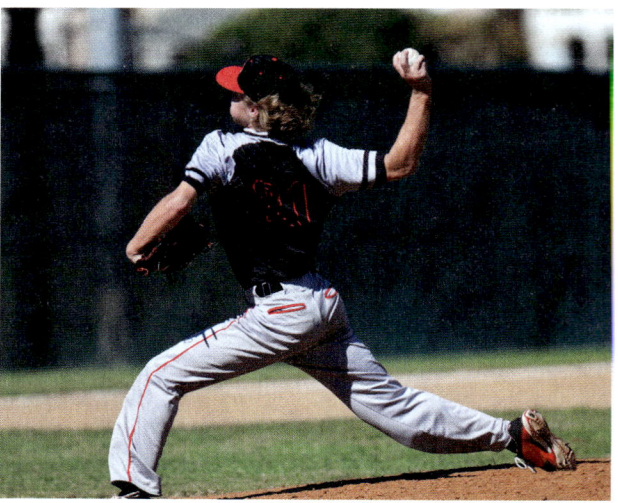

Figure 1.14 The correct pitching technique combined with limits on the number of pitches per week can spare Little Leaguers possible elbow damage.
© tammykayphoto/Shutterstock.

Commotio cordis A rare, lethal disruption of heart rhythm as a result of abrupt, blunt, nonpenetrating trauma to the chest/heart area.

Apophysis Bony outgrowth to which muscles attach.

Little League elbow Condition related to excessive throwing that results in swelling of the growth plate at the medial epicondyle of the elbow (i.e., medial humeral epicondylitis).

Little League shoulder Condition related to excessive throwing that results in pain and swelling in the growth plate in the upper humerus bone (i.e., proximal humeral epiphysitis).

between pitching outings (Rice & Congeni, 2012; Smucny et al., 2016). A critical finding to consider is that several studies that attempted to link curve balls with baseball elbow injuries failed to find a consistent link (Fleisig & Andrews, 2012). For example, pain in the **anterior** shoulder has been reported as a common symptom in softball pitchers and is associated with excessively high forces that are generated during the windmill pitch, which stresses the attachment of the long head of the biceps brachii to the glenoid labrum (Rojas et al., 2009). However, these shoulder injuries seem to be more linked to overuse, especially in female softball pitchers, who can pitch in as many as 6 games during a weekend softball tournament with a total of 1,200–1,500 pitches made over 3 days (Werner et al., 2006). Ultimately, the key to treatment of either of these conditions is prevention by all adults associated with the sports program, including parents (Fleisig & Andrews, 2012). Proper throwing mechanics need to be emphasized at an early age, and rest must be incorporated into an athlete's training regimen.

Wrestling

Wrestling is a growing sport, with an estimated 218,000 children ages 6–12 participating on a regular basis, which represents an increase of 14.2% since 2017–2018 (Aspen Institute, 2019). Wrestling at the high school level drew close to 270,000 boys and girls during the 2018–2019 season (NFHS, 2020). Forty-two states reported girls participating in wrestling (total = 21,124), with California, Texas, and Washington reporting the highest number of participants (NFHS, 2020). At the collegiate level, only men's wrestling is sanctioned, and there are around 7,300 participants (NCAA, 2020). Its continued popularity and growth are no doubt partly a result of the fact that both boys and girls can participate, and opponents are matched by body weight, thus allowing children of all body sizes to participate. However, given the nature of the sport, collisions/contact with opponents and mats do result in various injuries. In addition, joint injuries occur in takedown and escape maneuvers as well as in holds (**Figure 1.15**), which are essential parts of the sport.

Unfortunately, published data are inadequate regarding girls' wrestling injuries at the high school or youth level because the number of participants is less than 10% of the total. However, the HS RIO system

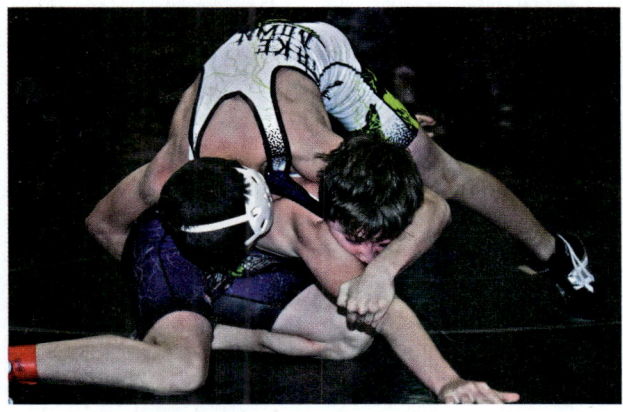

Figure 1.15 In wrestling, takedown and escape maneuvers can result in injuries.
© Susan Leggett/Shutterstock.

for boys' 2005–2006 to 2013–2014 wrestling seasons indicated 3,376 time-loss injuries during 1,416,314 AEs, and the NCAA ISP documented 2,387 time-loss injuries during 257,297 AEs. The injury rate was higher in college (9.28/1,000 AEs) than in high school (2.38/1,000 AEs; Kroshus et al., 2018). The injury rates between high school practices and competitions did not significantly differ; however, competitions were more associated with injuries at the collegiate level. Most orthopedic injuries for high school boys were sprains/strains or concussions. The top three injury locations were the head/face, neck, and shoulder for the period 2005–2014, but for the 2018–2019 year the top three injury locations were the head/face, knee, and shoulder. Most of the orthopedic injuries in high school boys were caused by contact with a person and occurred during takedowns or sparring (Comstock & Pierpoint, 2019; Kroshus et al., 2018). Most orthopedic injuries for collegiate men were sprains/strains or concussions. The top three injury locations were the knee, head/face, and shoulder/trunk for the period 2004–2014, and like high school the injuries were mostly caused by contact with takedowns and sparring (Kroshus et al., 2018).

Illnesses and infections are also common in wrestling; they accounted for 12.4% and 26% in high school and college athletes, respectively. Many skin infections are highly contagious through direct contact with an infected person or contaminated equipment, such as wrestling mats and clothing. Kroshus

Anterior Located before or in front of.

and colleagues (2018) reported that bacterial infections (e.g., impetigo, staphylococcus, and cellulitis) accounted for over 50% of infections in high school boys, followed by tinea lesions (e.g., ringworm and athlete's foot) and herpetic lesions at 38.5% and 7.5%, respectively. For collegiate athletes, herpetic lesions (44.1%) were most common, followed by bacterial infections (34.4%) and tinea lesions (6.6%; Kroshus et al., 2018). The differences between the types of infections in high school and collegiate settings are likely factors of experience and time spent wrestling. Collegiate wrestlers might be more aware of how to prevent and recognize bacterial infection, but they are also more likely to have had exposure to blood-borne herpes virus. However, wrestling rooms and wrestlers with good hygiene can mitigate the spread of infections, along with proper management. A critical factor is for coaches, athletes, and support personnel, such as ATs, to remain vigilant to identify potential skin infections and treat them accordingly before they can spread to others. Athletes with active skin infections should be removed from participation and referred to a physician for diagnosis; when necessary, these athletes should not return to participation until cleared to return by a physician. Wrestling mats should be cleaned daily after practice with an appropriate disinfectant product designed specifically to kill all common viral and bacterial pathogens (Kroshus et al., 2018). Of particular concern is community-acquired methicillin-resistant staphylococcus aureus (CA-MRSA) infections; around 5% of the population carries a colonized form of MRSA in their noses (Centers for Disease Control and Prevention [CDC], 2019). Cases often develop from person-to-person contact, shared soap and towels, or improperly cleaned athletic equipment (mats) or therapy devices (whirlpools). CA-MRSA often presents as a warm, red, swollen, painful pimple or pustule, and, if it is not treated, it can result in bloodstream infections, pneumonia, or myocarditis (heart muscle infection; CDC, 2019).

Other injuries common to wrestling are **friction** burns to the skin and irritation of the outer ear (sometimes referred to as cauliflower ear). Cauliflower ear (auricular hematoma) can result in permanent scaring, deformities, and even hearing

Friction Heat producing.

> **WHAT IF**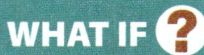
>
> Parents ask you for advice about which high school sport is the safest for their daughters. Based on available data, what would you tell them?

loss if not treated quickly and effectively (Patel, Skidmore, et al., 2017). Mandatory headgear that provides ear protection and improvements in mat surfaces have significantly reduced the incidence of these problems (Patel, Skidmore, et al., 2017). Another concern is disordered eating and complications related to lack of nutrients. Because wrestling incorporates specific weight categories, it has historically been plagued with problems associated with rapid and excessive weight loss by participants.

Volleyball

Volleyball (Figure 1.16) has continued to grow in popularity among children ages 6–12; around 846,000 participated in 2018, representing a 5.5% growth (Aspen Institute, 2019). It continues to be extremely popular at the high school level, and the latest participation figures show that, for the 2018–2019 season, it garnered 516,371 participants, most of whom were girls, with only 14% boys (NFHS, 2020). The NCAA reported 2,355 male athletes and 17,780 female athletes (NCAA, 2020).

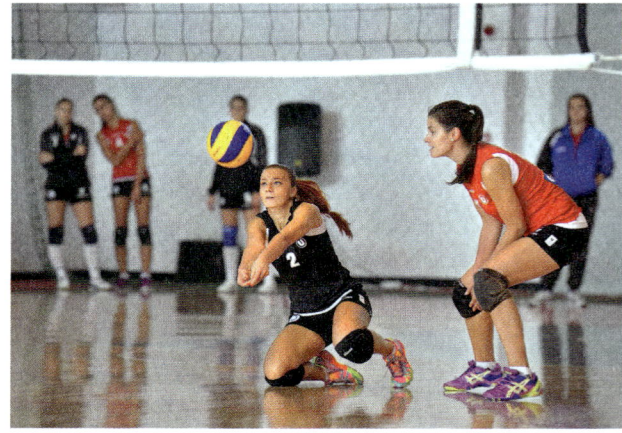

Figure 1.16 The most common injuries among volleyball players involve the ankle, head, and hand/wrist.
© paulinux/Shutterstock.

Volleyball involves jumping, diving, and overhand arm swinging (serves and spiking), and as such qualifies as a limited-contact sport. The HS RIO system for girls' volleyball for the 2005–2006 to 2013–2014 seasons indicated 1,634 time-loss injuries during 1,417,872 AEs, and the NCAA ISP (2004–2014) documented 2,149 time-loss injuries during 563,845 AEs. The injury rate was lower for high school (1.11/1,000 AEs) than college (3.81/1,000 AEs), and injuries were more common in competitions than practices in high school but not in college (Kerr, Gregory, et al., 2018). Most of the injuries were sprains/strains and concussions, with the top three injured areas being the ankle, head/face, and hand/wrist/knee in high school players and the ankle, knee, head/face/trunk in college players (Kerr, Gregory, et al., 2018). At the collegiate level, most of the injuries occurred in general play and resulted from noncontact or overuse mechanisms, but contact with players and playing surfaces was the third and fourth most common overall, respectively. In contrast, at the high school level, most of the injuries were noncontact, contact with another player, and contact with the playing surface during group play and blocking situations, with overuse injuries a distant fourth in the rankings (Kerr, Gregory, et al., 2018). Ankle sprains were the biggest concern for most players. However, those in the libero position experienced more concussions than ankle sprains because that position specializes in defensive skills and the concussions were linked to contact with the playing surface, and setters had more hand/wrist injuries than concussions. Therefore, it is important to take a preventive approach, such as taping and exercises to prevent ankle injuries in all players and teaching appropriate skills so liberos and setters can avoid situations that might lead to these common injuries.

Soccer

Soccer, commonly called football outside the United States (Figure 1.17), has grown in popularity throughout the United States, with recent estimates of nearly 2.2 million participants between the ages of 6–12 years old. According to the NFHS, during the 2018–2019 season, 459,077 boys and 394,105 girls, a total just under 1 million, participated in soccer programs at the high school level (NFHS, 2020). According to the NCAA, at the collegiate level during the 2018–2019

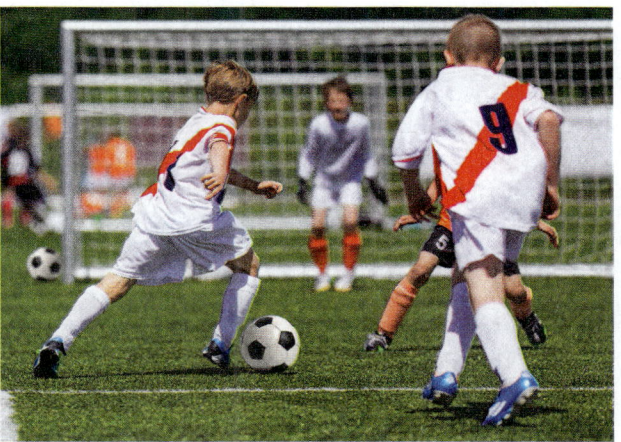

Figure 1.17 The most common injuries among soccer players involve the knee, shin, and ankle.
© matimix/Shutterstock.

season, the proportions are similar to those at the high school level, with 25,499 females and 28,310 males playing soccer (NCAA, 2020).

Although soccer does not involve intentional collisions between players, incidental collisions frequently occur; therefore, it is classified by the AAP as a contact/collision sport (Table 1.1). Protective equipment is limited, with most body areas exposed to external trauma. For girls' soccer, the HS RIO system documented 3,242 time-loss injuries during 1,393,753 AEs (DiStefano et al., 2018) and for boys' soccer, 2,912 time-loss injuries during 1,592,238 AEs over the 2005–2014 data collection years (Kerr, Putukian, et al., 2018). The NCAA ISP documented 5,092 time-loss injuries during 772,048 AEs for female soccer (DiStefano et al., 2018) and 4,765 time-loss injuries during 686,918 AEs for male soccer over the decade ending in 2014 (Kerr, Putukian, et al., 2018). For both genders, the injury rate was higher in college (females = 6.6/1,000 AEs; males = 6.64/1,000 AEs) than in high school (females = 2.33/1,000 AEs; males = 1.83/1,000 AEs), and the injury rate was higher in competitions than in practices for both groups of players (DiStefano et al., 2018; Kerr, Putukian, et al., 2018).

The top three types of injuries with the highest rates during practice for girls' soccer were ankle, hip/thigh, and knee, and they were mostly strains and then sprains. For collegiate women, the hip/thigh, ankle, and knee were the most common (DiStefano et al., 2018). However, in competitions, head/face injuries, including concussions, advance to the most commonly occurring injury. Trends are also different in the cause of injury in girls' soccer at the high school level, with noncontact and overuse mechanisms being the most common in practice, whereas contact with another player or the playing surface is the most common in competitions (DiStefano et al., 2018). For collegiate women's soccer, noncontact is still the most common cause, but collision with another player is more common than overuse. As with the high school level, contact situations become the more prevalent mechanism in competitions. Finally, overall, the largest proportion of injuries resulted in time loss of less than 1 week, and the most injuries occurred in general play in both practices and competitions. Goalkeepers and midfielders were more susceptible to concussions than forwards in games, but for defenders, the level of play determined injury occurrence because high school defenders had more concussions than ankle sprains and defenders at the NCAA level had more ankle sprains than concussions (DiStefano et al., 2018).

Boys' soccer also demonstrated more strains than sprains in practice, with the top three areas of injury being hip/thigh, ankle, and knee, whereas during competition the areas of injury shift just like in girls' soccer to head/face, followed by ankle, knee, and hip/thigh (Kerr, Putukian, et al., 2018). At the collegiate level, men continue to experience more strains than sprains at the hip/thigh, ankle, and knee, but during competitions head/face injuries take over the third spot, which moves knee injuries to the fourth spot. Ultimately, concussions are more common in both high school and college levels during games. Noncontact mechanisms cause the most injuries in practice for both high school and college males, but contact with another player or contact with the playing surface is the second most common, followed by overuse injuries. Regarding competitions, contact injuries with other players takes over the top spot followed by noncontact and playing surface contact (Kerr, Putukian, et al., 2018). Overall, most of the injuries occurred during general play and time loss was less than 1 week, just like females. Regarding position, forwards were more likely to sprain their ankle than suffer a concussion at both levels, and goalkeepers received more concussions than any other injury. Interestingly, the level of play and likely their experience dictated the percentage of injuries for defenders and midfielders, with high school players being diagnosed with more concussions than ankle sprains and college players, with more ankle sprains than concussions (Kerr, Putukian, et al., 2018).

Regarding knee injuries, specifically the ACL, available data indicate that female youth participants sustain higher numbers of these injuries than their male counterparts do. A recent systematic review revealed that female soccer players have a two to three times higher average risk of ACL injury than male soccer players and also seem to sustain the injuries at younger ages (Waldén et al., 2011). As mentioned earlier in the basketball section, the risk of anyone developing osteoarthritis within 10–15 years of an ACL injury and repair is over 60% (Cheung et al., 2020). However, another statistic of concern for female soccer players is that, after having an ACL injury and reconstruction, they have a nearly fivefold higher rate of receiving a new ACL injury to the ipsilateral or contralateral knee and a two- to fourfold higher rate of experiencing other types of knee injuries when they return to their sport (Fältström et al., 2019). Also, more than 60% of players with a previous ACL reconstruction quit soccer within 2 years compared to 36% of a noninjured population. Prevention programs designed to protect athletes from a variety of knee injuries, especially ACL injuries, have been instituted for over 25 years. Practitioners generally accept that a program should be sport specific and include flexibility, strength, power, and balance components and should involve coaches, parents, athletes, and medical professionals (Padua et al., 2014). Furthermore, a very thorough and scoping review related to the outcomes of different prevention programs for ACL injuries has determined that these programs decrease the risk of all ACL injuries by 50% and female noncontact ACL injuries by two-thirds (Webster & Hewett, 2018). Therefore, the wise thing to do is to incorporate a quality injury prevention program into any soccer program to improve athlete safety.

In addition to the occurrence of ACL injuries, a unique aspect of the game involves the skill known as heading, in which a participant contacts a ball with the head, in most cases after it has been kicked into the air. Some medical experts have hypothesized that this practice may lead to head injury. However, research has shown that, although heading the ball continues to result in concussion, collisions between players is the more common cause of concussion (Comstock et al., 2015). Contact with another player was the most common mechanism of injury among boys (78.1%) and girls (61.9%), whereas heading a soccer ball was responsible for 30.6% of boys' and 25.3% of girls' concussions in soccer (Comstock et al., 2015). Comstock and colleagues (2015) concluded that banning heading would limit effectiveness as a primary prevention mechanism unless a ban included efforts to reduce athlete-to-athlete contact in the game. In recent years, specialized helmets and headgear for soccer players have been introduced in to reduce the incidence of head injury. However, data based on sound science fail to support the use of soccer headgear because it did not reduce the incidence or severity of concussion in high school soccer players (McGuine et al., 2020).

Several deaths and severe injuries have been related to improperly constructed movable soccer goals. For the period from 1979 to 2014, at least 36 deaths were reported, and hundreds of nonfatal injuries occurred that were directly related to moveable goals (Consumer Product Safety Commission, 2014). The majority of these injuries and fatalities occurred when the goals tipped over and struck the victims. As a result, numerous soccer organizations (e.g., the Federation Internationale de Football, the NFSH, and the NCAA) have established strict criteria for the construction of soccer goals. In addition, the Consumer Product Safety Commission has published guidelines for the design and construction of movable soccer goals (https://www.cpsc.gov/safety-education/safety-guides/sports-fitness-and-recreation/guidelines-movable-soccer-goals).

Gymnastics

With the success of the U.S. Olympic women's and men's gymnastics teams, the sport has grown over the past few years, with over 4.81 million children over the age of 6 years old reported as participating in 2017 (Lock, 2020). In 2017, 3.1% of 6- to 12-year-olds participated regularly in gymnastics, which has grown over the past 3 years. Around 20,000 high school students participate in gymnastics (NFHS, 2020), and during the 2015 season, 1,418 women were on the NCAA women's gymnastics rosters at 82 member institutions over the three divisions.

The injury incidence and prevalence are substantial in artistic gymnastics, especially in athletes who train at highly competitive levels (Campbell et al., 2019). Females were reported to experience 3.7 injuries per 1,000 hours of practice/competition, whereas males experienced 0.7 injuries per 1,000 hours. Most injuries for females were reported as lower extremity related and included nonspecific pain, fractures, stress fractures, ankle sprains, lumbar soft-tissue strains, and lumbar pars defects (i.e., spondylolysis or spondylolisthesis; Figure 1.18). However, injuries to wrists/hands and elbow subluxation and dislocations were also prevalent. Not much data was available on specific injuries experienced by males, but trends point to more upper extremity injuries (Campbell et al., 2019). Acute injuries were more prevalent across gender (55–83%) compared to overuse injuries (23–44%), and the floor exercise routine was most commonly associated with acute injuries. Overall, the landing phase of a gymnastic skill was when most of the injuries occurred.

Cheerleading

Like gymnastics, cheerleading has seen growth over the past few years because of public recognition in movies and other TV dramas. As of 2018, around 775,000 children ages 6–12 years participated in

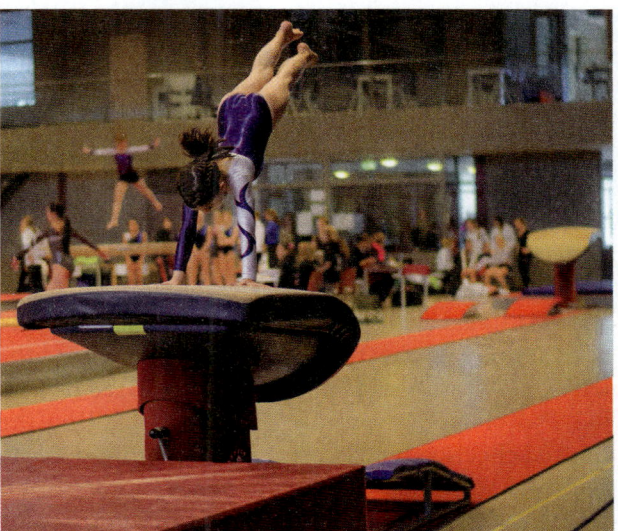

Figure 1.18 The most common injuries among gymnasts involve the foot, ankle, lower leg, knee, trunk, and shoulder.
© Sasha Samardzija/Shutterstock.

cheerleading, which was an 18.2% increase from 2017 (Aspen Institute, 2019). The NFHS estimates that about 400,000 high school students participate in cheerleading each year, including 123,386 participants in competitive spirit squads. Both cheerleading squads and competitive spirit squads rank in the top 10 of girls' sports in high school (Currie et al., 2016).

Catastrophic injuries have occurred in cheerleading, with 1 fatal, 24 nonfatal, and 43 serious injuries over 36 years of data collection by the NCCSIR (Kucera & Cantu, 2019). Although there have been far more fatal injuries in football ($n = 137$) over this period, the rate of nonfatal injuries in cheerleading was 0.98/10,000 AEs for girls and 1.71/100,000 AEs for boys, and the rate of serious injuries was 1.8/10,000 AEs for girls and 1.71/100,000 AEs for boys. In comparison, the rate of nonfatal injury was 1.41/10,000 AEs and serious injuries was 1.12/10,000 AEs, so the concern over cheerleading being a dangerous sport with the risk of head, neck, or organ injuries is valid (Kucera & Cantu, 2019). However, the noncatastrophic injury rates in cheerleading were lower than for most other high school sports, with an overall injury rate of 0.71/1,000 AEs. Performance injury rates were the lowest (0.49/1,000 AEs), and competition (0.85/1,000 AEs) and practice (0.76/1,000 AEs) injury rates were very close to one another. Most of the cheerleading injuries happen to girls, but boys have almost twice the chance of getting injured (rate ratio = 1.93). Most of the injuries occurred during stunts (53.2%), and, unfortunately, they are usually more severe. When injuries do occur, 40% of injuries result in time loss of 1–3 weeks, and 33% result in over 3 weeks of time loss. The top three injuries were concussions, ankle sprains, and knee sprains; however, the concussion rates are significantly lower than for all other high school sports (2.21/10,000 AEs vs. 3.78/10,000 AEs; Currie et al., 2016). Most concussions in cheerleading were in younger athletes (<17 years old) and were largely caused by falls (52.2%) or having another cheerleader fall on the injured cheerleader (13.6%; Jones & Hammig, 2020; Figure 1.19). The use of a pyramid or formation was the leading cause of the concussive injuries, so that fact provides information for athletes, coaches, and parents regarding safety practices (Jones & Hammig, 2020).

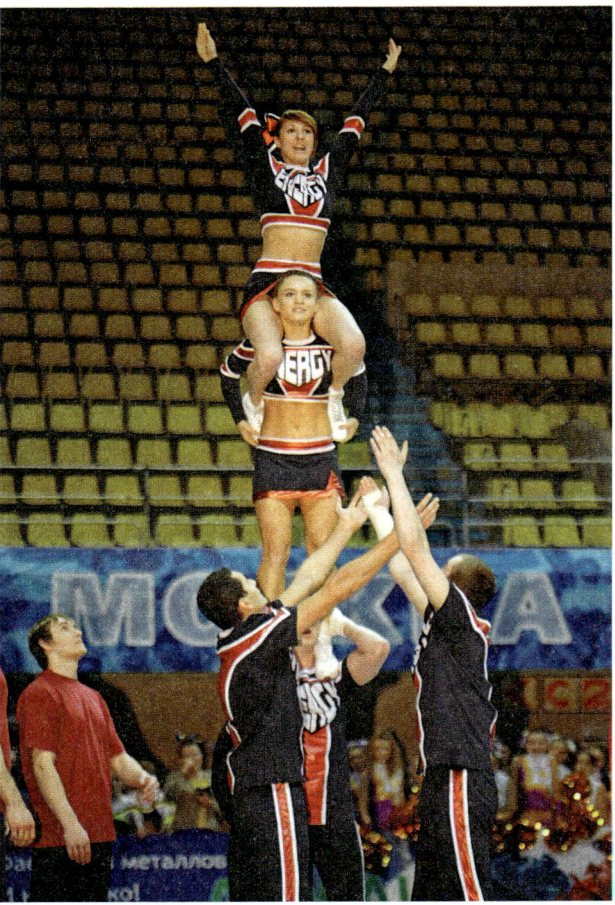

Figure 1.19 The most common injuries among cheerleaders involve concussions and ligament sprains.
© Pavel L Photo and Video/Shutterstock.

Recurrent Injuries

Research has been lacking regarding recurrent injuries across all boys' and girls' high school sports; however, Welton and colleagues (2018) reviewed epidemiological data during the 2005–2006 through 2015–2016 academic years and found that 10.5% of all high school sports–related injuries were recurrent. The good news is this rate has held steady over time when compared with other reviews. But the bad news is that recurrent injuries result in a higher likelihood of surgical intervention, an increased amount of time away from sports, and a higher likelihood of sports discontinuation as compared with new injuries (Welton et al., 2018). The ankle joint was the most commonly reinjured body part, with sprains being the most common type of injury. Recurrent knee sprains were both second and third most common in several sports, including boys' and girls' basketball, girls' gymnastics, girls' soccer, boys' wrestling, boys' ice hockey, and boys' and girls' lacrosse, respectively (Welton et al., 2018). These joint injuries that reoccur during key developmental time periods of growing adolescents can have long-term effects on growth and development and may lead to early onset of osteoarthritis. Head and facial injuries were also fairly common recurrent injuries, and concussions represented about 16.7% of all the recurrent injuries reported (Welton et al., 2018). The reoccurrence of concussions is concerning on multiple levels as we continue to learn about this complex functional brain injury and the potential long-term effects (Churchill et al., 2019). Recent evidence has pointed to an elevated risk of musculoskeletal injury when individuals demonstrate poor neurocognitive performances postconcussion, and a meta-analysis has determined that athletes with concussion have two times the odds of receiving a musculoskeletal injury when compared to control groups (McPherson et al., 2019). Therefore, recurrent concussions could have neurological and musculoskeletal consequences for a young athlete. Overall, these statistics may not seem important, but, unfortunately, the rate has not decreased as our knowledge of safety, prevention, rehabilitation, and return to play has increased and more high schools have medical coverage at practices and games.

Youth Sport Specialization

Reviewing the epidemiology of sports injuries and discussing recurrent injuries in boys' and girls' sports transitions nicely into a brief review of youth sports specialization. The paradox of youth sports participation is complicated and involves many dimensions (McKay et al., 2019). Clearly, youth sports participation provides many benefits, including physical, social, and mental development (Felfe et al., 2016; Merkel, 2013), yet concern exists that early sports specialization (ESS) may lead to adverse health and social effects (Jayanthi et al., 2019).

As youth sports participation has grown over the years, an unfortunate shift has taken place going from extolling the positive aspects of sports to being concerned about scholarships, playing time, and advanced skill development. Such as shift has resulted in many young athletes participating and specializing in a single sport while excluding all others (Bell et al., 2018). Myer and colleagues (2016b) defined sports specialization as having three components: (1) year-round training (i.e., more than 8 months per year) and/or participating in too many hours of training or competitions per week, (2) participating on multiple teams of the same sport, and (3) quitting all other sports to focus on one. Aspects of sports specialization can also include participating in several competitions across a variety of sports, participating in periods of intense training or practices, entering into competitive play at an early age, and developing sports technical skills at an early age (e.g., pitching or gymnastic stunts; Myer et al., 2016a). Fortunately, some sports organizations have limited early specialization or overtraining at young ages, such as the Women's Tennis Association, which has age eligibility rules, and USA Baseball, which has daily pitch limits and age-related pitch counts. However, adults (parents) often alter records to keep youth athletes out on the court, pitch, or field or do not enforce these rules (Myer et al., 2016b). Because over- or early specialization in sports can result in a variety of negative consequences, such as psychological (i.e., burnout) and physiological (i.e., overtraining syndrome and increased risk of injury), several medical and sports organizations, including the AAP, the American Medical Society for Sports Medicine (AMSSM), the American Orthopaedic Society for Sports Medicine (AOSSM), the Fédération Internationale de Médecine du Sport, the International Olympic Committee (IOC), the National Athletic Trainers' Association (NATA), and the National Strength and Conditioning Association (NSCA), have developed position statements that warn against the trend of youth sports specialization (Jayanthi et al., 2019). Outlining all the recommendations from these respected sports and medical groups is not possible here, but all of them have a position stance on youth sports specialization or overtraining, the physical and psychological risks of early specialization, and the benefits of early diversified training, as well as various other recommendations pertaining to age and training. Recently, the NATA (2019) made an official statement that supports six recommendations for adolescent and young athlete sports specialization as they relate to the participants' psychosocial health and well-being (**Time Out 1.1**).

> ### TIME OUT 1.1
>
> **Six Recommendations to Preserve the Psychosocial Health and Well-Being of Adolescent and Young Athletes**
>
> The NATA supports the following recommendations:
>
> 1. Adolescent and young athletes need to delay single-sport specialization as long as possible.
> 2. Adolescent and young athletes should participate in only one organized team at a time.
> 3. Adolescent and young athletes should not play a single sport more than 8 months in a year.
> 4. Adolescent and young athletes should limit the hours of participation in sports per week to their age (10-year-olds should not participate in more than 10 hours of specialized activity each week).
> 5. Adolescent and young athletes need 2 rest or recovery days from organized training each week.
> 6. Adolescent and young athletes should take a break from their organized sport at the end of the competitive season to prevent burnout or dropout.
>
> Modified from National Athletic Trainers' Association (NATA). (2019). *Sport specialization recommendations for adolescents and young athletes.* Retrieved from https://www.nata.org/news-publications/pressroom/statements/official

The odds of excelling to elite levels of sports glory do not appear to be increased by early sports specialization, and in many professional or Olympic sports the athletes were typically multisport athletes or crossed over to different sports to find hidden talents (i.e., former NCAA football player becoming a medal-winning bobsled athlete; Myer et al., 2016a). However, there are a few sports for which specializing during preadolescent ages is necessary because peak performances come before full maturation (i.e., gymnastics and diving). But regardless of the age of participation, overtraining or overemphasis in these sports can still be very counterintuitive because without sport diversification children may not completely develop neuromuscular coordination that might be protective of injury (Myer et al., 2016a).

As our understanding of youth sports specialization increases and the research literature is developed, three degrees of specialization (i.e., low, moderate, and high) have been identified so more complete conclusions can be made regarding the effects associated with sports specialization. Three characteristics (i.e., year-round training of greater than 8 months, choosing a single main sport, and quitting all other sports to focus on one sport) are used to set the degrees of specialization. A low degree of specialization has none or one of the three characteristics, a moderate degree of specialization has two characteristics, and a high degree of specialization has all three characteristics (Myer et al., 2016b). Bell and colleagues (2018) performed a systematic review and meta-analysis to determine whether sports specialization is associated with overuse musculoskeletal injuries. Those athletes with a high degree of specialization had a higher relative risk ratio (RR = 1.81) when compared to low and moderate degrees of specialization, and athletes with a moderate degree of specialization had a 1.39 relative risk ratio when compared to a low degree of specialization (Bell et al., 2018). Post and colleagues (2017) reported that highly specialized athletes were 1.59 times more likely to have experienced any previous injury and 1.45 times more likely to have had an overuse injury. Those athletes that played their main sport more than 8 months a year also had around 1.6 times the odds of developing upper and lower extremity injuries, and those that participated in more hours of training or competition than others of their age were 1.34 times more likely to report an injury of any type (Post et al., 2017).

Finally, two scoping reviews of the literature on youth sports specialization (Myer et al., 2016a, 2016b) used the Strength of Recommendation Taxonomy to develop six ranked clinical recommendations according to the evidence available in the literature at the time of their reviews. Important to note is that their conclusions have been supported

Table 1.2
Clinical Recommendations Regarding Youth Sports Specialization

Grade	Clinical Recommendation
B	Youth who participate in more hours of sports per week than their age and those that specialize in one sport need to be closely monitored for indicators of burnout, overuse injury, and performance decrements.
C	Youth need to be given opportunities for free and unstructured play to improve motor skills and encouraged to practice self-regulation to limit overuse injuries.
C	Parents and educators should help provide opportunities for free and unstructured play to improve motor skills and reduce injury risk during adolescence.
C	Youth should be encouraged to participate in a variety of sports so they can develop diverse motor skills and identify a sport or sports that they enjoy.
C	All youth can benefit from periodized strength and conditioning, including neuromuscular training, to help them prepare for sports participation.
C	Youth who do specialize in a single sport need to plan periods of focused integrative neuromuscular training so they can enhance diverse motor skills and reduce injury risks.

Data from Myer, G. D., Jayanthi, N., DiFiori, J. P., Faigenbaum, A. D., Kiefer, A. W., Logerstedt, D., & Micheli, L. J. (2016b). Sports specialization, part I: Does early sports specialization increase negative outcomes and reduce the opportunity for success in young athletes? *Sports Health, 7*(5), 437–442; and Myer, G. D., Jayanthi, N., DiFiori, J. P., Faigenbaum, A. D., Kiefer, A. W., Logerstedt, D., & Micheli, L. J. (2016a). Sports specialization, part II: Alternative solutions to early sport specialization in youth athletes. *Sports Health, 8*(1), 65–73.

by more recent research (Bell et al., 2018; Jayanthi et al., 2019; Jayanthi et al., 2020; Post et al., 2017). Five of the six recommendations were graded as a C, indicating consensus, disease-oriented evidence, usual practice, expert opinion, or case series evidence was available to support them, and one of the six recommendations was graded as a B, indicating that only limited-quality patient-oriented evidence was available (Myer et al., 2016a, 2016b; Table 1.2). Therefore, the advice is to continue education for coaches, parents, and youth regarding outcomes of sports specialization and to design current recommendations to prevent negative outcomes of youth participation in competitive sports.

Review Questions

1. What is the paradox associated with youth sports participation?
2. What did Title IX do to the participation numbers for sports across the United States?
3. What constitutes a catastrophic sports injury according to the National Center for Catastrophic Sports Injury Research (NCCSIR)?
4. What are the three criteria necessary for an injury to be classified as such under the HS RIO program and NCAA's Injury Surveillance Program (ISP)?
5. Briefly describe two major problems that arise regarding the most commonly used definitions of sports injury.
6. Define and differentiate between acute and chronic forms of injury.
7. What specific tissue types are involved in sprains and strains? How is the severity of these injuries defined, and how has it changed over time?
8. What makes a stress fracture unique when compared with other types of fractures?

9. What are the five types of Salter-Harris fractures?
10. Define and differentiate between *subluxation* and *luxation*.
11. What is the science of epidemiology?
12. Using the sports classification system presented in this chapter, what are the two classifications for the sport of basketball?
13. What are the most commonly injured areas of the body in tackle football at the high school level?
14. What are the most common ways that tackle football athletes suffer fatal or catastrophic nonfatal injuries?
15. How have head and neck injuries been reduced in tackle football over the years?
16. What type of catastrophic injury seems to affect male basketball players more than other athletes?
17. What are two concerning injuries for both baseball and softball players caused by sports equipment and the trend to pitch or throw too much?
18. What are the differences in the skin infections between high school wrestlers and collegiate wrestlers?
19. What area of the body do volleyball athletes seem to injure the most?
20. What do we know about ACL injuries and their occurrence rate between male and female athletes?
21. What is one of the major concerns regarding ACL injury and knee reconstruction surgery?
22. As a coach or parent, why should you be concerned about moveable soccer goals?
23. What is the major concern regarding female gymnastics relative to injury risk?
24. Why is cheerleading both a safer sport than many and also more dangerous?
25. Define *sports specialization*.
26. What are the six recommendations to preserve the psychosocial health and well-being of adolescent and young athletes?

References

Aicale, R., Tarantino, D., & Maffulli, N. (2018). Overuse injuries in sport: A comprehensive overview. *Journal of Orthopaedic Surgery and Research, 13*(1), 1–11.

American Medical Association. (1968). *Standard nomenclature of athletic injuries*. Chicago, IL: American Medical Association.

Aspen Institute. (2019). *State of play 2019: Trends and developments in youth sports*. Retrieved from https://www.aspeninstitute.org/wp-content/uploads/2019/10/2019_SOP_National_Final.pdf

Bell, D. R., Post, E. G., Biese, K., Bay, C., & McLeod, T. V. (2018). Sport specialization and risk of overuse injuries: A systematic review with meta-analysis. *Pediatrics, 142*(3).

Caine, C. G., Caine, D. J., & Lindner, K. J. (1996). The epidemiological approach to sports injuries. In D. J. Caine, C. G. Caine, & K. J. Lindner (Eds.), *Epidemiology of sports injuries* (pp. 2–3). Champaign, IL: Human Kinetics.

Caine, D., Maffulli, N., & Caine, C. (2008). Epidemiology of injury in child and adolescent sports: Injury rates, risk factors, and prevention. *Clinics in Sports Medicine, 27*(1), 19–50.

Campbell, R. A., Bradshaw, E. J., Ball, N. B., Pease, D. L., & Spratford, W. (2019). Injury epidemiology and risk factors in competitive artistic gymnasts: A systematic review. *British Journal of Sports Medicine, 53*(17), 1056–1069.

Centers for Disease Control and Prevention (CDC). (2019). *Methicillin-resistant staphylococcus infections (MRSA)*. Retrieved from https://www.cdc.gov/mrsa/community/index.html

Cheung, E. C., DiLallo, M., Feeley, B. T., & Lansdown, D. A. (2020). Osteoarthritis and ACL reconstruction—myths and risks. *Current Reviews in Musculoskeletal Medicine, 13*(1), 115–122.

Churchill, N. W., Hutchison, M. G., Graham, S. J., & Schweizer, T. A. (2019). Mapping brain recovery after concussion: From acute injury to 1 year after medical clearance. *Neurology, 93*(21), e1980–e1992.

Clifton, D. R., Hertel, J., Onate, J. A., Currie, D. W., Pierpoint, L. A., Wasserman, E. B., . . . Kerr, Z. Y. (2018). The first decade of web-based sports injury surveillance: Descriptive epidemiology of injuries in US high school girls' basketball (2005–2006 through 2013–2014) and National Collegiate Athletic Association Women's basketball (2004–2005 through 2013–2014). *Journal of Athletic Training, 53*(11), 1037–1048.

Clifton, D. R., Onate, J. A., Hertel, J., Pierpoint, L. A., Currie, D. W., Wasserman, E. B., . . . Kerr, Z. Y. (2018). The first decade of web-based sports injury surveillance: Descriptive epidemiology of injuries in US high school boys' basketball (2005–2006 through 2013–2014) and National Collegiate Athletic Association Men's basketball (2004–2005 through 2013–2014). *Journal of Athletic Training, 53*(11), 1025–1036.

Comstock, R. D., Currie, D. W., Pierpoint, L. A., Grubenhoff, J. A., & Fields, S. K. (2015). An evidence-based discussion of heading the ball and concussions in high school soccer. *JAMA Pediatrics, 169*(9), 830–837.

Comstock, R. D., & Pierpoint, L. A. (2020). *National High School Sports-Related Injury Surveillance Survey (2018-2019)*. Retrieved from https://coloradosph.cuanschutz.edu/research-and-practice/centers-programs/piper/research-practice/research-projects

Consumer Product Safety Commission. (2014). *Movable soccer goals can fall over on children*. Retrieved from https://www.cpsc.gov/s3fs-public/5118.pdf

Cooper, E. R., Grundstein, A. J., Miles, J. D., Ferrara, M. S., Curry, P., Casa, D. J., & Hosokawa, Y. (2020). Heat policy revision for Georgia high school football practices based on data-driven research. *Journal of Athletic Training, 55*(7), 673–681.

Coster, J. E., Turner, J. K., Bradbury, D., & Cantrell, A. (2017). Why do people choose emergency and urgent care services? A rapid review utilizing a systematic literature search and narrative synthesis. *Academic Emergency Medicine, 24*(9), 1137–1149.

Currie, D. W., Fields, S. K., Patterson, M. J., & Comstock, R. D. (2016). Cheerleading injuries in United States high schools. *Pediatrics, 137*(1), e20152447.

DiStefano, L. J., Dann, C. L., Chang, C. J., Putukian, M., Pierpoint, L. A., Currie, D. W., . . . Kerr, Z. Y. (2018). The first decade of web-based sports injury surveillance: Descriptive epidemiology of injuries in US high school girls' soccer (2005–2006 through 2013–2014) and National Collegiate Athletic Association women's soccer (2004–2005 through 2013–2014). *Journal of Athletic Training, 53*(9), 880–892.

DiStefano, L. J., Frank, B. S., Root, H. J., & Padua, D. A. (2017). Dissemination and implementation strategies of lower extremity preventive training programs in youth: A clinical review. *Sports Health, 9*(6), 524–531.

Edwards, W. B. (2018). Modeling overuse injuries in sport as a mechanical fatigue phenomenon. *Exercise and Sport Sciences Reviews, 46*(4), 224–231.

Endres, B. D., Kerr, Z. Y., Stearns, R. L., Adams, W. M., Hosokawa, Y., Huggins, R. A., . . . Casa, D. J. (2019). Epidemiology of sudden death in organized youth sports in the United States, 2007–2015. *Journal of Athletic Training, 54*(4), 349–355.

Fältström, A., Kvist, J., Gauffin, H., & Hägglund, M. (2019). Female soccer players with anterior cruciate ligament reconstruction have a higher risk of new knee injuries and quit soccer to a higher degree than knee-healthy controls. *American Journal of Sports Medicine, 47*(1), 31–40.

Felfe, C., Lechner, M., & Steinmayr, A. (2016). Sport and child development. *PloS One, 11*(5), e0151729. https://doi.org/10.1371/journal.pone.0151729

Findler, P. (2015). Should kids play (American) football? *Journal of the Philosophy of Sport, 42*(3), 443–462.

Fleisig, G. S., & Andrews, J. R. (2012). Prevention of elbow injuries in youth baseball pitchers. *Sports Health, 4*(5), 419–424.

Flint, J. H., Wade, A. M., Giuliani, J., & Rue, J. P. (2014). Defining the terms acute and chronic in orthopaedic sports injuries: A systematic review. *American Journal of Sports Medicine, 42*(1), 235–241.

Grundstein, A., Williams, C., Phan, M., & Cooper, E. (2015). Regional heat safety thresholds for athletics in the contiguous United States. *Applied Geography, 56*, 55–60.

Ingram, J. G., Fields, S. K., Yard, E. E., & Comstock, R. D. (2008). Epidemiology of knee injuries among boys and girls in US high school athletics. *American Journal of Sports Medicine, 36*(6), 1116–1122.

Jayanthi, N., Kleithermes, S., Dugas, L., Pasulka, J., Iqbal, S., & LaBella, C. (2020). Risk of injuries associated with sport specialization and intense training patterns in young athletes: A longitudinal clinical case-control study. *Orthopaedic Journal of Sports Medicine, 8*(6), 2325967120922764.

Jayanthi, N. A., Post, E. G., Laury, T. C., & Fabricant, P. D. (2019). Health consequences of youth sport specialization. *Journal of Athletic Training, 54*(10), 1040–1049.

Jones, C., & Hammig, B. (2020). Epidemiology of concussions among pediatric cheerleaders in the United States, 2009–2018. *Archives of Medical Research, 8*(5), 1–7.

Kerr, Z. Y., Comstock, R. D., Dompier, T. P., & Marshall, S. W. (2018). The first decade of web-based sports injury surveillance (2004–2005 through 2013–2014): Methods of the National Collegiate Athletic Association Injury Surveillance Program and High School Reporting Information Online. *Journal of Athletic Training, 53*(8), 729–737.

Kerr, Z. Y., Gregory, A. J., Wosmek, J., Pierpoint, L. A., Currie, D. W., Knowles, S. B., . . . Marshall, S. W. (2018). The first decade of web-based sports injury surveillance: Descriptive epidemiology of injuries in US high school girls' volleyball (2005–2006 through 2013–2014) and National Collegiate Athletic Association women's volleyball (2004–2005 through 2013–2014). *Journal of Athletic Training, 53*(10), 926–937.

Kerr, Z. Y., Putukian, M., Chang, C. J., DiStefano, L. J., Currie, D. W., Pierpoint, L. A., . . . Marshall, S. W. (2018). The first decade of web-based sports injury surveillance: Descriptive epidemiology of injuries in US high school boys' soccer (2005–2006 through 2013–2014) and National Collegiate Athletic Association men's soccer (2004–2005 through 2013–2014). *Journal of Athletic Training, 53*(9), 893–905.

Kerr, Z. Y., Wilkerson, G. B., Caswell, S. V., Currie, D. W., Pierpoint, L. A., Wasserman, E. B., . . . Marshall, S. W. (2018). The first decade of web-based sports injury surveillance: Descriptive epidemiology of injuries in United States high school football (2005–2006 through 2013–2014) and National Collegiate Athletic Association football (2004–2005 through 2013–2014). *Journal of Athletic Training, 53*(8), 738–751.

Knapik, J. J., Reynolds, K., & Hoedebecke, K. L. (2017). Stress fractures: Etiology, epidemiology, diagnosis, treatment, and prevention. *Journal of Special Operations Medicine, 17*(2), 120–130.

Kroshus, E., Utter, A. C., Pierpoint, L. A., Currie, D. W., Knowles, S. B., Wasserman, E. B., . . . Kerr, Z. Y. (2018). The first decade of web-based sports injury surveillance: Descriptive epidemiology of injuries in US high school boys' wrestling (2005–2006 through 2013–2014) and National Collegiate Athletic Association men's wrestling (2004–2005 through 2013–2014). *Journal of Athletic Training, 53*(12), 1143–1155.

Kucera, K. L., & Cantu, R. C. (2019). *Catastrophic sport injury research: Thirty-sixth annual report—Fall 1982–Spring*

2018. Retrieved from https://nccsir.unc.edu/wp-content/uploads/sites/5614/2019/10/2018-Catastrophic-Report-AS-36th-AY2017-2018-FINAL.pdf

Kucera, K. L., Klossner, D., Colgate, B., & Cantu R. C. (2019). *Annual survey of football injury research—1931-2018.* Retrieved from https://nccsir.unc.edu/wp-content/uploads/sites/5614/2019/02/Annual-Football-2018-Fatalities-FINAL.pdf

Leppänen, M., Pasanen, K., Kujala, U. M., Vasankari, T., Kannus, P., Äyrämö, S., . . . Parkkari, J. (2017). Stiff landings are associated with increased ACL injury risk in young female basketball and floorball players. *American Journal of Sports Medicine, 45*(2), 386-393.

Levine, B. D., Baggish, A. L., Kovacs, R. J., Link, M. S., Maron, M. S., & Mitchell, J. H. (2015). Eligibility and disqualification recommendations for competitive athletes with cardiovascular abnormalities: Task force 1: Classification of sports: Dynamic, static, and impact: A scientific statement from the American Heart Association and American College of Cardiology. *Journal of American College of Cardiology, 66*(21), 2350-2355.

Lewis, J. S. (2009). Rotator cuff tendinopathy. *British Journal of Sports Medicine, 43*(4), 236-241.

Lock, S. (2020). *Participants in gymnastics in the U.S. from 2006 to 2017.* Retrieved from https://www.statista.com/statistics/191908/participants-in-gymnastics-in-the-us-since-2006/

Lorimer, A. V., & Hume, P. A. (2014). Achilles tendon injury risk factors associated with running. *Sports Medicine, 44*(10), 1459-1472.

MacDonald, J., & Myer, G. D. (2017). 'Don't let kids play football': A killer idea. *British Journal of Sports Medicine, 51,* 1448-1449.

Maron, B. J., & Estes, N. M., III (2010). Commotio cordis. *New England Journal of Medicine, 362*(10), 917-927.

Maroon, J. C., Winkelman, R., Bost, J., Amos, A., Mathyssek, C., & Miele, V. (2015). Chronic traumatic encephalopathy in contact sports: A systematic review of all reported pathological cases. *PloS One, 10*(2), e0117338.

McCrory, P., Meeuwisse, W., Dvorak, J., Aubry, M., Bailes, J., Broglio, S., . . . Davis, G. A. (2017). Consensus statement on concussion in sport—The 5th International Conference on Concussion in Sport held in Berlin, October 2016. *British Journal of Sports Medicine, 51*(11), 838-847.

McGuine, T., Post, E., Pfaller, A. Y., Hetzel, S., Schwarz, A., Brooks, M. A., & Kliethermes, S. A. (2020). Does soccer headgear reduce the incidence of sport-related concussion? A cluster, randomised controlled trial of adolescent athletes. *British Journal of Sports Medicine, 54*(7), 408-413.

McKay, C. D., Cumming, S. P., & Blake, T. (2019). Youth sport: Friend or foe? *Best Practice & Research Clinical Rheumatology, 33,* 141-157.

McPherson, A. L., Nagai, T., Webster, K. E., & Hewett, T. E. (2019). Musculoskeletal injury risk after sport-related concussion: A systematic review and meta-analysis. *American Journal of Sports Medicine, 47*(7), 1754-1762.

Merkel, D. L. (2013). Youth sport: Positive and negative impact on young athletes. *Open Access Journal of Sports Medicine, 4,* 151-160.

Mickalide, A. D., & Hansen, L. M. (2012). *Coaching our kids to fewer injuries: A report on youth sports safety.* Washington, DC: Safe Kids Worldwide.

Montalvo, A. M., Schneider, D. K., Yut, L., Webster, K. E., Beynnon, B., Kocher, M. S., & Myer, G. D. (2019). "What's my risk of sustaining an ACL injury while playing sports?" A systematic review with meta-analysis. *British Journal of Sports Medicine, 53*(16), 1003-1012.

Mueller-Wohlfahrt, H. W., Haensel, L., Mithoefer, K., Ekstrand, J., English, B., McNally, S., . . . Ueblacker, P. (2013). Terminology and classification of muscle injuries in sport: The Munich consensus statement. *British Journal of Sports Medicine, 47*(6), 342-350.

Murtaugh, B., & Ihm, J. M. (2013). Eccentric training for the treatment of tendinopathies. *Current Sports Medicine Reports, 12*(3), 175-182.

Myer, G. D., Jayanthi, N., DiFiori, J. P., Faigenbaum, A. D., Kiefer, A. W., Logerstedt, D., & Micheli, L. J. (2016a). Sports specialization, part I: Does early sports specialization increase negative outcomes and reduce the opportunity for success in young athletes? *Sports Health, 7*(5), 437-442.

Myer, G. D., Jayanthi, N., DiFiori, J. P., Faigenbaum, A. D., Kiefer, A. W., Logerstedt, D., & Micheli, L. J. (2016b). Sports specialization, part II: Alternative solutions to early sport specialization in youth athletes. *Sports Health, 8*(1), 65-73.

National Athletic Trainers' Association (NATA). (2019). *Sport specialization recommendations for adolescents and young athletes.* Retrieved from https://www.nata.org/news-publications/pressroom/statements/official

National Collegiate Athletic Association (NCAA). (2020). *Estimated probability of competing in college athletics.* Retrieved from http://www.ncaa.org/about/resources/research/estimated-probability-competing-college-athletics

National Federation of State High School Associations (NFHS). (2020). *2018-19 High school athletics participation survey.* Retrieved from https://www.nfhs.org/sports-resource-content/high-school-participation-survey-archive/

National Safety Council (NSC). (1991). *First aid and CPR.* Boston, MA: Jones and Bartlett Publishers.

Padua, D. A., Frank, B., Donaldson, A., de la Motte, S., Cameron, K. L., Beutler, A. I., . . . Marshall, S. W. (2014). Seven steps for developing and implementing a preventive training program: Lessons learned from JUMP-ACL and beyond. *Clinical Sports Medicine, 33*(4), 615-632.

Patel, B. C., Skidmore, K., Hutchison, J., & Hatcher, J. D. (2017). *Cauliflower ear.* Treasure Island, FL: StatPearls Publishing, LLC.

Patel, D. R., Yamasaki, A., & Brown, K. (2017). Epidemiology of sports-related musculoskeletal injuries in young athletes in United States. *Translational Pediatrics, 6*(3), 160.

Post, E. G., Trigsted, S. M., Riekena, J. W., Hetzel, S., McGuine, T. A., Brooks, M. A., & Bell, D. R. (2017). The association of sport specialization and training volume with injury history in youth athletes. *American Journal of Sports Medicine, 45*(6), 1405-1412.

Prentice, W. E. (2017). *Principles of athletic training: A guide to evidence-based practice* (16th ed.). New York, NY: McGraw-Hill.

Reinking, M. F. (2016). Current concepts in the treatment of patellar tendinopathy. *International Journal of Sports Physical Therapy, 11*(6), 854–866.

Rice, S. G. (2008). Medical conditions affecting sports participation. *Pediatrics, 121*(4), 841–848.

Rice, S. G., & Congeni, J. A. (2012). Council on Sports Medicine and Fitness: Baseball and softball. *Pediatrics, 129*(3), e842–e856. https://doi.org/10.1542/peds.2015-3152

Rojas, I. L., Provencher, M. T., Bhatia, S., Foucher, K. C., Bach, B. R., Jr., Romeo, A. A., . . . Verma, N. N. (2009). Biceps activity during windmill softball pitching: Injury implications and comparison with overhand throwing. *American Journal of Sports Medicine, 37*(3), 558–565.

Rui, P., Ashman, J. J., & Akinseye, A. (2019). *Emergency department visits for injuries sustained during sports and recreational activities by patients aged 5-24 years, 2010-2016.* Retrieved from https://www.cdc.gov/nchs/data/nhsr/nhsr133-508.pdf

Sarmiento, K., Thomas, K. E., Daugherty, J., Waltzman, D., Haarbauer-Krupa, J. K., Peterson, A. B., . . . Breiding, M. J. (2019). Emergency department visits for sports- and recreation-related traumatic brain injuries among children—United States, 2010–2016. *Morbidity and Mortality Weekly Report, 68*(10), 237.

Scott, A., Squier, K., Alfredson, H., Bahr, R., Cook, J. L., Coombes, B., . . . Zwerver, J. (2020). Icon 2019: International scientific tendinopathy symposium consensus: Clinical terminology. *British Journal of Sports Medicine, 54*(5), 260–262.

Smucny, M., Kolmodin, J., & Saluan, P. (2016). Shoulder and elbow injuries in the adolescent athlete. *Sports Medicine and Arthroscopy Review, 24*(4), 188–194.

Stanford Children's Health. (n.d.) *Sports injury statistics.* Retrieved from https://www.stanfordchildrens.org/en/topic/default?id=sports-injury-statistics-90-P02787

Tee, J. C., McLaren, S. J., & Jones, B. (2020). Sports injury prevention is complex: We need to invest in better processes, not singular solutions. *Sports Medicine, 50*(4), 689–702.

Timpka, T., Alonso, J. M., Jacobsson, J., Junge, A., Branco, P., Clarsen, B., . . . Edouard, P. (2014). Injury and illness definitions and data collection procedures for use in epidemiological studies in athletics (track and field): Consensus statement. *British Journal of Sports Medicine, 48*(7), 483–490.

Timpka, T., Jacobsson, J., Bickenbach, J., Finch, C. F., Ekberg, J., & Nordenfelt, L. (2014). What is a sports injury? *Sports Medicine, 44*(4), 423–428.

Trojian, T. H. (2013). Muscle contusion (thigh). *Clinical Sports Medicine, 32*(2), 317–324.

Venes, D., & Taber, C. W. (2009). *Taber's cyclopedic medical dictionary* (21st ed.). Philadelphia, PA: F. A. Davis.

Waldén, M., Hägglund, M., Werner, J., & Ekstrand, J. (2011). The epidemiology of anterior cruciate ligament injury in football (soccer): A review of the literature from a gender-related perspective. *Knee Surgery, Sports Traumatology Arthroscopy, 19*(1), 3–10.

Walter, S. D., Sutton, J. R., McIntosh, J. M., & Connolly, C. (1985). The aetiology of sport injuries—A review of methodologies. *Sports Medicine, 2*, 47–58.

Wasserman, E. B., Sauers, E. L., Register-Mihalik, J. K., Pierpoint, L. A., Currie, D. W., . . . Kerr, Z. Y. (2019a). The first decade of web-based sports injury surveillance: Descriptive epidemiology of injuries in US high school boys' baseball (2005–2006 through 2013–2014) and National Collegiate Athletic Association men's baseball (2004–2005 through 2013–2014). *Journal of Athletic Training, 54*(2), 198–211.

Wasserman, E. B., Register-Mihalik, J. K., Sauers, E. L., Currie, D. W., Pierpoint, L. A., Knowles, S. B., . . . Kerr, Z. Y. (2019b). The first decade of web-based sports injury surveillance: Descriptive epidemiology of injuries in US high school girls' softball (2005–2006 through 2013–2014) and National Collegiate Athletic Association women's softball (2004–2005 through 2013–2014). *Journal of Athletic Training, 54*(2), 212–225.

Webster, K. E., & Hewett, T. E. (2018). Meta-analysis of meta-analyses of anterior cruciate ligament injury reduction training programs. *Journal of Orthopaedic Research, 36*(10), 2696–2708.

Welton, K. L., Kraeutler, M. J., Pierpoint, L. A., Bartley, J. H., McCarty, E. C., & Comstock, R. D. (2018). Injury recurrence among high school athletes in the United States: A decade of patterns and trends, 2005–2006 through 2015–2016. *Orthopaedic Journal of Sports Medicine, 6*(1), 2325967117745788.

Werner, S. L., Jones, D. G., Guido, J. A., Jr., & Brunet, M. E. (2006). Kinematics and kinetics of elite windmill softball pitching. *American Journal of Sports Medicine, 34*(4), 597–603.

Whatman, C., Walters, S., & Schluter, P. (2018). Coach and player attitudes to injury in youth sport. *Physical Therapy in Sport, 32*, 1–6.

Yeargin, S. W., Dompier, T. P., Casa, D. J., Hirschhorn, R. M., & Kerr, Z. Y. (2019). Epidemiology of exertional heat illnesses in National Collegiate Athletic Association athletes during the 2009–2010 through 2014–2015 academic years. *Journal of Athletic Training, 54*(1), 55–63.

CHAPTER 2

The Athletic Healthcare Team

MAJOR CONCEPTS

The cornerstone of optimal management of sports- and activity-related injuries is the athletic healthcare team (AHCT), which comprises a variety of highly trained medical and allied medical personnel, as well as other professionals, and coordinates on-site with nonmedical personnel, including coaches, administrators, parents, and the athletes. This chapter provides an overview of the principal members of the team and reviews the evolution of the field of sports medicine. In addition, it describes specific services provided by the athletic healthcare team, giving special attention to the team physician and the athletic trainer (AT) who is certified by the Board of Certification, Inc. (BOC). It also outlines educational requirements for BOC certification and employment options for certified ATs.

Effective delivery of health care to participants in sports and other physical activities is best achieved through a comprehensive AHCT approach, which includes BOC-certified ATs, a medical physician director, and emergency medical services (EMS) personnel, all of whom then work in concert with additional qualified medical personnel (QMP), such as other physician specialists, school nurses, physician assistants, dentists, and counselors (Cooper et al., 2019). This AHCT coordinates and functions in concert with coaches, administrators, athletes, and parents according to the accepted standards of good clinical practice (Cooper et al., 2019).

The AHCT integrates their services via effective communication (Gatchel et al., 2014). They treat the whole person by using the appropriate healthcare provider to address and achieve optimal health and healing. Ultimately, the members of the AHCT should be educated to deliver patient-centered care that emphasizes evidence-based practice (Knebel & Greiner, 2003). Several important elements comprise interprofessional care: (1) practitioners understanding their own roles and roles of other professionals; (2) practitioners from varying professions learning to communicate with each other in a collaborative, responsive, and respective manner; (3) practitioners learning to effectively deal with interprofessional conflict; (4) practitioners learning to work together with other professionals as well as patients, families, and communities to formulate, implement, and evaluate care and services to enhance health outcomes; and (5) practitioners understanding the principles of team dynamics and group processes to enable effective collaboration (Barwell et al., 2013). Therefore, the current healthcare providers and generations to come must be formally educated and encouraged to participate as interprofessional AHCTs to allow for the development of quality care based on the most current evidence.

Sports Medicine

Sports medicine generally refers to health care that is related to sports and physical activity; it typically includes a variety of healthcare specializations within performance enhancement, injury management, and injury care and rehabilitation (Prentice, 2017). Sports medicine delivery may be one of the first models of interprofessional care. The sports medicine umbrella of interprofessional care typically includes biomechanists, exercise physiologists, strength and conditioning specialists, sport psychologists, sports nutritionists, sports massage and manual therapists, sports dentists, osteopaths, orthotists (i.e., prosthetics/orthotics), emergency medical technicians, and podiatrists (Figure 2.1a–c).

Historically, those most often associated with the practice of sports medicine have included physicians who work directly with athletes, typically **orthopedic surgeons** and ATs. As the field of sports medicine has evolved over the past several decades, several related professionals have been added to the list of potential practitioners in the sports medicine field. These professionals include family care, internal medicine, and pediatric physicians; chiropractors; sports physical therapists; and, in school settings, school nurses. Those in the sports medicine field generally acknowledge that family practice, internal medicine, and pediatric physicians will likely continue to grow their offered services to the athletic community. Because medical schools typically do not provide specialized training in the care of sports- and activity-related injury to these disciplines within traditional medical education programs, additional

Sports medicine Branch of medicine concerned with the medical aspects of sports participation.

Orthopedic surgeon Physician who assesses and attempts to correct deformities and dysfunction of the musculoskeletal system.

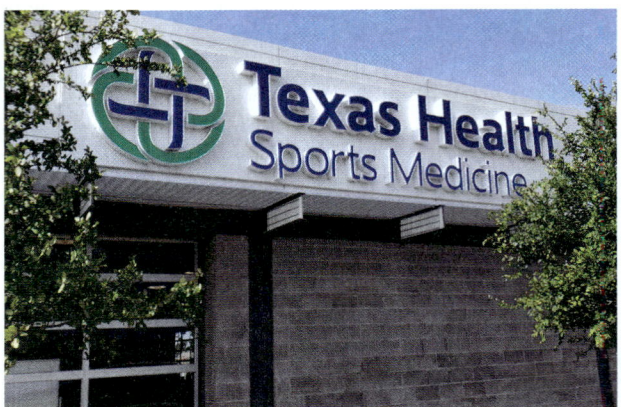

(a)

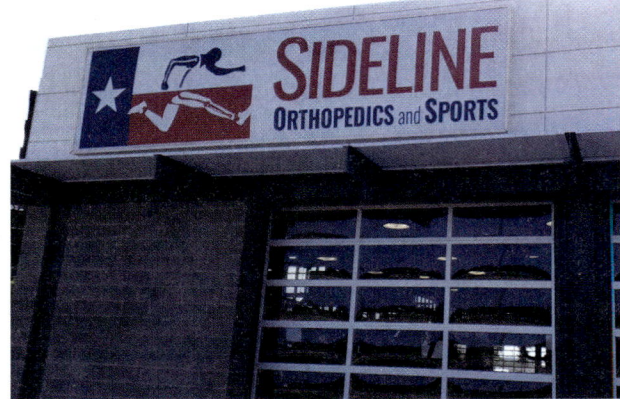

(b)

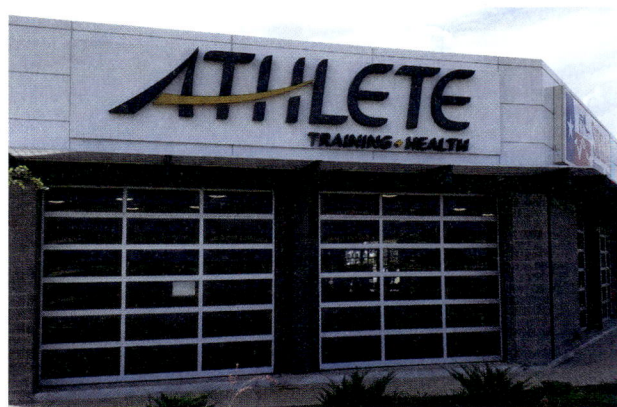

(c)

Figure 2.1 (a) Large hospital systems often provide the foundation for specialized care for the physically active. (b) Physician clinics that serve the physically active frequently employ athletic trainers as part of their healthcare team. (c) Performance centers connected to orthopedic and rehabilitation clinics provide prevention, performance, and return-to-play services.
Courtesy of Cindy Trowbridge.

postgraduate education is available to qualify different types of physicians in the sports medicine field. Sports medicine fellowships lasting a minimum of 1 year lead to an additional credential, the Certificate of Added Qualifications in Sports Medicine (CAQ). The CAQ is available to any primary care practitioner and is awarded on successful completion of the fellowship plus successful completion of an examination. The CAQ is offered annually to family physicians in conjunction with the American Board of Emergency Medicine, the American Board of Internal Medicine, and the American Board of Pediatrics (American Board of Family Medicine, 2013).

At the professional level of sports, today's athletes may have daily access to a wide variety of sports medicine services with access to all types of healthcare providers, including those trained in acupuncture, psychological assessments, and nutrition education and dietary management and counseling. Sports medicine services at the collegiate level involve a somewhat scaled-back version of the professional level, depending on the NCAA division or interscholastic level (e.g., junior college). However, at the secondary school level, in which nearly 8 million secondary school–aged students participate in athletics (National Federation of State High School Associations, 2018), participants often experience a lack of daily contact with sports medicine services, in particular a team physician and a BOC-certified AT.

Key Members of the Team

Although each member of the AHCT is important, three are essential: the coach, the team physician, and the BOC-certified AT.

Coaches

Although typically not recognized as experts in sports injury, coaches are critical in the process of injury prevention and, in many cases, function as a first responder when an athlete is injured. Regardless of their academic background, coaches in public schools should receive training in basic conditioning procedures; maintenance and fitting of protective equipment; first aid and CPR; operation of an automated external defibrillator (AED); and recognition and management of common sports injuries, including concussion and exertional heat illness. In addition, coaches should be competent to teach correct technique of sports skills to the athletes they train. Athletes' performing sports skills correctly is especially critical in contact/collision sports, which are inherently more dangerous than noncontact sports and can be made even more so by athletes' performing skills incorrectly.

Although the ideal situation would be for all public-school sports programs to have a team physician and a BOC-certified AT, the reality is that, in the majority of cases, coaches alone must provide basic sports medicine services to their athletes. Even when a school does employ a BOC-certified AT, for that AT to be physically present at all practices and games is impossible. Therefore, in many schools, when an injury occurs, coaches are the first ones on the scene of the injury, and they must make the initial decisions regarding the status of the athlete, including which first aid procedures to administer. Coaches must be good communicators and follow the recommendations of the AT and team physician regarding decisions about an injured athlete's recovery plan and return-to-play schedule. At the same time, the AT and team physician need to include the coach and other athletic department personnel in matters such as the development of the conditioning programs and emergency plans.

Team Physician

In 2000, the American College of Sport Medicine (ACSM, 2000) published the Team Physician Consensus Statement that outlined the roles and responsibilities required of the team physician. The ACSM consensus statement was updated in 2013 (Herring, Kibler, et al., 2013) and it provides a detailed listing of the team physician's qualifications and responsibilities. According to the latest update, a team physician must be either a medical doctor (MD) or a doctor of osteopathy (DO) and hold an unrestricted license, be knowledgeable about common sports-related medical emergencies (e.g., cardiac, heat-related, spinal, concussion), and have training in other common issues affecting the athlete (e.g., musculoskeletal, psychological), along with being trained in basic cardiopulmonary resuscitation and automated external defibrillator use.

> **Team physician** A medical doctor who agrees to provide at least limited medical coverage to a particular sports program or institution and ideally has additional training in sports medicine.

Team physicians agree to provide (either voluntarily or for pay) at least limited medical care to a particular sports program or institution. These services range in scope, for example, from a pediatrician who volunteers to be present for home football games at the local high school, to the other end of the continuum, a nationally prominent orthopedic surgeon who contracts with a Major League Baseball team to serve as its team physician. The team physician must be willing to commit the necessary time and effort to provide care to each athlete and team. In addition, team physicians must develop and maintain a contemporary knowledge base of the sports for which they are accepting responsibility. Qualified team physicians understand sports injuries that most other physicians simply do not. Furthermore, they generally know the common risk factors and epidemiology regarding illness and sports-injury prevention and treatment, are familiar with the athletes, and should have a genuine interest in the welfare of each participant. Team physicians can improve athletes' care by understanding and practicing methods of injury and illness prevention regarding specific sports medicine problems.

The ACSM helped developed a partner alliance with the American Academy of Family Physicians (AAFP), the American Academy of Orthopaedic Surgeons (AAOS), the American Medical Society for Sports Medicine (AMSSM), the American Orthopaedic Society for Sports Medicine (AOSSM), and the American Osteopathic Academy of Sports Medicine (AOASM), and together they created the Team Physician Consensus Conference (TPCC) group. The TPCC uses expert consensus and evidence-based research to annually produce an updated consensus statement related to different trending topics in sports medicine. Team physicians from a variety of settings serve as authors and panelists for these consensus statements. Over the years, topics have included sideline preparedness; mass participation event coverage; concussion; psychological concerns; strength and conditioning; load; overload; recovery; nutrition; adolescent, masters, and female athlete concerns; return to play; and pain management. These TPCC consensus statements are updated as new evidence emerges and are freely available at https://www.acsm.org/acsm-positions-policy/official-communications/team-physician-consensus-statements.

Acquiring the services of team physicians may not be an easy task, especially in rural communities and in situations where little or no money is available. Historically, team physicians have reported that the major reason they become involved with sports is because of a strong personal interest (Rogers, 1985). This likely remains the case today, and as such, obtaining team physicians on a volunteer basis may be possible, at least for the purposes of providing medical care at athletic events. To expect more will, in all likelihood, require that some sort of contractual payment plan and insurance matters be arranged. State medical associations or boards, as well as a college or university, may provide information on how to locate interested physicians.

A variety of continuing education programs are currently available to team physicians through workshops, seminars, and postgraduate courses offered by hospitals, medical schools, and professional groups. In addition, numerous medical organizations exist that promote the study of sports medicine through membership, including the AMSSM, the AAFP, the AOSSM, the ACSM, the AOASM, and the AAOS.

BOC-Certified Athletic Trainer

To provide comprehensive medical care for student-athletes (during practice and games), the general consensus within the sports medicine community is to hire a BOC-certified AT who works in conjunction with a team physician. The American Medical Association (AMA) recognizes athletic training as a healthcare profession. To be a BOC-certified AT, you must complete a master's degree with extensive academic and clinical training in the broad areas of the prevention, recognition, and management of sports injuries and then pass a national certification exam directed by the BOC.

The BOC (2017) defines ATs as:

healthcare professionals who render service or treatment, under the direction of or in collaboration with a physician, in accordance with their education and training and the states' statutes, rules and regulations. As a part of the healthcare team, services provided by ATs include injury and illness prevention, wellness promotion and education, emergent care, examination and clinical diagnosis, therapeutic intervention, and rehabilitation of injuries and medical conditions.

Including a BOC-certified AT on any AHCT can greatly enhance the overall quality of sports medicine

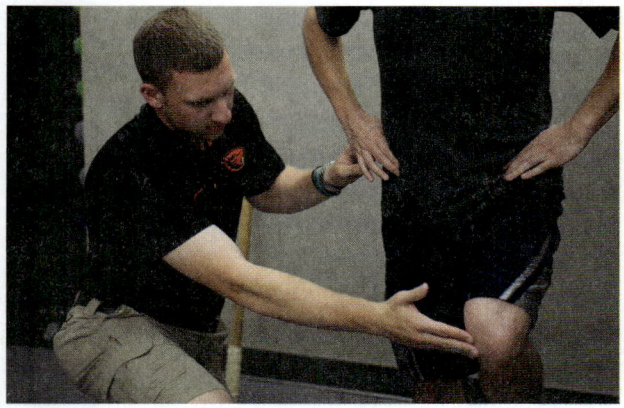

Figure 2.2 An athletic trainer helping to prevent injuries by improving knee joint position for an athlete.
Courtesy of Mark Hoffman.

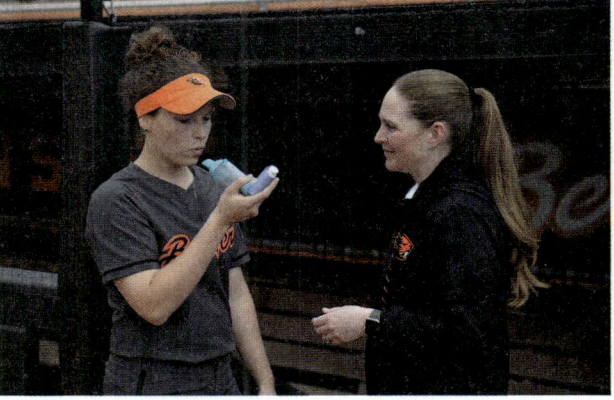

Figure 2.4 An athletic trainer assisting a softball player with a peak flow meter to assess lung capacity.
Courtesy of Mark Hoffman.

services and potentially save lives. The practice domains for athletic training, as described by the BOC (2017), are as follows:

- Risk Reduction, Wellness, and Health Literacy (Figure 2.2)
- Examination, Assessment and Diagnosis (Figure 2.3)
- Critical Incident Management (Figure 2.4)
- Therapeutic Intervention (Figures 2.5 and 2.6)
- Healthcare Administration and Professional Responsibility

Becoming a BOC-certified AT requires qualifying to sit for and then passing the BOC certification examination, which is an online exam that verifies knowledge of the practice domains with recall, application, and analysis questions. The certification exam is offered five times annually via a national network of computerized testing centers. To qualify to sit for the examination, the individual must have completed an educational program accredited by the Commission on Accreditation of Athletic Training Education (CAATE) and must be endorsed by their CAATE program director. In addition, they must have proof of current certification in emergency cardiac care. The *BOC Exam Candidate Handbook* and other details about the exam are available for review with a free download at the BOC website (https://bocatc.org/candidates/steps-to-become-certified/determine-eligibility/determine-exam-eligibility).

Founded in 1950, the National Athletic Trainers' Association (NATA) is the national professional

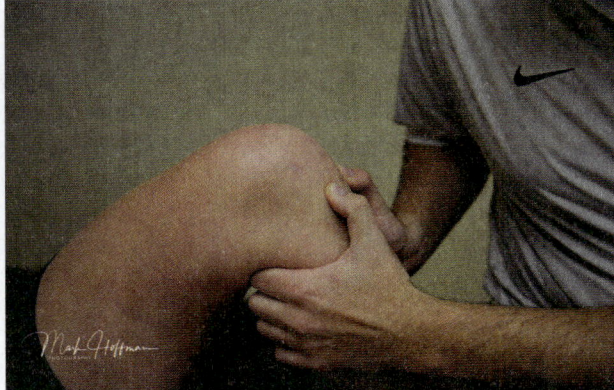

Figure 2.3 An athletic trainer examining a knee for ligament laxity.
Courtesy of Mark Hoffman.

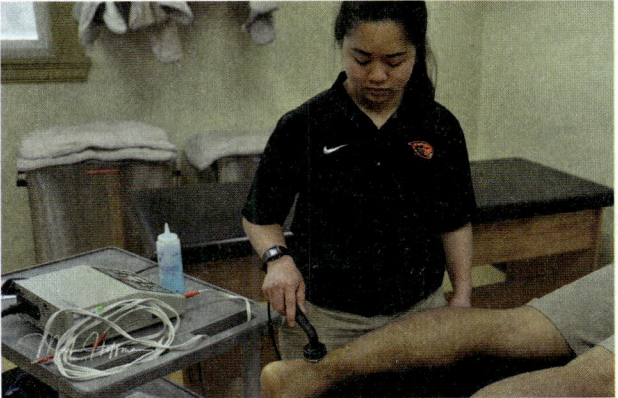

Figure 2.5 An athletic trainer providing therapeutic ultrasound to promote tissue healing.
Courtesy of Mark Hoffman.

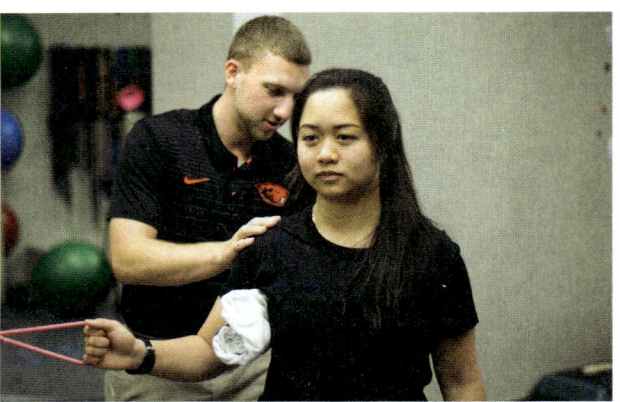

Figure 2.6 An athletic trainer instructing an athlete on therapeutic rehabilitation exercises.
Courtesy of Mark Hoffman.

membership association for the profession of athletic training in the United States. Its mission is to represent, engage, and foster the continued growth and development of the athletic training profession and ATS as unique healthcare providers. NATA's vision is for ATs to be globally recognized as vital practitioners in the delivery and advancement of health care through passionate provision of unique services and to be an integral part of the interprofessional AHCT. NATA is based in Carrollton, Texas, and currently has more than 40 full-time staff members who work to support NATA's vision and mission.

Guidelines for the development and implementation of education programs in athletic training have been developed by CAATE, whose mission is to define, assess, and continually improve AT education with a vision to assure accreditation excellence across the continuum of AT education to enhance clinical practice. In 2015, the professional membership (NATA), certification (BOC), and education (CAATE) organizations made the decision to transition from requiring an undergraduate to a graduate degree as the entry-level degree for the athletic training profession, which means that, by 2022, a candidate for the BOC certification exam must have a master's degree.

The CAATE is responsible for developing the Standards for Accreditation of Professional Athletic Training Programs (Standards). The most current edition of the Standards takes affect during the 2020–2021 academic year for all collegiate programs seeking continuing accreditation. The Standards are used to prepare professional ATs, and each accredited institution is responsible for demonstrating compliance with them to obtain and maintain recognition as a CAATE-accredited professional athletic training program (CAATE, 2018).

Educational programs in athletic training must be intensively reviewed for initial and continued accreditation via on-site visits and annual reports conducted by CAATE.

The CAATE Standards are designed to guide educational programs in the preparation of students through classroom instruction and clinical education in essential cognitive, affective, and psychomotor domains related to the practice of athletic training. The 94 Standards are broken down into several main categories and subcategories.

- Program design and quality
- Program delivery
- Institutional organization and administration
- Curricular content (prerequisites and foundational knowledge)
- Core competencies
  - Patient-centered care
  - Interprofessional practice and education
  - Evidence-based practice
  - Quality improvement
  - Healthcare informatics
  - Professionalism
- Patient/client care
  - Care plan
  - Examination, diagnosis, and intervention
  - Prevention, health promotion, and wellness
  - Healthcare administration

Clinical education involves students' acquiring skills under the direct supervision of clinical preceptors in a variety of settings and with a variety of patients, with the intent to provide students with guided autonomy to develop clinical reasoning and decision-making. Clinical settings are often in athletic training and medical facilities on the campus of the institution sponsoring the educational program, and via formal affiliations, students may gain additional clinical experience off campus in settings such as high schools, other colleges and universities, professional sports organizations, sports medicine clinics, and physician offices. Athletic training students must complete academic clinical education over the course of a minimum of 2 years, which must include clinical education hours with patient encounters across a wide spectrum of both illnesses and injuries and include both genders, various risk levels, different types of activity (i.e., upper

> **WHAT IF**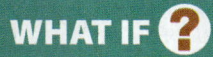
>
> High school seniors ask you for information on the academic requirements and certification process to become an athletic trainer. What do you tell them?

or lower extremity, contact, collision, and overuse), and different protective or sporting equipment.

To remain certified, an AT is required to earn continuing education units (CEUs) and report these activities to the BOC every 2 years by participating in activities such as attending professional meetings, writing articles for journals, making presentations, and enrolling in college classes that pertain to sports medicine. In addition, current certification in emergency cardiac care (ECC) must be maintained during each 2-year CEU cycle. Specifically, certification must include knowledge of adult and pediatric CPR, AED use, second-rescuer CPR, airway obstruction, and barrier devices. Organizations providing such training that are accepted by the BOC include the American Red Cross, the American Heart Association, and the American Academy of Orthopaedic Surgeons. For more information regarding the BOC certification examination as well as continuing education requirements, go to https://bocatc.org/athletic-trainers.

Settings of Employment for the Practice of Athletic Training

Athletic training provides an opportunity to engage in patient care while working in a dynamic, fast-paced, and challenging medical environment. Historically, the practice of athletic training was confined to collegiate sports, with an emphasis on caring for injuries in tackle football (Joseph, 2018). Employment situations have changed significantly over the decades since the organization of NATA in 1950. Athletic trainers now work in a variety of professional settings, including the following:

- Secondary schools
- Private K–12 institutions
- Intercollegiate athletics
- Professional and semiprofessional sports
- Sports medicine clinics
- Law enforcement and military
- Occupational, corporate, and industrial settings
- Performing arts
- Physician offices
- Rodeo
- Hospital emergency departments

Employment of ATs is projected to grow 19% from 2018 to 2028, much faster than the average for all other occupations (U.S. Bureau of Labor Statistics, 2020). As people become more aware of the effects of sports-related injuries and the middle-aged and older populations remain active, the demand for ATs is expected to increase. Today, the types of job settings for ATS continue to increase dramatically as the profession gains more public recognition. Growth continues in the secondary school setting, and ATs continue to find employment in settings such as clinics (private and hospital-based clinics) and occupational, corporate, and industrial settings. Major corporations and industries have found it beneficial and profitable to employ ATs to provide direct services to their employees involved in on-site health and fitness programs or in the area of ergonomics or treatment and rehabilitation of work-related injuries (**Time Out 2.1**).

NATA keeps a variety of membership statistics for its more than 45,000 members; however, an individual does not need to be a member to practice as an AT. All that is required in 48 states and the District of Columbia is BOC certification and an associated state licensure or registration. In California, the AT profession is not state regulated, and in Texas an individual must obtain state licensure, which can be done within or outside of BOC certification. Table 2.1 shows the statistics compiled at the end of 2018 for NATA members employed in various work settings and those unemployed. Females comprise 56% and males 44% of the total membership, with 17.7% of all members reported as being a minority.

To practice in the professional sports setting is often considered to be the dream job for many entering the profession of athletic training. Although the thrill of working with highly paid, marquee athletes may be attractive to some, working in this setting also has its less attractive aspects, such as the tremendous pressure to win that is placed on the coaching staff, which often affects the sports medicine staff; the lack of job security associated with changes in coaching staff that occur frequently at the professional level; and the travel and late hours associated with professional games. Forecasters do not anticipate that there will be any significant growth in employment in this setting in the near future.

TIME OUT 2.1

Industrial or Occupational AT

Musculoskeletal disorders (MSDs) are common occupational injuries affecting muscles, tendons, and ligaments that reduce employee morale, increase lost workdays, decrease retention rates, escalate health insurance costs, raise workers' compensation payouts, and promote potential personal injury litigation.[1] Occupational injuries related to MSDs account for approximately 30% of days off from work.[2] More than half of all MSDs occur in retail, manufacturing, health care and social assistance, and transportation and warehousing.[2]

As with athletes, industrial and occupational workers use mental and physical talents to perform their jobs across a variety of domains. Performing tasks in awkward positions, excessive contact stress, overexertion, and repetitive motions are primary causes of MSDs.[2]

ATs can apply their skill sets in injury and illness prevention and wellness promotion by being members of health and safety teams for industrial and occupational workers.

ATs benefit employees by:

- Having in-depth knowledge of injury prevention and the human body's capabilities and limitations
- Teaching workers to use proper body mechanics, such as when lifting, and correct posture when seated and standing
- Educating workers on safe labor practices
- Encouraging workers to practice healthy lifestyle and wellness habits
- Helping workers to be conditioned and work ready for physically demanding jobs
- Assisting workers with the return-to-work process after an injury or illness
- Advising the company in infection control, illness screening, and prevention
- Assisting in safety or compliance rounds for the company

Return on investment (ROI), reduction in medical costs, and maintenance of productivity are important reasons for the employment of ATs in the industrial setting.[3,4] For example:

- Companies reported a 100% positive ROI when an AT was employed.
- ROI was $1 to $10 per employee for every dollar invested.[3]
- Emergency room costs were reduced by 50% or more.[3]
- ATs helped to decrease restricted workdays and workers' compensation claims for MSDs by more than 25%.[3]
- ATs for a large county police force reduced overall medical costs by 22% and MSD costs by 21%.[4]
- Employee days away from work decreased by ≥ 25%.[3]

Information was adapted from National Athletic Trainers' Association[1,3,4] and the Bureau of Labor Statistics.[2]

[1] National Athletic Trainers' Association (NATA). (2022). *At your own risk.* Retrieved from https://www.atyourownrisk.org/employers/
[2] U.S. Bureau of Labor Statistics. (2020, May). *Occupational injuries and illnesses resulting in musculoskeletal disorders (MSDs).* Fact Sheet. Retrieved from https://www.bls.gov/iif/oshwc/case/msds.htm
[3] National Athletic Trainers' Association (NATA). (2003). *Certified athletic trainers deliver ROI in occupational work.* Retrieved from http://www.nata.org/sites/default/files/ROI_Occupational_Settings_2003.pdf
[4] National Athletic Trainers' Association (NATA). (2014). *Athletic trainers provide high return on investment in today's workplace.* Retrieved from https://www.nata.org/press-release/110414/athletic-trainers-provide-high-return-investment-today%E2%80%99s-workplace

The three settings that see the most overall employment of ATs are colleges and universities (20.7%), secondary schools (20.6%), and clinics and hospitals (combined 16.5%). The following sections will give a brief review of these settings for the practice of athletic training.

Colleges and Universities

Universities have three main divisions (i.e., I, II, and III), each with its own size; number of athletes; sports offered; athletic training and support staff; and

Table 2.1
NATA Membership Statistics End of 2018

Setting	Count	Percentage
Amateur/rec/youth	164	0.4%
Clinic	5,662	12.4%
College/university	9,468	20.7%
Corporate	275	0.6%
Health/fitness clubs	557	1.2%
Hospital	1,868	4.1%
Independent contractor	596	1.3%
Industrial/occupational	631	1.4%
Military/government/law enforcement	320	0.7%
Not given	1,620	3.5%
Other	2,156	4.7%
Pro sports	1,177	2.6%
Retired	1,372	3.0%
Secondary school	9,420	20.6%
Student	8,986	19.6%
Unemployed	1,516	3.3%

Modified from data from National Athletic Trainers' Association (NATA). (n.d.). Member resources. Retrieved from https://www.nata.org/membership/about-membership/member-resources

medical rules, such as sickle cell screening. The larger and more profitable universities tend to have large athletic facilities (e.g., fields, courts, and pools; healthcare facilities; locker rooms; and training areas). In these cases, healthcare and athletic operations may resemble professional levels, with traveling team physicians, team dentists, ATs, and other personnel as well as large budgets for equipment and supplies. In the smaller Division III universities, the number of medical and support staff; the size of athletic, healthcare, and training facilities; and size of their budgets may resemble those of a high school setting. In any university setting, adherence to the BOC standards of care and National Collegiate Athletic Association (NCAA) medical guidelines and rules is expected. The same pros and cons of working with professional sports applies to high-level Division I athletic teams.

Additionally, certain universities offer athletic training education programs, as discussed previously. ATs may be employed as educators (e.g., instructors, professors, or clinical instructors) to foster and mentor students who are studying athletic training. Many of these AT educators focus solely on teaching students and do not practice clinically as ATs in the same capacity as others in the same university; however, many function in both roles.

Secondary Schools

When asked the question of why their school does not employ an AT, most administrators respond that they cannot afford to hire such a person. In fact, only 66% of public and private U.S. secondary schools have access (full- or part-time) to an AT's services, and 31% of public and 45% of private secondary schools have no athletic training services (Huggins et al., 2019). However, the argument of an AT's being unaffordable is no longer as valid as it once may have been because schools now have a variety of options available to them if they want to hire a BOC-certified AT.

One option may be employing an individual as both teacher and AT. This person is typically hired as a teacher and in addition provides athletic training services after school. Ideally, classroom loads can be adjusted to give the teacher/AT time in the afternoons or mornings to see athletes before practice, which allows an opportunity for injury prevention, rehabilitation, evaluation of injury recovery, counseling, and any other tasks that cannot be effectively completed otherwise. Administrators may find this option appealing because the teacher/AT can be given a standard teaching contract to provide educational services to the general student population and the additional AT duties can be negotiated to pay for the services provided.

Another option for the school is to hire a full-time AT. This individual has no formal teaching responsibilities at the school but is responsible for implementing a comprehensive sports medicine program, which can include follow-up care and rehabilitation of injured athletes during the morning hours before practice (e.g., during study hall or athletic hours). In addition, full-time ATs may be able to arrange their schedules so that they more closely approximate the normal number of hours per week provided by other personnel at the school. Though this option often results in the best health care for student-athletes, school districts are generally reluctant to commit to the initial financial outlay necessary to develop such a position. Fifty-three percent of secondary schools with access to athletic training services had full-time services, but 47% received only part-time services usually via hospital or clinic contracts (Huggins et al., 2019).

ATs can be hired full- or part-time by a local hospital system or clinic to provide athletic training health care to nearby high school athletic programs. In this scenario, ATs may or may not have official responsibilities at the hospital; however, a majority if not all of their responsibilities will be at the high school or for the coverage of other sponsored events, such as marathons. The medical model for this approach is such that the high school contracts with the local hospital or clinic for athletic training services, which usually include the team physician and other rehabilitation specialists, who will receive referrals for treatment of injured athletes. This arrangement has grown in popularity over the years and is another way to gain athletic training health care at a high school. In some cases, this arrangement may allow for multiple ATs to provide care at the same high school.

Clinics and Hospitals

ATs are employed in clinics and hospitals and in family, pediatric, orthopedic, physiatry, and sports medicine office practices to help improve patient outcomes and satisfaction as well as productivity by helping patients engage more efficiently across the appointment, evaluation, and treatment processes. Ultimately, ATs assist physicians in increasing patient throughput and revenue generation by providing quality services to more patients in the same period of time (NATA, n.d.a). They provide a return on investment to the physician practice through their skills in taking patient histories, performing evaluations, and providing instruction and education on rehabilitation interventions.

ATs who work in clinics and hospitals often add to their overall competencies by learning basic business concepts, promotional strategies, third-party payer codes, diagnostic procedures techniques (e.g., X-ray, fluoroscopy, and musculoskeletal ultrasound), casting and bracing skills, and sterile procedures for both the orthopedic or sports medicine clinic and operating room environments.

AT Salaries

In the most recent NATA salary survey (NATA, 2019), the national average annual salary of ATs is $57,203, which represents a 4% increase since 2016. The degree level often determines the average salary: an AT with a bachelor's degree earns an average of $52,010; a master's degree, an average of $56,347; and a doctoral degree, an average of $79,418. ATs in New York, Pennsylvania, New Jersey, Delaware, Texas, Arkansas, California, Nevada, and Hawaii tend to have higher average salaries than those in other states (NATA, 2019). Those with over 15 years of employment are more likely to make over the average annual salary. Male ATS ($62,008) tend to earn more than female ATs ($53,240), but females are generally younger than males in this field. However, the gap is closing between genders as evidenced by female ATs' salaries increasing over $3,000 and male ATs' salaries increasing only $1,800 since the last salary survey was done in 2018. In Table 2.2, the average salary for the top 10 job settings for ATs is reported.

Importance of Athletic Training Services for Youth Athletes

Having a BOC-certified AT for youth athletes provides many indirect benefits to the school or organization. From a legal standpoint, the school is less vulnerable to tort claims related to sports injuries, many of which are based on the premise that the school failed to provide adequate medical care to athletes. From an organizational standpoint, ATs will likely bring membership in NATA with them, and thereby have access to a vast number of resources created to benefit youth athletes.

In a commitment to youth sport safety and protection of the secondary school athlete, NATA has been involved with federal advocacy and the establishment of several organizations that allow for the alliance of stakeholders interested in protecting youth athletes, educating the public and medical community, providing ATs to secondary schools, and recognizing schools that emphasize safety. Specific federal advocacy began in 2015 with the introduction of the Secondary School Student Athletes' Bill of Rights as a resolution to the U.S. House of Representatives (NATA, 2015). It offered 13 recommendations that any school could implement to make its student-athletes safer and recognized the best practices for

Table 2.2
Average Salary by Common Job Settings for Athletic Trainers

2018 Reported Average Salary	
College/University	
Faculty/Academic/Research	$73,540
NAIA–Professional Staff/Athletics/Clinic	$45,993
NCAA Division I–Professional Staff/Athletics/Clinic	$57,656
NCAA Division II–Professional Staff/Athletics/Clinic	$49,833
NCAA Division III–Professional Staff/Athletics/Clinic	$49,478
Secondary School	
High School–Athletic Only	$52,868
High School–Both Academic and Athletic	$58,603
Clinic	
Physician-Owned Clinic	$53,712
Secondary School Outreach	$45,786
Hospital	
Outreach	$52,496

Data from National Athletic Trainers' Association (NATA). (2019). NATA 2018 Salary Survey executive summary. Retrieved from https://members.nata.org/members1/salarysurvey2018/2018-Salary-Survey-Executive-Summary.pdf

maintaining a safe environment for youth sports. When the resolution was introduced, it had bipartisan support in both chambers of Congress but did not make it off the floor. However, current legislation designed to develop a federal law regarding youth sports concussion safety does include some of the bill of rights recommendations and has bipartisan support in the House and Democratic support in the Senate as of July 2020 (https://www.nata.org/advocacy/federal/federal-legislative-alert-center).

The Youth Sports Safety Alliance (YSSA) was created in 2010 to raise awareness, advance legislation, and improve medical care for young athletes across the country. The Alliance includes more than 230 organizations acting collectively to protect youth athletes. The Youth Sports Safety Summit is an annual event hosted by YSSA, which is designed to focus on current issues and scientific information to keep young athletes safe. The Collaborative Solutions for Safety in Sport supports the National Federation of State High School Associations by bringing stakeholders together to discuss strategies for developing and implementing life-saving policies for youth athletes. The NFL Athletic Trainer Initiative was created by the NFL Foundation, NATA, the Professional Football Athletic Trainers' Society, and Gatorade to provide AT coverage to underserved high schools. The groups also provide educational resources, hydration solutions, equipment, and other types of support to nurture and protect the youth athlete. The Safe Sports School award recognizes secondary schools for taking crucial steps to keep their athletes safe and free from injuries (https://www.nata.org/advocacy/youth-sports-safety).

For secondary schools, a qualified AT can offer many unique educational opportunities. For example, such an AT can teach classes in basic sports injury care, first aid and CPR, nutrition, and physical conditioning. The AT can also implement a student aide program at the school to provide educational opportunities for high school students interested in a career in sports medicine. Allowing secondary school students the opportunity to observe the duties and responsibilities of an AT is a valuable educational experience and may introduce them to the foundations of various health-related careers. However, regardless of practice setting, student aides must not act as if they are licensed and certified as an AT. Student aides must only observe and are not to be asked or permitted to make return-to-play decisions or act independently when evaluating, assessing, treating, or rehabilitating any injuries (NATA, 2014).

AHCT at the Secondary School Level

Major support for the placement of BOC-certified ATs in secondary schools was provided by the AMA's House of Delegates in June 1998 (NATA, 1998). BOC-certified ATs signify a marked improvement in the healthcare services provided to athletes, regardless of level of competition, partly because of the fact that even under the best of circumstances team physicians are typically available to athletes only on a part-time basis. The BOC-certified AT can provide a direct link between the injured athlete and the appropriate medical services.

All members of the AHCT must act according to established appropriate medical care standards for secondary school–aged athletes. Previous documents had addressed appropriate medical care standards for this population, but they had not been updated for over 12 years. In 2018, NATA formed a task force comprising secondary school ATs, administrators, researchers, and policy experts with a charge to review current guidelines related to the appropriate medical care standards for secondary school–aged athletes and to revise and update standards related to current research and scientific evidence (Cooper et al., 2019). The task force identified 12 standards, with supporting substandards, which encompassed the following:

- Readiness to participate in activity
- Practice and competition facilities and equipment
- Personal sports equipment fit and maintenance
- Protective materials
- Environmental policies
- Nutrition, hydration, and dietary supplementation
- Wellness and long-term health
- Comprehensive emergency action plans
- On-site immediate care
- On-site therapeutic interventions
- Psychological concerns
- Athletic healthcare administration

Although implementing the components outlined in this summary statement requires considerable investment of time and energy, the long-term results are improved, comprehensive healthcare services for secondary school–aged athletes. In addition, by having such a plan in place, the school and associated personnel can reduce the likelihood of litigation associated with sports-related injuries.

In conjunction with the summary statement, NATA (n.d.b) also developed an online tool called the Program Assessment for Safety in Sport (PASS), which was designed to help schools and organizations to continually prioritize the health and safety of their athletes. The PASS website (https://pass.nata.org) allows schools and organizations to benchmark their successes and opportunities against the 12 recommended standards, for visiting ATs to view documents such as emergency action plans and other key documents associated with the host school, and members of the public to view so they can learn about sports safety guidelines that should be in place at their local schools.

The AHCT was specifically addressed in Standard 12, with a focus on providing appropriate medical care under the guidance of a team or directing physician (MD or DO) who establishes the services provided. Because having a physician on campus daily in the high school setting to provide medical services to the athletes is not practical, a BOC-certified AT should be the QMP on campus daily and the individual in the position to observe, treat, and document injuries as soon as they occur. The AT coordinates the day-to-day operation and directives of the AHCT. At the very least, in cases when an AT is not present, coaches should be trained in first aid, blood-borne pathogens, CPR and AED, concussion management, and environmental preparation so they will be able to provide basic first aid and life-support services to the athletes in their charge.

Besides identifying the roles of all QMP and stakeholders, the AHCT standard covers several other key areas that should be addressed to coordinate its efforts regarding injury care and prevention. The following seven questions can be asked to determine the necessary steps for providing appropriate medical care.

- Does the organization ensure that a QMP properly documents athlete medical records according to professional and legal standards?
- Does the organization publish and make available its policy, procedures, and protocol manual to all stakeholders?
- Does the organization ensure that medical devices be maintained and calibrated according to manufacturer guidelines and government regulations?
- Does the organization provide appropriate storage of and security for medical records and require documented training for anyone accessing such records?
- Does the organization provide the necessary resources for a member of the AHCT to communicate professionally with athletes, parents, coaches, administrators, and the medical community?

Athletic Trainers SPEAK OUT

Why is it important for ATs to work alongside other healthcare providers?

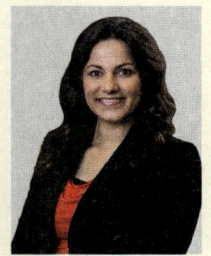

Courtesy of Michelle Holt, MA, LAT, ATC.

Working *with* other healthcare providers is essential in the AT role, but the opportunity for ATs to work *alongside* multiple care professionals in a daily, physical capacity may not occur consistently in some settings. In our sports medicine and orthopedic clinic, I have the privilege to work alongside physicians, physician assistants, nurses, radiology techs, medical assistants, and even clerical staff, all of whom are involved in the care process. In addition, our team collaborates with physical therapists and sports performance coaches, a joint venture of services located in one shared facility. These daily interactions provide learning experiences from a variety of healthcare professionals, which has evolved my perspective of the AT's important role. I learn something significant every day, growing my confidence in what I do know but also enhancing my discernment for what I do not know. This awareness of my own limitations will lead me to make correct decisions on behalf of the patient as to when it is best to refer or seek assistance and how to utilize the most appropriate resources.

Working alongside other providers is also beneficial to patient care because ATs are ideal teammates in a multidisciplinary medical model. They have the skill sets and work ethic to perform duties in the clinic more effectively, with the knowledge to explain the treatments and services they are providing the patient. By assisting in many forms of communication and spending the time in clinic to do so, ATs enhance patients' experiences and create a clearer understanding. Furthermore, communicating the treatment plan with those ATs refer to or receive referrals from creates a bridge for the continuum of quality care. Conducting this teamwork may be connecting acute care to follow-ups, from one specialty to another, or extending to ancillary services. Working together helps the patient navigate through a complex healthcare system to reach all the resources they need.

—**Michelle Holt, MA, LAT, ATC**

Michelle Holt is an AT at Sideline Orthopedics and Sports, a clinic in Arlington, Texas.

- Does the organization provide adequate funds for the supplies and equipment needed for a comprehensive athletic healthcare program?
- Does the organization provide adequate and equitable staffing of QMP to implement a comprehensive athletic healthcare program?

Constant dialogue regarding these seven areas will allow for the other 11 standards of care to be met. This dialogue should include key elements such as monitoring environmental conditions, conducting preparticipation health screenings, developing and implementing emergency action plans; and communicating with local emergency care providers, such as paramedics or emergency medical technicians, regarding access to game and practice facilities and specific procedures such as helmet removal in tackle football.

Review Questions

1. Define the term *sports medicine*.
2. What is the CAQ, and how does it relate to the team physician?
3. List the specific services that the team physician should provide the athlete.
4. List several professional medical organizations that promote the study of sports medicine.
5. What has been the largest employment market for ATs in recent years?
6. List the five practice domains for athletic training.

7. True or false? More females than males are members of NATA.

8. Name five areas that employ ATs.

9. What is the prediction for the athletic training profession according to the Bureau of Labor Statistics?

10. How many standards are proposed to provide appropriate medical care to the secondary school–aged athlete?

11. Name three skills that an AT would likely need to work in a healthcare administration setting.

12. Name and describe one of the ways that NATA is committed to protecting youth athletes.

References

American Board of Family Medicine. (2013). Certificates of added qualifications (CAQs). Retrieved from https://www.theabfm.org/caq/index.aspx

American College of Sports Medicine (2000). Team physician consensus statement. *Medicine & Science in Sports & Exercise, 32*(4), 87–96.

Barwell, J., Arnold, F., & Berry, H. (2013). How interprofessional learning improves care. *Nursing Times, 109*(21), 14–16.

Board of Certification, Inc. (BOC). (2017). What is an athletic trainer? Retrieved from https://bocatc.org/about-us

Commission on Accreditation of Athletic Training Education (CAATE). (2018). 2020 Standards for accreditation of professional athletic training programs: Master's degree programs. Retrieved from https://caate.net/wp-content/uploads/2018/09/2020-Standards-for-Professional-Programs-copyedited-clean.pdf

Cooper, L., Harper, R., Wham, G. S., Jr., Cates, J., Chafin, S. J., Jr., Cohen, R. P., . . . McLeod, T. C. V. (2019). Appropriate medical care standards for organizations sponsoring athletic activity for the secondary school–aged athlete: A summary statement. *Journal of Athletic Training, 54*(7), 741–748.

Gatchel, R. J., McGeary, D. D., McGeary, C. A., & Lippe, B. (2014). Interdisciplinary chronic pain management: Past, present, and future. *American Psychologist, 69*(2), 119–130.

Herring, S. A., Kibler, W. B., Putukian, M., Bergfeld, J. A., Boyajian-O'Neill, L. A., Chang, C. C., Franks, R. R., ... & Stanton, R. (2013). Team physician consensus statement: 2013 Update. *Medicine & Science in Sports & Exercise, 45*(8), 1618.

Huggins, R. A., Coleman, K. A., Attanasio, S. M., Cooper, G. L., Endres, B. D., Harper, R. C., . . . Casa, D. J. (2019). Athletic trainer services in the secondary school setting: The athletic training locations and services project. *Journal of Athletic Training, 54*(11), 1129–1139.

Joseph, R. (2018). *The history of athletic trainers*. Retrieved from https://insitehealthteam.com/history-of-athletic-trainers/

Knebel, E., & Greiner, A. C. (Eds.). (2003). *Health professions education: A bridge to quality*. Washington, DC: National Academies Press.

National Athletic Trainers' Association (NATA). (n.d.a). *Health care admin/rehab*. Retrieved from https://www.nata.org/professional-interests/emerging-settings/health-care-adminrehab

National Athletic Trainers' Association (NATA). (n.d.b). *Program assessment for safety in sport (PASS)*. Retrieved from https://pass.nata.org/

National Athletic Trainers' Association (NATA). (1998). *American Medical Association H-470.995 Athletic (sports) medicine*. Retrieved from https://www.nata.org/sites/default/files/ama_recommendation.pdf

National Athletic Trainers' Association (NATA). (2014). *Proper supervision of secondary school student aides official statement*. Retrieved from https://www.nata.org/professional-interests/job-settings/secondary-school/resources

National Athletic Trainers' Association (NATA). (2015, February 27). Student athletes' bill of rights introduced as a joint resolution in House and Senate. Retrieved from https://www.nata.org/press-release/022715/student-athletes%E2%80%99-bill-rights-introduced-joint-resolution-house-and-senate

National Athletic Trainers' Association (NATA). (2019). NATA 2018 salary survey executive summary. Retrieved from https://members.nata.org/members1/salarysurvey2018/2018-Salary-Survey-Executive-Summary.pdf

National Federation of State High School Associations (NFHS). (2018, September 11). High school sports participation increases for 29th consecutive year. Retrieved from https://www.nfhs.org/articles/high-school-sports-participation-increases-for-29th-consecutive-year/

Prentice, W. E. (2017). *Principles of athletic training: A guide to evidence-based practice* (16th ed.). New York, NY: McGraw-Hill.

Rogers, C. C. (1985). Does sports medicine fit in the new health care market? *Physician and Sports Medicine, 13*(1), 116–127.

U.S. Bureau of Labor Statistics. (2020). *Athletic trainers*. Retrieved from https://www.bls.gov/ooh/healthcare/athletic-trainers.htm

CHAPTER 3

The Law of Sports Injury

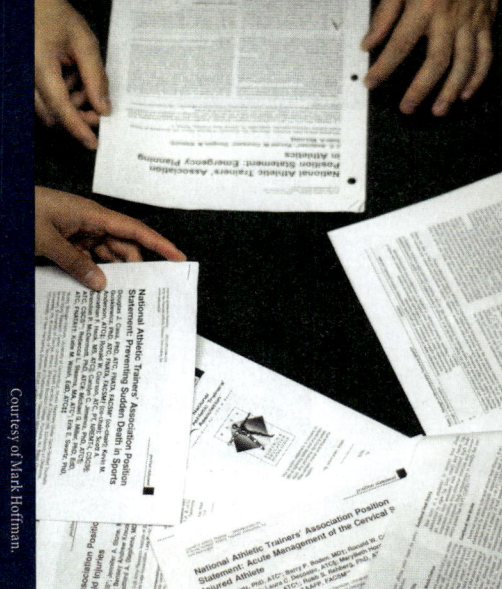

MAJOR CONCEPTS

As with medicine in general, the field of sports medicine has witnessed a dramatic increase in the amount of litigation over the past decade. This chapter introduces the reader to legal terminology and outlines what constitutes the physical education teacher's, coach's, and referee's duty during athletic activity. It provides a listing of the major forms of teaching, coaching, and refereeing liability along with information on how to reduce the risk of litigation. It also presents appropriate steps to take in the event of a lawsuit and concludes with a discussion on the ethics of sports-injury care. Finally, the definition and role of an athletic trainer (AT) is presented along with statistics regarding employment at the secondary school level.

The physical education teacher or coach is often the first on the scene when a sports injury occurs. Referees also may be called into action because of their proximity to the playing field. The physical education teacher's, coach's, or referee's decisions and actions at the time of the injury are critical to the athlete's welfare (Figure 3.1). These decisions and actions are based on the standards of care that a reasonably prudent person would perform in a similar circumstance to avoid harm to the athlete. Inappropriate or nonprudent decisions and actions may jeopardize the injured participant and lead to legal action by the athlete and/or parents or legal guardians (in the case of minors; Mirsafian, 2016). Perhaps at no other time in the history of sports has the potential for legal action against teachers, coaches, and other sports personnel been as great as it is today. Several recent tort cases are listed in **Time Out 3.1**.

Several reasons can be highlighted for this increase in lawsuits. According to Appenzeller (2000), one reason is the simple fact that, in the United States, people have the right to sue. Because a sports culture has been created in the United States whereby athletes expect that they should be able to participate without risk of injury, when they are injured they feel justified in suing for damages. As well, large monetary expenses are associated with many injuries; thus, those who are injured may sue to recover for medical expenses because many insurance companies will settle out of court by opting to pay a sum of money. Another reason is the sheer number of lawyers in the United States. According to the American Bar Association (2018), 1,338,678 licensed lawyers were practicing in 2018. Moreover, young athletes and parents have increased expectations relative to potential future financial gain of a successful sports career. If the athlete is injured,

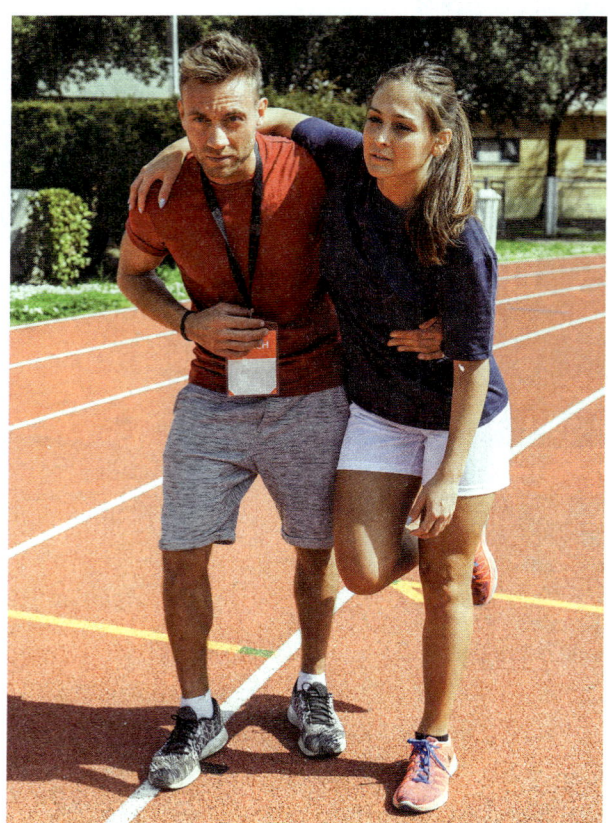

Figure 3.1 Coach assists an injured athlete.
© Marino Bocelli/Shutterstock.

affected parties may sue to recover their future financial losses. Other factors include the huge increase in the number of sports participants and increase in the severity of injuries, greater visibility of sports through the media, rising expectations regarding legal negligence, greater awareness of sports as a business because of the huge revenues of many athletic organizations, and consumer awareness about sports product manufacturing (Wong, 2010). In addition to a more litigious and sports-oriented culture, another reason for legal action is an injury whose cause can be attributed to having improper injury prevention measures and injury management in place.

Ethics of Sports-Injury Care

Thirty-two of 50 states and the District of Columbia require that coaches complete cardiopulmonary resuscitation (CPR) and first aid training before coaching (Student CPR, n.d.). In Oregon, such training is optional. The remaining 17 states do not have any laws requiring such training, but schools may require coaches to take training courses offered through the National Federation of State High Schools (NFHS), such as first aid or concussion education. Despite state laws, respected organizations, including

TIME OUT 3.1

Recently Settled Cases of Negligence in Sports

MACKENZIE CLAY (SEATTLE, WASHINGTON, 2007)

As a senior wrestler in high school, Mackenzie Clay suffered a spinal cord injury as a result of two wrestlers falling on him during a practice in the school's cafeteria. The injury left him in a wheelchair. Clay filed a negligence suit against the school district alleging the school's coaches lacked Washington Interscholastic Activities Association certification at the time and they failed to use the appropriate number and size of wrestling mats for the practice. Clay received a $1 million settlement from Seattle Public Schools and $14 million from Washington Schools Risk Management Pool, the district's insurance company (Cohen, 2009).

MAX GILPIN (LOUISVILLE, KENTUCKY, 2008)

Fifteen-year-old Max Gilpin died of heatstroke 3 days after a Louisville, Kentucky, high school football practice. The family filed a negligence lawsuit against the school district and head football coach alleging reckless disregard of safety requirements. The insurers settled for $1.75 million. The head football coach also became the first coach to be charged criminally with reckless homicide and wanton endangerment. The coach was acquitted in 2009 (Beahm, 2010).

ELISE CERAMI (SOUTHLAKE, TEXAS, 2016)

Thirteen-year-old Elise Cerami drowned at the Carroll Independent School District Aquatics Center during a routine swim practice while 30 teammates and two coaches were nearby. The swim coach, who had lifeguard training and other lifesaving skills, positioned herself 180 feet away from the pool for more than 9 minutes. No lifeguards were on duty at this practice, and two teammates were unable to pull Elise to safety. A jury determined that the swim coach had failed to watch Elise or to ensure that she was being supervised by someone else. The swim coach can no longer be certified as a swim coach and was charged with abandonment and endangering of a child by criminal negligence and sentenced to 3 years' probation.

UNIVERSITY OF IOWA FOOTBALL PLAYERS (IOWA CITY, IOWA, 2011)

An off-season football conditioning practice in January 2011 consisted of 100 back squats at 50% of the players' personal best weight within a certain period and sled work, followed by an intense upper body workout the following day and another intense workout 3 days later. Eventually, 13 practice participants were hospitalized and diagnosed with exertional rhabdomyolysis. Cases were filed against the university stating that coaches and ATs had failed to properly develop, implement, and supervise the workouts as well as offer prompt medical care after athletes had reported severe pain. Coaches were cleared of any wrongdoing, and one settlement of $15,000 was paid to one of the players.

JORDAN McNAIR (UNIVERSITY OF MARYLAND, 2018)

During an off-season practice in May 2018, Jordan collapsed during an intense afternoon practice and was hospitalized that evening, later to be airlifted to another hospital for an emergency liver transplant. He died 15 days later. Doctors determined that he had suffered heatstroke and the coach and ATs had failed to recognize early signs and symptoms, and therefore had not acted to treat him accordingly.

the Korey Stringer Institute (n.d.), recommend six coaching education requirements that should be implemented by each state's high school athletic association (Table 3.1).

The athlete's health and safety should be the ultimate priority for all those involved in organized sports. A coach's livelihood and career often depend on a win–loss record because sports are now viewed as a business with an increasing emphasis on winning and earning monetary rewards. In addition, athletes (and often their parents or legal guardians) will pressure coaches for an opportunity to play or return to play. Therefore, a coach may feel pressure to return an athlete to play without proper medical care or follow-up. Because many school districts determine their own policies and requirements for first aid, CPR, and automated external defibrillator (AED) certifications, most important is that coaches understand the intricacies of resuscitation and first aid care and the disposition of athletes after injury.

Research regarding whether coaches have adequate first aid knowledge in accordance with nationally recognized guidelines has produced discouraging results (Barron et al., 2009; McLeod et al., 2008; Ransone & Dunn, 1999). Thirty-six percent of 104 California high school athletic coaches passed a first

Table 3.1
Korey Stringer Institute Recommendations for Coaches' Education

1. Coaches should be certified in first aid, CPR, and AED use and be required to renew these certifications regularly.
2. Coaches should be required to participate in ongoing education in coaching techniques and renew CPR, first aid, and AED certifications regularly.
3. Coaches should be educated to recognize serious injuries and emergency situations.
4. Coaches should be aware of the school's policies and procedures, especially the emergency action plan and the availability of emergency equipment.
5. Coaches should annually practice implementation of the school's emergency action plan.
6. Coaches should follow NFHS requirements and complete any certifications supported by NFHS relative to their sport.

Adapted from Korey Stringer Institute. (n.d.). *Coaching education*. Retrieved from https://ksi.uconn.edu/prevention/coaching-education

aid test based on nationally recognized guidelines (Ransone & Dunn, 1999). In Arizona, only 3% of 156 youth sports coaches (McLeod et al., 2008) passed the same first aid assessment test used by Ransone and Dunn. The positive news is that those coaches who reported they had first aid or CPR certification scored higher on the assessment test, which indicates that education does help (Ransone & Dunn, 1999). Similar results were also achieved through a study done in Michigan; only 5% of 290 coaches in youth sporting leagues passed a first aid assessment quiz (Barron et al., 2009). Overall, coaches are likely to withhold an injured young athlete from competition (McLeod et al., 2008; Ransone & Dunn, 1999). However, researchers analyzed specific data from the Game Situation Data Sheet (GSDS), and the results indicated that coaches can still be aggressive in returning injured youth to competition if the game is "on the line" (Ransone & Dunn, 1999). The GSDS questionnaire asks questions related to specific game situations (e.g., 5 minutes left in the championship game), different types of injuries (e.g., mild pain in ankle), and player position (e.g., starting forward or bench player) in an effort to assess a coach's decision-making process regarding return to play after an injury. Researchers from both studies (McLeod et al., 2008; Ransone & Dunn, 1999) reported that, when a close game was at stake, more than 50% of all surveyed coaches reported a conflict of interest when a starting player was injured and wanted to return to the game. Perhaps even more alarming was that 75% of the first aid–knowledgeable coaches (i.e., higher score on assessment test) made incorrect return-to-play decisions in high-stakes games (Ransone & Dunn, 1999). Therefore, the coach must resist the temptation to circumvent the standards of first aid care. An objective and unbiased opinion is critical when decisions are made regarding the return of an injured athlete to participation. Under no circumstance should an injured athlete be allowed to resume sports without the consent of a qualified medical professional (QMP), such as a certified AT or medical doctor. Unethical behavior by a coach will in all probability be considered negligence by a court of law, so all individuals involved in the supervision or instruction of youth in sports need to understand the concepts of liability and tort law applied to sports.

The Concept of Tort

A **tort** is a private or civil wrong or injury suffered by an individual as a result of another person's conduct (Ray & Konin, 2011; Wong, 2010). There are two general categories of torts: intentional and unintentional (Wong, 2010). The difference between the two types of torts lies in the intent to harm. **Negligence** is a type of tort defined as the failure to do what a reasonably careful and prudent person would have done under the same or similar circumstances, or, conversely, as doing something that a reasonably careful and prudent person would not have done under the same or similar circumstances (Ray & Konin, 2011; Wong, 2010). The conduct of a reasonable person is not always perfect but will be considered to match the level of skills possessed by similar members of the community (Wong, 2010). Therefore, a team doctor is held to different standards of reasonable care than a coach or physical education teacher. In the context of sports, an injured athlete may argue that an injury resulted from someone else's behavior, such as that of an opponent, an official, a physical education teacher, or a coach. These torts are likely unintentional torts where there was no intent to harm but rather a failure to exercise reasonable care (Wong, 2010); however, intentional torts are not uncommon if the **plaintiff** feels the injury was caused with an intent to harm (player vs. player; Wolohan, 2008). Tort cases involving sports-related injuries generally seek to recover money to compensate the athlete for damages (medical expenses) that resulted from the defendant's alleged negligence.

Essential to proving a negligence tort is establishing that someone other than the athlete (injured party) acted in a negligent manner and this behavior resulted in an injury. Wong (2010) and Mirsafian (2016) identified the four elements that must be present to prove

---

Tort A private wrong or injury, suffered by an individual as a result of another person's conduct.

Negligence The failure to do what a reasonably careful and prudent person would have done under the same or similar circumstances or doing something that a reasonably careful and prudent person would not have done under the same or similar circumstances.

Plaintiff The individual who was injured and brings the lawsuit.

TIME OUT 3.2

Four Elements of Negligence

1. **Duty of care:** An obligation recognized by the law requiring a person to conform to a certain standard of conduct for the protection of others against unreasonable risks. There is a duty to act in a reasonable manner and a duty not to act in an unreasonable manner.
2. **Breach of duty:** Violation of the established duty (direct evidence), a failure to conform to the standard required, or inference from circumstantial evidence.
3. **Actual or proximate causation:** A reasonably close causal connection between the conduct (breach of duty) and the resulting injury.
4. **Damage:** Actual losses that are considered compensatory (e.g., medical expenses, future income, and mental stress).

negligence, which are listed in **Time Out 3.2**. Negligence involves either an act of **omission** (i.e., failure to act or nonfeasance) or an act of **commission** (i.e., acting in an improper way). An act of commission can be further divided into **misfeasance** or **malfeasance**. The essence of negligence is proving the proximate cause or causal connection between the resultant damage, duty of care, and breach of duty.

An example of negligence by an act of commission (i.e., misfeasance) is the high school football player (i.e., plaintiff) who claims that a significant knee injury resulted from the head coach throwing a tackling dummy at his legs to simulate illegal blocking and the techniques needed to avoid these tackles. In such a case, the athlete might claim the coach's actions caused the knee injury unnecessarily. The athlete would argue that the coach's actions constituted negligence because the coach acted in a way that he had the legal right to do (i.e., teach tackling techniques) but he did it with reckless behavior and incorrect techniques. The question that will be asked is, "Was the throwing of the tackling dummy at the legs of players a reasonable action by the coach in an attempt to teach a football technique?" This is known as the determination of reasonable care or the general desire to avoid creating risks that might result in an injury (Wong, 2010). An example of negligence by an act of omission (i.e., nonfeasance) is when the local high school failed to provide a certified lifeguard at the pool during a physical education swimming class and a student drowns. The defendant (i.e., local school) would then be judged in part on the basis of what other school districts routinely do at their aquatic facilities. Physical education teachers, coaching staffs, and school districts are held to a predetermined standard of care for all those under their supervision. The question that will be asked is, "Should the school district have anticipated the risk of death by drowning to a participant in the swimming class or swimming practice?" This is known as the "foreseeability" of the injury and, in essence, determines whether the school district and physical education teacher or coach provided the appropriate standard of care to the members of the swimming class or practice. If not, then the defendants may be found to have been negligent.

In school sports cases, tort claims often name as many defendants as possible. For example, in the scenarios given, the list of defendants might include the physical education teacher, head coach, assistant coach, school principal, athletic director, and school district administration and perhaps even the state high school athletic association. Tort claims generally ask

Omission A legal liability arising when a person does not perform a necessary action.

Commission A legal liability arising when individuals perform acts that are not legally theirs to perform.

Misfeasance An act of commission in which lawful conduct is improperly performed.

Malfeasance An act of commission in which wholly unlawful conduct is performed.

for monetary rewards; therefore, defendants' being selected in part based on their ability to pay such awards is only logical. Naming such defendants in lawsuits is commonly referred to as "going for the deepest pocket."

According to Wong (2010), showing proof of one of the following legal doctrines is the best way to defeat a negligence suit. However, each state has laws that may or may not allow one of these defenses, especially in the cases of minors.

- **No negligence.** The defendant disputes the claim of negligence by attacking one of the four elements of negligence as outlined in Time Out 3.2. In this case, the defendant did not have a duty or did not breach the applicable duty of care. An act of God (i.e., act of nature) is also used in a no negligence defense because it concedes that the injury occurred as a result of factors beyond the control of the defendant and could not have been prevented by the exercise of prudence, care, or diligence. For example, being injured or killed by an earthquake that occurs during a cross-country running event would, in all probability, be considered an act of God.
- **Contributory negligence.** The plaintiff is found to be in part or totally responsible for the injury. Therefore, the defendant must prove that the plaintiff failed to exercise due care for his or her own safety.
- **Comparative negligence.** This provides a basis of recovery for the injured plaintiff while assigning fault to both parties. It allows for the plaintiff to receive partial compensation on a prorated basis, dependent on a judgment regarding the extent of *contributory negligence*. In other words, if a monetary reward is given, it is based only on the percentage of negligence assigned to the plaintiff.
- **Assumption of risk.** This means that the plaintiff has voluntarily consented to assume responsibility for injury. The two types of assumption of risk are *expressed* and *implied*. Expressed risk is when a plaintiff gives advance notice (i.e., signs a waiver) to take the chances of known risks. Implied risk is an inference that, by participating in a risky event where negligence is possible, the plaintiff is releasing the defendant from a duty of care. Assumption of risk defenses can be used only in states that do not have comparative negligence laws. Also, know that signing an assumption of risk form does not always remove the defendant from responsibility because there are many legal issues that surround these forms.
- **Statute of limitations.** Plaintiffs must adhere to specific limitations of time (i.e., statutes) in which they can file lawsuits. Most are based on a period relative to the time of discovery of the harm.
- **Immunity.** Immunity is a condition that protects defendants from tort actions because of their position related to their capacity or relationship with the plaintiff. Each state determines types of conditions for establishing immunity. Sovereign immunity is when local government entities have immunity from many tort cases. However, coaches or teachers employed by local governments (e.g., state universities) cannot assume sovereign immunity because of their position because each state's laws may vary.
- **Good Samaritan laws.** This type of immunity is specific to those who attempt to aid another person who was put into a dangerous situation by a third party. Most states have Good Samaritan laws in place, which serve to protect citizens (even medical personnel) who voluntarily provide first aid to an injured person. Such laws were developed in part to encourage the average citizen or medical personnel to render first aid in an emergency, even though these individuals do not have a duty to provide such care. These laws protect most caregivers if the care was not reckless or did not worsen the condition of the injured person. Good Samaritan laws vary greatly from state to state regarding the categories of people the statutes protect and the circumstances in which they apply (Quandt et al., 2009). However, coaches and other school personnel do have a duty to provide appropriate emergency care, and, as a result, they typically do not enjoy immunity from tort claims under the tenets of Good Samaritan laws.

What Is the Physical Educator's or Coach's Liability?

Anyone serving in a coaching capacity, whether voluntarily or paid, bears considerable responsibility for the health and safety of athletes (Mirsafian, 2016). Historically, a coach employed by government institutions, such as school districts or universities, has enjoyed a certain degree of immunity from tort litigation under the doctrine of sovereign immunity. This in essence protects government institutions and their personnel from liability claims. However, some states have determined through legislative action that tort litigation against such agencies may be possible, depending on the specific circumstances (Wong, 2010). Consequently, more injury liability cases are now being contested successfully against coaching personnel. Therefore, protection under the doctrine of sovereign immunity is no longer guaranteed (Wong, 2010).

The coach must always use reasonable care to avoid creating a foreseeable risk of harm to others (Wong, 2010). The legal mechanisms by which coaches and physical educators can protect themselves have evolved over time. Whether they are staff members or volunteers, coaches and others should familiarize themselves with the duties they owe to their participants (McCaskey & Biedzynski, 1996) and understand any written job duties or contractual agreements afforded by their employer or local entity. The best way for coaches to prevent exposure to liability is to know the attendant risks of the sport and to be knowledgeable and prepared so that foreseeable consequences can be anticipated (McCaskey & Biedzynski, 1996). However, coaches and physical educators are not insurers of a participant's safety and will not be held liable for injuries resulting from the inherent dangers of the sport or activity provided they satisfied their duties as coaches or educators (McCaskey & Biedzynski, 1996). Wong (2010), Quandt and colleagues (2009), and McCaskey and Biedzynski (1996) present several specific duties for coaches and physical educators to use to minimize risk of injury for participants. These are explained in **Time Out 3.3**.

TIME OUT 3.3

Potentially Negligent Actions by Coaches

- **Failure to provide adequate supervision.** The coach is required to supervise activities to an extent that is determined, in part, by the age, skill, and experience of the participants. Thus, inexperienced children involved in a high-risk sport, such as football, require a higher level of supervision than do senior varsity athletes in the same sport. Any time children are involved, regardless of the activity, the coach is responsible for providing proper supervision. Leaving children unattended for any amount of time involves risk. For example, although swimmers are capable of swimming, at any time in the water they can present with an unfound underlying condition, panic attack, or a simple hiccup that causes distress and potential drowning. Proper supervision may not be required only during practices and games but also when athletes are in other settings, such as locker rooms or buses. Coaches should also be aware that encouraging violent conduct, unsafe conduct outside of the scope of the sport, or belligerent acts by players or other personnel can be considered as a failure to supervise.

- **Failure to provide competent personnel.** When a head coach hires an assistant or an administrator hires a physical education teacher, he or she assumes some responsibility for the competence of that assistant or teacher. If the assistant coach or teacher fails to give proper instruction or supervision to the athlete, the head coach or administrator could be found to be negligent.

- **Failure to provide appropriate training and instruction.** Coaches and physical education teachers should be qualified to teach the particular activity they are supervising. Such teaching involves providing proper instruction on the fundamental and advanced skills required for participation as well as injury prevention techniques. The coach must make sure that the participants receive adequate conditioning exercises geared toward sports performance and must instruct athletes on the rules and regulations regarding participation. Using established guidelines provided by governing bodies and keeping a log of all practice activities is the best way to prevent negligence.

- **Failure to provide proper use of safe equipment.** Because the coach may be responsible for the selection and purchase of protective, sports, and training equipment, he or she must make sure that any such equipment does not place an athlete in jeopardy. The coach or physical education teacher may also be held responsible

(continues)

> **TIME OUT 3.3** *(continued)*
>
> for failure to maintain or replace damaged sports equipment. Procedures need to be established for the regular inspection of personal protective gear and sports or training equipment. For example, large pieces of equipment, such as soccer goals, are typically moved on and off a shared field for practices and games. Ensuring that soccer goals are properly set up and free of damage to prevent them from falling is a necessity.
>
> - **Failure to warn of latent dangers.** The coach has the obligation to warn participants of any dangers that may not be obvious. Coaches and physical education teachers have a duty to warn about the nature of the activity and the techniques involved, the condition of the playing surface, and the use of equipment. For example, a coach has a duty to warn about adverse field conditions and is responsible for preventing those under his or her supervision from competing on a dangerous field. When dealing with minors, any warnings should also be given to parents or guardians.
>
> - **Failure to provide prompt and competent medical care.** The coach should know what medical personnel are present and determine accessibility in advance. If no medical personnel are available, the coach is required to provide medical care to an injured athlete. Given this mandate, the prudent coach should have basic training in proper first aid procedures for common athletic injuries. Coaches have been found liable for failing to provide appropriate first aid, moving an injured athlete incorrectly, not providing reasonable care in sending an athlete for advance medical treatment, and applying correct procedures but doing so inappropriately. That a coach remove an athlete from participation is critical if he or she has any doubt about the athlete's immediate health status. Many states have now passed laws mandating that all athletic events have QMP present (see the discussion of ATs later in this chapter).
>
> - **Failure to prevent injured athletes from competing.** Although the decision for return to play needs to be made by QMP, under no circumstances should injured players be allowed to play if the risk of further injury exists.
>
> - **Failure to match athletes of similar competitive levels.** Coaches and physical educators have a duty not to mismatch players by matching players of unequal skill, size, weight, or strength against one another in practices or games. Reducing the risk of serious injury should always be at the forefront of decisions regarding matchups. Coaches must also be careful that they do not injure players during practices because of their higher skill levels.
>
> Data from McCaskey, A. S., & Biedzynski, K. W. (1996). A guide to the legal liability of coaches for a sports participant's injuries. *Seton Hall Journal of Sports and Entertainment Law, 6*(1), 8–97; Quandt, E. F., Mitton, M. J., & Black, J. S. (2009). Legal liability in covering athletic events. *Sports Health, 1*(1), 84–90; and Wong, G. (2010). *Essentials of sports law* (2nd ed.). Santa Barbara, CA: Praeger.

Are Coaches and Physical Educators Protected?

The best protection a coach or physical educator can have against the risk of litigation is to avoid the problems listed in Time Out 3.3. Today's coaches and teachers must be constantly aware of potential risks to participants and must take appropriate action to reduce or eliminate those risks. This ongoing process of risk management involves being ever vigilant for potential risks to participants and will help reduce the chances of successful litigation because it indicates the staff has met the standard of care by eliminating all foreseeable risks for injury. Remember that some limits apply to immunity and the Good Samaritan laws because coaches and other school personnel have a duty to provide appropriate emergency care.

Because most tort claims seek monetary rewards, a coach's personal assets may be in jeopardy in the event of an unfavorable court decision. Therefore, the coach must be protected by liability insurance (McCaskey & Biedzynski, 1996). A coach in an interscholastic or intercollegiate setting is generally covered by insurance provided by the employer. However, coaches would be wise to ascertain the specific type of coverage provided and potentially acquire additional personal liability insurance to cover any gaps in employer coverage.

A good rule of thumb is for coaches, including volunteer coaches, never to assume that they

Athletic Trainers SPEAK OUT

What is the role of the AT in the establishment and maintenance of ethical behavior within athletic departments?

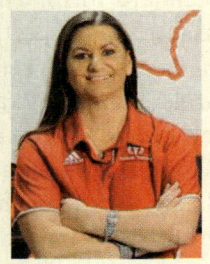

Courtesy of Catherine M. Marr, MEd, LAT, ATC.

Any ethics discussion can be a complicated matter, drawing on our morals, values, and upbringing as well as the legal system; basically, the difference between right and wrong isn't always black and white. Establishing an ethically solid foundation within the athletic department starts with administration (top down); the athletic director and head coaches are vital in setting the standards and behaviors. However, I believe that ATs end up being the moral compass and conscience in their place of employment not only regarding medical decisions but often overall. We are a sounding board and a confidant for coaches, staff, and athletes. They often ask for our leadership, advice, or guidance concerning all types of issues.

I personally try to lead by example, be reliable, and always respect my position as an AT and healthcare professional. As a result, I am often asked how I make the tough decisions that need to be made (and not be pressured to follow the easy road!). My response encompasses the idea that, as an AT, making those decisions is not only my job but also my privilege to put the health and safety of athletes above everything else (National Athletic Trainers' Association Code of Ethics). We must weigh the possibilities and rely on our training, our experience, and even our gut instinct. My thought process always includes the whole picture regardless of a game outcome (e.g., What is in athletes' best interest medically? What is best for their future?). Always document your professional medical advice and be able to back up what you believe is the best course of action. These decisions are not easy, but the more you practice, the more confident you will become. Even if you never intended to be a role model, as you grow in the profession, you will likely become the ethical example in your setting by default and not necessarily by designation.

—**Catherine M. Marr, MEd, LAT, ATC**

Catherine Marr is the head athletic trainer at Tomball High School in Tomball, Texas.

---

are covered. Before beginning the playing season, coaches should contact their employer, sponsoring organization, or an insurance company representative to determine which type of coverage they have and whether it offers the best protection and consider personal liability insurance to cover any gaps (McCaskey & Biedzynski, 1996).

How to Reduce the Chances of Going to Court

Following is a list of several important preventive steps a coach can implement to reduce the chances of being sued:

1. **Written contract.** This document should state in detail the expectations and limitations of the coach's service. (Having an attorney examine any contract is advisable, to determine what liabilities may be included.)

2. **Certification in basic or advanced first aid, CPR, and the use of an AED.** Coaches should ensure that their certification is current and that they periodically practice their skills. Such training is available through a variety of agencies, such as the American Heart Association, the American Red Cross, and the National Safety Council. Several youth or high school sports associations also offer training designed to help coaches review techniques.

3. **Emergency action plans.** Having formal emergency action plans is essential for both home and out-of-town contests. These plans should be in written form and posted publicly. All parties involved with their implementation should also have copies. Furthermore, the emergency plans should be periodically rehearsed to ensure that they will function effectively during a real crisis (Casa et al., 2013; Cooper et al., 2019).

4. **Parental consent form (for athletes younger than 18 years of age).** These forms provide an excellent opportunity to inform the athletes and their parents or guardians about the potential risk for injury that is inherent in participation. However, these signed forms do not typically release sports personnel from legal liability in cases where negligence may have occurred (Wong, 2010).

5. **Mandatory comprehensive preparticipation physical examination (PPE).** A PPE must be a requirement for all participants. A medical doctor (MD or DO) should administer the examination, and all pertinent information should be recorded on an appropriate form. Athletes should not be allowed to participate in sports activities until they have undergone the PPE (Conley et al., 2014). Most school districts, colleges, and universities have standard forms for these PPEs. The National Athletic Trainers' Association has a support statement titled Appropriate Medical Care Standards for Organizations Sponsoring Athletic Activity for the Secondary School Age Athlete, which includes a standard that emphasizes that an athlete's readiness to participate in activity should be determined through a standardized PPE process (Cooper et al., 2019). Information collected should be on file with the athletic administrator and handled confidentially. Whenever possible, the PPE should include some sort of neuropsychological or postural stability testing to establish a baseline for comparative purposes later if the athlete sustains a head injury at some point in the future (Osborne, 2001).

    Comprehensive guidelines for the PPE have been published by a consortium of medical groups, including the American Academy of Pediatrics, the American Academy of Family Physicians, the American Medical Society for Sports Medicine, the American Orthopaedic Society for Sports Medicine, the American College of Sports Medicine, and the American Osteopathic Academy of Sports Medicine. The fifth edition of the *Preparticipation Physical Evaluation* is a monograph that the medical societies contributed to so that system-by-system guidelines would be available for the PPE process and standard forms. The monograph is a valuable resource and is recommended reading because requiring a PPE that follows these guidelines will likely be interpreted by the courts as reasonable care toward athletes.

6. **Documentation of all injuries.** Regardless of severity, a detailed description of the initial care and treatment—as well as the causes—of all injuries must be recorded on a standard form. The school personnel should make sure that all pertinent information regarding an injury be collected and placed on file with the athletic administrator. If an AT is not on staff and keeping medical records, the administration should maintain an athlete's history of injuries. In this way, coaching and medical personnel are aware of all recent injuries a given athlete may have sustained.

    Federal regulations known as the Health Insurance Portability and Accountability Act (HIPAA) and Family Educational Rights and Privacy Act (FERPA) have had a dramatic effect on the health care of adolescents, including in the sports medicine field (Quandt et al., 2009). Although a comprehensive discussion of HIPAA or FERPA is beyond the scope of this chapter, coaches, physical education teachers, and other members of the athletic healthcare team should be familiar with those aspects of these regulations that can affect their place of employment or professional practice. For example, these regulations place strict limitations on the release of personal health information to third parties, such as family, teammates, and the media. Because sports are of great interest to the general public and sports injuries are often somewhat public by their very nature, school personnel must carefully monitor how information regarding an athlete's injury is distributed, if at all.

7. **Completion of seminars or postgraduate classes.** Owing in large part to the increased concern regarding sports-injury litigation, many states now require specific safety training for all personnel associated with youth athletes. This training often includes topics such as heat illness and concussions. School districts often meet this requirement by conducting training on the topic of the care and prevention of athletic injuries or requiring school personnel to complete online training offered by various groups. NFHS (n.d.) offers one of the more comprehensive groupings of educational modules. For volunteer coaches, the National Alliance for

Youth Sports offers online training videos that include injury prevention, first aid, and concussion management modules. These modules can be found at http://www.nays.org. In addition, school administrators often encourage coaches to enroll in postgraduate classes pertaining to the care and prevention of sports injuries. Completion of voluntary training or courses demonstrates a willingness on the part of coaching personnel to remain informed regarding current standards of care and prevention of sports injury.

8. **Inspections of facilities and equipment.** Foresee accidents before they happen by conducting routine inspections to ensure that any potential hazards are corrected. All equipment should be inspected before every use. Athletes are generally responsible for their own personal protective equipment; however, coaches and physical educators are responsible for facility and general equipment inspections. In addition, coaches should notify the athletic administrator, in writing, of any hazards that remain uncorrected.

9. **Development and maintenance of effective lines of communication.** Communication with athletes, parents, athletic administrators, and medical personnel is essential to providing safe activity for sports participants.

10. **Enforce rules and regulations, especially those that are designed to safeguard student athletes.** Inform participants of the inherent risks associated with specific sports. Use teachable moments on the practice field to prevent the risk of injury in game situations.

11. **Be aware of laws that govern sports and injury.** Any person involved in coaching, teaching, or refereeing sports should review all state policies and laws regarding regulations governing participation and potential liability. Environment-based activity modification policies, heat acclimatization policies, and concussion laws are good examples. Environment-based and heat acclimatization policies vary significantly across the United States. Twenty-seven states have heat activity modification policies, but only eight of these policies meet all the evidence-based guidelines related to heat acclimatization, including day-by-day progressive time and equipment exposure for all athletes and the presence of an AT at all preseason activities (Adams et al., 2018). Concussion laws typically provide guidelines for the removal of an athlete from play; the personnel who can provide return-to-play permission; and the education of coaches, parents, and athletes, but they vary from state to state. For example, all 50 states and the District of Columbia have passed laws on concussions in sports for young athletes, and each law requires some type of concussion awareness or education; however, the laws vary significantly regarding who can clear and when an athlete can be returned to play. As of 2019, only Arizona and South Carolina still allow athletes to return on the same day if they are cleared by healthcare professionals (Harris et al., 2019), and eight states allow only MDs or DOs to clear athletes for return to play (Society of Health and Physical Educators, 2017).

> **WHAT IF**
>
> You are asked to take a part-time position coaching girls' volleyball at a local junior high school. What specific steps can you take to protect yourself from a potential lawsuit if an injury occurs to one of your athletes?

What Coaches or Physical Educators Can Do If They Are Sued

If coaches or physical educators are about to be sued in a tort case, they must take the appropriate steps to protect themselves. The recommendation is for them to first contact their lawyer and call their insurance company (Appenzeller, 2000). Doing so allows them to obtain proper advice about how to further protect themselves. Furthermore, all pertinent facts related to the case can then be recorded while events are still recent.

Coaches and physical educators should write a detailed description of all events leading up to and immediately following the injury and include signed statements by eyewitnesses if possible. They also should not make any statements to the media or to other parties without the advice of an attorney (Appenzeller, 2000). In this way, they can avoid compromising their position during a subsequent trial or appeal.

Role of the AT

ATs are a vital part of the healthcare team; their services include injury and illness prevention, wellness promotion and education, emergent care, examination and clinical diagnosis, therapeutic intervention, and rehabilitation of injuries and medical conditions (Board of Certification [BOC], 2017). Several types of state regulation of ATs are presently in place in 49 of the 50 states and the District of Columbia; only California has refused to regulate the practice of ATs to licensed individuals. Licensure is considered the gold standard for professional regulation of ATs, and the majority of states (45 of 48) with regulations in place have incorporated some form of licensing. The intent of state regulation is to protect the public from incompetent practitioners. Other forms of state regulation include registration and certification. In general, state regulation defines the scope and practice of athletic training in a particular state. Anyone certified by BOC who is planning to practice in a state with regulations must contact the state regulatory body to determine the steps necessary for eligibility to practice in that state. Most often an application process is required and will be strictly enforced. The best interests of coaches or school personnel are served when they have an AT on staff who is certified nationally and has the appropriate state regulation paperwork.

Ideally, coaches, physical educators, student-athletes, school nurses, and administrators should have direct access to ATs within their school or district; however, only 66% of U.S. secondary schools have access to such services (Huggins et al., 2019). Fifty-three percent of secondary schools with access to athletic training services had full-time services, but 47% received only part-time services (Huggins et al., 2019). Thirty-one percent of public and 45% of private secondary schools had no athletic training services at all (Huggins et al., 2019). ATs can assist school personnel in maintaining safe environments for athletes and students, adhering to state laws pertaining to medical care of student-athletes, and preventing acts of negligence. Only a few states mandate having ATs at the secondary school level. However, more attention is being focused on the need for youth safety at all levels of athletic participation as evidenced by the fact that all 50 states and the District of Columbia have passed laws regarding concussion management and 27 states have activity modification plans related to heat. Legislation encouraging schools to develop and adopt best practices and standards to prevent and address student-athlete injury is being moved forward by organizations such as the National Athletic Trainers' Association, Korey Stringer Institute, and National Alliance for Youth Sports.

Sudden death occurs in 10 main areas in athletics, all of which require proper administration of medical care standards to prevent loss of life: cardiac incidents, catastrophic brain injuries, cervical spine injuries, diabetes, exertional heat illnesses, asthma, exertional sickling, exertional hyponatremia, head down contact in football, and lightning incidents (Casa et al., 2013). From July through December 2015, 14 high school football athletes died during sports participation, 7 of whom had survivable conditions if there had been appropriate recognition, treatment, and care (Kucera et al., 2016). Several evidence-based practice recommendations serve as the gold standard for medical treatment of sudden death scenarios, such as following heat acclimatization policies, removing a player from participation on the same day after sustaining a concussion, assessing core temperature via rectal thermometer to determine appropriate management, cooling via immediate cold-water immersion when exertional heat illness is occurring, and accessing an AED within 3 minutes after cardiac arrest.

The most qualified individual to plan, implement, and manage such emergencies is an AT or another QMP. In the event an AT or QMP cannot be hired at the high school level, the responsibilities of proper medical care and prevention of injury are then passed along to the coaches, other school staff, and administrators. School districts and administrators should keep in mind that state laws and medical standards need to be upheld and they need to be aware of each state's policies. Adams and colleagues (2018) recently reviewed state high school association laws across all 50 states and the District of Columbia to examine the best-practice health and safety policies pertaining to the leading causes of sudden death in sports. Their review included policies on emergency preparedness, sudden cardiac arrest and AEDs, exertional heatstroke, and head and neck injuries. A limited number of states require public secondary school athletics programs to follow all best-practice recommendations related to exertional heatstroke (16%), head injuries (6%), emergency preparedness (8%), and sudden cardiac arrest and AEDs (14%) (Adams et al., 2018). This means that, if an AT or QMP is not present during athletic activity, then the coaches, school nurses, and administrators may not be implementing gold standard medical policies regarding the prevention of sudden death in sports. Therefore, the responsibility and the potential liability of an unexpected and often preventable sports-related death or catastrophic injury of a young student-athlete may lie directly in their hands.

Review Questions

1. Briefly describe the two types of negligence discussed in the chapter, acts of commission and acts of omission.
2. Define the terms *tort* and *negligence* as discussed in the chapter.
3. What are the four elements that must be present to prove negligence?
4. Briefly describe the ways that a negligence suit may be defeated.
5. Does liability differ for a paid versus a volunteer coach?
6. Do Good Samaritan laws protect school personnel, such as coaches, from litigation?
7. List and describe the reasons a coach or physical educator may be found negligent.
8. Outline the steps that can reduce a coach's chances of being sued.
9. What are the first two things a coach should do when notified of an impending lawsuit?
10. Elaborate on the sociological pressures exerted on today's coaches that may challenge their sense of professional ethics.
11. True or false? The courts have found that a coach is liable for the injury or death of a student-athlete.
12. What do ATs provide to the secondary school setting?
13. What is the purpose of state regulation of ATs, and how many states presently regulate the profession?
14. Why is having an AT or a QMP associated with school-sponsored and youth sport activities so important?

Recommended Reading

Bernhardt, D. T., & Roberts, W. O. (Eds). (2019). *Preparticipation physical evaluation* (5th ed.). Itasca, IL: American Academy of Pediatrics.

References

Adams, W. M., Scarneo, S. E., & Casa, D. J. (2018). Assessment of evidence-based health and safety policies on sudden death and concussion management in secondary school athletics: A benchmark study. *Journal of Athletic Training, 53*(8), 756–767.

American Bar Association. (2018). *New ABA data reveals rise in number of U.S. lawyers, 15 percent increase since 2008.* Retrieved from https://www.americanbar.org/news/abanews/aba-news-archives/2018/05/new_aba_data_reveals/

Appenzeller, T. (2000). *Youth sport and the law.* Durham, NC: Carolina Academic Press.

Barron, M. J., Powell, J. W., Ewing, M. E., Nogle, S. E., & Branta, C. F. (2009). First aid and injury prevention: Knowledge of youth basketball, football, and soccer coaches. *International Journal of Coaching Science, 3*(1), 55–67.

Beahm, J. (2010). *Max Gilpin school football death suit settles.* Retrieved from http://blogs.findlaw.com/injured/2010/09/max-gilpin-school-football-death-suit-settles.html

Board of Certification, Inc. (BOC). (2017). *What is an athletic trainer?* Retrieved from https://bocatc.org/about-us

Casa, D. J., Almquist, J. L., Anderson, S. A., Baker, L., Bergeron, M. F., Biagioli, B., . . . Valentine, V. (2013). The Inter-Association

Task Force for Preventing Sudden Death in Secondary School Athletics Programs: Best-practices recommendations. *Journal of Athletic Training, 48*(4), 546–553.

Cohen, A. (2009). High school to pay $15 million settlement to paralyzed wrestler. *Athletic Business, 33*(6), 24.

Conley, K. M., Bolin, D. J., Carek, P. J., Konin, J. G., Neal, T. L., & Violette, D. (2014). National Athletic Trainers' Association position statement: Preparticipation physical examinations and disqualifying conditions. *Journal of Athletic Training, 49*(1), 102–120.

Cooper, L., Harper, R., Wham, G. S. Jr., Cates, J., Chafin, S. J. Jr., Cohen, R. P., . . . McLeod, T. C. V. (2019). Appropriate medical care standards for organizations sponsoring athletic activity for the secondary school–aged athlete: A summary statement. *Journal of Athletic Training, 54*(7), 741–748.

Harris, E., Rangarajan, S., & Miner, C. (2019, February 9). *Concussion laws: How does your state stack up?* Retrieved from https://www.revealnews.org/article/concussion-laws-how-does-your-state-stack-up/

Huggins, R. A., Coleman, K. A., Attanasio, S. M., Cooper, G. L., Endres, B. D., Harper, R. C., . . . Casa, D. J. (2019). Athletic trainer services in the secondary school setting: The athletic training locations and services project. *Journal of Athletic Training, 54*(11), 1129–1139.

Korey Stringer Institute. (n.d.). *Coaching education.* Retrieved from https://ksi.uconn.edu/prevention/coaching-education/#

Kucera, K. L., Yau, R., Thomas, L. C., Wolff, C., & Cantu, R. C. (2016). Catastrophic sports injury research: Thirty-third annual report, Fall 1982–Spring 2015. Retrieved from https://nccsir.unc.edu/files/2013/10/NCCSIR-33rd-Annual-All-Sport-Report-1982_2015.pdf

McCaskey, A. S., & Biedzynski, K. W. (1996). A guide to the legal liability of coaches for a sports participant's injuries. *Seton Hall Journal of Sports and Entertainment Law, 6*(1), 8–97.

McLeod, T. C. V., McGaugh, J. W., Boquiren, M. L., & Bay, R. C. (2008). Youth sports coaches do not have adequate knowledge regarding first-aid and injury prevention. *Applied Research in Coaching and Athletics Annual, 23*, 130–146.

Mirsafian, H. (2016). Legal duties and legal liabilities of coaches toward athletes. *Physical Culture and Sport Studies and Research, 69*(1), 5–14.

National Federation of State High School Associations (NFHS). (n.d.). *Interscholastic education, made easy.* Retrieved from http://www.nfhslearn.com/StatePricingRegs.aspx

Osborne, B. (2001). Principles of liability for athletic trainers: Managing sport-related concussion. *Journal of Athletic Training, 36*(3), 316–321.

Quandt, E. F., Mitton, M. J., & Black, J. S. (2009). Legal liability in covering athletic events. *Sports Health, 1*(1), 84–90.

Ransone, J. W., & Dunn, L. R. (1999). Assessment of first aid knowledge and decision-making of high school coaches. *Journal of Athletic Training, 34*(3), 267–271.

Ray, R., & Konin, J. (2011). *Management strategies in athletic training* (4th ed.). Champaign, IL: Human Kinetics.

Society of Health and Physical Educators. (2017, June). *Concussion: State legislation and policy.* Retrieved from https://www.shapeamerica.org/standards/guidelines/Concussion/state-policy.aspx

Student CPR. *States where CPR training is mandatory for coaches.* (n.d.). Retrieved from https://schoolcpr.com/requirements/coaches/

Wolohan, J. T. (2008). By the boards. *Athletic Business, 32*(10), 28–32.

Wong, G. (2010). *Essentials of sports law* (2nd ed.). Santa Barbara, CA: Praeger.

CHAPTER 4
Sports-Injury Prevention

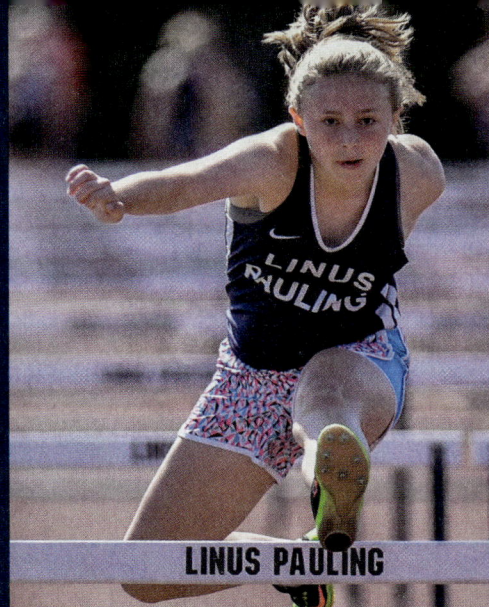

MAJOR CONCEPTS

Prevention of sports-related injuries must be a priority for everyone involved in organized sports, particularly coaches, physical educators, officials, administrators, sports medicine personnel, and athletes and their parents. This chapter describes the critical steps that must be taken to minimize risk factors that may lead to injury and maximize strategies that athletes can use to ensure physical preparation for their activity or sport of choice. First, the chapter differentiates between two major categories of injury risk factors—extrinsic (e.g., equipment, environment, and sport) and intrinsic (i.e., anatomical characteristics, age, gender, and skill). The chapter continues with a description of the major factors to be considered to modify the common extrinsic risk factors related to sports injuries. It then distinguishes between two essential prevention strategies related to intrinsic risk factors: the preparticipation physical examination and physical conditioning with an emphasis on periodization of training. As outlined in this chapter, periodization of the training program optimizes the performance objectives of the conditioning program while avoiding training-induced injuries and ensuring that the training done by the athlete is beneficial and not detrimental. Finally, the chapter concludes with various sport-specific injury considerations, including overuse injuries, and provides an overview of the importance of emergency action plans and return-to-play criteria.

There are more than 11 million students participating in organized secondary school athletics and performing arts in the United States alone (National Federation of State High School Associations [NFHS], 2016). Athletics add to the overall growth of an adolescent, and those involved in athletics with proper coaching learn lifelong lessons for success and demonstrate better academic achievements (NFHS, 2016). The burden of sport-related injury in youth sports is significant as it effects physical, psychological, mental, and financial domains of the athlete and family (Emery & Pasanen, 2019). Therefore, it is in the best interest of not only the participants but also the coaches, parents, and sports medicine staff to reduce the number of injuries and contribute to the athletes' ability to participate in athletics through a well-planned, coordinated program of injury risk reduction and prevention. However, before such an endeavor can be effective, causative factors must be identified that contribute to injuries. Because of the risk and scope of sports injuries and the legal implications of catastrophic injuries, all parties involved, including the athletic

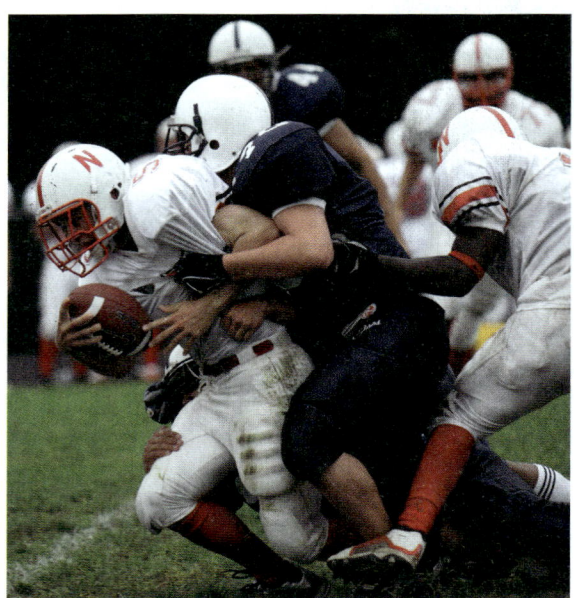

Figure 4.1 In some sports, the cause of an injury might seem obvious, but other factors may also contribute.
© Larry St. Pierre/Shutterstock.

healthcare team, coaches, physical educators, officials, parents, school or league administrators, and athletes, should take steps to eliminate or at least reduce the risk and/or the severity of injury. At first, this may seem to be a simple process with regard to common sports injuries. For example, when a football running back collides with a linebacker and sustains a sprained knee ligament, the cause of the injury would seem to be related to the force of the collision or playing field conditions (see Figure 4.1). However, other factors may have played a role in creating the injury, including the player's skill and/or technique, age, strength-to-weight ratio, shoe type, fatigue, and/or previous injuries.

Causative Factors in Injury

Sports scientists and other researchers have collected considerable information regarding injuries, and some have conducted research to identify causative factors

Extrinsic injury risk factors Anything outside the body that can affect an individual, such as environmental temperature.

Intrinsic injury risk factors Anything inherent to the body that cannot be changed, such as age or bony characteristics, or that is changeable, such as fitness level, both of which can affect the individual.

of not only acute but also chronic or overuse injuries that are suffered by participants. They propose two general categories of injury risk factors: extrinsic and intrinsic. **Extrinsic injury risk factors** are characteristics outside the body that can affect an individual and include sports equipment, environment, type of activity, and playing field conditions. **Intrinsic injury risk factors** are characteristics inherent to the body and include age, gender, body size, history of injury, fitness, muscle strength (especially imbalances), ligamentous laxity, skill, psychological status, and perhaps even overall intelligence (Emery & Pasanen, 2019; Nauta et al., 2017; Theisen et al., 2014). For example, the type of injury has been linked with sex in collegiate athletes. Males had a higher acute injury rate compared to females, whereas female athletes had a higher rate of overuse injury than male athletes (Yang et al., 2012).

To delineate between extrinsic and intrinsic factors, several studies have sought to investigate risk factors for particular sports (Badgeley et al., 2013; Steinberg et al., 2012) and body areas (Alentorn-Geli et al., 2014; Bayer et al., 2020; Murphy et al., 2003). For example, Badgeley and colleagues (2013) identified two extrinsic factors, player–player contact and player–surface contact, as the leading mechanisms of injury for high school football players. Conversely, young dancers' mechanisms of injury were more often related to intrinsic factors, including joint hypermobility, anatomical anomalies, and technique (Steinberg et al., 2012). Both investigations also found that "sport" position played a significant role in the type of injury because dancers who spent more time *en pointe* had more injuries (Steinberg et al., 2012) and offensive football players suffered more heat illnesses (Badgeley et al., 2013). In relation to body area, Murphy and colleagues (2003) identified 5 extrinsic and more than 18 intrinsic risk factors that typically lead to injury in the lower extremities. The extrinsic factors included playing surface, protective equipment, and level of competition, and the intrinsic factors included tight or weak muscles, limb dominance, joint malalignments, poor muscle conditioning, and ineffective rehabilitation postinjury. Alentorn-Geli et al. (2014) reported in a systematic review that male athletes' risk for noncontact anterior cruciate ligament (ACL) injury is a complicated combination of intrinsic (i.e., anatomical factors) and extrinsic (e.g., dry weather and artificial turf) factors. The upper

Table 4.1

Extrinsic and Intrinsic Factors Associated With Injury

	Extrinsic Factors (Outside the Body)	Intrinsic Factors (Inside the Body)
Unchangeable	Environment; equipment; field conditions; officiating	Age; height; sex; previous injury
Changeable	Sport; position; level of competition; contact with player or surface; coaching; rules	Weight; muscle strength, endurance, and flexibility; ligament laxity; limb dominance; coordination; skill level, technique, fitness level, fatigue, balance, psychological status

Based on Theisen, D., Malisoux, L., Seil, R., & Urhausen, A. (2014). Injuries in youth sports: Epidemiology, risk factors, and prevention. *Deutsche Zeitschrift Fur Sportmedizin, 65*(9), 248–252.

extremities also had similar intrinsic risk factors associated with injury, including range of motion (ROM) and strength differences between nondominant and dominant limbs, age, gender, and injury mechanism (e.g., fall, contact, or no contact; Hjelm et al., 2012; Sytema et al., 2010).

It is clear that not all of these factors can be eliminated or changed. However, it is certainly possible to reduce or eliminate problems such as poor or faulty equipment, inadequate muscle strength, poor skills, and training errors (Table 4.1).

Intervention Strategies

All members of the athletic healthcare team, coaching staff, and athletic administration share the responsibility to remain vigilant to identify causative factors before an injury occurs. Many of the extrinsic factors are more recognizable than intrinsic factors; however, there are techniques and methods that can be employed to prevent injury. For example, regular inspections of protective equipment and athletic facilities alert personnel to potential problems, and adequate physical exams before athletic participation are convenient ways to help minimize risk. Regular inspection of equipment and facilities is specific to the type of personal or sports equipment and facilities. As to personal protective equipment, regular inspection often involves daily assessment of safety, whereas athletic facilities may require inspection only prior to competitions or monthly to semiannual inspection by maintenance staff. Other strategies may include wearing protective devices or bracing above and beyond the minimum required equipment for the rules of the sport.

Extrinsic Factors

Extrinsic risk factors for sports injuries include the practice/competition environment, facilities, protective equipment, and officiating and coaching. It is critical that coaching personnel; physical educators; athletic program or school administrators; and, if on staff, Board of Certification–certified athletic trainers monitor the extrinsic factors to identify and eliminate any potential risks to the athletes. Currently, no state has a mandate for a certified athletic trainer at all secondary schools. Recently the Korey Stringer Institute (KSI) and the National Athletic Trainers' Association (NATA) completed the Athletic Training Locations and Services (ATLAS) Project and reported that approximately 66% of all public and private secondary schools have access to a certified athletic trainer, but only 35% of all secondary schools have a full-time athletic trainer on site (Huggins et al., 2018). Overall, public secondary schools employ more athletic training (AT) services than private secondary schools by 14%. AT services are also more prevalent in cities or suburbs then towns or rural districts (Huggins et al., 2018). For even more detailed information, the 1st annual ATLAS report contains detailed information about the type of athletic trainer services across all 50 states and the District of Columbia.

> For more information about athletic training, go to the National Athletic Trainers' Association website at **www.nata.org**

Practice/Competition Environment

Whether outdoors or indoors, the environment must be assessed to determine whether it represents a potential health risk. If electrical storms (i.e., lightning; Walsh et al., 2013), cold weather conditions (Cappaert, 2008; Madden & Fudge, 2018), or high relative heat and humidity (Casa et al., 2015; Hosokawa et al., 2021) conditions are present in the outdoor environment, athletic participation is unsafe.

Note that if an electrical storm is in the area lightning can strike in the absence of rain and when skies are blue. It is important to establish safety criteria from lightning safety guidelines (National Weather Service, n.d.) and adhere to recommendations for the safety of athletic participants and spectators. Conservatively, athletic participation should stop at the first sight of lightning or sound of thunder and resume 30 minutes after the last sight of lightning or sound of thunder (Walsh et al., 2013). Participants and spectators should take cover indoors and not seek shelter in dugouts or picnic areas when an electrical storm is nearby. The slogan "When thunder roars, go indoors" is a helpful reminder and can be used to educate individuals by posting signs in the athletic complex (Walsh et al., 2013).

Preventing thermal injuries from cold or heat and humidity conditions is also a consideration of environmental conditions. Organizations such as the KSI are devoted to researching ways to prevent heat-related illness. It is important to remember that indoor activity can also pose a significant risk of thermal injury, particularly if the participant is not properly hydrated or the indoor temperature and humidity are high. Monitoring the weather for air temperature, humidity, wind speed, and electrical storms is imperative to prevent injuries and allow a safe participation environment.

> For more information about maximizing safety for participants, please visit the Korey Stringer Institute at **https://ksi.uconn.edu**

Facilities

All sports facilities, regardless of the sports played in them, must be designed, maintained for safe activity and cleanliness, and frequently inspected for the well-being of the participants. Existing facilities should have the same emphasis put on them to minimize injury risk of the participants as new facilities or those being designed and built. Budgets and local building codes must be considered; however, these factors should never be allowed to supersede safety. Shared facilities are common; for example, a school may build a multiuse facility where many sports (i.e., football, lacrosse, soccer, and track and field) will be played depending on the time of the year. These types of facilities may have a game field that is surrounded by an outdoor running track with field event equipment (e.g., landing pits for long jump, high jump, and pole vault and shot-put ring) either on the playing field or on the ends of the field. Baseball fields may be located next to a soccer or softball field or perhaps even share some of the same ground, causing excessive overuse of natural surfaces, potentially resulting in dirt patches and/or divots and holes. Some complexes are built with multiple fields in close proximity to each other intended for use by the same sport. Regardless of the specific situation, it is critical that care be taken that all facilities meet the minimum requirements for safe participation (Figure 4.2). These requirements include such things as integrity of field conditions, safety fences, and batting cages; location of dugouts in baseball and softball; type of bases used (i.e., breakaway or fixed); correctly constructed and anchored soccer goals; location of water and sanitation facilities; and integrity of emergency medical services (EMS) access routes. It is important

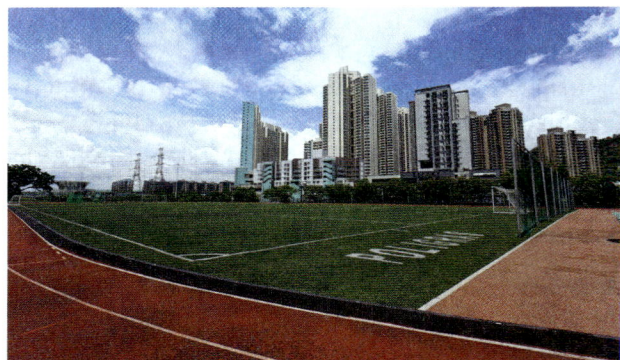

Figure 4.2 Multiuse facilities may play a role in injury.
© coloursinmylife/Shutterstock.

for coaches, physical educators, sports medicine staff personnel, and administrators to remember that several deaths have been attributed to faulty integrity of sports equipment, including soccer goals and batting cages.

With respect to indoor facilities, primary concerns center on lighting, playing surfaces, ventilation, and room dimensions. Poor lighting may contribute to accidents resulting from poor visibility. A floor that is not cleaned regularly or is improperly finished may become slippery and thus contribute to collisions and falls. Budgetary constraints may dictate some gymnasiums' dimensions, which do not provide adequate space between the basketball baskets and the adjacent wall or between the sidelines and the bleachers or walls. Junior high and elementary school facilities are often not built with the same safety designs as those used for adults due to the building designers not seeing safety issues of younger and smaller participants equal to those of older and larger participants. In such situations, it is critical that items such as protective padding be placed on the walls behind the basketball backboards to reduce players' collisions with the walls. If there are other facility-specific items that may not be as safe as they could be, the athletic administrator along with the coaching and sports medicine staffs may want to create protective rule modifications for the facility.

Locker rooms and shower facilities should be designed to enable participants to move around safely, with adequate ventilation, lighting, and nonskid floors. It is imperative that medical equipment, such as whirlpool baths, and other therapeutic modalities, such as ultrasound or diathermy machines, not be available for use in the locker room. Such equipment represents a significant safety risk and greatly increases the legal liability of the school.

Protective Equipment

Protective equipment plays a vital role in the prevention of injuries. This is especially true in sports such as tackle football, ice hockey, lacrosse, baseball, and softball. However, virtually all sports can benefit from the use of some form of safety equipment, even something as simple as shin guards in soccer, mouth guards in basketball or wresting, or additional protective guards in baseball or softball (i.e., elbow guards for batters). Most equipment companies provide instructions for the fitting and maintenance of protective equipment, including helmets. National associations also govern the regular inspection and recertification of sports helmets and other protective equipment. It is important to regularly inspect and adhere to manufacturer and national association guidelines to maintain safe equipment (Table 4.2). Lastly, protective equipment should be clean at all times to prevent the spread of viruses, bacteria, and fungi.

Intrinsic Factors

Although one cannot change biological factors, such as age and height, many of the intrinsic factors that can lead to injury can be changed. For example, individuals who have muscle imbalances may be at increased

Table 4.2
Common Sports and Medical Equipment Organization Websites

Organization	Website
National Operating Committee on Standards for Athletic Equipment	http://nocsae.org
International Organization for Standardization	http://www.iso.org/iso/home.htm
ASTM International	http://www.astm.org
Hockey Equipment Certification Council	http://www.hecc.net
Safety Equipment Institute	http://www.seinet.org
American National Standards Institute	http://www.ansi.org

risk of muscle strains. Also, athletes in high-risk sports must be informed of the potential hazards and prevention strategies; for example, in tackle football, players should be taught proper blocking and tackling techniques to avoid using the helmeted head as a weapon. It has been found that the incidence of serious head and neck injuries can be greatly reduced in this way (Champagne et al., 2019; Evans et al., 2020; Swartz et al., 2022). Together a preparticipation physical examination and proper conditioning may reduce the risk of injury by identifying and rectifying preexisting problems.

Preparticipation Physical Examination

Athletes must also undergo a **preparticipation physical examination (PPE)** designed to identify individual risk factors associated with sport participation. The primary purposes of the PPEs are to identify preexisting risk factors for injury, ascertain injuries or diseases that may create problems for the student-athlete as a result of sport participation, and identify any preexisting conditions that may disqualify the individual from participation permanently or at least until follow-up with another medical professional has been done (Douglas & Siddiqi, 2021; Khodaee et al., 2018).

PPEs are a necessary part of any athletic organization, including schools and youth sports, because the number of sport participants has grown significantly and U.S. society has become increasingly more litigious over the years. It has become ever more difficult for school officials (i.e., coaches, athletic administrators) or youth sports directors (i.e., club coaches, regional directors, parents) to monitor the health of all of their incoming youth or student-athletes on an annual basis, and there is a greater fear of being sued if an athlete is injured as a result of inadequate health screening. Therefore, the PPE is an important tool for all concerned.

Historically, PPEs often only consisted of a quick check of the major physiological systems. As a result, to improve the overall quality of PPEs nationally, a consortium of professional medical organizations (American Academy of Family Physicians [AAFP] in association with American Academy of Pediatrics [AAP], American College of Sports Medicine [ACSM], American Medical Society for Sports Medicine, American Orthopaedic Society for Sports Medicine, and American Osteopathic Academy of Sports Medicine) developed and published a comprehensive set of guidelines in 1992, titled "Preparticipation Physical Evaluation (PPE)." The guidelines have since been updated several times, and the latest monograph is the fifth edition, published in 2021 (MacDonald et al., 2021).

In 2014, the NATA released a position statement on the PPE and disqualifying conditions (Conley et al., 2014). This position statement outlines what is strongly recommended and emphasized in the PPE. The cornerstone of the examination is obtaining and reviewing a comprehensive medical and family history. Typical physical examinations involve an assessment of general appearance, eyes/vision, cardiac auscultation (i.e., listening to the heart with a stethoscope) and blood pressure measurement, respiratory assessment, abdominal palpation, skin assessment, hernia check (males only), and musculoskeletal assessment, including ROM, general strength, and joint laxity (Douglas & Siddiqi, 2021; Khodaee et al., 2018). The NATA position statement also recommends a thorough investigation of musculoskeletal injuries and prior surgeries.

In particular, the cardiac portion of the PPE and the potential mandatory inclusion of routine electrocardiogram (EKG, aka ECG) have received considerable attention over the last decade because sudden cardiac arrest is the leading cause of death in athletes during sports (Drezner et al., 2019; Williams et al., 2019). It has been reported that up to 36 sudden cardiac deaths occur annually in youths under 18 years of age (Maron, 2015). However, debate still exists among many medical professionals regarding the inclusion of routine EKGs within the PPE despite scientific advances and extensive research (Douglas & Siddiqi, 2021; Petek & Baggish, 2020; Roberts et al., 2015; Van der Wall, 2015). Proponents of routine EKGs point to the fact that abnormal findings on an EKG will increase the medical professional's ability to detect an underlying cardiac condition that may cause sudden cardiac death (Brandt & O'Keefe, 2019; Van der Wall, 2015). While that may

---

Preparticipation physical examination (PPE)
A clinical examination performed by a physician on physically active individuals to assess their physical and mental health before participation in sports or physical activities to determine their physical readiness.

be true, correct interpretation of the EKG results is critical, and many false-positive tests are received, which often results in expensive medical visits that ultimately provide no evidence for concern (Roberts et al., 2015). Assuming that accurate testing with mass screening is limited, the American Heart Association (AHA) recommends against mandating EKG in conjunction with the PPE because sufficient infrastructure within the U.S. medical community does not exist to produce consistently accurate results (Williams et al., 2019). The AHA recommends that 14 specific areas related to the heart should be evaluated within the PPE (Williams et al., 2019), including personal cardiac history (7 elements), family cardiac history (3 elements), and heart-specific physical exam (4 elements; Maron et al., 2014). In essence, particular attention should be given to the physical exam results, as well as the answers given to the cardiac-related questions within the medical history. The **Time Out 4.1** includes the ten questions used for personal and familial cardiac medical history and the four cardiac physical exam tests.

The NCAA, NFHS, and NATA have developed and implemented either mandated or suggested guidelines regarding medical evaluations of student-athletes. The NCAA guidelines require that all student-athletes receive a PPE upon their initial entrance into the institution's athletic program. The initial PPE should include a comprehensive medical history, an immunization history (defined by the Centers for Disease Control and Prevention [CDC]), and a physical examination that includes an emphasis on musculoskeletal, neurological, and cardiovascular evaluation (Douglas & Siddiqi, 2021). Ideally, the PPE is performed a minimum of 4–6 weeks before the first workout to allow time for potentially needed follow-up. Thereafter,

TIME OUT 4.1

Ten questions related to personal and family history regarding cardiac medical conditions

1. Do you experience chest pressure, discomfort, pain, or tightness related to exercising or exertion?
2. Do you experience unexplained fainting or almost fainting?
3. Do you experience unexplained fatigue, heart palpitations, or painful/excessive breathing related to exercising or exertion?
4. Have you had a heart murmur diagnosed by a physician?
5. Do you have high blood pressure?
6. Have you ever been restricted from participating in physical activity?
7. Have you ever had testing for the heart prescribed by a physician?
8. Has anyone in your family died prematurely (unexpected, sudden, or other) before age 50 and it is attributable to heart issues?
9. Has anyone in your family less than 50 years old experienced disability due to a heart condition?
10. Has anyone in your family experienced significant arrhythmias, long-QT syndrome, hypertrophic/dilated cardiomyopathy, Marfan syndrome, or genetic/acquired defects within the ion channels of the heart?

Diagnoses from Physical Examination by Qualified Medical Professional

1. Are there physical signs of Marfan syndrome (i.e., tall and slender build, disproportionately long arms, legs, fingers, protruding or concave breastbone)?
2. Are there weak pulses in the femoral arteries?
3. Is there a nonorganic heart murmur or left ventricular outflow obstruction?
4. Is there abnormal brachial artery blood pressure in both arms while sitting?

Modified from Maron, B. J., Friedman, R. A., Kligfield, P., Levine, B. D., Viskin, S., Chaitman, B. R., Okin, P. M., . . . Thompson, P. D. (2014). Assessment of the 12-lead electrocardiogram as a screening test for detection of cardiovascular disease in healthy general populations of young people (12–25 years of age). *Journal of the American College of Cardiology, 64*(14), 1479–1514.

an annual updated medical history is required, unless an additional medical examination is warranted based on the updated history or a new medical condition (Douglas & Siddiqi, 2021).

The NFHS continues to recommend a yearly medical evaluation before participation in interscholastic sports, and many high schools abide by this recommendation; however, the NFHS does not mandate that every state require this. As such, the requirement for participants in secondary school athletics varies greatly among the states (Caswell et al., 2015). There are many factors that cause state associations not to require a PPE on an annual basis. These factors include, but are not limited to, rising costs of a medical examination, lack of access to qualified medical personnel who can perform the examinations, or simply the belief that an annual PPE is not warranted. It should be noted that, whenever an athlete has sustained a more serious injury, such as head or spinal trauma, or undergone surgery, he or she should receive a complete physical evaluation by a physician before being allowed to return to participation. The AAFP, along with five other consensus groups, recommends that younger secondary school or middle-school athletes receive a comprehensive PPE biannually and at 2- to 3-year intervals for older athletes. In addition, NFHS recommends that a comprehensive PPE be administered for athletes entering either middle or high school or those transferring to a new school. Further, all athletes should receive annual updates that consist of a comprehensive medical history along with assessment of height, weight, and blood pressure. Follow-up examination for any problems detected in the history is also recommended (Douglas & Siddiqi, 2021).

A well-administered PPE provides a great deal of information about the athlete's readiness for participation by evaluating cardiac, neurological, and musculoskeletal systems using history questions and physical examination techniques. Commonly identified conditions include congenital disorders, such as spina bifida occulta (i.e., incomplete closure of the vertebral neural arch); absence of one of a paired set of organs (i.e., eye, kidney, or testicle); postural problems, such as abnormal spinal curvatures or abnormalities of the upper and lower extremities; muscle imbalances; obesity; high blood pressure; cardiac defects or disorders of cardiac rhythm; respiratory conditions, such as asthma; drug allergies; skin infections; vision problems; and general medical concerns, such as diabetes and sickle cell trait. NCAA Division I–III institutions are required to screen for sickle cell trait before participation unless documented results are provided to the institution (Mitchell, 2018). The NATA recommends confirming sickle cell trait status of all athletes (Conley et al., 2014).

Two PPE formats are currently recommended for obtaining the medical examination. One option is for the athlete's personal physician to perform the PPE in the physician's office; this option is considered the ideal. However, with the increased numbers of sports participants since the 1990s, the demand on the medical community for these services has increased. Obviously, as the costs of health care in general have escalated, so have the costs of undergoing a PPE. As a result, many young athletes simply cannot afford to visit a personal physician (assuming they have one) each year for such an evaluation. The other option accommodates groups of athletes in one screening session and is called the "coordinated medical team" approach (Khodaee et al., 2018).

Both formats can be highly effective tools for the delivery of the PPE. The advantages of the individual PPE performed by the athlete's personal physician include familiarity of the physician with the athlete's medical history and immediate access to medical records that include such information as immunization history. In addition, the athlete's personal physician in all likelihood has established a relationship of trust with the athlete that will allow for some discussion regarding health risk behaviors, such as concealing concussion symptoms, drug use, and sexual behavior. In some situations, however, the office visit with a personal physician may not be possible. For example, when a group of athletes, such as a basketball or volleyball team, all need PPEs, the team physician may prefer to arrange for the team members to be evaluated by a team of clinicians that includes primary care physicians, athletic trainers, physical therapists, exercise physiologists, and nutritionists. According to the AAFP, this approach to the administration of the PPE does have some advantages over the office visit format. Its advantages include possible cost savings to the athletes and provision of PPEs to athletes who do not have a personal physician. To expedite the PPE process, it is recommended that the athlete complete a PPE medical history in advance of the actual evaluation. Whenever possible, the medical history should be done with the athlete and parent(s) or guardian(s) together. In the coordinated medical team approach of administering PPEs, it should be noted that the convenience of administering multiple PPEs in a near-simultaneous nature does not override the importance of doing the PPEs in a thorough fashion.

Regardless of which type of PPE administration is employed, the procedure can provide valuable information relative to an athlete's readiness for participation. Coaches and sports medicine personnel must be aware of any preexisting conditions that may make the athlete vulnerable to specific medical problems. A thorough medical history, including previous injuries, represents information essential to the welfare of the athlete.

Athletes with medical conditions, such as asthma; diabetes; epilepsy; drug, food, and/or environmental allergies; cardiac conditions; blood disorders; and other illnesses/diseases, should be identified in case of subsequent injury or other problems related to their condition. Special populations need to be evaluated on the basis of injury risk factors that may not be present in the general population. It is recommended that physicians who are familiar with the unique medical implications of each specific disorder evaluate special populations.

The results of the PPE will fall into one of three categories in relation to sport participation: An athlete will be cleared, not be cleared, or be in need of further evaluation for clearance. The most confusing outcome is when further evaluation is needed. Needing further evaluation usually occurs due to orthopedic injury, concussion, systemic illness (e.g., mononucleosis), or a found medical problem. All athletes who receive an "in need of further evaluation" status must then be referred via a coordinated approach with the family and associated sports medicine team (Douglas & Siddiqi, 2021; Khodaee et al., 2018).

To determine whether an athlete with an abnormality or condition is cleared to play sports, physicians should calculate the risk for future injury to the athlete and other athletes, assess whether the athlete can safely participate with treatment (e.g., padding, bracing, or medicine), and consider which sports and positions (i.e., noncontact vs. contact sports) would best suit the situation (Conley et al., 2014). Concern has been raised in the sports medicine community regarding the safety of participation for athletes who are missing one of a paired set of organs, for example, those who have only one eye, kidney, or testicle. This issue is addressed by the AAP in its updated policy statement, which presents guidelines to physicians when considering an array of medical conditions that could affect sport participation (Khodaee et al., 2018; Rice, 2008). The AAP recognizes that this is a complex issue and a number of variables must be considered, including the relative risk associated with a particular sport; for example, collision versus limited-contact sports. The amount of contact may be an important factor when considering an athlete who is missing one of a paired set of organs. As such, the AAP policy statement gives a "qualified yes" to these athletes, based on the premise that, with proper protection, participation in limited-contact and even collision sports may be acceptable when appropriate protective equipment remains in place (Khodaee et al., 2018; Rice, 2008).

Legally, physicians and institutions have the right to restrict an athlete from participating in a sport after carefully considering the individual's situation backed up by sound medical evidence (Conley et al., 2014). The AAP policy statement also recommends that, if the physician advises against participation for medical reasons and the family chooses to allow the child to participate, a signed informed consent document, preferably in a parent's or guardian's own handwriting, be obtained that verifies he or she has been advised of the risks. Further, it is advised that the athlete and parent or guardian also sign the document accepting that he or she understands these risks (Khodaee et al., 2018; Rice, 2008). Obviously, all information obtained during a physical examination should be handled confidentially according to the Family Educational Rights and Privacy Act (FERPA) and Health Insurance Portability and Accountability Act (HIPPA; Conley et al., 2014; Table 4.3).

WHAT IF ❓

A parent asks you, the soccer coach at the local high school, your recommendation for whether he should take his child to the family doctor or to a mass evaluation screening for the required preparticipation physical examination that is required by the state high school association. What would you recommend?

Table 4.3
Preparticipation Physical Examination Components

1. History—acquire medical and family history of injury and illness/disease provided by the athlete and parent. Focus on cardiac, heat and humidity, concussion, and sickle cell concerns.
2. Screening
   a. General health—assess vitals, visual acuity, pulmonary, skin, and abdomen.
   b. Cardiovascular—auscultate the heart, followed up with electrocardiography, echocardiography, and/or stress test if warranted.
   c. Neurological—assess ability to feel and distinguish touch and assess reflexes (e.g., patellar at knee).
   d. Orthopedic—assess ROM, joint stability, muscle strength.
   e. Special conditions—screen for subclinical symptoms and complications of existing disease/conditions (i.e., conditions associated with anemia, diabetes, sickle cell trait, high cholesterol). Screening may include blood tests or urinalysis.
   f. Medications—review proper administration and dosage.
   g. Nutrition—review diet and screen for eating disorders.
   h. Mental health—screen for mental health.

Based on Conley, K. M., Bolin, D. J., Carek, P. J., Konin, J. G., Neal, T. L., & Violette, D. (2014). National Athletic Trainers' Association position statement: Preparticipation physical examinations and disqualifying conditions. *Journal of Athletic Training, 49*(1), 102–120.

Injury Prevention by Conditioning

An essential aspect of any injury prevention program is the optimal development of physical fitness in the athlete because many of the intrinsic risk factors can be significantly modified as a result of effective conditioning programs. The role of a coach cannot be underestimated when it comes to injury prevention via appropriate conditioning programs because recent estimates indicate that young athletes can spend an average of 326 hours of practice time under the supervision of a coach, which is far more than the time spent with teachers, physicians, or other allied healthcare professionals (Koester, 2000).

School-age youths are encouraged to participate in 60 minutes or more of moderate to vigorous physical activity each day (CDC, 2017), including vigorous physical activity at least 3 days a week. Current public health recommendations indicate that physical education (PE) within the school setting helps to accomplish this activity goal (Hills et al., 2015). In fact, 150 minutes per week of PE for elementary school children and 225 minutes per week of PE for secondary school children are recommended (Hills et al., 2015). These activities should be developmentally appropriate, enjoyable, and safe. Children can safely participate in aerobic activities, such as swimming, running, and bicycling, and increasing evidence indicates that strength training can also be a safe and effective activity for children. Additionally, the 60 minutes should include muscle and bone strengthening activities, such as push-ups and jumping (CDC, 2017). A significant body of evidence also exists supporting the premise that injury prevention strategies should focus on preseason conditioning and training throughout the season that includes strength, balance, and functional sport-specific skills (Emery & Pasanen, 2019). It has also been demonstrated that supervised training programs that focus on developing neuromuscular control of the lower extremities via plyometric, strengthening, and proprioception exercises can prevent a variety of musculoskeletal injuries, including ACL injuries (Donnell-Fink et al., 2015; Emery & Pasanen, 2019). Most "off-season" conditioning programs at the secondary school level have several components in them. One is improvement of skill level of the individual, but the second and equally important component is increasing strength and flexibility in an attempt to minimize future injuries.

For all individuals, the components of fitness include cardiorespiratory (aerobic) fitness, muscular strength and endurance, flexibility, and body composition (Armstrong & McManus, 2017; Haskell, 2019). Athletes in any sport are well advised to develop a total conditioning program that addresses all these components and also nutrition. By doing so, the athlete benefits in two ways—improved performance and injury reduction. It is important to remember that a conditioning program consists of two primary components: general conditioning and sport-specific conditioning. The general conditioning program focuses on the major fitness components listed earlier in addition to *specificity* and *overload*. Specificity refers to specific adaptations that occur by performing activities that engage muscle groups and energy systems similar to competition activity. For example, a sprinter becomes a better sprinter by running at a high velocity over short distances (Powers & Howley, 2015, pp. 280, 477) and by the principle of overload, which refers to exercising at a level beyond what the individual is accustomed to. Progressively overloading a system or tissue will show improvements in performance over time (Powers & Howley, 2015, p. 280). Beyond this, sport-specific conditioning focuses on any aspect of a particular sport or activity that is unique to it. For example, the shoulder girdle and glenohumeral joint muscles in a tennis player need to receive special attention to avoid overuse injuries related to repetitive overhand strokes, which are inherent to the sport. To be effective, the conditioning program should allow for general conditioning and strength training on a year-round basis. This is best accomplished by incorporating the concept of **periodization** in the total conditioning program, which is the process of arranging training around specific goals and objectives with predetermined amounts of time spent training and resting. The purpose of periodization is to tailor the training program to meet the specific needs of an athlete to maximize performance at the time of competitions and avoid training-related injury (Haff, 2016, pp. 584–604). The process of periodization is discussed later in this chapter. Optimally, the program that an athlete is on to improve his or her strength and conditioning should be done by an individual who is certified by the National Strength and Conditioning Association (NSCA) as a **Certified Strength and Conditioning Specialist (CSCS)**.

Aerobic Fitness

Aerobic fitness, also commonly termed *aerobic power*, is defined as the amount of work that can be accomplished using the oxidative system of converting nutrients into energy. Aerobic power (VO_2 max) can be tested in the laboratory and is normally expressed in a formula that states the volume of oxygen consumed per unit of body weight per unit of time. The most common expression is in milliliters of oxygen per kilogram of body weight per minute (mL/kg/min^{-1}). A high VO_2 max is important for successful aerobic performance; however, other factors, such as good exercise economy (expend less energy at a given velocity), fuel substrate use (i.e., fat use vs. glucose use), muscle fiber type (i.e., Type I), and high lactate threshold, can also contribute to successful performance in aerobic events (Reuter & Dawes, 2016, p. 560). Continuous activities with durations in excess of a minute or longer rely on the

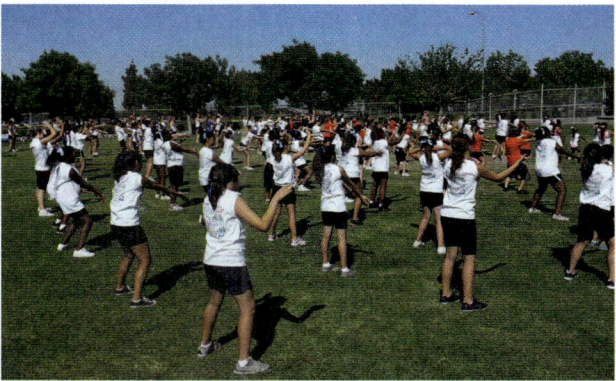

Figure 4.3 Summer camps and conditioning programs help athletes prepare for their upcoming season.
© Richard Thornton/Shutterstock.

aerobic energy system. However, athletes involved in short-duration, high-intensity anaerobic (energy production in the absence of oxygen) activities can benefit indirectly from having a high level of aerobic fitness. Poor physical fitness is a risk factor for sports-related injury in addition to having negative health consequences (Emery & Pasanen, 2019). It has been shown that aerobic fitness can assist in injury avoidance by preventing general fatigue, which decreases muscle strength, reaction time, and neuromuscular coordination (Emery & Pasanen, 2019).

In short, regardless of the sport, athletes who enter the season with a high level of aerobic fitness are less prone to injury. This is one of the main reasons coaches encourage athletes to participate in some type of preseason conditioning activities (Figure 4.3). Aerobic fitness can be enhanced by regular participation in activities such as running, bicycling, swimming,

---

Periodization The organization of training into a cyclical structure to attain the optimal development of an athlete's performance capacities.

Certified Strength and Conditioning Specialist (CSCS) Professional who trains athletes in order to improve athletic performance by using scientific knowledge of many disciplines such as exercise physiology to design testing and workout sessions, strength training and coordination programs, and provide nutrition and injury prevention guidance.

Aerobic fitness The amount of work that can be accomplished using the oxidative system of converting nutrients into energy. Also called aerobic power.

cross-country skiing, in-line skating, stairstepping, and aerobic dancing. However, any aerobic program needs to be tailored to the strengths, weaknesses, and needs of the individual athlete. As a general rule, training programs designed to improve aerobic fitness must overload the physiological system beyond what it is accustomed to at rest or low levels of activity (Reuter & Dawes, 2016, p. 560). Besides the mode or type of aerobic activity, four primary program design variables—training intensity, frequency, duration, and progression—are essential for success (Reuter & Dawes, 2016, p. 561).

Exercise mode refers to the specific activity being performed (e.g., running, swimming, or cycling). Individuals should select modes of exercise that closely mimic the movements of competition to create beneficial physiological adaptations (Reuter & Dawes, 2016, p. 562). **Training intensity** is the effort expended during a training session; it is most commonly assessed by heart rate or rate of perceived exertion (RPE), which is a 1–10 scale with 10 representing maximal effort. Percentages greater than 60% of maximal heart rate are most often used to elicit training adaptations (Powers & Howley, 2015, p. 360; Reuter & Dawes, 2016). **Training frequency** is the number of workouts per day or per week and will fluctuate depending on the season (i.e., preseason, in-season, off-season) or time period before a competition. **Training duration** is the time to complete a workout or exercise session. Training intensity, frequency, and duration have unique interactions and vary in relation to one another. In training periods when intensity is high, the frequency and duration are likely lower. Typically, athletes who are not participating in an aerobic sport should include some sort of aerobic training at least 3 days per week. **Exercise progression** involves gradually increasing the frequency, intensity, and/or duration to achieve set goals. A general rule is that frequency, intensity, and duration should not increase by more than 10% in 1 week (Reuter & Dawes, 2016, p. 566).

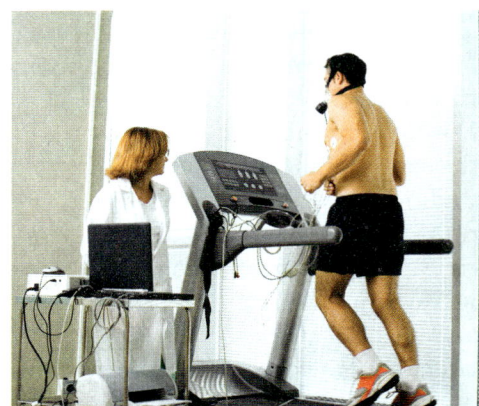

VO_2 max aerobic test for determining maximal aerobic power.
© IT Stock/Polka Dot/Getty Images.

Anaerobic Fitness

Anaerobic fitness is defined as the amount of work that can be accomplished using the creatine-phosphate or glycogen systems (nonoxidative) to produce energy. Anaerobic training typically consists of resistance training; plyometrics; speed; agility; and speed–endurance training, which is short in duration and high in intensity (Haff, 2016). Our focus in this chapter is on resistance training. It is widely accepted that muscle and connective tissues (i.e., fascia, tendons, and ligaments) undergo physiological and morphological changes and tissue becomes stronger as a result of resistive exercise (Haff, 2016, pp. 87–114). Furthermore, bone density increases and bone becomes less susceptible to both trauma and fractures related to overuse (French, 2016, pp. 98–99). Improved muscle strength has also been found to be helpful in reducing the chances of musculoskeletal injury because strengthening the muscles that surround a joint helps to protect the joint from injury. Improving the strength ratio between opposing muscle groups, such as hamstrings and quadriceps, continues to be a generally well-accepted technique for preventing injury (Sheppard & Triplett, 2016, p. 445).

Exercise mode Refers to the specific activity being performed (e.g., running, swimming, or cycling).

Training intensity The effort expended during an exercise session.

Training frequency The number of training sessions per week or day.

Training duration The length of time of the training session.

Exercise progression Involves gradually increasing the frequency, intensity, and/or duration of training to achieve set goals.

Anaerobic fitness The amount of work that can be accomplished using nonoxidative pathways to produce energy.

On a side note, special attention and education regarding youths and resistance exercise should occur before working with youth conditioning programs. Coaches and physical educators are encouraged to use the Youth Resistance Training position statement developed by the NSCA (Faigenbaum et al., 2009) when designing strength training programs for young athletes. Faigenbaum and colleagues (2009) reported that a properly designed and supervised resistance training program is relatively safe for youths and can improve muscular strength and power, cardiovascular risk profile, and motor skill performance. Additionally, it may contribute to enhanced sport performance of youths by increasing their resistance to sports-related injuries, improving psychosocial well-being, and helping to promote and develop exercise habits during childhood and adolescence. Recent scientific evidence has also dispelled the following myths: (a) strength training will stunt the growth of children, (b) children will experience bone growth plate damage as a result of strength training, and (c) children, specifically boys, cannot increase strength because they do not have enough testosterone (Lloyd & Faigenbaum, 2016, pp. 136–144).

Having a PPE before beginning a resistance training program is also recommended. Minimally, any youth with signs or symptoms suggestive of injury or disease or with known injury or disease should have a medical examination performed by his or her personal physician (Faigenbaum et al., 2009). Understanding the unique physical and psychosocial needs of children and adolescents is important in the instruction and supervision of resistance training programs. Coaches are encouraged to obtain additional training specific to youths through various resources offered by local and national youth sports coaching associations.

Muscle Strength, Power, and Endurance

Strength (resistance) or weight training refers to a systematic program of exercises designed to increase an individual's ability to exert or resist force (Kraemer et al., 2018). **Muscle strength** is defined as the maximum amount of force that can be produced in one repetition, often referred to as one-repetition maximum (1-RM). **Muscle power** is defined as "the time rate of performing work" and expressed in the following equation (McBride, 2016, p. 28; McGuigan, 2016, p. 260):

$$\text{Power} = \text{Force} \times \text{Velocity}$$

For most athletic applications, muscle power is much more important to performance than is pure strength because performance is most often time dependent. That is, to be effective, athletes need to be quicker and more explosive in their performance. **Muscle endurance**, in contrast to strength, is defined as the ability to sustain a muscle activity. Muscle strength, power, and endurance are typically improved with some form of resistance training. Each of these muscle attributes requires distinctly different types of training and must be based on a needs analysis or assessment of an individual (Sheppard & Triplett, 2016). Effective training is achieved by manipulation of the training volume, training intensity, training frequency, frequency and duration of rest (recovery) periods, exercise selection, and exercise order (Sheppard & Triplett, 2016, p. 465).

Training volume can be calculated by repetition volume or load volume. **Repetition volume** represents the number of repetitions the weight is lifted; it is calculated by multiplying the number of sets by the number of repetitions to calculate the total number of repetitions. However, another volume term may be more important: load volume. **Load volume** is defined as the total amount of weight lifted in a given workout session. The calculation includes the amount of weight lifted in addition to the repetitions and the sets (Sheppard & Triplett, 2016). The load volume for an exercise of three sets of 10 repetitions (reps) using a progressively increasing weight value of 175, 185, and 195 pounds would be calculated by multiplying the

---

Muscle strength The maximal amount of force that can be generated by muscles.

Muscle power The ability to generate force as quickly as possible, or a rate of work.

Muscle endurance The ability to sustain repeated contractions against a submaximal load.

Training volume The amount of work performed during a training session or period of time (i.e., number of repetitions multiplied by the amount of weight used, number of miles).

Repetition volume The number of repetitions a weight is lifted.

Load volume The total amount of weight lifted in a given workout session.

total number of sets and repetitions by the amount of weight lifted in each set. Therefore, the first set would have 175 pounds × 10 reps = 1,750 units; the second set, 185 pounds × 10 reps = 1,850 units; and the third set, 195 pounds × 10 reps = 1,950 units, for a total training volume of 1,750 + 1,850 + 1,950 = 5,550 units (Sheppard & Triplett, 2016, p. 451). To calculate the average weight lifted per repetition per workout session, divide the load volume by the repetition volume. As a general rule, the average weight will represent quality of work performed in the training session. The higher the average weight is in a given workout, the higher the true intensity is for the total workout (Sheppard & Triplett, 2016, p. 451).

Training intensity for an exercise in a resistance training session is most often defined as the amount of weight lifted per repetition; thus, a lift of 50 pounds for 10 reps (5 intensity units) would be one-half the intensity of a lift of 100 pounds for 10 reps (10 intensity units). Typically, intensity is represented as a percentage of the maximum amount of weight an athlete can lift only one time (1-RM). The number of times (training volume) an exercise can be performed is inversely related to the load lifted. Sets completed with heavy loads will have fewer repetitions, and sets completed with lighter loads will have more repetitions (Sheppard & Triplett, 2016). It is the training goal that dictates the training intensity. When the goal is primarily strength, the training intensity is usually ≥ 85% 1-RM, and, when the goal is primarily endurance, the training intensity is usually ≤ 65% 1-RM (Sheppard & Triplett, 2016). Therefore, athletes training for more muscle strength will use heavier loads and fewer repetitions (~6–12), whereas athletes training for more muscular endurance will use lighter loads and more repetitions (≥ 12). Another way to define training intensity is in terms of velocity of movement; that is, the faster the repetition is performed, the higher the intensity is (Sheppard & Triplett, 2016). Exercises performed at high speeds are commonly known as muscular power exercises. Explosive power training should be performed only under the guidance of someone with expertise in program design because inappropriate forms of explosive power training can result in injury.

Training frequency is the number of training sessions completed in a given period of time (Sheppard & Triplett, 2016). The most common way to express frequency is by recording the number of workouts per week or, in some cases, number of workouts per day. A number of factors must be considered when determining the training frequency. These considerations include the training goal and current fitness status of the athlete, the training volume and intensity, and the specific types of exercises planned (Sheppard & Triplett, 2016). As a general rule, most strength training programs incorporate between three and five workouts per week. As programs become more sophisticated and complex, frequency can be increased; however, such programs usually divide the training into segments, such as legs, trunk, or arms, so that each area is developed in separate workouts throughout the week. It is critical to remember that, physiologically, there are limits on how quickly muscle tissue can adapt to a given workout. In general, moderate- to high-intensity training requires 24 to 48 hours for full recovery to occur. The amount of time allowed for the body or specific muscle group to recover between training sessions is as important as the frequency of training sessions used in an athlete's program. Failure to consider these physiological adaptations may result in overuse injuries related to the training program.

Rest periods are usually specific to the amount of time allowed between sets in a given training session. However, rest can be used in a broader sense to describe the recovery between training days. The rest period allowed between sets of lifts in a given training session can, to a great extent, determine the specific effects of that session. For example, when the goal of the training session is absolute strength or muscle power, the training intensity will be high; therefore, the rest period between sets should be relatively long, for example, 2 to 5 minutes (Sheppard & Triplett, 2016). Conversely, when training for muscle endurance, the rest periods between sets can be shorter, sometimes as short as 15 to 30 seconds. Another way is to use a work-to-rest ratio to help calculate rest periods between sets. A work-to-rest ratio determines the amount of time a person works and rests. For example, a 1:1 ratio means that a person works and rests for the same

---

Rest periods Usually specific to the amount of time allowed between sets in a given training session; can be used in a broader sense to describe the recovery between training days.

amount of time; a 1:3 ratio can be accomplished by doing 15 seconds of work followed by 45 seconds of rest. Because strength exercises are usually done for fewer repetitions with near maximal loads, athletes need longer rest for muscle regeneration, so the work-to-rest ratio is usually 1:5–1:12. For muscle endurance exercises with light loads for many repetitions, the rest period is approximately less than 30 seconds, and the work-to-rest ratio is usually 1:1–1:3 (Sheppard & Triplett, 2016, pp. 465–467).

Exercise selection is defined as choosing a resistance training exercise based on the movement and the muscular requirements of the sport. It is also based on an athlete's experience, available equipment, and amount of time available for training (Sheppard & Triplett, 2016). Exercises typically fall into two categories—core/structural and assistance. Core exercises are focused on the larger muscle group areas (i.e., hip, back, chest, and shoulder), and assistance exercises are focused on smaller muscle groups (i.e., upper arm, calves/shins, and abdominals). Core exercises are usually multijoint exercises, and assistance exercises are usually single-joint exercises that isolate a specific muscle or muscle group. When planning a training session, core exercises take priority and should be done when an athlete is not fatigued (Sheppard & Triplett, 2016). Muscle balance must also be maintained within a program; therefore, both agonists and antagonists should be trained in relative proportion based on sport demand (Sheppard & Triplett, 2016, p. 445).

Exercise order refers to the sequence of the resistance training exercises within one training session (Sheppard & Triplett, 2016). Adaptation of muscles requires overload; however, fatigue of muscle groups too early in a resistance training session can hamper an athlete's ability to produce maximal force throughout the workout. There are several common methods for ordering resistance exercises in a training session—alternating upper and lower body exercises, performing multijoint before single-joint exercises, alternating push and pull exercises, or performing pairs of exercises among agonists or agonist/antagonist groups (Sheppard & Triplett, 2016, pp. 448–450).

Flexibility

Flexibility is a measure of the ROM of a joint or combination of joints (Jeffreys, 2016). Flexibility has both static and dynamic components. Static flexibility is the ROM of a joint and its surrounding muscles as a result of passive (nonvoluntary) movement; it is achieved by the manipulation of a joint by another person while the muscles are relaxed. Dynamic flexibility requires voluntary muscle activity and refers to the ROM during active motions; it is typically greater than static flexibility (Jeffreys, 2016). Several factors determine the ROM of a given joint—age; sex; bone structure; tissue mass surrounding the joint; and extensibility of tendons, ligaments, muscles, and skin surrounding the joint. In general, flexibility decreases with age, although maintaining an active lifestyle may greatly reduce such changes. In addition, females have been found to be more flexible than their male counterparts. The temperature of the tissue, which is mediated by metabolism, local blood flow, and external (ambient) temperature, can also significantly affect joint ROM. Warm-up exercises that increase heart rate above resting levels have been found to be effective in increasing tissue temperatures temporarily (Jeffreys, 2016, pp. 318–320).

Static and dynamic stretching have been demonstrated to improve ROM at targeted joints; however,

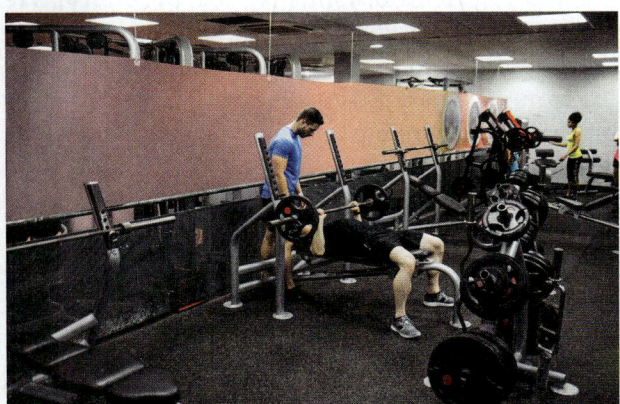

Developing muscle strength and endurance is critical to injury prevention.
© wavebreakmedia/Shutterstock.

> **Exercise selection** Choosing a training exercise based on the movement and the muscular requirements of the sport.
>
> **Exercise order** Specific order in which exercises should be performed within a session.
>
> **Flexibility** The range of motion in a given joint or combination of joints.

it takes significant amounts of time to create permanent or plastic changes in muscle and surrounding connective tissue (McHugh & Cosgrave, 2010). Elastic, or nonpermanent, changes in ROM are evident after both static and dynamic stretching protocols, but these changes are time limited; the tissue will return to its normal resting length soon after the activity is discontinued (McHugh & Cosgrave, 2010). Therefore, stretching protocols can be valuable in improving ROM right after their application, but there is limited evidence that the application of brief stretching bouts prior to activity can actually improve ROM over the long term. Therefore, controversy exists among coaches, physical educators, and fitness professionals as to the effectiveness of stretching in reducing injury. However, a scientific review of research on the effectiveness of stretching on injury prevention by Jamtvedt and colleagues (2010) demonstrated that stretching before and after physical activity does not appreciably reduce all-injury risk but seems to reduce the risk of some injuries to muscles, ligaments, and tendons. The evidence suggested that long-duration (12-week) stretching programs were more likely to reduce the chance of injury than any other application. Stretching activities were also determined to reduce the risk of bothersome soreness (Jamtvedt et al., 2010) when compared to exercisers who did not stretch as a part of their activity plan. Therefore, stretching activities before and after sports participation should be continued; however, its limitations in preventing all sports injury must be understood.

Stretching exercises can be grouped into four categories based on the method employed. **Ballistic stretching** involves powerful contractions of muscles to force a joint to a greater ROM. A typical example is what is commonly called a standing toe touch; the athlete bends over and makes an effort to force the hands down to touch his or her toes. The athlete typically repeatedly extends the trunk back up and then forcefully bends downward again (i.e., bouncing) to get the hands closer to the feet. The muscles presumably being targeted in this stretch are the hamstrings as well as the trunk extensors (erector spinae). Ballistic stretching is not recommended because it triggers a muscle protective mechanism that defeats the purpose of stretching (Jeffreys, 2016; Shrier, 2018). **Static stretching**, as the name implies, involves moving a joint to a position where tension can be felt in the target muscles being stretched, with the position being sustained (held) for a time period ranging from 30 seconds up to a minute or longer (Jeffreys, 2016). The length of time one should hold a static stretch has often been debated; however, static stretches need to be held at least 30 seconds for tissue length to appreciably change (McHugh & Cosgrave, 2010; Shrier, 2018). Static stretching can be done passively by having another person move the athlete's limbs or actively by the athlete moving their own limbs to a stretched position. **Dynamic stretching** involves mobility drills and places an emphasis on the sport activity that will be performed. Drills are used to mimic sport movements that an athlete may experience during participation and include taking joints through controlled full ROM activities designed to prepare the body for the activity to come (Jeffreys, 2016). Examples include knee lifts, marching drills, arm swings, and torso twists. The key difference between dynamic and ballistic stretching is that there is no bouncing and full ROM of joints is used. **Proprioceptive neuromuscular facilitation (PNF)** involves a technique originally developed for use with patients suffering from paralysis. Essentially, PNF uses the body's proprioceptive system to stimulate muscles to relax. A variety of manual techniques have been developed, all using PNF principles. To use PNF techniques effectively, specialized training is required. However, basic PNF techniques for muscles that commonly benefit from stretching, such as the hamstrings, can be taught to nonmedical professionals and executed effectively by teammates during the warm-up before practice or competitions.

Research comparing these techniques continues to produce varied results as to the effectiveness of the different stretching techniques on improving ROM and not affecting subsequent performance. Static

Ballistic stretching Stretching technique that uses quick, sudden, and repetitive bouncing motions.

Static stretching Passively stretching a muscle by placing it in a maximal lengthened position and holding it there for extended periods of time (anywhere from 10 to 60 seconds or longer).

Dynamic stretching A voluntary stretching technique that uses full-range, sport-like motions to warm up.

Proprioceptive neuromuscular facilitation (PNF) Stretching techniques that involve combinations of alternating contractions and stretches.

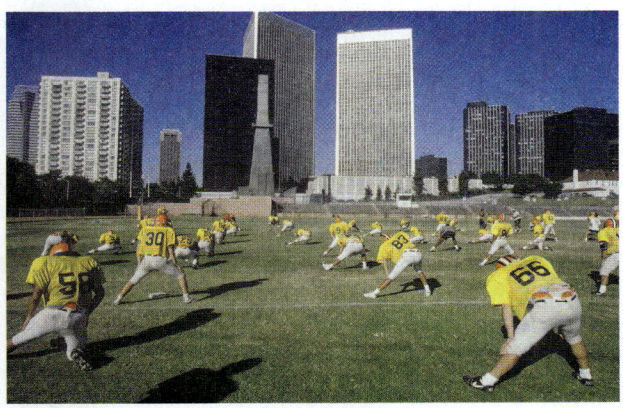

Figure 4.4 Stretching before an activity has been shown to increase range of motion at a given joint.
© Joseph Sohm/Shutterstock.

stretching is probably the most effective for improving ROM and achieving permanent changes in flexibility (Figure 4.4). It should be performed for overall fitness and wellness independent of other training workouts or at the end of a workout when the tissues are warmer as a result of increased blood flow (Shrier, 2018). Dynamic stretching is likely the most effective for performance when performed after a submaximal aerobic activity warm-up and before a workout that involves strength, high-speed, explosive, or reactive activities (Shrier, 2018). Ballistic stretching is considered the least effective method and may even result in injury.

Body Composition

The dietary habits and body composition of any athlete, regardless of the sport, have a profound influence on overall performance and recovery from injury. Maintaining a healthy composition between lean mass (i.e., bones, muscles, and organs) and fat mass is essential for optimal performance. Nutrition plays an important role in maintaining appropriate body compositions for age, sex, and sport. The body responds to a conditioning program in a more positive manner when adequate amounts of essential nutrients are consumed in the daily diet. Two conditions on opposite spectrums of the body composition scales are affecting young sport participants in today's society. Many boys and girls are reporting to school-sponsored sports with body compositions over the recommended level for healthy maturation. There are also groups of young athletes who are exposed to an overemphasis on leanness, especially in performance sports such as gymnastics, diving, and weight lifting. General statistics indicate that 1 in 5 children and adolescents in the United States experience obesity (CDC, 2021) and the occurrence of disordered eating and body dysmorphia in an attempt to control body size has also increased in both boys and girls over the last decade due to the increase in social media (Marks et al., 2020).

Periodization

As mentioned earlier in this chapter, a conditioning program should be designed to develop all fitness components to an optimal level while also allowing adequate intervals for rest and recovery. The periodization model includes several components that represent increasingly smaller units of training time. The largest unit is known as a **macrocycle** and typically encompasses 1 calendar year. The macrocycle can then be divided into smaller units known as **mesocycles**, which last from several weeks to a month or more, depending on the number of competitive seasons in the macrocycle. The components of a macrocycle are determined by the number of competitive seasons contained in a given calendar year. For an athlete who competes in one sport per year with one competitive season, the macrocycle typically includes postseason, off-season, preseason, and in-season components. Conversely, for an athlete with more than one competition season in the same calendar year, there may be two or more groups of training cycles composed of an off-season, a preseason, and an in-season. This would be a model for the college-level football player who has two seasons each year, like spring ball and the regular season.

The smallest component is called a **microcycle** and consists of 2 to 4 weeks of training with fluctuations in intensity, duration, and frequency (Haff, 2016). A mesocycle consists of several successive microcycles leading to a specific conditioning goal,

> **Macrocycle** The largest unit of time (i.e., 1 year) when planning exercise to achieve a particular goal.
>
> **Mesocycle** Smaller units of time in a macrocycle (i.e., weeks to months).
>
> **Microcycle** Smallest units of time in a macrocycle (i.e., 2–4 weeks).

for example, **hypertrophy** of leg muscles. A **transition phase** is a period of 2 to 4 weeks that occurs between training seasons or between successive mesocycles. During a transition phase, training is adjusted gradually either to bring an athlete to peak fitness or to allow the athlete to rest and recover after the competitive season. In short, the function of the transition phase is to give the body time to recover from the previous cycle to be ready for the next segment of the training season.

Periodized programs that include a goal of developing muscle power have a preparatory period, normally placed in the off-season portion of the training year, which progresses the athlete through three phases: hypertrophy/endurance, strength, and power. The rationale for this progression is based on sound science of muscle physiology. The purpose of the hypertrophy/endurance phase is to strengthen the connective tissue surrounding the muscle fibers and the tendons attaching the muscles to bones. This development of connective tissue enables the athlete to progress safely to the higher-intensity training that follows without risking training-related injury. The intensity levels in the hypertrophy/endurance phase are generally low with higher volumes, which equates to more repetitions completed per session with a smaller percentage of the 1-RM weight for each exercise. The strength phase is next and represents a significant change in both the objectives and the protocol. The objective of this phase is obviously to increase the strength of the involved muscle groups. The exercise intensity levels are increased progressively to as high as 80% of 1-RM for each exercise. Conversely, volume is decreased to several sets of 5-RM to 8-RM levels (five to eight repetitions per set; Haff, 2016). The final phase, known as the power phase, focuses on the development of higher-velocity movements. By definition, the intensity during the power phase is very high, often as high as 90% of 1-RM for each exercise with lower training volumes.

A typical application of periodization for a two-season-per-year athlete can be illustrated with a collegiate-level football lineman preparing for the spring football season. During the preseason phase, he may spend the first 3 weeks working on muscle strength and hypertrophy (microcycle), followed by 3 weeks of high-intensity, low-volume strength training to develop muscle power (microcycle). These two microcycles constitute a mesocycle with the goal of improving lower extremity power. A transition phase is then inserted just prior to the onset of the competitive season. During the spring season, the player reduces his weekly frequency of weight training to maintain the gains achieved during the preseason phase. This player would have a similar program established for his preparation for the regular season as well, and it would build on the gains made in the program just described (Haff, 2016).

Sport-Specific Injury Prevention Considerations

In addition to proper training and conditioning specific to a sport, injury prevention considerations should be incorporated to ensure safety. First, there are several recommendations and guidelines that organizations publish to assist in injury prevention beyond the PPE and physical conditioning. Additionally, being prepared in the event of an emergency is another way to prevent an injury/illness from becoming worse. Lastly, once an injury occurs, common return-to-play criteria need to be met before an athlete can resume full activities.

Overuse Injuries

In today's society, there are an increasing number of athletes who do not simply play the sport that is in season but rather specialize in one sport and do so at an early age. Once the athlete makes the decision to specialize in one sport, he or she then plays only that sport and may do so on a year-round or almost year-round basis. The perceived benefit of playing only one sport and doing so year-round is that the individual will improve the skills needed for that sport at a higher rate than that of their peers. Often, the individual or his or her parents imagine that a collegiate scholarship or lucrative professional career is on the line and the best way to reach that goal is to play only one sport and do so regardless of the time of year and whether the sport is in season.

The benefit of playing only one sport is increased skill development at a higher rate than that of their peer group. The drawbacks of playing only one sport and doing so year-round are many (**Figure 4.5**). Athletes

---

Hypertrophy Enlargement of a body part caused by an increase in the size of its cells.

Transition phase 2–4 weeks of adjusted exercise to bring an athlete to peak performance or the next phase of the plan.

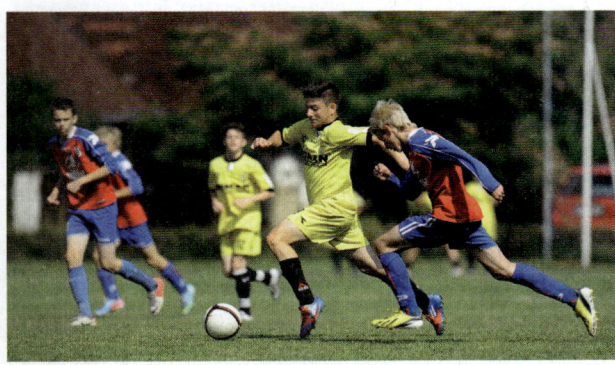

Figure 4.5 Early sport specialization may have more drawbacks than benefits.
© muzsy/Shutterstock.

who specialize early on in their athletic careers run the risk of overuse injuries because they do not use different muscle groups on a regular basis but rather use the same muscle groups repeatedly without rest or change. Recent research indicates that parents are concerned about the risk of injury, especially overuse injuries, and they do consider sport specialization a potential problem, but parents do not know the specific recommendations associated with youth sport participation (Bell et al., 2018).

An overuse injury is defined as "an injury that occurs due to repetitive submaximal loading of the musculoskeletal system when rest is not adequate to allow for structural adaptation to take place" (DiFiori et al., 2014, p. 7). Oftentimes, once a student specializes in one sport, there is little to no differentiation from the practice and training schedules of the younger, less-skilled athlete than that of the higher-level elite athlete. It should also be noted that specialization at a younger age may not let athletes determine which sport is actually their favorite or one that their skill set is best suited for as they mature (Goodway & Robinson, 2015) and it may lead to unnecessary sport injuries (DiFiori et al., 2014). Overuse injuries include, but are not limited to, tendinitis, stress fractures, and ligament tears. Another possible result of early specialization is emotional burnout (DiFiori et al., 2014). A simple definition of burnout is continued and repetitive emotional stress that leads to the athlete's ceasing participation in his or her sport which was previously enjoyable (DiFiori et al., 2014). Noted sports medicine orthopedist, James Andrews, MD, developed the STOP sports injuries initiative in an attempt to decrease the number of overuse injuries that are suffered by younger and younger participants (https://www.stopsportsinjuries.org/). Dr. Andrews stated on the Andrews Institute for Orthopaedic & Sports Medicine website, "I have seen my patient population and surgical cases get increasingly younger. Children, parents and coaches need to realize that kids need to take a break from playing one sport year round. Sports should be fun for children. Overuse injuries in children is a concerning trend." (Andrews, 2019, front page).

Guidelines

Several organizations publish guidelines, position statements, consensus statements, and public infographics to assist individuals with safely planning and carrying out exercise and sports activities. Providing the details of the guidelines of the many professional organizations that discuss prevention strategies is beyond the scope of this chapter. However, one of the major organizations to make exercise recommendations is the ACSM. All current position stands and joint position statements are available online free to the public at www.acsm.org/acsm-positions-policy. There, you will find the most current exercise recommendations incorporating specifics on intensity, duration, and other important exercise considerations for several populations, including younger and older individuals.

Another organization to provide guidelines is the NATA. Free access to its position statements and consensus statements can be found at www.nata.org/news-publications/pressroom/statements. These documents provide in-depth details for athletic trainers, coaches, and administrators to properly prepare for sports activities. Specifically, there are statements concerning many aspects of prevention, such as PPE, lightning, sudden death, heat acclimatization and illness, pediatric overuse injuries, eating disorders, football tackling techniques, sickle cell trait, and best practices for managing health care in the athletic setting.

Some examples of guidelines set forth by various organizations are briefly described here. The first example is baseball pitch count recommendations for pitchers of all ages. If a well-conditioned baseball pitcher exceeds his or her training preparations by pitching too much (higher volume), too soon (not enough time to build up to volume or intensity), or too intense during an outing or over the course of many days or weeks in games/tournaments/practices, injury may result (American Sports Medicine Institute, 2013; Valovich McLeod et al., 2011). Likewise, in the sport of wrestling, weight class guidelines and rules have been established to keep wrestlers safely competing at appropriate weight classes (Stanzione & Volpe, 2019; Turocy et al., 2011). Last but not least, football acclimatization guidelines and rules have been established to keep players safely participating in the heat and humidity, especially during preseason practices (Hosokawa et al., 2021). These are just a few examples of sports-specific injury prevention considerations.

Emergency Action Plan

An emergency action plan (EAP) is a well-thought-out strategy for handling emergency situations, such as asthma attacks, head injuries, heat-related illnesses, cardiac emergencies, and other catastrophic injuries. The purpose of an EAP is to ensure the best care is provided in a timely manner in the event of an emergency. A written document as to how emergency situations will be handled at each venue with specific equipment needed, routes of transport, and the responsibilities of each person, including local EMS personnel and their contact information, should be included in this document. Not only does it serve as a legal document, but it also should be reviewed once per year with all involved personnel and offer first aid and CPR training for those in need (Courson et al., 2014; NATA, n.d., pp. 38–45).

Return-to-Play Criteria

Once an athlete or physically active individual is injured, he or she should allow time for healing and recovery usually with assistance from a rehabilitation program that safely restores his or her function. An individual will most likely be very eager to resume his or her activities before it is safe to do so. Return-to-play (RTP) or return-to-activity (RTA) criteria formalize the athletic requirements needed to safely return to a sport or activity; however, criteria are rarely general and often are specific to the injury (Ardern et al., 2016). The decision for a return to sport or activity also must be made in a collaborative manner between the athlete, clinicians, and coaches (Ardern et al., 2016). For example, an individual may have regained full concentric (muscle-shortening) strength but may still lack eccentric (muscle-lengthening) strength, which may put the individual at risk for reinjury if he or she were to return to his or her sport. Most orthopedic injuries have functional criteria an injured person needs to meet in order to return to activity. For example, a person who has torn his or her ACL should demonstrate he or she has at minimum 80% functional performance and control with the injured limb compared to the uninjured limb with field tests, such as single-leg hopping, balance tests, and change-of-direction tasks (Kaplan & Witvrouw, 2019). Additionally, mental state should be considered when determining RTP because a poor perception of function can cause exaggerated caution on the field or court, which may lead to further injury (Kaminski et al., 2013). Ultimately, guidelines are constantly being updated, and readers are encouraged to seek out the most up-to-date evidence. For example, there are unique RTP criteria associated with concussions (Berry et al., 2019), exertional heat illness (Gauer & Meyers, 2019), and COVID-19 infection (Dores & Cardim, 2020).

WHAT IF ?

One of your cross-country runners, who suffers from chronic hamstring tightness, comes to you for advice on how to improve flexibility. What would you advise?

Athletic Trainers SPEAK OUT

What are the best ways to prevent injuries for professional athletes?

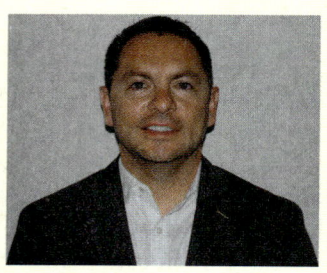

Courtesy of Matthew Lucero.

Catching an injury before it completely presents itself can be a very tricky obstacle for an athletic trainer. In the professional setting it is crucial that we take every step possible and explore all avenues to keep our players on the field giving us the best chance to win each night.

There are many variables involved in heading off a potential injury and recognizing injury risk. Knowing your athlete and getting them to have trust and confidence in you may be the most important factor. Daily communication with our players is a must in gathering all necessary information on how a player feels. This is similar to taking a good history on a chronic injury. We also rely on several other tools to supplement what the player communicates to us.

We do preseason and in-season upper body, lower body, and trunk /core measurements (range of motion and strength). This allows us to document any changes that might be occurring during the season that our players often do not recognize. We also receive daily handouts from our analytics department with measurements that indicate what each position player did the previous day as well as the week's workload. This allows us to discuss with our strength coaches the amount of work a player should do in the weight room as well as make recommendations to coaches in regards taking days off games.

With the information we have we implement a plan that can include several maintenance (preventative) techniques including modalities, various soft tissue massage techniques, flexibility programs, and customized position-specific strengthening programs. Since we are one of the few sports that play games daily we constantly pay particular attention to recovery tools, including compression pants, electrical stimulation, contrast baths, and cryo-sauna.

Athletic trainers are excellent resources for education, and the ultimate lessons you can teach your athletes are independent techniques on how to keep their body balanced in both strength and flexibility as well as a daily routine of dynamic warm-ups. These are tools that they can take with them for a lifetime of good health.

—Matthew Lucero, ATC, LAT

Matt Lucero is the Head Athletic Trainer for Texas Rangers MLB Baseball in Arlington, Texas.

Review Questions

1. Differentiate between intrinsic and extrinsic types of causative factors leading to sports injuries. Provide several examples of both types.
2. List four types of intrinsic factors related to sports injuries that a medical doctor might identify during a preparticipation physical examination.
3. What are two disadvantages to using an individual format for a preparticipation physical examination?
4. List the components of fitness as described in the chapter.
5. Briefly describe the relationship between volume, intensity, and frequency of training as they relate to periodization.
6. Describe how exercise order and selection can influence the outcomes of resistance training programs.
7. Define the terms *macrocycle, mesocycle*, and *microcycle* as they relate to sports training programs.
8. True or false: According to the chapter, athletes, regardless of their sport, can benefit from possessing a relatively high level of aerobic fitness.
9. What is the meaning of the acronym ROM?
10. Discuss the advantages and disadvantages of the major categories of stretching exercises.
11. Why is it important to take a thorough and accurate medical history when a preparticipation physical examination is performed?
12. What could be a negative result of early sport specialization?

References

Alentorn-Geli, E., Mendiguchia, J., Samuelsson, K., Musahl, V., Karsson, J., Cugat, R., & Myer, G. (2014). Prevention of anterior cruciate ligament injuries in sports—Part 1: Systematic review of risk factors in male athletes. *Knee Surgery, Sports Traumatology, Arthroscopy, 22*(1), 3–15.

American Sports Medicine Institute. (2013). Position statement for youth baseball pitchers. Retrieved from http://www.asmi.org/research.php?page=research&section=positionStatement

Andrews, J. R. (2019). Andrews Institute teams up with community to STOP sports injuries. *Andrews Institute for Orthopaedics & Sports Medicine.* Retrieved from http://www.andrewsinstitute.com/InjuryPrevention/STOPSportsInjuries.aspx

Ardern, C. L., Glasgow, P., Schneiders, A., Witvrouw, E., Clarsen, B., Cools, A., ... & Bizzini, M. (2016). 2016 consensus statement on return to sport from the First World

Congress in Sports Physical Therapy, Bern. *British Journal of Sports Medicine, 50*(14), 853–864.

Armstrong, N., & McManus, A. M. (2017). Development of the young athlete. In N. Armstrong & W. Van Mechelen (Eds.), *Oxford textbook of children's sport and exercise medicine* (pp. 413–424). New York, NY: Oxford University Press.

Badgeley, M. A., McIlvain, N. M., Yard, E. E., Fields, S. K., & Comstock, R. D. (2013). Epidemiology of 10,000 high school football injuries: Patterns of injury by position played. *Journal of Physical Activity and Health, 10*(2), 160–169.

Bayer, S., Meredith, S. J., Wilson, K. W., Pauyo, T., Byrne, K., McDonough, C. M., & Musahl, V. (2020). Knee morphological risk factors for anterior cruciate ligament injury: A systematic review. *Journal of Bone and Joint Surgery, 102*(8), 703–718.

Bell, D. R., Post, E. G., Trigsted, S. M., Schaefer, D. A., McGuine, T. A., & Brooks, M. A. (2018). Parents' awareness and perceptions of sport specialization and injury prevention recommendations. *Clinical Journal of Sport Medicine: Official Journal of the Canadian Academy of Sport Medicine, 30*(6), 539–543.

Berry, J. A., Wacker, M., Menoni, R., Zampella, B., Majeed, G., Kashyap, S., ... & Miulli, D. (2019). Return-to-play after concussion: Clinical guidelines for young athletes. *Journal of Osteopathic Medicine, 119*(12), 833–838.

Brandt, A., & O'Keefe, C. (2019). Integration of 12-lead electrocardiograms into preparticipation screenings to prevent sudden cardiac death in high school athletes. *Journal of Pediatric Health Care, 33*(2), 153–161.

Cappaert, T. A., Stone, J. A., Castellani, J. W., Krause, B. A., Smith, D., & Stephens, B. A. (2008). National Athletic Trainers' Association position statement: Environmental cold injuries. *Journal of Athletic Training, 43*(6), 640–658.

Casa, D. J., DeMartini, J. K., Bergeron, M. F., Csillan, D., Eichner, E. R., Lopez, R. M., . . . Yeargin, S. W. (2015). National Athletic Trainers' Association position statement: Exertional heat illnesses. *Journal of Athletic Training, 50*(9), 986–1000.

Caswell, S. V., Cortes, N., Chabolla, M., Ambegaonkar, J. P., Caswell, A. M., & Brenner, J. S. (2015). State-specific differences in school sports preparticipation physical examination policies. *Pediatrics, 125*(1), 26–32.

Centers for Disease Control and Prevention (CDC). (2017). Youth physical activity guidelines toolkit. Retrieved from https://www.cdc.gov/healthyschools/physicalactivity/guidelines_backup.htm

Centers for Disease Control and Prevention (CDC). (2021). Childhood overweight & obesity. Retrieved from https://www.cdc.gov/obesity/childhood/

Champagne, A. A., DiStefano, V., Boulanger, M., Magee, B., Coverdale, N. S., Gallucci, D., ... & Cook, D. J. (2019). Data-informed intervention improves football technique and reduces head impacts. *Medicine and Science in Sports and Exercise, 51*(11), 2366.

Conley, K. M., Bolin, D. J., Carek, P. J., Konin, J. G., Neal, T. L., & Violette, D. (2014). National Athletic Trainers' Association position statement: Preparticipation physical examinations and disqualifying conditions. *Journal of Athletic Training, 49*(1), 102–120.

Courson, R., Goldenberg, M., Adams, K. G., Anderson, S. C., Colgate, B., Cooper, L., ... Turbak, G. (2014). Inter-association consensus statement on best practices for sports medicine management for secondary schools and colleges. *Journal of Athletic Training, 49*(1), 128–137. Retrieved from http://natajournals.org/doi/pdf/10.4085/1062-6050-49.1.06

DiFiori, J. P., Benjamin, H. J., Brenner, J., Gregory, A., Jayanthi, N., Landry, G., & Luke, A. (2014). Overuse injuries and burnout in youth sports: A position statement from the American Medical Society for Sports Medicine. *Clinical Journal of Sport Medicine, 24*(1), 3–20.

Donnell-Fink, L. A., Klara, K., Collins, J. E., Yang, H. Y., Goczalk, M. G., Katz, J. N., & Losina, E. (2015). Effectiveness of knee injury and anterior cruciate ligament tear prevention programs: A meta-analysis. *PLOS ONE, 10*(12), 1–17.

Dores, H., & Cardim, N. (2020). Return to play after COVID-19: A sport cardiologist's view. *British Journal of Sports Medicine, 54*(19), 1132–1133.

Douglas, W., & Siddiqi, A. R. (2021). Preparticipation evaluation. In G. Miranda-Comas, G. Cooper, J. Herrera, & S. Curtis (Eds.), *Essential sports medicine* (pp. 45–73). New York, NY: Springer, Cham.

Drezner, J. A., O'Connor, F. G., Harmon, K. G., Fields, K. B., Asplund, C. A., Asif, I. M., ... & Roberts, W. O. (2017). AMSSM position statement on cardiovascular preparticipation screening in athletes: Current evidence, knowledge gaps, recommendations, and future directions. *British Journal of Sports Medicine, 51*(3), 153–167.

Drezner, J. A., Peterson, D. F., Siebert, D. M., Thomas, L. C., Lopez-Anderson, M., Suchsland, M. Z., ... & Kucera, K. L. (2019). Survival after exercise-related sudden cardiac arrest in young athletes: Can we do better? *Sports Health, 11*(1), 91–98.

Emery, C. A., & Pasanen, K. (2019). Current trends in sport injury prevention. *Best Practice & Research Clinical Rheumatology, 33*(1), 3–15.

Evans, A. E., Curtis, M., & Beidler, E. (2020). Behavioral tackling interventions decrease head impact frequency in American football players: A critically appraised topic. *International Journal of Athletic Therapy and Training, 26*(2), 89–95.

Faigenbaum, A. D., Kraemer, W. J., Blimkie, C. J., Jeffreys, I., Micheli, L. J., Nitka, M., Rowland, T. W. (2009). Youth resistance training: Updated position statement paper from the National Strength and Conditioning Association. *Journal of Strength and Conditioning Research, 23*(5 Suppl), S60–S79.

French, D. (2016). Adaptations to anaerobic training programs. In G. G. Haff & N. T. Triplett (Eds.), *Essentials of strength training and conditioning* (4th ed., pp. 87–114). Champaign, IL: Human Kinetics.

Gauer, R., & Meyers, B. K. (2019). Heat-related illnesses. *American Family Physician, 99*(8), 482–489.

Goodway, J. D., & Robinson, L. E. (2015). Developmental trajectories in early sport specialization: A case for early sampling from a physical growth and motor development perspective. *Kinesiology Review, 4*(3), 267–278.

Haff, G. G. (2016). Periodization. In G. G. Haff & N. T. Triplett (Eds.), *Essentials of strength training and conditioning* (4th ed., pp. 583–604). Champaign, IL: Human Kinetics.

Haskell, W. L. (2019). Guidelines for physical activity and health in the United States: Evolution over 50 years. *ACSM's Health & Fitness Journal, 23*(5), 5–8.

Hills, A. P., Dengel, D. R., & Lubans, D. R. (2015). Supporting public health priorities: Recommendations for physical education and physical activity promotion in schools. *Progress in Cardiovascular Diseases, 57*(4), 368–374.

Hjelm, N., Werner, S., & Renstrom, P. (2012). Injury risk factors in junior tennis players: A prospective 2-year study. *Scandinavian Journal of Medicine & Science in Sports, 22*(1), 40–48.

Hosokawa, Y., Adams, W. M., Casa, D. J., Vanos, J. K., Cooper, E. R., Grundstein, A. J., ... & Tripp, B. L. (2021). Roundtable on preseason heat safety in secondary school athletics: Environmental monitoring during activities in the heat. *Journal of Athletic Training, 56*(4), 362–371.

Huggins, R. A., Attanasio, S. M., Endres, B. D., Coleman, K. A., Casa, D. J. (2018, July 24). Athletic Training Locations and Services (ATLAS) Project. 1st annual report. *Korey Stringer Institute*. Retrieved from http://www.ksi.uconn.edu/nata-atlas/

Jamtvedt, G., Herbert, R. D., Flottorp, S., Odgaard-Jensen, J., Håvelsrud, H., Barratt, A., . . . Oxman, A. D. (2010). A pragmatic randomised trial of stretching before and after physical activity to prevent injury and soreness. *British Journal of Sports Medicine, 44*(14), 1002–1009.

Jeffreys, I. (2016). Warm-up and flexibility training. In G. G. Haff & N. T. Triplett (Eds.), *Essentials of strength training and conditioning* (4th ed., pp. 317–350). Champaign, IL: Human Kinetics.

Kaminski, T. W., Hertel, J., Amendola, N., Docherty, C. L., Dolan, M. G., Hopkins, J. T., . . . Richie, D. (2013). National Athletic Trainers' Association position statement: Conservative management and prevention of ankle sprains in athletes. *Journal of Athletic Training, 48*(4), 528–545.

Kaplan, Y., & Witvrouw, E. (2019). When is it safe to return to sport after ACL reconstruction? Reviewing the criteria. *Sports Health, 11*(4), 301–305.

Khodaee, M., Putukian, M., & Madden, C. C. (2018). The pre-participation physical examination. In C. C. Madden, M. Putukian, E. C. McCarty, & C. C. Young (Eds.), *Netter's sports medicine* (2nd ed., pp. 8–22). Philadelphia, PA: Elsevier.

Koester, M. C. (2000). Youth sports: A pediatrician's perspective on coaching and injury prevention. *Journal of Athletic Training, 35*(4), 466–470.

Kraemer, W. J., Thomas, G. A., & Hatfield, D. L. (2018). Resistance training. In C. C. Madden, M. Putukian, E. C. McCarty, & C. C. Young (Eds.), *Netter's sports medicine* (2nd ed., pp. 133–137). Philadelphia, PA: Elsevier.

Lloyd, R. S., & Faigenbaum, A. D. (2016). Age- and sex-related differences and their implications for resistance exercise. In G. G. Haff & N. T. Triplett (Eds.), *Essentials of strength training and conditioning* (4th ed., pp. 135–154). Champaign, IL: Human Kinetics.

MacDonald, J., Schaefer, M., & Stumph, J. (2021). The preparticipation physical evaluation. *American Academy of Family Physicians, 103*(9), 539–546.

Madden, C. C., & Fudge, J. R. (2018). Exercise in the cold and cold injuries. In C. C. Madden, M. Putukian, E. C. McCarty, & C. C. Young (Eds.), *Netter's sports medicine* (2nd ed., pp. 152–160). Philadelphia, PA: Elsevier.

Marks, R. J., De Foe, A., & Collett, J. (2020). The pursuit of wellness: Social media, body image and eating disorders. *Children and Youth Services Review, 119*, 105659.

Maron, B. (2015). Historical perspectives on sudden deaths in young athletes with evolution over 35 years. *American Journal of Cardiology, 116*(9), 1461–1468.

Maron, B. J., Friedman, R. A., Kligfield, P., Levine, B. D., Viskin, S., Chaitman, B. R., Okin, P. M., . . . Thompson, P. D. (2014). Assessment of the 12-lead electrocardiogram as a screening test for detection of cardiovascular disease in healthy general populations of young people (12–25 years of age). *Journal of the American College of Cardiology, 64*(14), 1479–1514.

McBride, J. M. (2016). Biomechanics of resistance exercise. In G. G. Haff & N. T. Triplett (Eds.), *Essentials of strength training and conditioning* (4th ed., pp. 19–42). Champaign, IL: Human Kinetics.

McGuigan, M. (2016). Principles of test selection and administration. In G. G. Haff & N. T. Triplett (Eds.), *Essentials of strength training and conditioning* (4th ed., pp. 249–258). Champaign, IL: Human Kinetics.

McHugh, M. P., & Cosgrave, C. H. (2010). To stretch or not to stretch: The role of stretching in injury prevention and performance. *Scandinavian Journal of Medicine & Science in Sports, 20*(2), 169–181.

Mitchell, B. L. (2018). Sickle cell trait and sudden death. *Sports Medicine-Open, 4*(1), 1–6.

Murphy, D. F., Connolly, D. A. J., & Beynnon, B. D. (2003). Risk factors for lower extremity injury: A review of the literature. *British Journal of Sports Medicine, 37*(1), 13–29.

National Athletic Trainers' Association (NATA). (n.d.). Emergency action plans. Retrieved from http://www.nata.org/sites/default/files/white-paper-Emergency-Action-Plan.pdf

National Federation of State High School Associations (NFHS). (2016). The case for high school activities. Retrieved from https://www.nfhs.org/articles/the-case-for-high-school-activities/

National Weather Service. (n.d.). Lightning safety. Retrieved from https://www.weather.gov/safety/lightning-safety

Nauta, J., van Mechelen, W., & Verhagen, E. A. L. M. (2017). Epidemiology and prevention of sports injuries. In N. Armstrong & W. van Mechelen (Eds.), *Oxford textbook of children's sport and exercise medicine* (pp. 541–546). New York, NY: Oxford University Press.

Petek, B. J., & Baggish, A. L. (2020). Pre-participation cardiovascular screening in young competitive athletes. *Current Emergency and Hospital Medicine Reports, 8*(3), 77–89.

Powers, S. K., & Howley, E. T. (2015). *Exercise physiology: Theory and application to fitness and performance* (9th ed.). New York, NY: McGraw-Hill Education.

Reuter, B. H., & Dawes, J. J. (2016). Program design and technique for aerobic endurance training. In G. G. Haff & N. T. Triplett (Eds.), *Essentials of strength training and conditioning* (4th ed., pp. 559–581). Champaign, IL: Human Kinetics.

Rice, S. G. (2008). Medical conditions affecting sports participation. *Pediatrics, 121*(4), 841–848.

Roberts, W. O., Asplund, C. A., O'Connor, F. G., & Stovitz, S. D. (2015). Cardiac preparticipation screening for the young athlete: why the routine use of ECG is not necessary. *Journal of electrocardiology, 48*(3), 311–315.

Sheppard, J. M., & Triplett, N. T. (2016). Program design for resistance training. In G. G. Haff & N. T. Triplett (Eds.), *Essentials of strength training and conditioning* (4th ed., pp. 439–470). Champaign, IL: Human Kinetics.

Shrier, I. (2018). Flexibility. In C. C. Madden, M. Putukian, E. C. McCarty, & C. C. Young (Eds.), *Netter's sports medicine* (2nd ed., pp. 138–140). Philadelphia, PA: Elsevier.

Stanzione, J. R., & Volpe, S. L. (2019). Nutritional considerations for wrestlers. *Nutrition Today, 54*(5), 207–212.

Steinberg, N., Siev-Ner, I., Pelegi, S., Dar, G., Masharas, Y., Zeev, A., & Hershkovitz, I. (2012). Extrinsic and intrinsic risk factors associated with injuries in young dancers aged 8–16 years. *Journal of Sports Science, 30*(5), 485–495.

Swartz, E. E., Register-Mihalik, J. K., Broglio, S. P., Mihalik, J. P., Myers, J. L., Guskiewicz, K. M., ... & Hoge, M. (2022). National Athletic Trainers' Association position statement: Reducing intentional head-first contact behavior in American football players. *Journal of Athletic Training, 57*(2), 113–124.

Sytema, R., Dekker, R., Dijkstra, P., ten Duis, H. J., & van der Sluis, C. K. (2010). Upper extremity sports injury: Risk factors in comparison to lower extremity injury in more than 25,000 cases. *Clinical Journal of Sport Medicine, 20*(4), 256–263.

Theisen, D., Malisoux, L., Seil, R., & Urhausen, A. (2014). Injuries in youth sports: Epidemiology, risk factors, and prevention. *Deutsche Zeitschrift für Sportmedizin, 65*(9), 248–252.

Turocy, P. S., DePalma, B. F., Horswill, C. A., Lauale, K. M., Martin, T. J., Perry, A. C., . . . Utter, A. C. (2011). National Athletic Trainers' Association position statement: Safe weight loss and maintenance practices in sport and exercise. *Journal of Athletic Training, 46*(3), 322–336.

Van der Wall, E. E. (2015). ECG screening in athletes: optional or mandatory? *Netherlands Heart Journal, 23*(7–8), 353–355.

Valovich McLeod, T. C., Decoster, L., Loud, K. J., Micheli, L. J., Parker, J. T., Sandrey, M. A., & White, C. (2011). National Athletic Trainers' Association position statement: Prevention of pediatric overuse injuries. *Journal of Athletic Training, 46*(2), 206–220.

Walsh, K. M., Cooper, M. A., Holle, R., Rakov, V. A., Roederll, W. P., & Ryan, M. (2013). National Athletic Trainers' Association position statement: Lightning safety for athletics and recreation. *Journal of Athletic Training, 48*(2), 258–270.

Williams, E. A., Pelto, H. F., Toresdahl, B. G., Prutkin, J. M., Owens, D. S., Salerno, J. C., ... & Drezner, J. A. (2019). Performance of the American Heart Association (AHA) 14-point evaluation versus electrocardiography for the cardiovascular screening of high school athletes: A prospective study. *Journal of the American Heart Association, 8*(14), e012235.

Yang, J., Tibbetts, A. S., Covassin, T., Cheng, G., Nayar, S., & Heiden, E. (2012). Epidemiology of overuse and acute injuries among competitive collegiate athletes. *Journal of Athletic Training, 47*(2), 198–204.

CHAPTER 5

The Psychology of Athletes and Sports Injury

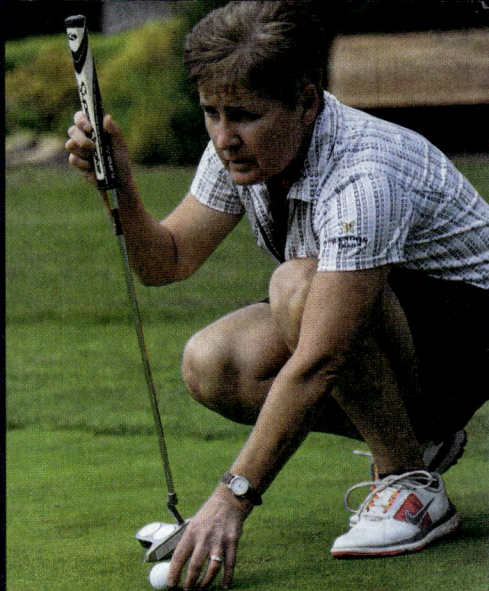

MAJOR CONCEPTS

Sports injuries and decreased performance can be caused by more than physical reasons and often involve more than damaged ligaments, tendons, and muscles. An athlete's mental health before injury and his or her perception of and reaction to an injury will play a major role in the recovery process. This chapter introduces the reader to the psychology of athletes. It begins with an examination of the psychology of competition such that the relationship between athletes and their social and athletic environment along with normal life stressors can predispose athletes to physical or mental exhaustion, sports injury, or decreased performance. The chapter will also touch upon the psychology of the injured athlete and how to handle feelings and behavior associated with injury and rehabilitation. Furthermore, mental health issues, specifically anxiety, mood, and behavioral disorders, are also presented along with their implications for the athletic community. The chapter also discusses attention deficit hyperactivity disorder as it affects today's athletes. Lastly, it outlines a plan to recognize and refer athletes with mental health concerns.

To be clear, in this chapter, the use of the term "mental illness" is reserved for credentialed mental healthcare professionals, such as psychologists, psychiatrists, and licensed/certified counselors. For other allied healthcare professionals, the terms that can be used are "psychological concerns" and "mental health issues/concerns."

Psychology of Competition

Not only are athletes under physical stress of training, but athletes may also be under psychological stress associated with competition, which may lead to physical injury and mental health concerns. This is a multifaceted topic ranging from the pressure and expectations athletes put upon themselves to the pressure and expectations put upon them from others, such as parents, coaches, and teammates. Additionally, an athlete's personality traits may also contribute to the stress of competition.

Competitive Stress and the Athlete

Sports are one of the most popular achievement domains for children, adolescents, and college-age athletes (National Collegiate Athletic Association [NCAA], 2016). It is probable that the majority of children, even today, get involved in sports for recreational and social reasons. However, it is also true that the intensity of competition has been increased dramatically in some sports at exceedingly early ages. Sports such as women's gymnastics, tennis, figure skating, bicycle motocross (BMX), and professional skateboarding routinely produce regional and national champions under the age of 16 years. It is highly suspected that competitive sports teams requiring intense physical activity for young athletes may have negative psychological impacts, such as social isolation, problems with identity formation, maladaptive internal and external factors (e.g., perfectionism, unrealistic expectations), mood disturbances, and burnout (Jayanthi et al., 2019). Because many young athletes perceive losing as failure and winning as success, many professionals in psychology and sociology have raised serious concerns regarding the psychological impact of competition on youths.

The pressure to win can come from parents, coaches, peers, sponsors, and even the media. However, parents are highly involved and visible in youth sports and can influence their children positively and negatively.

Although the immediate effects of such pressure on children may be difficult to gauge, it is safe to assume that children and adolescents do not possess the psychological coping skills of adults. Consequently, the stress of competition may result in significant problems for some youths. Young athletes may be more prone to injury, psychosomatic illnesses, emotional burnout, and other stress-related afflictions. Parents and coaches must be cognizant to not force children beyond their ability to cope with an activity. It is a sad commentary on the values of today's society to think that some children may be driven from a sport that they love simply because they were pushed too hard, too early.

It is important for coaches to recognize their behavior toward children and adolescents, but parents also need to be aware of their behavior. A number of resources are available for coaches and parents regarding minimizing competitive stress in the adolescent. According to the Association for Applied Sport Psychology, the following are some warning signs that athletes may be having trouble at home and experiencing stress related to their participation in athletics: Concern should be raised if conversations at home are dominated by sport discussions, the child is allowed little time to spend with friends, the child's education becomes a distant second priority to competition and talent development, and the child is overly nervous about competing, especially when parents are watching (Lauer, n.d.). To help coaches and parents, several dos and don'ts related to youth sport participation are listed here (Porter, n.d.).

The Dos:
- Do allow children to be interested in and play whatever sport they choose.
- Do teach children to respect their coaches and parents.
- Do be willing to let children make their own mistakes and learn from them.
- Do be interested and supportive, light and playful, understanding and openhearted, and accepting and tolerant of children's learning process and their physical abilities.
- Do model flexibility of your own opinions.

The Don'ts:
- Don't try to relive your youth through children and adolescents.
- Don't blame the equipment, team members, referees, or even the weather if the team does not do well or win.
- Don't "push, push, push." Children and adolescents who are pushed beyond their capabilities may lose their self-confidence, become resistant and resentful toward their parents, become unsure of themselves and their abilities, and stop trying.
- Don't expect perfection or tie your ego or image to the young person's performance.

Just because an athlete is over 18 years old and in college doesn't mean potential parental or other pressures are erased. Rather, collegiate athletes not only feel many pressures, such as maintaining scholarships and managing time effectively between sports and academics, but also often base their self-worth on their performance. Collegiate athletes have the same challenges as nonathlete students in addition to the challenges of being a student-athlete, yet they may be conditioned to demonstrate mental toughness and not admit weakness or struggles. They will even go to great lengths not to disclose mental health information to medical personnel or the coach. Many young adults have experienced life adversity, such as parents' divorce, economic hardship, or loss that affects mental health and may be correlated to physical health and/or use of substances. For these reasons and many others, it is important to properly recognize and handle mental health concerns (NCAA, 2014).

Personality Variables and Competition

Trait theory assumes that individual personalities are composed of broad dispositions that are stable over time and influence behavior. Traits are permanent personality characteristics, whereas personality states are temporary changes in personal characteristics. There are five personality traits that are consistently used to capture the general dimensions of trait personality: extraversion, agreeableness, conscientiousness (dependability), neuroticism (emotional stability), and openness. There are conflicting reports as to personality and sport choice. The most common belief is that extroverted athletes typically choose team sports, whereas introverted athletes often choose individual sports. Personality traits are complex and might only be part of what determines sports disposition (Guo et al., 2021).

Psychology of Injury

Personality Traits and Injury

Regarding sports injury, both state and trait aspects of personality are important for the athlete. The complex interaction of these personality aspects is what is likely to cause injury. For example, athletes who tend to be anxious and feel they do not have strong resources for success in participating in a sporting event that has high demands and big consequences may be more likely to suffer injury (Cagle et al., 2017). Williams and Andersen (1998) developed the stress-injury model, which integrates state and *trait variables* into the occurrence of injury. According to the model, when a person recognizes a potentially stressful situation, a stress response will be generated that is influenced by a cognitive appraisal (i.e., it is serious) and physiological/attentional changes (e.g., heart rate and focus). When the stress response results in an appraisal of harm and there are physiological changes that cause performance decrements, then an injury is likely to occur. Williams and Andersen (1998) proposed that an athlete's personality traits, history of stressors, and coping resources determined whether the athlete's response to the stressful situation would result in injury. Three areas of personality—trait anxiety, locus of control, and self-concept—are often explored in their relation to the stress response.

Trait anxiety is associated with the personality trait of neuroticism (emotional stability) and is connected with a person's general disposition or tendency to perceive certain situations as threatening and to react with an anxiety response (physiological and emotional). Sports injury trait anxiety is the widely indefinite concern or worry about sustaining an injury in a sport. In a critically appraised topic, Cagle and colleagues (2017) found that higher levels of trait anxiety tended to increase the risk of injury in athletes; however, it is only one of many psychosocial characteristics that predicted injury.

Locus of control has to do with people's belief, or lack thereof, of being in control of events occurring in their lives. Two types of individuals have been identified—those with an external locus of control and those with an internal locus of control. The former feel they have very little control over events in their lives. These people believe factors such as destiny, luck, or fate determine life events. Individuals with an internal locus of control feel they are responsible for what happens to them; that is, they are in charge. Research that has attempted to link incidence and/or severity of injury to locus of control has yielded inconclusive results. There is evidence that such connections, if they do exist, may be sport specific; that is, locus of control and trait anxiety may play a role in injury in only certain types of sports.

Self-concept (image of the self that is constructed from the beliefs one holds about oneself) may also be a risk factor in injury. Athletes with a low self-concept may suffer with sports injuries as athletes with a low self-concept are less able to deal effectively with the high stress of competition, especially when there is pressure to succeed. The inability to cope may even result in behavior that leads to injury. In extreme cases, being injured may become an attractive alternative to participation because it gives the athlete a legitimate excuse to avoid playing.

Trait anxiety A general disposition or tendency to perceive certain situations as threatening and to react with an anxiety response.

Locus of control People's belief, or lack thereof, of being in control of events occurring in their lives.

Self-concept The image of the self that is constructed from the beliefs one holds about oneself.

Athletes identified as having a low self-concept may be aided by a variety of intervention strategies. There is evidence that self-concept can be raised through a program of individualized counseling and exercise. Once identified, athletes with low self-concepts should be advised to consult a professional sports psychologist, a guidance counselor, or even a clinical psychiatrist for help ("Psychological Issues Related to Illness and Injury," 2017).

> **WHAT IF?**
>
> You are coaching wrestling in a northern Michigan high school. It is early December, and one of your athletes comes to you complaining of chronic fatigue, a craving for sweets, and a loss of interest in the sport. Could these complaints be symptoms of a psychological disorder, and, if so, what would you do to help this athlete?

Psychosocial Variables and Injury

We live in a time of changing social environments as a result of increased economic and family stresses; therefore, it is important to consider these ever-changing psychosocial variables in the injury equation. Specifically, attention has been given to studying the effects of stressful life events on athletes. Stressful life events have been defined as positive or negative episodes that usually evoke an adaptive or coping behavior or significant change in the ongoing life pattern of the individual. This theory holds that life events can be very stressful, even those that most people would consider positive, such as getting married, taking a vacation, or winning the lottery. Researchers have endeavored to study the effects of life events on different populations, including athletes.

The stress-injury model proposed by Williams and Andersen (1998) indicated that two psychosocial variables—a history of stressors and coping resources—play a significant role in the cognitive appraisal and physiological responses to stressful situations and that both of them may influence the occurrence of injuries. A number of studies have revealed relationships between stressful life events and sports injuries (Guo et al., 2021; "Psychological Issues Related to Illness and Injury," 2017; Williams & Andersen, 1998).

Evidence suggests that, when an athlete is experiencing significant personal changes, especially those seen as negative, the chances of injury increase. As was the case with determination of self-concept status, the care providers may find it helpful to assess the life-stress status of athletes before the season begins and on a follow-up basis. In this way, athletes who are at high risk—that is, those with high life-stress scores—can be identified and referred to a counselor to help improve their coping skills. A variety of questionnaires (Table 5.1) have been developed and can be implemented during a preparticipation physical examination (PPE) or at any time as needed, such as recovery from injury. The administration and interpretation of psychometric tests are most effectively conducted by sports psychologists and other trained professionals (Guo et al., 2021; "Psychological Issues Related to Illness and Injury," 2017).

Psychological Stress and Injury

A wide variety of psychological factors might affect the mental and physical health of an individual as high levels of stress may make an individual more prone to illness. To relate these findings to athletes, sports scientists have been investigating the possible relationship between psychological variables and sports injuries (Figure 5.1). Major injuries were associated with greater perceived stress and less perceived social support and life satisfaction. Perceived stress, levels of social support, and fatigue may be connected to

Table 5.1
Psychological Questionnaires

Social Readjustment Rating Scale (SRRS)
Social and Athletic Readjustment Rating Scale (SARRS)
Life Event Scale for Adolescents (LESA)
Life Event Questionnaire (LEQ)
Life Event Survey for Collegiate Athletes (LESCA)
Athletic Life Experience Survey (ALES)
Generalized Anxiety Disorder 7-Item Scale (GAD-7)
Sport Competition Anxiety Test (SCAT)
Sport Anxiety Scale-2
Athletic Coping Skills Inventory 28 (ACSI-28)
Tennessee Self-Concept Scale (TSCS)

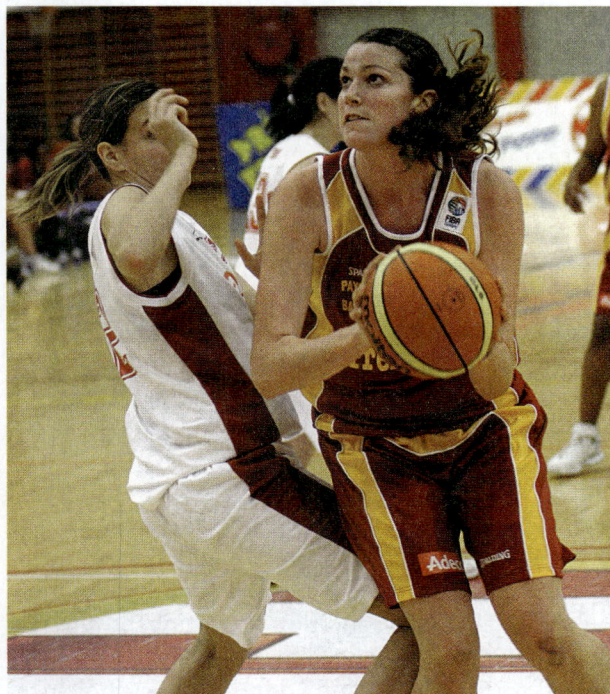

Figure 5.1 Competition can create a great deal of psychological stress.
© Pétur Ásgeirsson/Shutterstock.

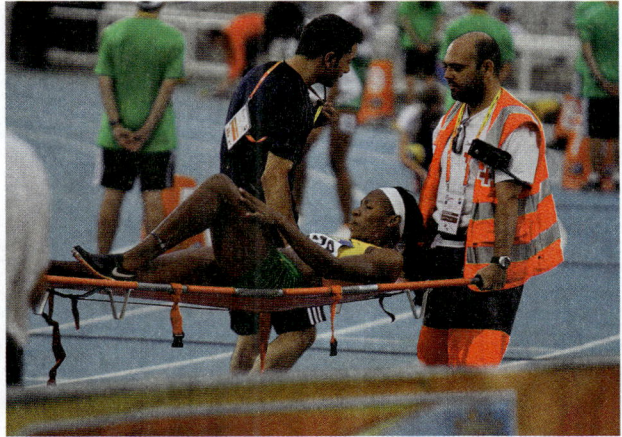

Figure 5.2 The potential for injury is an ever-present fear for most athletes.
© Denis Kuvaev/Shutterstock.

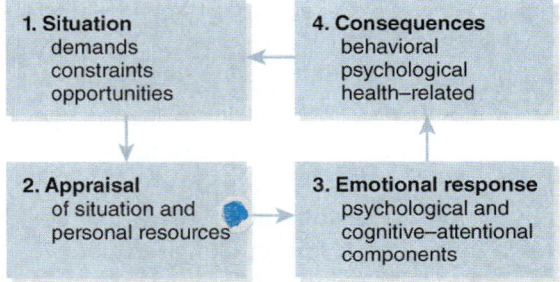

Figure 5.3 The stress process.
Data from Weiss, M. R., & Troxel, R. K. (1986). Psychology of the injured athlete. *Journal of Athletic Training*, 21(2), 104–109.

sports injury and need to be addressed because they present problems for athletes in their sport and life. It is important to understand there are complex interactions between life situations, personality, current situations, sociocultural factors, and psychological factors. Stress changes attention, which can affect athletic performance by increasing muscle tension and influencing coordination (Guo et al., 2021; "Psychological Issues Related to Illness and Injury," 2017).

Psychology of the Injured Athlete

An injury itself represents a potent form of psychological stress for the athlete. For most athletes, the possibility of being sidelined by a traumatic episode is an ever-present fear (Figure 5.2). For most athletes, an injury produces a predictable psychological response. Research by Weiss and Troxel (1986) reported that an injury could cause a psychophysiological reaction in the athlete that follows the classic stress-response model originally formulated by Selye (Figure 5.3).

As depicted in Figure 5.3, in phase 1, the injury serves as a potent **stressor** (i.e., anything that affects the body's physiological or psychological condition and upsets the homeostatic balance) and requires the athlete to adapt to a restriction of normal activity. Phase 2 involves an appraisal of the significance of the injury in both a short- and long-term sense. Weiss and Troxel (1986) reported that this phase is when an athlete may engage in negative self-doubt ("What if I can't recover by the next game?"). Phase 3 of the stress model involves an emotional response, which can precipitate a host of physical and psychological reactions, ranging from

Stressor Anything that affects the body's physiological or psychological condition and upsets the homeostatic balance.

> **TIME OUT 5.1**
>
> **Guidelines for Working With an Injured Athlete**
>
> 1. Treat the person, not just the injury.
> 2. Treat the athlete as an individual.
> 3. Be empathetic and listen.
> 4. Understand the psychological response to injury.
> 5. Communicate with coaches about problematic response to injury and how to be supportive.
> 6. Seek the help of a mental health professional if psychological responses to injury are worsening.
>
> Reproduced from Weiss, M. R., & Troxel, R. K. (1986). Psychology of the injured athlete. *Journal of Athletic Training, 21*(2), 104–109; and National Collegiate Athletic Association (NCAA). (2014). Mind, body and sport. Reprinted with permission.

severe anxiety, depression, and anger to increased muscle tension, blood pressure, and heart rate. It is important to note that the stages described by Kübler-Ross, which are denial, anger, bargaining, depression, and acceptance, can be skipped altogether or experienced in various orders in cases of sports injury (Kübler-Ross, 1969). The fourth stage of the stress model involves the long-term consequences of the emotional response in phase 3. If an athlete fails to respond to an injury in a positive manner, he or she may suffer from a wide variety of problems, including sleep disorders, loss of appetite, and decreased motivation (Weiss & Troxel, 1986). As a result of the development of these injury-response models, recommendations have been made regarding how best to assist the injured athlete in coping with an injury. Weiss and Troxel (1986) developed a list of guidelines for personnel to follow when working with an injured athlete. These guidelines, in addition to the strategies outlined by the NCAA, are enumerated in **Time Out 5.1**.

Several themes have emerged from interviews with injured collegiate athletes, including fluctuations in emotions characterized by feelings of loss, decreased self-esteem, frustration, **anxiety**, and anger. Psychological symptoms persist even after athletes are cleared to play. Even though they may be ready physically, they are not prepared mentally to return.

Therefore, coaches, parents, and athletic trainers must be aware that, in addition to treating the physical aspects of injury, they need to protect athletes' physical and mental health and address the psychological aspects of injury recovery (Guo et al., 2021; "Psychological Issues Related to Illness and Injury," 2017).

It is important to note that how athletes respond to injury may differ and the response to minor or severe injury or unpredictable recovery can be from the time of injury through rehabilitation to return to activity. The certified athletic trainer, team physician, coaches, and administrators should be aware of the symptoms presented in **Table 5.2** that either do not resolve or worsen over time. For example, an athlete with a significant injury that restricts participation may go on a diet with the mentality that she does not deserve to eat (NCAA, 2014). The care providers need to be aware of such responses and act accordingly.

Table 5.2

Emotional Responses to Injury

Sadness
Isolation
Irritation
Anger
Frustration
Sleep disturbances
Altered appetite

Anxiety Feelings of apprehensiveness, powerlessness, and impending danger along with physical symptoms of increased heart rate and breathing rate, sweating, and trembling to the point where it interferes with one's ability to perform daily functions.

Recommendations

Several suggestions have come from applied sports psychologists for addressing the psychological needs of athletes after injury and during rehabilitation. Rehabilitation adherence is complex and multidimensional; therefore, providing multiple treatment options is important. Social support has been identified as a key component of psychological recovery from injury. Applied sports psychologists suggest helping athletes by providing a connection to their team during rehabilitation, comfort during the hard work of returning to play, an understanding of the injury and what to expect from the rehabilitation process, and support for completing day-to-day rehabilitation tasks (Shelley et al., 2003). Social support should be emotional, educational, and tangible (Hedstrom, n.d.). Although more research is needed in this area, sports injuries may well be responsible for lingering psychological effects in young athletes.

Also, psychological skills, such as goal setting, imagery, relaxation techniques, and positive self-talk, have been found to be helpful for athletes to enhance performance, regulate emotions, increase confidence, decrease stress, and recover from injury (Madrigal, 2015). A meta-analysis conducted in 2015 confirmed that psychological skills training most likely reduces the severity of the stress response, decreases muscle tension, and increases perceptual ability leading to the reduced risk for injuries (Tranaeus et al., 2015). Care providers can work in conjunction with mental health professionals to implement these strategies into injury prevention and recovery.

Mental Health Concerns

Mood Disorders

Depression

Everyone feels sad at some time or another; however, when that feeling and others last a long time, for example, for most days for 2 weeks, or is too intense, a mood disorder may be present. Together, the biological, psychological, and social factors may contribute to mood disorders. The most common mood disorder is depression. According to the U.S. Department of Health and Human Services (n.d.), approximately 12.5% of youths ages 12–17 and 6.7% of adults experienced a major depressive episode in 2015. Wolanin, Hong, Marks, Panchoo, and Gross (2016) reported that almost 25% of NCAA student-athletes experienced clinical levels of depression, which is comparable to the general college population. And, according to the National Alliance on Mental Illness (n.d.), LGBTQ (lesbian, gay, bisexual, transgender, and queer) individuals are up to three times more likely to suffer depression and anxiety than others due to social stresses and biases, such as being discriminated against or feeling isolated.

Depressive illnesses come in various forms, and the number, severity, and duration of symptoms also vary. Depression is more than the "blues" or other letdowns related to daily hassles (NCAA, 2012). Major depression, dysthymia, and bipolar disorder are the most common forms of depression. **Major depression** is more severe than dysthymia but is often short term, **dysthymia** is less severe than major depression but more chronic, and **bipolar disorder** is characterized by manic episodes. Depressive illnesses can involve the signs and symptoms as presented in Table 5.3 and affect general health and performance.

Athletes may have depression before an injury or as a result of an injury. For example, a volleyball player may lack concentration due to depression and land from a jump awkwardly, causing injury (NCAA, 2014). In the college student population, women are twice as likely to experience depression as men, and 1 in 10 students will suffer from depressive symptoms in a 1-year time frame (NCAA, 2012). Data also indicate that student-athletes experience depressive symptoms and illness at similar or increased rates compared to nonathlete students (NCAA, 2012). Even though athletes typically have higher levels of self-esteem and

---

Major depression Characterized by a combination of five or more symptoms and noticeable changes in usual functioning, such as sleep, eating, work, or school.

Dysthymia Characterized by nondisabling depressive symptoms that are chronic but do not cause changes in usual functioning.

Bipolar disorder A manic-depressive illness that involves cycling mood swings from major depression to mania, during which individuals feel full of energy.

Table 5.3
Signs and Symptoms of Depression

Individuals May Feel	Individuals May Present With
Sad	Lack of energy, depressed, low mood
Anxious	Loss of interest in activities previously enjoyed (hanging out with friends, practice, school, sex)
Hopeless	Loss of appetite or eating more than normal, resulting in weight loss of weight gain
Worthless	Decreased performance in school and sport or recurring thoughts of death, suicide, or suicide attempts
Helpless	Problems falling asleep, staying asleep, or sleeping too much or unusual crying
Guilty	Problems concentrating, remembering information, or making decisions
	Obsessing over your shamefulness and being self-critical or paranoid
Irritable	Quick to anger or easily frustrated and upset
Restless	Feeling "on edge" or having an "uncomfortable urge to move"
Aches, pains, headaches, cramps	The physical symptoms of aches, pains, headaches, cramps

Reproduced from Neal, T. L., Diamond, A. B., Goldman, S., Liedtka, K. D., Mathis, K., Morse, E. D., . . . Welzant, V. (2015). Inter-association recommendations for developing a plan to recognize and refer student-athletes with psychological concerns at the secondary school level: A consensus statement. *Journal of Athletic Training, 50*(3), 231–249.

social connectedness when compared to nonathletes, it is interesting to note that these positive psychosocial attributes were not significant deterrents to depressive symptoms; therefore, coaches, parents, and athletic trainers need to be aware of depressive symptoms and provide athletes with referrals for help as necessary. Furthermore, depression can be a double-edged sword for athletes in that, if their athletic identity is taken away because of depression, their depression may increase even more. Likewise, forcing a depressed athlete to perform may decrease performance or cause injury leading to increased depression (NCAA, 2014).

Athletes may experience events that possibly trigger or even worsen their emotional health, including concussions, poor sports performance, lack of playing time, being cut from the team, and/or injuries with time loss (NCAA, 2012). It is also important to know that anxiety and depression can occur simultaneously, especially in the case of concussions. First, the timeline to heal from a concussion is unknown, and, oftentimes, athletes miss academic work, both of which can create anxiety. Second, concussions usually require a period of inactivity, which is the opposite of what athletes are used to. Third, some athletes may worry about future consequences of a concussion due to the heightened media attention around concussions, specifically chronic traumatic encephalopathy (CTE). Some concussed athletes experience emotions due to the concussion itself, others may have a mental health issue not directly related to the concussion, and still others experience depression as a reaction to the concussion (NCAA, 2014). Athletic trainers treating athletes during the acute and subacute phases of an injury may play a valuable role in the recognition of depressive symptoms.

If depression becomes too severe and a feeling of hopelessness is experienced, it can lead to suicidal thoughts and unfortunate actions. It is important to know that depression does not always lead to suicide but, when people are suicidal, the situation needs to be taken seriously and acted upon by immediately referring them to a mental health professional in a counseling center or hospital emergency room. Most importantly, do not leave them alone until they are in the care of a mental health professional (NCAA, 2014). Table 5.4 lists the symptoms of suicidal thoughts.

Table 5.4
Warning Signs of Suicide

Talking about wanting to die
Looking for a way to kill oneself
Talking about feeling trapped or in unbearable pain
Talking about being a burden to others
Talking about feeling hopeless or having no purpose
Increasing the use of alcohol or drugs
Sleeping too little or too much
Withdrawing or feeling isolated
Showing rage or talking about seeking revenge
Acting anxious, agitated, or recklessly
Displaying extreme mood swings

Suicidal behavior. (n.d.). Retrieved from https://www.mentalhealth.gov/what-to-look-for/suicidal-behavior

Mental health checkups can be as simple as providing empathetic listening and encouraging student-athletes to talk about situations that may trigger depressive episodes. Check-ups can also include the repeated use of screening tools (Table 5.1) with athletes. However, caution must be used when interpreting any screening tools; it is essential that a licensed professional (e.g., physician, psychiatrist, or counselor) be consulted if there is any concern that an athlete may be suffering from depression. Several self-help strategies can also be provided to student-athletes to help them improve mild depressive symptoms ("Psychological Issues Related to Illness and Injury," 2017). **Time Out 5.2** lists several recommended self-help strategies.

Seasonal Affective Disorder

Seasonal affective disorder (SAD) is a psychiatric disorder that affects the general population, including athletes, primarily in the fall and winter seasons. Previously, SAD was classified as a mood disorder. However, SAD is a distinct category within major depressive disorder and is linked to the colder months of fall and winter, when there is less sunlight. SAD has a higher prevalence in northern latitudes, where there is less sunlight, a shift in circadian rhythm, and lower activity levels. In addition, those who have more negative attitudes to weather seem to be more at risk for SAD.

A wide array of symptoms, including a loss of physical capacity and energy, increased appetite (especially carbohydrate craving), decreased libido, hypersomnia (excessive sleep or drowsiness), anhedonia (lack of interest in normally pleasurable activities), and impaired social activity, are common in SAD.

Considering the fact that many of the symptoms of this disorder may negatively affect performance or, worse, predispose some to injury, it seems prudent for parents, coaches, and athletic trainers to become familiar with the specific signs and symptoms of SAD. Although subsyndromal SAD represents a less-severe form of the affliction, the potential for problems is high given that athletes may fail to seek medical attention. Accurate diagnostic tests are available for SAD, and anyone exhibiting such symptoms as described herein

---

TIME OUT 5.2

Self-Help Strategies to Improve Mild Depressive Symptoms

- Increase positive thinking.
- Let family, friends, coaches, and athletic trainers help you.
- Break large tasks into smaller ones; set realistic goals.
- Eat regular and nutritious meals.
- Engage in regular and adequate sleep habits.
- Reduce consumption of alcohol.
- Participate in activities that make you feel better.

Data from National Collegiate Athletic Association (NCAA). (2012). *2012–2013 NCAA sports medicine handbook* (pp. 79–80). Retrieved from http://www.ncaapublications.com/productdownloads/MD12.pdf; and National Institute of Mental Health. (2016). Depression basics. Retrieved from https://www.nimh.nih.gov/health/publications/depression/index.shtml

should be referred to a specialist for evaluation. Regarding treatment, promising results have been shown using light therapy (phototherapy), lifestyle interventions, medication, and cognitive behavior therapy (Galima et al., 2020).

Anxiety Disorders

Anxiety disorders are not uncommon in athletics. In fact, 31% of teens are affected, and about 58% of college-certified athletic trainers believe anxiety is an issue with student-athletes (NCAA, 2014). Anxiety disorders include several types, such as general anxiety disorder, panic attacks, obsessive-compulsive disorder, phobias, and posttraumatic stress disorder. The signs and symptoms of anxiety disorders are presented in Table 5.5 and can intensify when under stress. They also happen frequently or intensely enough to affect the ability to function socially, academically, and athletically. For athletes, it is usually a future event that causes anxiety and the cognitive and physiological symptoms. It is important to recognize these symptoms early and refer the athlete to a mental health professional (NCAA, 2014).

Behavioral Disorders

Athletes, just like nonathletes, may adjust their behavior to deal with stress in a way that they feel more in control of their lives; they are subjected to societal and cultural pressures through media and other sources to look a certain way. In addition, an athlete deals with extra challenges related to sports participation, such as dealing with relationships with coaches and teammates, missing school work, and managing time, which may weigh heavily on their minds. For these reasons and more, athletes may suffer from eating disorders and sleep disturbances (NCAA, 2014).

Eating Disorders

With few exceptions, all sports impose an extremely narrow set of parameters for the appropriate body type required for success. It is difficult to imagine, for example, a world-class gymnast who is 6 feet tall and weighs 240 pounds or a successful long-distance runner or figure skater who is obese.

Biomechanics Branch of study that applies the laws of mechanics, internal or external, to the living body.

Table 5.5
Signs and Symptoms of Anxiety

Feeling apprehensive
Having a sense of impending danger, panic, or doom
Having an increased heart rate
Breathing rapidly
Sweating
Trembling
Feeling powerless
Feeling weak or tired
Feel depressed, have trouble with drugs or alcohol, or have other mental health concerns
Feel anxiety is related to physical health problems
Worrying too much may interfere with work, relationships, other parts of life
Have suicidal thoughts or behaviors
Muscle tension
Sleep disturbances
Restlessness

Anxiety disorders. (2018, May 4). Retrieved from https://www.mayoclinic.org/diseases-conditions/anxiety/symptoms-causes/syc-20350961. Used with permission of Mayo Foundation for Medical Education and Research, all rights reserved; Psychological issues related to illness and injury in athletes and the team physician: A consensus statement-2016 update. (2017). *Medicine in Sports and Exercise, 49*(5), 1043–1054.

Reality dictates that specific sports require specific body types for athletes to be competitive. Some sports, such as those mentioned, demand leanness for at least two reasons. First, the **biomechanics** of the sport may require a lean and muscular body for the athlete to effectively perform highly complex skills. Second, the sports community and society as a whole have come to expect that successful athletes look lean and muscular. In recent years, media exposure of many top athletes has focused as much on physical appearance as on performance. Such scrutiny on physical appearance has created the need for many aspiring athletes to conform to a certain narrowly defined body type (Figure 5.4). This is especially true for female athletes, but male athletes also suffer from distorted body images.

Psychologists are aware that this emphasis on the ideal body has resulted in serious negative effects on the athletic community. An increasing number

Athletic Trainers SPEAK OUT

Why is addressing the psychology of an injury important in the rehabilitation and recovery process? How can athletic trainers best do this?

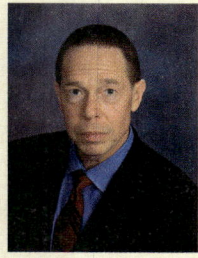

Courtesy of Timothy Neal.

The growing prevalence in the types, severity, and percentage of mental illness within the age group of secondary school and intercollegiate athletes is being recognized. Being an athlete does not provide immunity from mental illness. While some studies suggest that sports participation is a protective measure against mental illness, other studies outline the unique and at times overwhelming stressors that athletes face (e.g., time spent on sport, isolation from the rest of the student body, academic requirements to remain eligible) that could start or worsen an existing mental illness. The still present stigma of experiencing a mental health condition can inhibit an athlete from seeking assistance. Having an awareness that mental health illnesses are present in one to every four to five adolescents and young adults, and that athletes can suffer from a mental health concern are important first steps in helping an athlete with a mental health concern.

Two key areas where an athlete's mental health is challenged are physical overtraining and experiencing an injury. Physical overtraining, whether by design by a coach, or by the individual athlete, can set the athlete up for psychological stress. Overtraining results in poor outcomes in daily fatigue, sleep disturbances, dehydration, and perhaps chronic pain from a lingering injury that doesn't get the proper rest or treatment to recover. The mix of these elements can leave the athlete frustrated and at risk for developing a mental health condition such as anxiety and depression. The other area that can expose the athlete to a mental health condition is an injury. Most athlete's identities are that as an athlete. Once that identity is at risk as a result of a significant injury, or is challenged through surgery and long-term rehabilitation, the athlete can experience challenges that result in, or worsens a preexisting, mental health condition. The athlete experiences a loss with an injury, similar to the grieving process.

Athletes can experience mental health disorders. Unique stressors of being an athlete, overtraining, and injury are just some of the areas that could put the athlete at risk for a mental health condition. Awareness of these factors and approaching the athlete with a concern is important step in referring the athlete for help by a mental healthcare professional.

— **Timothy Neal, MS, AT, ATC, CCISM**

Timothy Neal is program director of athletic training education and assistant professor of health and human performance at Concordia University in Ann Arbor, Michigan.

---

of athletes demonstrate abnormal eating behaviors (disordered eating) or even **pathogenic** eating behaviors that may have deeper psychological origins. These pathogenic eating behaviors are on the increase within the athletic community and include **bulimia nervosa** and **anorexia nervosa**, with the former being more prevalent. Overall, abnormal eating behaviors are higher in adolescent elite athletes than matched controls and higher in female athletes than male athletes (Marinsen & Sundgot-Borgen, 2013). Even though the majority of athletes with eating disorders are female, recent studies demonstrate that males are also affected and should not be excluded from continuing discussions (Chatterton & Petrie, 2013). To better understand eating disorders and their ramifications, readers are encouraged to learn more at the website of the National Eating Disorders Association (**www.nationaleatingdisorders.org**) or

> **Pathogenic** Causing disease.
>
> **Bulimia nervosa** A disorder characterized by repeated bouts of binge eating followed by some form of purging, such as vomiting, use of laxatives, fasting, and vigorous and excessive exercise.
>
> **Anorexia nervosa** A disorder characterized by a pattern of self-starvation with a concomitant obsession with being thin and an overwhelming fear of being fat.

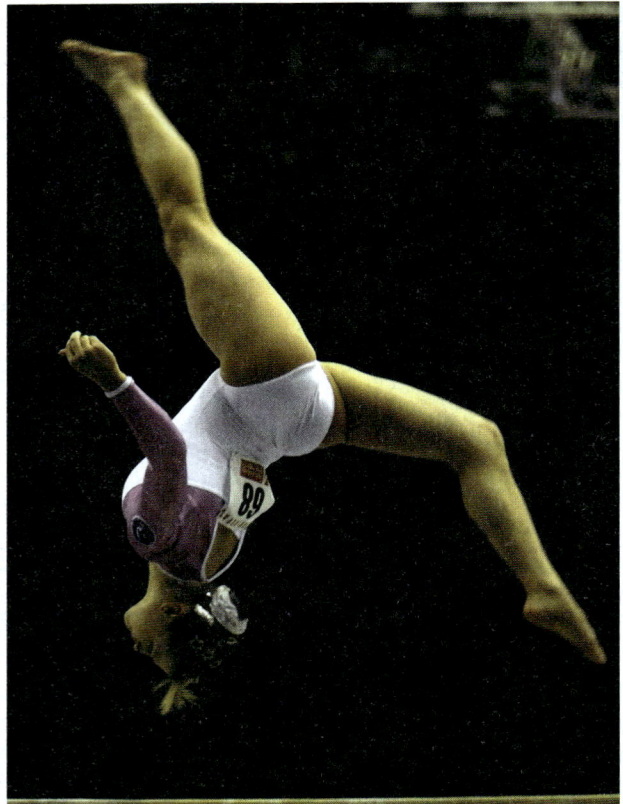

Figure 5.4 Many athletes feel compelled to conform to a certain body type.
© John Lumb/Shutterstock.

self-control as vulnerabilities to disordered eating behaviors. Interestingly, the ability to tolerate pain and enjoy hunger pains were shown to increase vulnerability to disordered eating ("Psychological Issues Related to Illness and Injury," 2017; Stirling & Kerr, 2012).

Anorexia Nervosa and Bulimia Nervosa

It is important to note that disordered eating behaviors are not always represented by a clinical diagnosis of anorexia nervosa or bulimia nervosa. Many subclinical eating disorders (eating disorders otherwise nonspecified) are associated with a variety of warning signs. These warning signs are presented in Table 5.6.

Anorexia nervosa is the third most common illness for adolescents and is characterized by a pattern of self-starvation motivated by an obsession with being thin and an overwhelming fear of being fat (ANAD, 2013). An intake of only a few hundred

the website of the National Association of Anorexia Nervosa and Associated Disorders (ANAD) (**www.anad.org**). Additionally, readers can access the National Athletic Trainers' Association "Position Statement: Preventing, Detecting, and Managing Disordered Eating in Athletes" (Bonci et al., 2008). Four factors have been identified as having the greatest effect on the risk of athletes developing disordered eating: (1) features of the *sport task*, such as revealing uniforms or being physically evaluated; (2) the *sport environment*, which can include comments from teammates, coaches, parents, or judges, as well as the audience; (3) *biological characteristics*, such as metabolism and physical size; and (4) *psychological characteristics* of the individual, which can include self-esteem, body image, and anxiety about being evaluated by others (also known as social physique anxiety). Stirling and Kerr (2012) have also described personal qualities of perfectionism, achievement motivation, self-absorption, competitiveness, and

Table 5.6
Warning Signs of Nonspecific Disordered Eating

- Dieting obsessively when not overweight
- Claiming to feel "fat" when overweight is not a reality
- Preoccupation with food, calories, nutrition, and cooking
- Being overly active
- Frequent weighing
- Strange food-related behaviors
- Rapid weight loss
- Depression
- Slowness of thought/memory difficulties
- Hair loss
- Fatigue and irritability
- Loss of menstrual period (females)
- Normal, overweight, or low body weight
- GI upset
- Arrythmia
- Depression/anxiety
- Low self-esteem

Data from Psychological issues related to illness and injury in athletes and the team physician: A consensus statement-2016 update. (2017). *Medicine in Sports and Exercise, 49*(5), 1043–1054.

calories a day is regular practice. It is very common for those with this illness to have a grossly distorted body image in which they think of themselves as being fat when they are, in fact, abnormally lean. Several warning signs, including deliberate self-starvation with weight loss, persistent fear of gaining weight, refusal to eat or highly restrictive eating, sensitivity to cold, and absent or irregular menstruation, are characteristic of anorexic individuals (Bonci et al., 2008). Anorexic individuals typically refuse to maintain weight at 85% of their ideal body weight (Bonci et al., 2008).

Bulimia nervosa is characterized by repeated bouts of binge eating followed by some form of purging, for example, vomiting; taking laxatives; fasting; or undertaking vigorous, excessive exercise (Bonci et al., 2008). The bingeing and purging must occur more than twice a week for at least 3 months to be considered bulimia nervosa. Because those persons suffering from bulimia nervosa often have normal weight, it is important to pay attention to several specific warning signs, including preoccupation with food, secret eating and purging, gastrointestinal problems, laxative addiction, tooth decay, swollen salivary glands, and broken blood vessels in the eyes (ANAD, 2013). Both anorexia and bulimia are considered to be serious psychological problems and are classified as psychological disorders by the American Psychological Association ("Psychological Issues Related to Illness and Injury," 2017).

Research of Eating Habits

Research indicates that athletes are at a greater risk to develop eating disorders than nonathletes, and up to 20% of elite female athletes met the criteria for eating disorders, compared with up to 10% in collegiate male athletes. Eating disorders were found to have increased incidence in lean or weight-controlled sports. Most individuals diagnosed with eating disorders experience remission within 5 years and the mortality rate is up to 5% ("Psychological Issues Related to Illness and Injury," 2017).

In a study ($n = 204$), 25% of females were classified as having symptoms and patterns of clinical disordered eating, and 2% were classified as needing a clinical diagnosis of an eating disorder. Aesthetic and power sports, including gymnastics, diving, cheerleading, crew, power lifting, and downhill skiing, had the most symptomatic athletes (33–40%), and cross-country, swimming, track, and ball sports had 21–27% (Greenleaf et al., 2009).

Even though the prevalence is increasing, little is known about pathogenic eating behaviors and disordered eating among male athletes. However, Chatterton and Petrie (2013) identified that most eating disturbances in males occur at the subclinical level and that athletes who participate in weight-class sports are more likely to be classified as symptomatic and engage in pathogenic eating, weight control, or excessive exercise behaviors when compared to endurance-sport or ball-game male athletes. Research also indicates that, in aesthetic sports (e.g., diving, dance, or gymnastics), sports where low body fat is advantageous (e.g., distance running), or sports where athletes need to "make weight" (e.g., wrestling and horse racing), there is a danger of pathogenic eating behaviors in males ("Psychological Issues Related to Illness and Injury," 2017). Historically, the sport of wrestling has received the most attention regarding this problem. It is common knowledge that many wrestlers routinely practice a variety of strange eating and training behaviors, especially just before competition. Such behaviors include fasting, restricting fluids, using laxatives, vomiting, and sweating off weight by wearing a rubber suit in the sauna. Obviously, all of these practices are to be discouraged. At best, they result in a short-term water loss; at worst, they can cause severe illness and even death. More research is needed to determine whether male athletes are vulnerable to the same pressures as their female counterparts when it comes to maintaining body build and leanness. Additionally, it needs to be determined whether the reported low incidence of clinical eating disorders in male athletes is an accurate reflection of the true incidence in this population.

Sport Specificity and Eating Disorders

It has been well documented that aesthetic sports carry a high risk that participants will develop eating disorders. These sports include gymnastics, ballet, swimming, diving, and figure skating. All these activities place a heavy emphasis on lean, muscular body builds. Greenleaf and colleagues (2009) surveyed female athletes from a variety of university sports and found that power and aesthetic sports did have the highest percentages (40% and 33%, respectively) but there were no statistical differences between the sports.

The same study (Greenleaf et al., 2009) also reported a 28% incidence of disordered eating in ball sports and a 22% incidence in endurance sports (including swimming); therefore, recent research confirms these findings.

A variety of physical and psychological problems are associated with subclinical eating disorders, anorexia nervosa, and bulimia nervosa. Athletes with eating disorders run the risk of esophageal inflammation, erosion of tooth enamel, and hormone imbalances. These physiological changes can lead to **osteoporosis**, **amenorrhea**, and electrolyte imbalances, which can cause kidney and heart problems. The use of the word *triad* to describe the linked physiological changes that are associated with disordered eating behaviors has been prevalent in the medical literature since the early 2000s because the primary conditions associated are (1) low energy availability (disordered eating), (2) declines in bone health (bone loss), and (3) hormonal imbalances (Aerni & Knapp, 2018). Both the *female athlete triad*, which links low energy availability to the occurrence of osteoporosis and amenorrhea, and the *male athlete triad*, which includes a connection between low energy availability, bone loss, low sperm counts, and hormonal changes associated with low testosterone, low estradiol, and high glucocorticoids (Chatterton & Petrie, 2013) are often used to describe the health consequences of disordered eating behaviors. Both sexes should be educated on the health and performance consequences of hormonal irregularities (i.e., low testosterone, amenorrhea) and the importance of seeking timely medical intervention at the first sign of abnormalities (Chatterton & Petrie, 2013; Marinsen & Sundgot-Borgen, 2013). In fact, the International Olympic Committee (IOC) has recently concluded that the clinical phenomenon of physiological changes associated with the imbalance between dietary energy intake and energy expenditure is not a triad of just the three entities, but rather a syndrome that affects many aspects of physiological function including metabolic rate, menstrual/hormonal function, bone health, immunity, protein synthesis, cardiovascular and psychological health (Mountjoy et al., 2014). The more current term for this syndrome is *Relative Energy Deficiency in Sport (RED-S)*, which is considered a more comprehensive, broader term for the overall syndrome resulting from an imbalance in the amount or quality of energy taken in and the amount of energy expended (Mountjoy et al., 2014). Education efforts should focus on the broad array of signs and symptoms. As the scientific understanding of RED-S syndrome improves, three sport risk assessment categories (high, moderate, and low) for beginning sport participation and three return-to-play plans (red light, no participation; yellow light, cautious participation; and green light, full participation) have been identified (Mountjoy et al., 2014). Return-to-play decisions are based on the evaluation of athlete's health status, evaluation of athlete's participation risk, and inclusion of decision modifications (e.g., time in season, conflicts of interest; Mountjoy et al., 2014).

Prevention

Prevention of disordered eating, including bulimia and anorexia nervosa, must be the goal of all those involved with organized sports. Coaches need to place less emphasis on body weight and fat when working with athletes. Referring to weight in a negative manner, requiring mandatory weigh-ins, or publicly ostracizing an athlete for being overweight are practices to be condemned. Negative body image has also been identified as a precursor to disordered eating. Body image refers to the thoughts, feelings, and perceptions an individual has about his or her body appearance and shape (Greenleaf et al., 2009). Negative self-perceptions should be of concern because they are detrimental to the health and wellness of athletes. Athletes suffering from poor body image are encouraged to engage in positive body talk, focus on what their body can do, and accept the idea that healthy and happy bodies come in all shapes and sizes.

Coaches and parents need to be alert to the early warning signs of disordered eating (Table 5.6). Screening for athletes who may be at risk for disordered eating can commence at the time of the PPE. The athlete can complete a simple questionnaire, the Eating Disorder Examination Questionnaire (EDE-Q), or an online screening tool (www.nationaleatingdisorders.org/screening-tool) during the PPE. If an athlete achieves a score indicative of someone who may be at risk, he or she can be referred for psychological counseling. However, two research projects have suggested physiological screening and clinical interviews are superior to self-report measures. Marinsen and Sundgot-Borgen (2013) indicated that the clinical interview might be better than other

---

Osteoporosis When the body loses too much bone, makes too little bone, or both, then the bones become porous and weak, making them more likely to fracture.

Amenorrhea Absence or suppression of menstruation.

> ### TIME OUT 5.3
>
> #### Advice for Coaches
>
> 1. Be aware that you are a role model for your athletes. Your influence goes a long way in their lives.
> 2. If an athlete has signs of an eating disorder, do not become the "food police." Refer the individual for help.
> 3. Be sensitive in making comments about your athlete and/or team expectations and how you address body image.
> 4. Avoid discriminating against athletes because of their weight. Refrain from weigh-ins and asking athletes to lose weight or diet.
> 5. Provide educational resources concerning nutrition, growth and development, exercise, and disordered eating.
> 6. Be positive and empathetic.
>
> Courtesy of Eva Monsma, Ph.D., Associate Professor, Developmental Sport Psychology, University of South Carolina; Psychological issues related to illness and injury in athletes and the team physician: A consensus statement-2016 update. (2017). *Medicine in Sports and Exercise, 49*(5), 1043–1054; Chang, C., Putukian, M., Aerni, G., Diamond, A., Hong, G., Ingram, Y., Reardon, C. L., & Wolanin, A. (2020). Mental health issues and psychological factors in athletes: Detection, management, effect on performance and prevention: American Medical Society for Sports Medicine Position Statement-Executive Summary. *British Journal of Sports Medicine, 54*(4), 216–220.

screening tools, especially in an athletic population. It is suggested that a physiological screening, including skinfold body fat assessment, waist-to-hip ratio, standing diastolic blood pressure, and parotid (salivary) gland size, is a potentially better alternative than self-reported measures and similar tests because the physiological screening is designed for females. The performance of these assessments is less obvious especially if it is included in the PPE (Costello, 2018; "Psychological Issues Related to Illness and Injury," 2017).

Tips for coaches are provided in **Time Out 5.3**. However, coaches should encourage the adoption of peer-led programs, such as Athletes Targeting Healthy Exercise & Nutrition Alternatives (ATHENA). This program has been very successful in encouraging lifelong skills directed toward sustainable dietary habits. Overall, researchers conclude that education about health, performance-related nutrition, and body composition should be administered before high school (Marinsen & Sundgot-Borgen, 2013).

Treatment

Treatment of eating disorders ranges from simple counseling and education (when diagnosed in early stages) to hospitalization in severe cases. It must be remembered that, in many cases, an eating disorder may be a symptom of a psychological problem, such as depression or anxiety. Despite improved treatment programs, experts report that at least one-third of these cases do not respond to therapy. It is hoped that continued research will improve the prognosis for these individuals.

> ### WHAT IF ❓
>
> You are coaching high school track and field, and one of your players demonstrates strange eating behaviors and excessive workout patterns. Other members of the team tell you that she also weighs herself all the time. What could such behavior imply? What would be your best course of action?

Neurodevelopmental Disorders

Attention deficit hyperactivity disorder (ADHD) is abnormal levels of inattention, hyperactivity, or impulsiveness or a combination of all three that affect normal function. The disorder has mild to severe categories depending on the number of symptoms and level of impaired social and work function. Because

> **Attention deficit hyperactivity disorder (ADHD)**
> A disorder characterized by an abnormal level of inattentiveness, hyperactivity, and/or impulsiveness that interferes with social and academic function.

the symptoms of ADHD (Table 5.7) can be present in other medical conditions, it is important to accurately diagnose it (Neal et al., 2015). It should be noted that ADHD maybe treated with medications just for academics or sports or both. Even though exercise may improve ADHD symptoms, both the International Olympic Committee and World Anti-Doping Agency do not allow certain ADHD medications even though the medication is used as a therapy. Similarly, the NCAA allows an athlete to participate in sports but requires an exemption form completed by the treating physician. Lastly, certain ADHD medications may increase the risk of heat injury when participating in hot and humid environments (Putukian et al., 2011) and/or warrant the screening for anxiety and depression (Paul et al., 2018).

Table 5.7
Symptoms of Attention Deficit Hyperactivity Disorder

- Having difficulty focusing on one thing
- Easily distracted, missing details, forgetting things, and frequently switch from one activity to another
- Become bored with a test after only a few minutes unless they are doing something enjoyable
- Having difficulty focusing attention on organizing and completing a task or learning something new
- Having trouble completing or turning in homework assignments, often losing things needed to complete tasks or assignments
- Daydream, become easily confused, and move slowly
- Not appearing to listen when spoken to
- Having difficulty processing information as quickly and accurately as others
- Struggle to follow instructions
- Hyperactivity symptoms:
  - Fidget constantly
  - Be constantly in motion
  - Talk nonstop
  - Trouble sitting still during dinner, school, or traveling
  - Dash around, touching or playing with anything and everything in sight

Data from Neal, T. L., et al. (2015). Interassociation recommendations for developing a plan to recognize and refer student-athletes with psychological concerns at the secondary school level: A consensus statement. *Journal of Athletic Training, 50*(3), 231–249.

Adjustment disorder An emotional or behavioral reaction in response to specific events. It is considered unhealthy if the reaction lasts longer than 3 months.

Plan to Manage Mental Health Concerns and Role of Care Provider

Identification, referral, and treatment for depression or other mental illnesses are extremely important yet may be inhibited within athletic culture because physical injury is easier to detect, history and tradition prevent change, athletic departments may not have adequate resources, and the high-profile status of athletes may prevent them from reporting symptoms. Team dynamics also may be a factor in the recognition of mental health concerns because seeking help is often seen as a sign of weakness or failure rather than one of strength (NCAA, 2012). Athletics departments are encouraged to stay in tune with student-athletes' mental well-being by including mental health checkups, especially around high-risk times, such as the loss of a coach or teammate, significant injury, being cut from the team, or other catastrophic events.

According to the consensus statements for secondary school (Neal et al., 2015) and collegiate settings (Neal et al., 2013) published in the *Journal of Athletic Training*, it is recommended to develop a plan to address psychological concerns in athletes (Table 5.8). Developing a mental health action plan is important, especially for collegiate athletic departments because many athletes experience an **adjustment disorder** when they report to school and are away from home. Acquiring mental health histories within the overall medical history is ideal and can be accomplished during the PPE. If mental health concerns are identified during the PPE, they can be discussed with the team physician, just as would be done for a physical injury.

As mentioned previously, there are several behaviors to look out for that reflect psychological responses to events in an athlete's life (Table 5.3). If these responses are long-lasting or too intense, a timely referral to a mental health professional is warranted. It is recommended to approach athletes

Table 5.8
Plan for Managing Athletes with Mental Health Concerns

1. A mental health team, which includes the team physicians, athletic trainers, campus counseling service, community-based mental healthcare professionals, school nurses, and administrators
2. A point of contact for the counseling center
3. Guidelines for staff members who are considered mandatory reporters
4. An emergency action plan for emergent mental health referrals, such as calling the local or campus police and seeking assistance
5. A predetermined confidentiality plan to notify certain individuals under various circumstances when a referral takes place
6. Communication about this plan to athletes, parents, coaches, and others as appropriate

Data from Neal, T. L., Diamond, A. B., Goldman, S., Klossner, D., Morse, E. D., Pajak, D. E., ... Welzant, V. (2013). Inter-association recommendations for developing a plan to recognize and refer student-athletes with psychological concerns at the collegiate level: An executive summary of a consensus statement. *Journal of Athletic Training, 48*(5), 716–720; and Neal, T. L., et al. (2015). Interassociation recommendations for developing a plan to recognize and refer student-athletes with psychological concerns at the secondary school level: A consensus statement. *Journal of Athletic Training, 50*(3), 231–249.

who are displaying behaviors of mental health concerns only after facts concerning their behavior are gathered. The interaction should be empathetic and focus on the athletes as persons to encourage them to consider a mental health visit. Questions that can be asked during meetings with athletes are "How are you feeling?" "Tell me about what is going on." "Perhaps you would want to talk to someone about this." "I want to help, but this issue is beyond my education and training; I know how to refer you to someone who can help." (Neal et al., 2013). Also, during these meetings, the limits of confidentiality should be explained so the athletes understand that, if they mention emergent psychological concerns, then state laws need to be followed. Under nonemergent circumstances, a referral to a mental health professional should occur as soon as the athletes agree to be psychologically evaluated.

Review Questions

1. Briefly define several of the personality variables described in the chapter.
2. Discuss the relationship between an athlete's self-concept and the risk of sports injury.
3. Briefly describe the relationship between psychosocial variables and the risk of sports injury.
4. Discuss the possible relationship between high levels of competitive stress and the psychology of the adolescent athlete.
5. How can parents and coaches increase the psychological stress an adolescent athlete experiences?
6. Discuss the psychological impact of a sports injury on an athlete in terms of the stress model shown in the chapter.
7. List five common signs or behaviors that may indicate the development of a depressive disorder.
8. Define the acronym SAD, and discuss its implications for competitive athletes.
9. List the recommended guidelines for dealing with an injured athlete.
10. Define anorexia nervosa and bulimia nervosa.
11. True or false: Nonathletes show a greater percentage of disordered eating behaviors than do athletes.
12. True or false: Male athletes do not show significant patterns of disordered eating.
13. List several common forms of disordered eating behaviors practiced by athletes.
14. What are the female athlete triad and the male athlete triad?
15. List three ways a coach can help prevent eating disorders.

References

Aerni, G. A., & Knapp, J. (2018). The female athlete. In C. C. Madden, M. Putukian, E. C. McCarty, & C. C. Young (Eds.), *Netter's sports medicine* (2nd ed., pp. 77–84). Philadelphia, PA: Elsevier.

Bonci, C. M., Bonci, L. J., Granger, L. R., Johnson, C. L., Malina, R. M., Milne, L. W., . . . Vanderbunt, E. M. (2008). National Athletic Trainers' Association position statement: Preventing, detecting, and managing disordered eating in athletes. *Journal of Athletic Training, 43*(1), 80–108. Retrieved from http://www.nata.org/sites/default/files/Preventing DetectingAndManagingDisorderedEating.pdf

Cagle, J. A., Overcash, K. B., Rowe, D. P., & Needle, A. R. (2017). Trait anxiety as a risk factor for musculoskeletal injury in athletes: A critically appraised topic. *International Journal of Athletic Therapy and Training, 22*(3), 26–31.

Chang, C., Putukian, M., Aerni, G., Diamond, A., Hong, G., Ingram, Y., Reardon, C. L., & Wolanin, A. (2020). Mental health issues and psychological factors in athletes: Detection, management, effect on performance and prevention: American Medical Society for Sports Medicine Position Statement-Executive Summary. *British Journal of Sports Medicine, 54*(4), 216–220.

Chatterton, J. M., & Petrie, T. A. (2013). Prevalence of disordered eating and pathogenic weight control behaviors among male collegiate athletes. *Eating Disorders, 21*(4), 328–341.

Costello, L. (2018). Eating disorder in athletes. In C. C. Madden, M. Putukian, E. C. McCarty, & C. C. Young (Eds.), *Netter's sports medicine* (2nd ed., pp. 191–196). Philadelphia, PA: Elsevier.

Galima, S. V., Vogel, S. R., & Kowalski, A. W. (2020). Seasonal affective disorder: Common questions and answers. *American Family Physician, 102*(11), 668–672.

Greenleaf, C., Petrie, T. A., Carter, J., & Reel, J. (2009). Female collegiate athletes: Prevalence of eating disorders and disordered eating behaviors. *Journal of American College Health, 57*(5), 489–495.

Guo, C., Xiao, B., Zhang, Z., Dong, J., Yang, M., Shan, G., & Wan, B. (2021). Relationships between risk events, personality traits, and risk perception of adolescent athletes in sports training. *International Journal of Environmental Research and Public Health, 19*(1), 445.

Hedstrom, R. (n.d.). With a little help from my friends: Using your social support network when dealing with injury. Retrieved from http://www.appliedsportpsych.org/resource-center/injury-rehabilitation/with-a-little-help-from-my-friends/

Jayanthi, N. A., Post, E. G., Laury, T. C., & Fabricant, P. D. (2019). Health consequences of youth sport specialization. *Journal of Athletic Training, 54*(10), 1040–1049.

Kübler-Ross, E. (1969). *On death and dying*. New York, NY: Macmillan.

Lauer, L. (n.d.). Keeping perspective in youth sport. Retrieved from https://appliedsportpsych.org/resources/resources-for-parents/keeping-perspective-in-youth-sport

Madrigal, L. (2015). Psychological skills for injury prevention and recovery. *Women in Sport and Physical Activity Journal, 23*(2), 79–84.

Marinsen, M., & Sundgot-Borgen, J. (2013). Higher prevalence of eating disorders among adolescent elite athletes than controls. *Medicine & Science in Sports & Exercise, 45*(6), 1188–1197.

Mountjoy, M., Sundgot-Borgen, J., Burke, L., Carter, S., Constantini, N., Lebrun, C., . . . Ljungqvist, A. (2014). The IOC consensus statement: Beyond the female athlete triad—Relative Energy Deficiency in Sport (RED-S). *British Journal of Sports Medicine, 48*(7), 491–497.

National Alliance on Mental Illness. (n.d.). LGBTQ. Retrieved from https://www.nami.org/find-support/lgbtq

National Association of Anorexia Nervosa and Associated Disorders (ANAD). (2013). Eating disorder statistics. Retrieved from http://www.anad.org/get-information/about-eating-disorders/eating-disorders-statistics/

National Collegiate Athletic Association (NCAA). (2012). 2012–2013 NCAA sports medicine handbook. Retrieved from http://www.ncaapublications.com/productdownloads/MD12.pdf

National Collegiate Athletic Association (NCAA). (2014). Mind, body, and sport. Retrieved from http://www.ncaapublications.com/productdownloads/MindBodySport.pdf

National Collegiate Athletic Association (NCAA). (2016). Mental health best practices. Retrieved from http://www.ncaa.org/sites/default/files/HS_Mental-Health-Best-Practices_20160317.pdf

Neal, T. L., Diamond, A. B., Goldman, S., Klossner, D., Morse, E. D., Pajak, D. E., . . . Welzant, V. (2013). Inter-association recommendations for developing a plan to recognize and refer student-athletes with psychological concerns at the collegiate level: An executive summary of a consensus statement. *Journal of Athletic Training, 48*(5), 716–720.

Neal, T. L., Diamond, A. B., Goldman, S., Liedtka, K. D., Mathis, K., Morse, E. D., . . . Welzant, V. (2015). Inter-association recommendations for developing a plan to recognize and refer student-athletes with psychological concerns at the secondary school level: A consensus statement. *Journal of Athletic Training, 50*(3), 231–249.

Paul, S. R., John-Daniel, B., & Helming, B. (2018). Sports pharmacology and psychiatry and behavioral medicine. In C. C. Madden, M. Putukian, E. C. McCarty, & C. C. Young (Eds.), *Netter's sports medicine* (2nd ed., pp. 55–60). Philadelphia, PA: Elsevier.

Porter, K. (n.d.). Do's and don'ts for parents of young athletes. Retrieved from http://www.appliedsportpsych.org/resource-center/resources-for-parents/dos-and-donts-for-parents-of-young-athletes/

Psychological issues related to illness and injury in athletes and the team physician: A consensus statement-2016 update. (2017). *Medicine and Science in Sports and Exercise, 49*(5), 1043–1054.

Putukian, M., Kreher, J. B., Coppel, D. B., Glazer, J. L., McKeag, D. B., & White, R. D. (2011). Attention deficit hyperactivity disorder and the athlete: An American Medical Society for Sports Medicine position statement. *Clinical Journal of Sport Medicine, 21*(5), 392–400.

Selye, H. (1956). *The Stress of Life*. New York, NY: McGraw-Hill.

Shelley, G. A., Trowbridge, C. A., & Detling, N. (2003). Practical counseling skills for the athletic therapist. *Athletic Therapy Today, 8*(2), 57–63.

Stirling, A., & Kerr, G. (2012). Development of disordered eating behaviours. *European Journal of Sport Science, 12*(3), 262–273.

Tranaeus, U., Ivarsson, A., & Johnson, U. (2015). Evaluation of the effects of psychological prevention interventions on sports injuries: A meta-analysis. *Science & Sports, 30*(6), 305–313.

U.S. Department of Health and Human Services. (n.d.). Mental health and mental disorders. Retrieved from https://www.healthypeople.gov/2020/data-search/Search-the-Data#objid=4813

Weiss, M. R., & Troxel, R. K. (1986). Psychology of the injured athlete. *Journal of Athletic Training, 21*(2), 104–109.

Williams, J. M., & Andersen, M. B. (1998). Psychological antecedents of sport injury: Review and critique of the stress and injury model. *Journal of Applied Sport Psychology, 10*(1), 5–25.

Wolanin, A., Hong, E., Marks, D., Panchoo, K., & Gross, M. (2016). Prevalence of clinically elevated depressive symptoms in college athletes and differences by gender and sport. *British Journal of Sports Medicine, 50*(3), 167–171.

CHAPTER 6
Nutritional Considerations

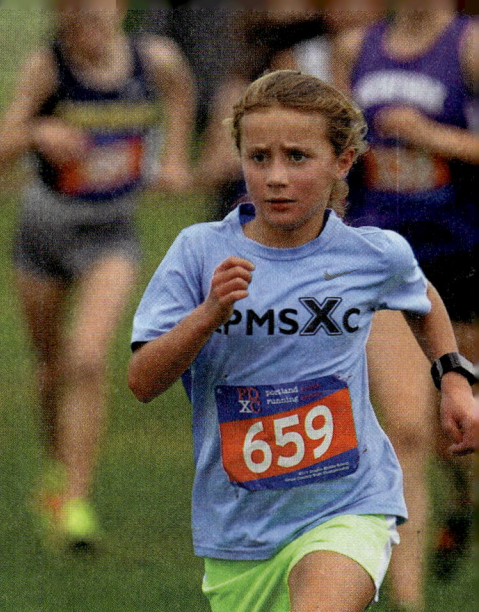

MAJOR CONCEPTS

Research shows that, regardless of the sport, an athlete's diet plays a critical, if not essential, role in performance, yet misinformation and misconceptions persist among coaches and athletes regarding what constitutes an adequate diet. This chapter first examines available evidence concerning the dietary knowledge and practices of coaches and athletes. It next outlines dietary recommendations for healthy eating, including the roles of carbohydrate, protein, fat, vitamins, and minerals. Precompetition, competition, and postcompetition nutrition are also explored, as well as the nutritional requirements during injury rehabilitation. Special attention is given to females, endurance, strength/power, and team sport athletes, as well as the sport of wrestling. Wrestling has been plagued with the problem of athletes attempting to lose body weight rapidly by dehydration, so a simple method is provided to assess an athlete's ability to maintain a healthy weight and rehydrate adequately. This chapter concludes with a brief discussion regarding ergogenic aids (i.e., nutritional supplements and pharmacological substances) commonly used in sports.

Proper nutritional knowledge is imperative for all individuals but especially for those involved in athletic competitions (Fink & Mikesky, 2021). An athlete's diet has a direct impact on performance; recovery from training and competition; resistance to environmental extremes; recovery from injury; immune system function; and, to some extent, likelihood of injury. In essence, diet influences virtually all aspects of sports participation.

Yet research over time has demonstrated that both coaches and athletes are largely uneducated regarding proper nutrition (Riviere et al., 2021; Torres-McGehee et al., 2012). Torres-McGehee and colleagues (2012) reported that only 39.5% of Division I coaches scored above 75% on a nutritional knowledge test that included questions about macronutrients, micronutrients, hydration, supplements and performance, and weight control and eating disorders. These data support the premise that many coaches are ill-prepared to provide good nutritional counsel to their athletes. Torres-McGehee and colleagues (2012) further substantiated these reports and opinions by demonstrating that, in a sample of 185 Division I, II, and III athletes, only 9% scored above the correct answer benchmark (75% of questions correct) on a nutritional knowledge test. The good news is that there are knowledgeable individuals within athletic departments. Board of Certification (BOC)–certified athletic trainers and certified strength and conditioning specialists were the most knowledgeable regarding nutrition (Torres-McGehee et al., 2012). In a narrative review, Riviere et al. (2021) suggest that sports nutritional knowledge among college athletes is poor, as athletes tend to look to coaches for knowledge and their knowledge does not meet current recommendations. Although the number of registered dietitians in collegiate settings has quadrupled in the last several years, more knowledgeable athletes and improved outcomes is the goal.

Nutrients: An Overview

The following section provides an overview of the fundamental concepts of nutrition and is presented as a basis for the chapter content that follows. According to the Academy of Nutrition and Dietetics, eating correctly for sports performance will (a) help the athlete train longer and at a higher intensity, (b) delay the onset of fatigue, (c) promote recovery, (d) help the athlete's body adapt to workouts, (e) improve body composition and strength, (f) enhance concentration, (g) help maintain healthy immune function, (h) reduce the chance of injury, and (i) reduce the risk of heat illness.

Although a comprehensive investigation of all topics related to nutrition is beyond the scope of this chapter, an overview of caloric intake and the cost of activity plus a review of both **macronutrients** (required in large amounts) and **micronutrients** (required in small, or trace, amounts) is provided. Carbohydrate, protein, and fat are the macronutrients, and each of them is important in the diet. The mix of these macronutrients may change based on the type of sport, fitness levels, exercise goals, and personal food preferences. Vitamins and minerals are the micronutrients that contribute to metabolic reactions and tissue structure. And, finally, water, which is essential for substrate transport, waste removal, and joint health, is also discussed (Fink & Mikesky, 2021).

Energy Expenditure

Energy expenditure is the energy needed to sustain (a) **resting metabolic rate (RMR)**, or the energy used for basic physiology during rest, such as breathing; (b) **thermal effect of food (TEF)**, or the energy used to process food; and (c) **thermal effect of activity (TEA)**, or the energy used for nonrest activities. Approximately 60–75% of total energy expenditure is used to maintain basic functions, or the RMR. Oftentimes **basal metabolic rate (BMR)**, or the amount of energy needed to sustain functioning at rest, is used interchangeably with RMR; however, BMR is typically calculated 12–18 hours after no exercise and tends to be slightly lower than RMR (Fink & Mikesky, 2021). Those with larger surface areas and increased lean muscle mass tend to have a higher RMR. RMR is usually consistent for an individual but varies greatly between individuals. During periods of injury, growth, illness, and extreme temperature environments, energy expenditure increases (Fink & Mikesky, 2021).

A proper nutrition plan begins with an assessment of the athlete's **total daily energy expenditure (TDEE)** based on his or her age, height, and current weight and should include the extra energy needed to sustain physical activity. To begin, the athlete's baseline energy needs should be calculated using a standardized equation. The goal of the calculation is to predict the energy needs for 24 hours in kilocalories (kcal), or **Calories**. The two most commonly used

---

Macronutrients Carbohydrates, proteins, and fats that provide calories for our energy needs.

Micronutrients Essential vitamins and minerals required in very small amounts for our body functions but that do not have caloric value or provide direct energy.

Resting metabolic rate (RMR) The minimal amount of energy needed to meet the body's demands at rest (calculated hours after a meal or exercise and is usually slightly higher than BMR).

Thermal effect of food (TEF) The energy used to process food.

Thermal effect of activity (TEA) The energy used for nonrest activities.

Basal metabolic rate (BMR) The amount of energy needed to sustain functioning at rest (calculated after 12–18 hours of no exercise).

Total daily energy expenditure (TDEE) An estimation of calories burned per day when exercise is taken into account.

Calorie Kilocalorie; unit of energy equal to 1,000 calories.

equations are the **Harris–Benedict equation** or the World Health Organization (WHO) equation. The product of these equation is called the **resting energy expenditure (REE)**, or the basic energy needs, which accounts for approximately 60–75% of energy expenditure. The following equation is the Harris-Benedict method for adult males and females:

Female REE = 655 + (9.6 × weight [kg]) + (1.8 × height [cm]) − (4.7 × age [years])

Male REE = 66.5 + (13.7 × weight [kg]) + (5 × height [cm]) − (6.8 × age [years])

The following equation is the WHO method for males and females ages 19–30 years:

Male REE = (15.3 × weight [kg]) + 679

Females REE = (14.7 × weight [kg]) + 496

The REE value is the Calories needed to maintain physiological function at rest. A Calorie, commonly referred to as a kilocalorie (kcal), is the energy equivalent required to raise the temperature of 1 kg of water through 1°C, whereas a calorie (lowercase c) is the energy required to raise the temperature of 1 g of water through 1°C.

After acquiring the REE value, the next step is to calculate the TDEE, which is the REE adjusted relative to the level of general activity or exercise. To adjust the REE by accounting for the energy used by nonrest activity, multiply the REE value by an activity factor. The activity factor is based on a person's lifestyle (extremely inactive, sedentary, moderately active, vigorously active, or extremely active), and the values typically range from 1–2.4. The lower the value, the more sedentary an individual is; the higher the value, the more active an individual is (Fink & Mikesky, 2021). Lastly, the TEF is estimated and added to the calculated TDEE. The TEF is determined by taking 10% of TDEE. If a person's TDEE is 3,000 Calories, then the TEF would be 300 Calories per day (Fink & Mikesky, 2021). Therefore, the total Calories needed per day would be 3,300 (TDEE + TEF).

For example, a 24-year-old male athlete who weighs 180 lb (81.8 kg) and is 5 ft 11 in. (180.3 cm) tall would require 1,925.46 Calories a day at rest: [1,925.46 = 66.5 + (13.7 × 81.8) + (5 × 180.3) − (6.8 × 24)] (Fink & Mikesky, 2021). Our 24-year-old male athlete is highly active, doing 1–1.5 hours/day of high-intensity training. His activity factor would be 2.0, and his daily Caloric need is 3,850 [1,925.46 × 2]. After calculating his TEF, his total daily Calories needed are 4,235 (3,850 + 385). Remember that this is just an estimate for his current weight and activity level because there are many prediction formulas as well as direct and indirect calorimetry methods used in hospitals and research labs. It is important to also remember that this is just one part of the nutrition plan that needs to be personalized to meet the athlete's unique needs for his or her sport, goals, food preferences, medical conditions, and lifestyle (ACSM, 2016; Fink & Mikesky, 2021).

Weight Loss

Weight loss for athletes and nonathletes includes a plan of calorie deficit, increased exercise, or both, and the loss should be slow, 1–2 pounds per week (Fink & Mikesky, 2021) or 1% of body weight per week (ACSM, 2016), with the end weight goal falling within 5–10% loss of their current body weight. This loss should be maintained for 3–6 months before additional weight loss is attempted. Specific to athletes, the weight loss program should occur out of season or before the season starts, and include a good balance of macronutrients with a slight increase in protein. Additionally, the portion and timing of meals is also important to the athlete during weight loss (Aragon et al., 2017; Hector & Phillips, 2018).

Unfortunately, weight-sensitive sports such as gymnastics and wrestling may use rapid, short-term weight loss strategies that are not ideal. These strategies include hypohydration (water deficit), decreased glycogen stores, and pathological methods (e.g., purging, starving, and excessively exercising) (ACSM, 2016).

Once weight loss is determined to be the plan for the athlete, a goal weight or body fat percentage should be calculated by nutrition professionals based on the individual's **body mass index (BMI)**, waist-to-hip ratio

---

Harris–Benedict equation Equation used to calculate resting energy expenditure.

Resting energy expenditure (REE) Energy used to maintain basic physiologic function, which accounts for approximately 60–75% of energy expenditure.

Body mass index (BMI) A value derived from a person's height and weight that indicates nutritional status.

(WHR), and other factors such as body fat percentage, sport, position, medical conditions, and lifestyle (Fink & Mikesky, 2021). BMI is a measurement based on height and weight (mass [kg]/ height [cm]^2) to determine health status. BMI is not gender specific; however, it correlates well to body fatness. BMI values of 18.5–24.9 kg/cm^2 are considered healthy and a value of 25 kg/cm^2 or greater is considered overweight or obese. The distribution of body fat is also valuable information for the nutrition professional, and one way of assessing this is WHR, where abdominal circumference is compared to hip girth and a description of body shape (i.e., apple [WHR > 1] or pear [WHR < 1]) is assigned. Athletes with apple shapes have more body fat located around the abdominal area and are at higher risk for cardiovascular disease, diabetes, and hypertension then people with pear shapes (i.e., more body fat located in the hip region).

While BMI and WHR are noninvasive, inexpensive, and may be the only tools most athletes have at their disposal, those athletes with higher muscle mass will have an elevated BMI because muscle weighs more than fat. Therefore, body fat percentage and fat distribution data will provide more accurate analysis of their overall health and sport needs (Fink & Mikesky, 2021).

There are various ways to measure **body composition**, or how much of the body is made of muscle, fat, or minerals. Most of these methods need expensive equipment to perform, and a full discussion of them is beyond the scope of this textbook. Skinfold assessment is the most affordable method; it estimates subcutaneous fat by measuring a pinch of skin and fat in several areas of the body and then utilizes prediction equations to determine overall percentage of body fat. These values have been found to accurately predict percent body fat within 3–4% of other sophisticated methods (Fink & Mikesky, 2021; Thomas et al., 2016).

Healthy body fat ranges for normal, nonathletic populations have been suggested to be 10–20% for males and 20–30% for females, and athletic populations tend to have lower percentages, such as 5–19% for males and 7–20% for females, depending on the sport. It must be emphasized that there is no ideal percentage of body fat for a specific sport but success in certain sports may benefit from having low or high body fat percentages (Fink & Mikesky, 2021). Two athletes can have very different percentages of body fat but weigh the same on the scale and be the same height, and an athlete trying to lose weight may not see a change on the scale but is changing his or her body composition. For these scenarios and others, monitoring percentage of body fat is valuable information.

Ideally, current percentage of body fat data should be used to determine goals, but BMI data can be used as well by using a BMI chart and choosing the weight that represents one or more points below the athlete's current BMI. The goal value should also adhere to the general guidelines of 5–10% loss of current body weight.

To calculate goal weight, athletes should be encouraged to use the following formulas from the NATA position statement (Turocy et al., 2011):

Current % body fat — Desired % body fat = Nonessential body fat %

Current body weight × Nonessential body fat (decimal format) % = Nonessential fat (lb)

Current body weight — Nonessential fat (lb) = Ideal body weight (lb)

Once the goal weight and body fat percentage are decided, energy needs are determined as described in the previous section. Next, reduce the value of the caloric needs by 250–1,000 Calories per day. This caloric restriction has a large range to allow flexibility in the weight loss plan based on how the athlete feels and what he or she can accomplish in the given scenario. According to Aragon et al. (2017) and Hector and Phillips (2018), athletes may need to increase their protein intake beyond recommended standards to support weight loss and improve athletic performance during calorie restriction. This is best accomplished by consuming protein throughout the day, as opposed to a large amount during a meal. Many athletes and nonathletes assume cutting a lot of calories will result in greater and faster weight loss; however, this will typically cause hunger, leading to reduced adherence to the program, and a change in metabolic rate making it harder to lose weight. Creating the calorie deficit from increased exercise may lead to injury. Therefore, calorie reduction of 250–500 calories per day and increased exercise is likely to result in weight loss of 1–2 pounds per week

Body composition The makeup of the body divided into lean body weight, or fat free mass, and fat.

(Fink & Mikesky, 2021). Athletes can monitor their weight weekly and their body fat percentage monthly so appropriate changes and guidance can be made.

Energy Systems

A very important topic related to nutrition is the energy systems or ways humans consume food to create energy. The plants use the sun to create carbohydrate, protein, and fat; when humans consume plants, they break them down, more specifically, break the chemical bonds of molecules so they can be absorbed and transported into our cells to make **adenosine triphosphate (ATP)**. ATP is stored energy for our bodies, so the more ATP in our bodies, the more potential energy for activity. When ATP is broken down, energy is released. There are three ways the body creates energy, or ATP. The first is called the **immediate energy system**; it is the fastest and easiest way to create energy, but it does not yield plentiful amounts of ATP. Our muscle cells store small amounts of ATP for quick bursts of activity lasting a few seconds, such as bursting out of the starting blocks. As a protective mechanism, our muscle cells will fatigue or decrease activity to spare levels of limited ATP storage, but our bodies have ways of replenishing these ATP stores. It is important to note that poor nutrition negatively affects ATP stores (Fink & Mikesky, 2021).

Activity lasts longer than a few seconds, so the body must find another way to create energy. The next two energy systems take more time to create ATP, but they will yield more ATP than the immediate energy system. The second energy system is called the **anaerobic system**; it uses only carbohydrate without utilizing oxygen to create ATP. This system will fuel activity for about 1–3 minutes, such as a 400-m run. The third way to create ATP is called the **aerobic system**; it uses carbohydrate, protein, fat, and oxygen. The aerobic system takes the longest to create ATP, but it provides fuel for resting metabolic needs and long-duration exercise because it can make unlimited amounts of ATP (Fink & Mikesky, 2021). The body prefers to use carbohydrate and fat for most energy production, whereas protein is not a normal source of energy unless not enough energy can be made from carbohydrate (Fink & Mikesky, 2021). Because carbohydrate is used in both the anaerobic and aerobic systems, it is important for athletes of all types. It is also important to note that these three systems work in concert with each other, meaning that while one system may be working more than the others, depending on the intensity and duration of exercise, the other systems are still working (Fink & Mikesky, 2021).

Carbohydrate

Carbohydrate consists of carbon, hydrogen, and oxygen atoms, with the number of carbon atoms ranging from three to seven. Carbohydrate consists of molecules that, by way of their metabolic breakdown, provide energy for high-intensity exercise. The specific forms of carbohydrate used within the body are glucose, found in the blood, and glycogen (the storage form of glucose), found in the liver and skeletal muscle. Carbohydrates fall into three categories based on the complexity of the molecule. The simplest forms of carbohydrate are the **monosaccharides** (a single molecule), which include sugars such as fructose, glucose, and galactose. The next group is the **disaccharides** (two monosaccharide molecules combined), which include commonly known sugars such as lactose (milk sugar), sucrose (the most common form of sugar in the diet), and maltose. And, last, the **polysaccharides**,

---

Adenosine triphosphate (ATP) The molecule that is the body's direct source of energy.

Immediate energy system The energy system that produces ATP at the fastest rate. Also known as the phosphagen system.

Anaerobic system An energy system that makes ATP and lactic acid without oxygen.

Aerobic system An energy system that makes ATP with the use of oxygen.

Carbohydrate A macronutrient consisting of carbon, hydrogen, and oxygen atoms that provides energy for high-intensity exercise.

Monosaccharide Simplest form of sugar and the basic unit of carbohydrate. Includes fructose, glucose, and galactose.

Disaccharide Two monosaccharide molecules combined; include lactose (milk sugar), sucrose, and maltose.

Polysaccharide Many, up to thousands, of monosaccharides linked together; examples include glycogen, starch, and cellulose (fiber).

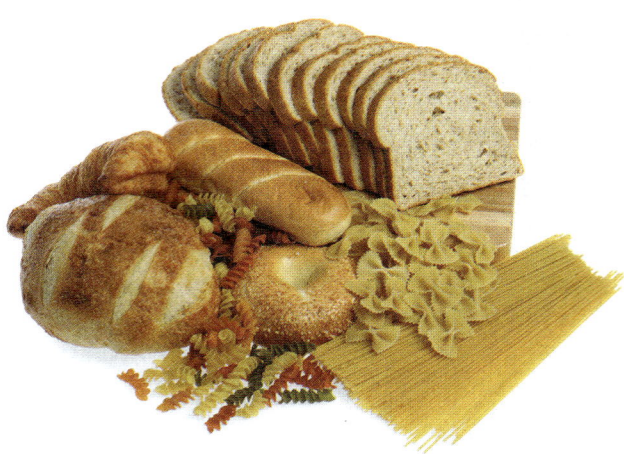

Figure 6.1 Carbohydrate primarily comes from grains, beans, fruits, and vegetables.
© Hurst Photo/Shutterstock.

which are 10 to thousands of monosaccharides linked together and include compounds such as glycogen, starch, and cellulose (dietary fiber).

The majority of dietary carbohydrate is derived from plant sources, primarily grains, seeds, fruits, and vegetables (Figure 6.1). In a practical context, carbohydrate is classified as either simple (monosaccharides) or complex (di- or polysaccharides). The most common form of dietary carbohydrate intake for some is from simple sugars, primarily from foods high in sucrose, such as soft drinks, candies, and cereals (high in sugar). Although high in caloric content, these foods stimulate insulin release, cause fluctuations in blood glucose (blood sugar) levels, and provide little in the way of other nutrients; therefore, they are often referred to as "empty calorie" foods.

In general, **complex carbohydrates** contain more nutrients and fiber than **simple carbohydrates**.

Complex carbohydrates Polysaccharides that contain more nutrients and fiber compared to simple carbohydrate.

Simple carbohydrates Monosaccharides.

Fiber Nondigestible carbohydrate.

Glycemic index (GI) A rating based on how quickly carbohydrates are digested and absorbed into the bloodstream. The quicker the blood glucose rises, the higher the rating.

A superior form of dietary carbohydrate is derived from eating more complex carbohydrates from sources such as whole grains, vegetables, and fruits. The carbohydrate in these foods is in the form of starch found in the cereals and breads or cellulose found in leaves, stems, roots, seeds, and coverings of plants. An added benefit of consuming complex carbohydrate is that it typically contains **fiber** (nondigestible carbohydrate), which may lower cholesterol absorption and is beneficial to the digestive tract. Daily fiber intake should be between 21 and 38 grams (g) depending on gender and age. When fiber is consumed in excess, it may cause bloating and flatulence, which can interfere with training and competition (Fink & Mikesky, 2021).

Another excellent source of carbohydrate is fruit, which can provide a significant amount of carbohydrate in the form of fructose. Fructose, a monosaccharide, is much sweeter than sucrose; however, the benefit of fructose is that it does not stimulate pancreatic insulin secretion and, as a result, helps to stabilize blood-glucose and insulin levels (Fink & Mikesky, 2021). An added benefit of whole grains, fruits, and vegetables is that they typically contain a wide variety of other nutrients and, as such, help provide a balanced diet.

Although the classifications of simple and complex carbohydrate often are suitable to describe foods containing carbohydrate, these classifications do not represent the ways simple and complex carbohydrates are hydrolyzed and absorbed by the body. Foods are also classified as producing either high, moderate, or low glycemic response or impact on the body, and are often classified regarding how fast they are oxidized. Foods classified as having a high glycemic response are quickly oxidized (~60 g/hour) and typically result in a large and rapid rise in blood glucose and insulin, followed by a rapid decrease in blood glucose. Foods with a slower oxidation rate (~30 g/hour) and a lower glycemic response cause a steadier rise and decline in blood glucose and insulin. Low glycemic index carbohydrate improves diabetes management, reduces the risk of heart disease, reduces hunger, reduces gastrointestinal distress during exercise, and prolongs physical endurance, whereas high glycemic carbohydrate helps refuel carbohydrate stores after exercise and may cause gastrointestinal distress during exercise. Table 6.1 provides a short list of foods sorted according to **glycemic index (GI)** (rating

Table 6.1

Glycemic Index (GI) for Foods

High Glycemic Index Foods (GI > 70)		
White bread	Muesli	Baked or mashed potatoes
Rice cakes, English muffin, or bagel	Pretzels	Watermelons
Grape Nuts™, Corn Flakes™, Cheerios™	Sport drinks	Hard candy
Moderate Glycemic Index Foods (GI = 56–69)		
100% whole-wheat bread, pita bread	Brown or wild rice	Bananas (ripe)
Sweet potato	Oatmeal (quick oats)	Sweet corn
Mini Wheats™, Raisin Bran™, Froot Loops™	Raisins	Popcorn
Low Glycemic Index Foods (GI < 55)		
Oatmeal (rolled or steel cut)	Barley and bulgur	Carrots
Most fruits, including apples, grapes, oranges, and pears	Peas, legumes, and lentils	Milk (all types)
Yam	All Bran™ cereal	Yogurt (most types)

Glycemic index data from Glycemic index. (2017). Retrieved from http://www.glycemicindex.com; and American Diabetes Association. (2014). Glycemic index and diabetes. Retrieved from http://www.diabetes.org/food-and-fitness/food/what-can-i-eat/understanding-carbohydrates/glycemic-index-and-diabetes.html?loc=ff-slabnav

based on white bread = 100). It has been established that consuming lower glycemic index foods is associated with a lower risk of cardiovascular disease (Jenkins et al., 2021). For more information, please refer to the 4th Edition of the International Tables of Glycemic Index and Glycemic Load Values.

Muscles require carbohydrate as a fuel source during exercise. For the general population, the recommended proportion of carbohydrate in the diet should range between 45% and 65% of the total calories consumed daily. Active children and adolescents ages 8–18 are advised to intake 1800–3200 kcals/day (Dietary Guidelines Advisory Committee, 2018). Exercise frequency and intensity, competitive event schedule, environment, personal preference, and medical conditions can increase or decrease these amounts (Fink & Mikesky, 2021). Regardless of the type of carbohydrate consumed (Table 6.1), it all provides approximately 4 kcal per gram of carbohydrate. The average person stores approximately 1,600–2,400 kcal of carbohydrate, the majority of which is in the form of muscle and liver glycogen, with a small portion available as blood glucose (Fink & Mikesky, 2021). All individuals need to consume carbohydrate to maintain body functions and support exercise; however, athletes engaging in intense activities need to consume carbohydrate at greater levels than sedentary individuals. Recommendations have also included the type of carbohydrate (rapid or slow oxidizing) and the importance of nutritional counseling. See recommendations for intake based on exercise duration in Table 6.2.

Carbohydrate (Glycogen) Loading

As stated earlier, the majority of carbohydrate in the body is stored in the skeletal muscles and liver in the form of glycogen. Physiologically, it is to the athlete's advantage if the total amount of stored glycogen can be increased before a competition. Athletes involved in aerobic sports, especially those with durations in excess of 60 minutes, benefit the most from an increased level of stored glycogen and may carbohydrate load to prepare for competitions.

Table 6.2
Recommended Carbohydrate Intake Based on Exercise Duration

Exercise Duration	Amount/Type of Carbohydrate Needed During Exercise
More than 45–75 minutes of high-intensity exercise	Very little needed above daily needs. During exercise a mouth rinse of a carbohydrate solution (e.g., sports drink) is even effective.
1–2.5 hours of endurance or aerobic sports	30–60 g carbohydrate/hour of exercise
More than 2.5–3 hours of ultra-endurance exercise	Up to 90 g carbohydrate/hour of exercise

Data from Thomas, D. T., Erdman, K. A., & Burke, L. M. (2016). American College of Sports Medicine joint position statement: Nutrition and athletic performance. *Medicine & Science in Sports & Exercise, 48*(3), 543–568.

Early procedures for **carbohydrate loading** were particularly Spartan in nature, requiring multiple days of intense exercise (depletion phase) combined with dietary restriction of carbohydrate intake. Ironically, although such protocols often did result in an increase in stored glycogen, the negative impacts often outweighed the benefits to performance. The adverse effects included severe physical fatigue associated with the depletion phase along with negative emotional changes, such as hyperirritability. Modified, less draconian versions of carbohydrate loading have been developed and found to be highly effective in elevating stored glycogen levels well above what can be achieved by consuming a high-carbohydrate diet. Research verifies that a properly executed regimen of carbohydrate loading can boost the level of stored glycogen from the normal of 1.7 g of glycogen per 100 g of muscle tissue to 4 to 5 g of glycogen per 100 g of muscle tissue. A typical modified regimen begins approximately 1 week before the competition and includes a gradual tapering of physical activity accompanied with a slight increase in carbohydrate ingestion. Exercise (75% maximal oxygen consumption [VO_2 max]) over the first 3 days follows a steady decline in total time (1.5 hours/day to 40 minutes) while carbohydrate consumption is maintained at 50% of total caloric intake. Over the next 3 days, exercise time is decreased to about 10–15 minutes while carbohydrate consumption is increased to 75% of total caloric intake. A normal protein and fat intake is maintained. A high-carbohydrate meal is then consumed on the day of the competition (McArdle et al., 2009). However, a problem related to carbohydrate loading is that, for every gram of carbohydrate stored, an additional 3 g of water is also stored. As such, the process of carbohydrate loading results in an overall increase in body weight that, in sports, such as distance running, may represent a performance detriment. For this reason, some athletes may consume 50–70% of calories from carbohydrate daily close to an event to fill muscle stores without changing eating habits (Fink & Mikesky, 2021).

Protein

As with carbohydrate, **protein** also contains carbon, hydrogen, and oxygen atoms in its molecules and provides 4 kcal per gram of protein. However, protein also includes nitrogen, and, as such, it is a unique molecule compared to the other nutrients. Protein molecules are assembled by combining **amino acids** using peptide bonds to form large, complex molecules. There are 20 amino acids available in the body. The majority of the body's amino acids build protein that is mostly found in muscle and connective tissues.

The body builds protein from the amino acids that are available from the protein that is consumed in the diet. Of the 20 amino acids required to construct the body's protein, 9 of them cannot be synthesized by the body and must, therefore, be ingested in the diet;

Carbohydrate loading A nutritional technique used to maximize the volume of stored carbohydrate in the muscle and liver to improve performance.

Protein In terms of the diet, a macronutrient consisting of carbon, hydrogen, oxygen, and nitrogen; mainly found in connective and muscle tissue, there are 20 different types of amino acids which can be combined to form a protein.

Amino acids Building blocks of proteins.

they are known as the **essential amino acids**—histidine, isoleucine, leucine, lysine, methionine, phenylalanine, threonine, tryptophan, and valine. They are also called **branched chain amino acids (BCAAs)**. The best dietary sources of the essential amino acids are eggs, meats, and dairy products, all known as **complete proteins** (Figure 6.2). **Incomplete proteins** are those that lack one or more of the essential amino acids, yet it does not mean they are inadequate. They include plant foods (e.g., legumes, grains, fruits, vegetables, nuts, and seeds). However, soy is a complete plant protein. Athletes who are on vegetarian diets must eat foods in the correct combination to provide all the essential amino acids. A solution to the problem is for vegetarian athletes to include soy products or either eggs (ovo vegetarian), milk products (lacto vegetarian), or both (ovo-lacto vegetarian) to ensure adequate supplies of essential amino acids. Vegans, who do not eat any animal products, need to complement their protein to ensure essential amino acids are consumed in the same meal or the same day. To do this, foods lacking in a specific amino acid are paired with other foods containing the needed amino acid so the combination of the two results in consumption of the essential amino acids. For example, eating grains and beans is a common combination, as is beans and nuts and seeds. For example, a spinach salad with garbanzo beans and sunflower seeds will have complementary protein (Fink & Mikesky, 2021).

Other than building muscle and contributing to structures of nails, bones, ligaments, and hormones, protein regulates cell function, assists in maintaining fluid and acid-base balance, transports substances, makes enzymes, assists in immune function in the form of antibodies, and serves as an energy source when absolutely needed. Only about 5% of protein is converted for energy during exercise, and up to 10–15% of protein is converted for energy during ultra-long endurance events (Fink & Mikesky, 2021). Without adequate protein in the diet, cellular structures and enzymes cannot be maintained, immune function is compromised, swelling occurs, lactic acid is not buffered, and hemoglobin levels are lowered. The body prefers to use carbohydrate and fat for energy at rest and during exercise, but, if that energy is low or depleted with high-energy expenditure and/or inadequate calorie intake (starvation or low-calorie diets), protein is converted to glucose for energy. To avoid using protein for energy, adequate amounts of protein should be consumed based on body weight, age, diet composition, exercise intensity and duration, and training status. Generally, strength athletes and youths/teens need more protein in their diet than others need (Fink & Mikesky, 2021; Table 6.3).

Protein Supplementation

Today, there is a huge commercial market for what are commonly known as protein supplements, often sold at health-food stores, grocery chains, and sporting goods stores and through mail order and the internet. Most of these products consist of meat by-products (e.g., whey, casein, egg, and beef), which are processed into a powder form that is then mixed with water or some other liquid and consumed orally. Unfortunately, because these products are marketed as food supplements, their purity is not monitored by the U.S. Food and Drug Administration (FDA). In addition, many of them are extremely expensive on a per-pound basis, often exceeding the cost of more common sources of protein, such as meat and dairy products, as well as contain additional ingredients, such as artificial sweeteners and colors, that may not only be harmful

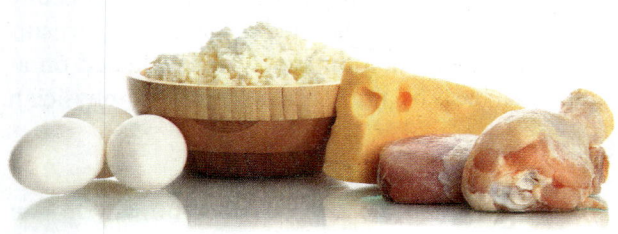

Figure 6.2 Protein comes from both animal and plant sources.
©Africa Studio/Shutterstock.

Essential amino acids Nine amino acids (histidine, isoleucine, leucine, lysine, methionine, phenylalanine, threonine, tryptophan, and valine) that the body cannot make and therefore must obtain from the diet.

Branched chain amino acids (BCAAs) Essential amino acids.

Complete protein A protein that contains all 9 essential amino acids (e.g., meat, dairy, eggs, and soy).

Incomplete protein A protein that lacks one or more of the essential amino acids. This does not imply that they are inadequate or not needed in the diet.

Table 6.3
Recommended Daily Protein Intake

Type Person	Daily Protein Intake
Vegetarians (sedentary)	0.9–1 g/kg of body mass (0.41–0.45 g/lb of body weight); usually calculate needs on higher end of range due to incomplete protein intake
General population (sedentary)	0.8–1 g/kg of body mass (0.36–0.45 g/lb of body weight)
Team sport athletes	1.2–1.6 g/kg of body mass (0.55–0.72 g/lb of body weight)
Endurance athletes	1.2–2 g/kg of body mass (0.55–0.9 g/lb of body weight)
Strength athletes	1.4–2 g/kg of body mass (0.64–0.9 g/lb of body weight); 2 g/kg maximum

Data from Torres-McGehee, T., Pritchett, K., Zippel, D., Minton, D., Cellamare, A., & Sibilia, M. (2012). Sports nutrition knowledge among collegiate athletes, coaches, athletic trainers, and strength and conditioning specialists. *Journal of Athletic Training, 47*(2), 205–211. Retrieved from http://www.natajournals.org/doi/pdf/10.4085/1062-6050-47.2.205; and Fink, H. H., & Mikesky, A. E. (2021). *Practical applications in sports nutrition* (6th ed.). Burlington, MA: Jones & Bartlett Learning.

to health (allergies) but also produce positive drug tests (Fink & Mikesky, 2021).

Because dietary protein is associated with building muscle mass, many athletes are curious about the benefits of extra protein consumption beyond that found in their regular diets, in part, due to heavy marketing by companies. However, at least two problems are associated with the practice of consuming additional protein. The first is that many sources of dietary protein also contain a large amount of saturated fat, such as beef and pork products. The second problem is that in certain cases the body may be unable to eliminate the by-products of excess protein breakdown efficiently, and, as a result, organs such as the liver and kidney are stressed (Fink & Mikesky, 2021). Muscle mass does not increase simply by eating high-protein foods or special preparations of amino acids. To gain muscle mass and strength, muscles need to be exercised against resistance for a period of time as well as consuming proper nutrition (e.g., carbohydrate and protein; Hector & Phillips, 2018). At present, available research indicates athletes involved in intense training, particularly strength training, need to consume between 1.2 g and 2 g of protein per day for each kilogram of body mass (Fink & Mikesky, 2021), whereas the sedentary person or light exerciser needs to consume only 0.83–1.2 g per kilogram. A more complete listing is provided in Table 6.3. To put this into a practical context, the calculated protein requirement for a 60-kg (132-lb) athlete involved in moderate to heavy training would be 72–108 g per day. Eight ounces of broiled salmon provides approximately 62 g of protein, 8 oz of lean sirloin steak provides approximately 65 g of protein, and 8 oz of skinless chicken breast yields a little over 70 g of protein. It can be seen that adequate protein to meet the daily requirements of an athlete in heavy training can easily be achieved through meals without the need of additional supplements. Protein intake should be 12–20% of total daily calories and should not exceed 35% of total daily calories (Fink & Mikesky, 2021). Growing infants and children, pregnant or nursing women, or adults suffering from certain disease or injury states likely may need to consume more than the recommended amount. Protein supplement implementation should be evaluated on an individual basis by a registered dietician or physician.

Fat A macronutrient consisting of carbon, hydrogen, and oxygen atoms that provides energy for low-intensity, long-duration exercise.

Lipids Fat molecules classified as triglycerides, phospholipids, and sterols.

Fat

Fat, like carbohydrate, consists of carbon, hydrogen, and oxygen atoms; however, the ratio of hydrogen to oxygen is far greater in fat than in carbohydrate. Fats are molecules called **lipids** and are classified as triglycerides, phospholipids, and sterols based on their molecular structure. **Triglycerides**, or simple lipids made of glycerol and three fatty acids, make up 98% of lipids found in food and are the most common in the body. They provide a major source of stored energy primarily in adipose tissue and are also found in muscle and liver, where their energy is faster to access during exercise. Beyond providing energy, triglycerides provide protection to organs, by thermally insulating the body as subcutaneous fat, and carry substances throughout the blood. These simple fats can be either saturated or unsaturated. **Saturated fat** means that a hydrogen atom occupies all the available bonding sites on the fatty acid molecule. Most dietary sources of saturated fat are derived from animal sources (e.g., beef, pork, poultry, and dairy products) and are generally solid at room temperature. **Unsaturated fat**, as the term implies, is structured in such a way as to prevent all the available bonding sites from being occupied by a hydrogen atom. The majority of unsaturated fat exists as a liquid at room temperature. Unsaturated fat exists in two forms, monounsaturated and polyunsaturated. **Monounsaturated fat** molecules include a single site on the carbon chain where a double bond exists, thus preventing hydrogen atoms from bonding at that site. **Polyunsaturated fat** has two or more double bonds and, as such, has at least two sites that cannot be occupied by hydrogen atoms. Last, the food industry may add additional hydrogen atoms to unsaturated fat in a process called **hydrogenation** to make unsaturated oils more desirable for baking and cooking. The result of this process is a fat called **trans fat**; it should be kept to a minimum because of its negative association with cardiovascular health (Fink & Mikesky, 2021).

Phospholipids are found in foods such as egg yolks, peanuts, and soybeans; they are not essential to the diet because the body can make them if needed. Their unique molecular structure allows them to be both water and fat soluble, and they are located mostly in cell membranes of the body that provide transport functions.

Last are **sterols**, which do not contain fatty acid chains like the other lipids; rather, they are primarily made of carbon and hydrogen atoms. The most notable sterol is **cholesterol**. Cholesterol has important functions, such as in the production of vitamin D and steroid hormones such as estrogen, and providing cell membrane structure, especially in brain and nervous tissue. Cholesterol is also a nonessential nutrient because the body can make it, but it is commonly associated with heart disease. Sampling a person's blood for values of total cholesterol and other cholesterol markers, such as **high-density lipoprotein (HDL)**, **low-density lipoprotein (LDL)**, triglycerides,

Triglycerides Simple lipids made of a glycerol molecule and three fatty acids that are stored in muscles and the liver; protect organs and insulate the body as well as carry substances through the blood.

Saturated fat A fatty acid molecule in which hydrogen atoms occupy all the available bonding sites; solid at room temperature.

Unsaturated fat A fatty acid molecule in which the available bonding sites are not occupied by hydrogen; liquid at room temperature.

Monounsaturated fat A fatty acid molecule with one double or triple bond per molecule that prevents hydrogen from bonding.

Polyunsaturated fat A fatty acid molecule with many double or triple bonds that prevents at least two hydrogen atoms from bonding.

Hydrogenation A process where hydrogen atoms are added to unsaturated fat to make unsaturated oils more conducive to baking and cooking.

Trans fat The result of hydrogenation; has a negative association with cardiovascular health.

Phospholipids Lipids that are both fat and water soluble; located in the cell membranes of the body.

Sterols Lipids primarily made of carbon and hydrogen.

Cholesterol A sterol or fat-like substance found in cell membranes that helps produce vitamin D, steroid hormones, and bile.

High-density lipoprotein (HDL) A substance that transports lipids in the blood and lymph. Also referred to as "good cholesterol" because it is considered protective against cardiovascular disease. Levels should be >60 mg/dL.

Low-density lipoprotein (LDL) A substance that transports lipids in the blood and lymph. Also referred to as the "bad cholesterol" because it is considered to increase risk of cardiovascular disease. Levels should be <100 mg/dL.

Table 6.4
Cholesterol Levels

Normal Cholesterol Ranges (mg/dL)	Adults 20 Years and Older		19 Years and Younger
	Male	Female	
Total	125–200	125–200	≤ 170
LDL	≤ 100	≤ 100	≤ 100
HDL	≥ 40	≥ 50	≥ 45
Triglycerides*	≤ 150	≤ 150	≤ 150

*Not a cholesterol but often performed with cholesterol screening.
U.S. National Library of Medicine. (2019, April 18). Cholesterol Levels: What You Need to Know. Retrieved from https://medlineplus.gov/cholesterollevelswhatyouneedtoknow.html

Table 6.5
Energy and Composition of Fat-Containing Foods

Food	Serving Size	Energy (kcal)	Fat (g)
Milk, whole	8 oz	150	8.2
Milk, 1%	8 oz	102	2.6
Cheese, cheddar	1 oz	111	9.1
Peanut butter	1 tbsp	95	8.2
Cookies, Oreos	3 cookies	160	7.0
Mayonnaise, regular	1 tbsp	100	1.0
Apple	1 medium	81	0.5
Avocado	1 medium	324	29.0
Egg	1 large	80	5.5
Strawberries	1 cup	45	1.0
Ground beef	3 oz	231	15.5
Flounder	3 oz	80	1.0
Chicken breast	3 oz	140	3.1

Data from Manore, M. M., Meyer, N. L., & Thompson, J. (2009). *Sport nutrition for health and performance* (2nd ed.). Champaign, IL: Human Kinetics; and NaturoDoc. (n.d.). Fat calories in foods. Retrieved from https://naturodoc.com/fatcontent/

and **very low-density lipoprotein (VLDL)**, can provide information about risk for heart disease (Table 6.4). Cholesterol is found only in animal products and can be lowered by reducing or avoiding them (Fink & Mikesky, 2021).

The recommended percentage of fat for adults should be 20–35% of the total calories consumed daily (Fink & Mikesky, 2021). It is recommended that saturated fat make up only 7–10% of total fat; therefore, the majority of fat consumed should be unsaturated. This helps avoid the problems attributed to excessive consumption of saturated fat, including high cholesterol and cardiovascular disease. Dietary sources of fat, as stated earlier, are animal products, such as beef, poultry, and pork. Other sources include dairy products, such as milk, butter, and cheese. In addition, plant sources of fat include nuts and plant oils, such as corn oil, olive oil, and soybean oil. See Table 6.5 for common foods and their fat and caloric content.

Like carbohydrate, fat is an important source of energy during rest and exercise. Carbohydrate and fat are oxidized for energy at the same time. The proportion of energy that comes from carbohydrate and fat is dependent on the duration, intensity, and type of exercise as well as the athlete's fitness level and the meal eaten before exercise. Typically, endurance athletes consume lower-fat and higher-carbohydrate foods compared to short-distance runners. Regardless of the type of fat consumed, all forms provide approximately 9 kcal per gram; therefore, fat is calorie dense. One tablespoon of butter has the same kilocalories as 4 cups of chopped broccoli (100 kcal). The available amount of energy in the form of stored body fat is significantly greater than what is available from carbohydrate. For example, the available energy in a 70-kg person who has 18% body fat is calculated to be around 113,400 kcal (70 kg of body

Very low-density lipoprotein (VLDL) A substance that transports lipids in the blood and lymph. Currently there is no recommended level.

weight × 0.18 body fat = 12.6 kg of fat; 12.6 kg of fat × 1,000 g/kg = 12,600 g of fat; 12,600 g of fat × 9 kcal/g of fat = 113,400 kcal; Fink & Mikesky, 2021).

Vitamins

Vitamins are chemicals needed by the body in relatively small amounts and, therefore, are classified as micronutrients. This should not be interpreted, however, to mean that vitamins have little importance nutritionally. On the contrary, adequate amounts of vitamins are essential to health and performance. Vitamins serve a multitude of functions in the body, essentially helping to regulate biochemical reactions, such as energy metabolism and cell and tissue generation, as well as serving as **antioxidants** (antioxidants protect structures, such as cell membranes, from the damaging effects of free radicals, which are released during vigorous exercise). Vitamins contain no caloric value and, as such, do not directly provide energy for muscle contraction (Figure 6.3).

So far, 13 vitamins have been identified; they are divided into two groups, water soluble and fat soluble. The **water-soluble vitamins** include vitamin C (i.e., ascorbic acid), the B vitamins (i.e., B_1, B_2, B_6, B_{12}, niacin, folic acid, biotin, and pantothenic acid), and choline. Water-soluble vitamins, with the exception of B_{12}, are easily transported in the blood and are not stored in the body. These vitamins are used on an as-needed basis; thus, excess amounts are excreted via the kidneys and urine, making regular intake of these vitamins important. **Fat-soluble vitamins** are vitamins A, D, E, and K; because of their solubility, they are stored in the fat tissues of the body. Consumption of fat-soluble vitamins beyond what is recommended in the U.S. Department of Agriculture's (USDA) **Recommended Dietary Allowance (RDA)**, **Adequate Intake (AI)**, or **Dietary Reference Intake (DRI)** (Table 6.6) can result in buildup of and eventual toxic reaction to the stored vitamin. The DRI typically includes the RDA and AI that are sufficient to meet the nutrient requirements of nearly all (97–98%) healthy people. Toxicity usually results from supplementation and not from dietary intake (Fink & Mikesky, 2021).

To date, there is no evidence that taking any vitamin in an amount greater than the recommended level

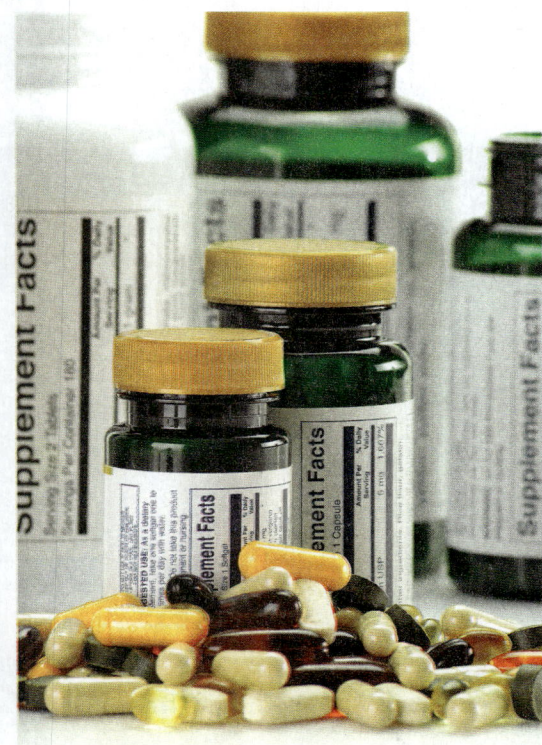

Figure 6.3 Various vitamin and mineral resources.
Monticello/Shutterstock.

> **Vitamins** Thirteen micronutrients that must be consumed regularly because they are essential to health and performance but have no caloric value nor provide direct energy.
>
> **Antioxidants** Protective compounds that fight against free radicals or highly reactive molecules.
>
> **Water-soluble vitamins** Vitamins B and C, which are easily transported through the blood but are not stored in the body and are excreted through the kidneys and urine.
>
> **Fat-soluble vitamins** Vitamins A, D, E, and K, which are stored in the fat tissue; can be toxic to the body if they are in excess.
>
> **Recommended Dietary Allowance (RDA)** Average daily intake sufficient enough to meet daily nutrient requirements.
>
> **Adequate Intake (AI)** The daily intake level based on observed or experimentally determined estimates of nutrient intake by a group(s) of apparently healthy people.
>
> **Dietary Reference Intakes (DRI)** This value includes the Recommended Dietary Allowance (RDA) and average daily level of intake sufficient to meet the nutrient requirements of nearly all (97–98%) healthy people.

Table 6.6
Dietary Reference Intakes* (DRI) for Vitamins

Group (years old)	Vitamin A (μg/d)	Vitamin C (mg/d)	Vitamin D (μg/d)	Vitamin E (mg/d)	Vitamin K (μg/d)	Thiamin (mg/d)	Riboflavin (mg/d)
Males							
9–13	600	45	15	11	60	.9	.9
14–18	900	75	15	15	75	1.2	1.3
19–30	900	90	15	15	120	1.2	1.3
31–50	900	90	15	15	120	1.2	1.3
51–70	900	90	15	15	120	1.2	1.3
> 70	900	90	20	15	120	1.2	1.3
Females							
9–13	700	65	15	15	75	1	1
14–18	700	75	15	15	90	1.1	1.1
19–30	700	75	15	15	90	1.1	1.1
31–50	700	75	15	15	90	1.1	1.1
51–70	700	75	15	15	90	1.1	1.1
> 70	700	75	20	15	90	1.1	1.1

Group (years old)	Niacin (mg/d)	Vitamin B_6 (mg/d)	Folate (μg/d)	Vitamin B_{12} (μg/d)	Panthothenic Acid (mg/d)	Biotin (μg/d)	Choline (mg/d)
Males							
9–13	12	1	300	1.8	4	20	375
14–18	16	1.3	400	2.4	5	25	550
19–30	16	1.3	400	2.4	5	30	550
31–50	16	1.3	400	2.4	5	30	550
51–70	16	1.7	400	2.4	5	30	550
> 70	16	1.7	400	2.4	5	30	550
Females							
9–13	14	1.2	400	2.4	5	25	400
14–18	14	1.3	400	2.4	5	30	425

Group (years old)	Niacin (mg/d)	Vitamin B_6 (mg/d)	Folate (µg/d)	Vitamin B_{12} (µg/d)	Panthothenic Acid (mg/d)	Biotin (µg/d)	Choline (mg/d)
19–30	14	1.3	400	2.4	5	30	425
31–50	18	1.3	400	2.4	5	30	425
51–70	18	1.5	400	2.4	5	30	425
> 70	18	1.5	400	2.4	5	30	425

Data from National Institutes of Health (NIH). (n.d.). Nutrient Recommendations: Dietary Reference Intakes (DRI). Retrieved from https://ods.od.nih.gov/Health_Information/Dietary_Reference_Intakes.aspx
*DRI: An updated method to quantify nutrient needs for nearly all healthy individuals.
mg/d = milligram (1/1,000 g) per day; µg/d = microgram (1/1,000,000 g) per day

provides any performance enhancement. Athletes who consume balanced diets most likely are getting adequate amounts of vitamins through their food and beverage consumption. Excessive cooking may destroy water-soluble vitamins; therefore, to maximize the benefits of the vitamin B complex and vitamin C, foods should be eaten raw or cooked for short periods of time, with the exception of meats (Fink & Mikesky, 2021). Vitamins that are particularly important to athletes are B_1 (thiamine), B_2 (riboflavin), B_3 (niacin), B_6, and B_{12} because of their role in energy production. In particular, B_{12}, found only in animal products, is important to vegan, vegetarian, and older athletes because B_{12} plays a role in the health of the cardiovascular and nervous systems and in energy production. These individuals need to consume foods fortified with vitamin B_{12} or take a daily supplement to avoid deficiency. Additionally, athletes may need vitamin C in higher amounts than the DRI because of oxidative stress from training and competition (Fink & Mikesky, 2021). Last, vitamin D has recently received attention from the medical community. The body synthesizes vitamin D as sunshine reaches the skin. The primary role of vitamin D is to regulate calcium, which affects bone growth. Vitamin D is also considered a hormone important for immune and muscle function and controlling inflammation and more. Deficiency in vitamin D is a concern across the globe, and athletes have the same predisposition to low levels of vitamin D as the rest of the population, especially in winter months. Being deficient in vitamin D is associated with autoimmune diseases, osteomalacia, and osteoporosis (de la Puente Yagüe et al., 2020; Fink & Mikesky, 2021) and can be mistaken for orthopedic symptoms, such as muscle weakness (Hildebrand et al., 2016), pain, chronic injury, and bone pain. In fact, a study done on National Football League (NFL) players concluded that professional football players with higher vitamin D levels were more likely to acquire a contract position in the NFL and those deficient in vitamin D may be at greater risk of fractures (Maroon et al., 2015). Because many athletes may be insufficient or deficient in vitamin D, especially if they are an indoor athlete (Fishman et al., 2016) or have a poor diet, nutritional professionals are now recommending blood tests for vitamin D levels in athletes (de la Puente Yagüe et al., 2020). Ways to improve vitamin D levels are to spend 15 minutes a day outside exposed to the sun during mid-day (around noon) and eating fortified foods, such as milk, orange juice, and cereals, and supplementing if needed (de la Puente Yagüe et al., 2020; Fink & Mikesky, 2021).

Minerals

Minerals, like vitamins, are substances that must be consumed regularly to ensure normal body functions such as maintaining normal heart rhythm, assisting with muscle contractility, promoting neural conductivity, and regulating metabolism. A typical over-the-counter (OTC) daily vitamin and mineral supplement usually includes all the **major minerals** and

> **Minerals** Micronutrients that lack carbon, are made of a variety of elements, and must be consumed regularly for proper body function.
>
> **Major minerals** Minerals needed in quantities greater than 100 mg daily (i.e., calcium, phosphorus, magnesium, sodium, chloride, potassium, and sulfur).

minor, or trace, minerals, as listed in Table 6.7. As is the case with vitamins, there is no scientific evidence that consuming minerals in excess of the DRI provides any advantage in performance. In addition, a well-balanced diet can provide all the necessary dietary minerals.

Calcium is metabolically associated with normal bone and dental health, but it is also the most prevalent mineral in the body and easily obtained in the diet by consuming dairy products; other foods/beverages that have been artificially fortified with calcium; or green leafy vegetables, such as spinach. Athletes with poor nutrition may be at increased risk of calcium deficiency. Diets high in sodium, fiber, animal protein, and phosphorus can negatively affect calcium absorption (Fink & Mikesky, 2021). Female athletes involved in aerobic running sports and female gymnasts have been found to be consuming too little calcium, which places them at risk for inadequate bone development and can contribute to osteopenia or osteoporosis in later life. In these high-risk groups, calcium supplementation is most certainly warranted. Again, it is important to note that a supplement that provides the DRI is appropriate because consuming calcium in excess of this level may lead to other problems. Also, supplements greater than 500 milligrams (mg) are not well absorbed, so consuming calcium should be done throughout the day (Fink & Mikesky, 2021) with meals and not be taken with other supplements. Individuals should avoid supplements from oyster

Minor, or trace, minerals Minerals needed in quantities of less than 100 mg daily (i.e., iron, zinc, chromium, fluoride, copper, manganese, iodine, molybdenum, and selenium).

Table 6.7
Dietary Reference Intakes* (DRI) for Major and Trace Minerals (mg/d or μg/d)

Group (years old)	Calcium (mg/d)	Chromium (μg/d)	Copper (μg/d)	Flouride (mg/d)	Iodine (μg/d)	Iron (μg/d)	Magnesium (mg/d)	Manganese (mg/d)
Males								
9–13	1,300	25	700	2	120	8	240	1.9
14–18	1,300	35	890	3	150	11	410	2.2
19–30	1,000	35	900	4	150	8	400	2.3
31–50	1,000	35	900	4	150	8	420	2.3
51–70	1,000	30	900	4	150	8	420	2.3
> 70	1,200	30	900	4	150	8	420	2.3
Females								
9–13	1,300	21	700	2	120	8	240	1.6
14–18	1,300	24	890	3	150	15	360	1.6
19–30	1,000	25	900	3	150	18	310	1.8
31–50	1,000	25	900	3	150	18	320	1.8
51–70	1,200	20	900	3	150	8	320	1.8
> 70	1,200	20	900	3	150	8	320	1.8

Group (years old)	Molybdenum (μg/d)	Phosphorus (mg/d)	Selenium (μg/d)	Zinc (mg/d)	Potassium (g/d)	Sodium (g/d)	Chloride (g/d)
Males							
9–13	34	1,250	40	8	4.5	1.5	2.3
14–18	43	1,250	55	11	4.7	1.5	2.3
19–30	45	700	55	11	4.7	1.5	2.3
31–50	45	700	55	11	4.7	1.5	2.3
51–70	45	700	55	11	4.7	1.5	2.0
> 70	45	700	55	11	4.7	1.3	1.8
Females							
9–13	34	1,250	40	8	4.5	1.5	2.3
14–18	43	1,250	55	9	4.7	1.5	2.3
19–30	45	700	55	8	4.7	1.5	2.3
31–50	45	700	55	8	4.7	1.5	2.3
51–70	45	700	55	8	4.7	1.3	2.0
> 70	45	700	55	8	4.7	1.2	1.8

Data from National Institutes of Health (NIH). (n.d.). Nutrient Recommendations: Dietary Reference Intakes (DRI). Retrieved from https://ods.od.nih.gov/Health_Information/Dietary_Reference_Intakes.aspx

*DRI: An updated method to quantify nutrient needs for nearly all healthy individuals.

mg/d, milligram (1/1,000 g) per day; μg/d, microgram (1/1,000,000 g) per day.

shells or bone meal due to potential lead contamination. The recommended daily intake for adolescent females is 1,300 mg (Fink & Mikesky, 2021).

Sodium helps with regulation of blood pressure, muscle contraction, and nerve transmission. Most notably, a high-sodium diet is linked to high blood pressure in the general population, but athletes may need more than previously thought due to its role during exercise. It is a key ingredient in sports drinks because sodium is one of the body's main electrolytes, along with chloride and potassium, and is lost in sweat. Excessively low sodium concentration in the blood can lead to a serious condition called **hyponatremia**. This condition can occur from prolonged diarrhea or vomiting or exercising for a long period of time with excessive sweat loss. Drinking too much water and not enough sports drinks during exercise can also cause hyponatremia. Supplementing with sodium may be required in events lasting longer than 4 hours (Fink & Mikesky, 2021).

Chloride is mostly involved in fluid balance, but it can merge with sodium to make sodium chloride, or table salt, or merge with hydrogen to make hydrochloric acid, which is found in the stomach to keep bacteria at bay. Although chloride is an electrolyte and lost in sweat, athletes do not need to supplement with chloride (Fink & Mikesky, 2021).

Potassium, working with sodium, is involved in regulating blood pressure and fluid balance. If sodium intake is too high and potassium is too low, high blood

Hyponatremia Low blood sodium levels due to too much water consumption and/or sodium deficiency.

pressure will result. Athletes who sweat a lot may also sweat large amounts of potassium. For these individuals, paying attention to a proper diet is important (Fink & Mikesky, 2021).

Phosphorus works in conjunction with calcium for bone and teeth health and combines with lipids to provide structure to cell membranes. It is also a component of ATP, which provides energy (Fink & Mikesky, 2021).

Magnesium assists with enzyme reactions for energy, bone health, blood clotting, and blood pressure regulation. Decreased levels of magnesium may occur during long-duration events and lead to muscle cramping (Fink & Mikesky, 2021).

Iron is associated with red blood cell formation, oxygen storage and transport, and enzymatic reactions related to protein and carbohydrate metabolism. Iron is available from plant (nonheme) and animal (heme) sources, but it is best absorbed from animal sources. The DRI for iron is 8 mg for adult males, 18 mg for adult females, and is 1.8 times higher for vegetarians (Fink & Mikesky, 2021). Iron is lost through skin, hair, sweat, and the intestinal tract. Along with vegetarians and distance runners, females are at greatest risk for altered iron in the body. Females require more iron than males because of their menstrual cycles (DRI increases to 20 mg). During menstruation, female athletes may lose as much as 2 mg of iron daily. Inadequate intake of iron or limited rates of iron absorption can cause anemia, resulting in decreased performance, low-energy levels, and cold intolerance. Physically active individuals need include only the DRI levels of iron in their daily diet; they should steer clear of supplements, unless a deficiency exists, because excess iron can be very toxic to the body. However, endurance, vegetarian, and female athletes may want to consult a physician for assessment and maintenance of proper iron balances. Current thought among sports scientists is that iron deficiency is common in athletes involved in endurance sports (Fink & Mikesky, 2021). As mentioned previously, iron is lost through sweating and menstrual bleeding as well as gastrointestinal bleeding and excessive red blood cell destruction (hemolysis) in the blood vessels. This loss may be offset by a dietary adjustment of iron-rich foods, such as organ meats or enriched whole-grain products. A convenient method of supplementation is a daily multivitamin and mineral tablet. Numerous products are available OTC that provide the adult DRI of iron. The bottom line is that athletes should eat adequate nutrients from a variety of foods, especially during high-intensity and/or long-duration training, and thus no vitamin and mineral supplements are required. However, some athletes do not eat well-balanced diets due to weight loss goals, illness, disease, food allergies, tight schedules, or injury; therefore, they should be evaluated by a nutritional professional. Also, as athletes progress through training (i.e., preseason, competition season, and postseason), their nutrition needs change; thus, it is important to seek counsel from a nutrition professional during training. With that said, single-nutrient supplements may be more appropriate than a daily vitamin and mineral supplement in athletes' diet, depending on their circumstances (Thomas et al., 2016). It must be emphasized that megadoses of vitamin and mineral supplementation beyond the DRI values usually prove physiologically and economically wasteful and could adversely affect health, but, for those athletes in need of nutrients, consulting with a registered dietician and/or physician is warranted.

Water

There is virtually no debate in the sports medicine community regarding the importance of water not only to human performance but also to survival because a person can die from water restriction in a few days, depending on the situation. A person's body weight is 55–60% from water, and muscle tissue is up to 70% water. Water serves myriad functions in the body because the molecule is necessary for cellular function, heat regulation, and elimination of waste products. Water is housed in the body in two locations—**extracellular fluids** (those fluids outside of the cells, commonly called interstitial fluid) and **intracellular fluids** (those fluids contained in the cell). Water is constantly being lost through normal body functions, such as breathing, elimination of wastes, and sweating.

At rest, the daily requirement for water is approximately 3 liters (L) for adult men and 2.2 L for adult women (Fink & Mikesky, 2021). Water is lost through urine; feces; sweat due to exercise; insensible perspiration; and respiration, especially if at high altitude. Under conditions of heavy exercise, especially in a high ambient–temperature environment, water requirements can escalate up to 5 L to 10 L daily. The

Extracellular fluid Fluid outside of cells; also called interstitial fluid.

Intracellular fluid Fluid contained inside the cell.

process of controlling the body's core temperature during exercise is known as **thermoregulation**. A significant amount of body water is lost during exercise to eliminate metabolic heat. The circulatory system transports the excess heat via the blood to the skin, where, in harmony with the body's sweat glands, heat is carried from the surface by way of evaporation. The process of sweat evaporation from the skin surface can easily result in an hourly water loss from the body of 2 L or more for each hour of exercise. The most serious consequence of profuse sweating is the loss of body water. A reduction in body weight of 2–5% can result in reduced performance and stress on internal organs. To calculate the percentage of reduction in body weight due to fluid loss, weigh the athlete before and after practice. Then, divide the number of pounds lost in activity by the prepractice weight and multiply by 100. This fluid must be replaced, or serious, even life-threatening, consequences can result.

Water needs should be determined on an individual basis. The goal before exercise starts is to be properly hydrated. During exercise, the goal is to maintain hydration by consuming beverages to match the individual's sweat rate. The American College of Sports Medicine (ACSM) states that 1 liter (L) of sweat loss is equal to 1 kg in body weight loss (Thomas et al., 2016). After exercise, the goal is to replace fluid and electrolyte losses. Carbohydrates and electrolytes should be included in this process, depending on exercise duration and intensity and environment. Ideally, beverages should be 50–59°F, and sports drinks should have 6–8% carbohydrate solution. Avoiding caffeine, alcohol, a high-protein diet and certain OTC medications will help maintain hydration. Also, monitoring urine color will help determine hydration status. Ideally, urine color should be pale yellow to clear. It is important not to overconsume fluids such that the athlete's preexercise weight is more than his or her postexercise weight. Athletes should eat and drink within 2 hours postexercise to replace fluid, electrolytes, carbohydrate, and protein (McDermott et al., 2017; Thomas et al., 2016). Current recommendations by the NATA and ACSM are outlined in Table 6.8.

> **Thermoregulation** The processes involved in order to maintain an optimal physiological range of core body temperature.

Table 6.8
NATA and ACSM Fluid Recommendations

Before Exercise	During Exercise	After Exercise
Consume 5–7 mL/kg 4 hours before, or take weight and consume as needed.	Consume 30–60 g/hour. Consider CHO and sodium, or consume as needed as per thirst. Per NATA fluid replacement guidelines: Fluid replacement is an individualized process that is determined by many factors. Athletes should monitor their weight before and after exercise to ensure they did not lose or gain too much weight. Ideally, athletes should lose no more than 2% of their body weight after exercise and/or sweat trial	Take weight and consume as needed. Eat and drink within 2 hours after exercise to replace fluid, electrolytes, CHO, and protein or consume 1.5 L/kg lost.
Check urine; if dark, increase consumption (3–5 mL/kg 2 hours before); consider CHO and sodium.	Volume determined by sweat rate.	Replace fluid and electrolyte balance.

CHO, carbohydrate.
Based on McDermott, B. P., Anderson, S. A., Armstrong, L. E., Casa, D. J., Ceuvront, S. N., Cooper, L., ... Roberts, W. O. (2017). National Athletic Trainers' Association position statement: Fluid replacement for the physically active. *Journal of Athletic Training, 52*(9), 877–895; and Thomas, D. T., Erdman, K. A., & Burke, L. M. (2016). American College of Sports Medicine joint position statement: Nutrition and athletic performance. *Medicine & Science in Sports & Exercise, 48*(3), 543–568.

NATA Fluid Replacement Guidelines

Fluid replacement is an individualized process that is determined by age, weight, gender, exercise intensity and duration, environment, sweat rate, medical conditions, acclimatization, gastric emptying rate, and diet/preferences. Athletes should monitor their weight before and after exercise to ensure they did not lose or gain too much. Ideally, athletes should lose no more than 2% of their body weight after exercise.

WHAT IF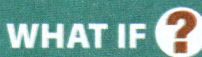

A female high school gymnast (17 years old, 110 lb, 5 ft 1 in., and 14% body fat) asks you for recommendations for her training diet. How many kilocalories would you suggest she consume on a daily basis to remain competitive, and what is the breakdown for carbohydrate, protein, and fat?

Athletic Trainers SPEAK OUT

How can athletic trainers assist with the challenges physically active individuals have to meet their nutritional needs?

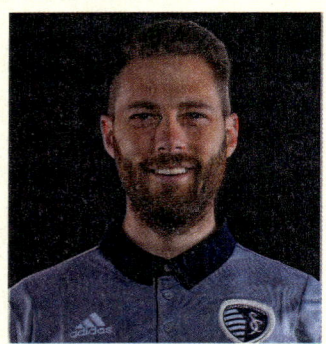

Courtesy of Kurt Andrews.

As athletic trainers (ATs), we are constantly looking for ways to improve the health and performance of our athletes. One of biggest developing areas of athlete care is sports nutrition. Following changes in 2014 to National Collegiate Athletic Association (NCAA) bylaws governing the provision of meals and snacks to student athletes, there is a race to fuel student-athletes across the country like never before. The professionals behind well-fueled student-athletes are registered dietitians, and they work in collaboration with ATs to maximize health, training, performance, and recovery.

Providing nutritional guidance is not only a job important for NCAA student-athletes, professional athletes across the spectrum of sport are in need of assistance, too. At Sporting KC, we work with a registered dietitian to oversee sports nutrition for our first team, United Soccer Leagues (USL) team, and youth academy teams. This includes providing healthy breakfast options; designing daily lunch menus; planning meals for the team while on the road; providing individualized recovery protein shakes after training sessions and games; one-on-one nutrition consultations; providing individualized supplement recommendations; regular body fat testing; blood testing and analysis; and hydration management.

While there are still few registered dietitians working in collegiate and professional sports and zero in the secondary school system, it is important that athletic trainers understand the importance of incorporating nutrition professionals into the care of their athletes. Is it efficient for us to spend time utilizing different therapeutic modalities to help players recover after practice and games if they don't consume the appropriate post training fuel to repair and replenish their muscles? Could we ameliorate an athlete's constant struggle with colds after team travel with maximized nutrition to strengthen their immune system rather than scramble to make them feel better with medicine after the fact? As athletic trainers, it's important we have a thorough understanding of basic nutritional concepts but have a qualified professional to contact to help our athletes get nutritional advice to help with their performance, recovery, sleep, and overall health goals.

The future of sports medicine is one in which registered dietitians are present in larger and larger numbers in both university athletic departments and professional sports teams' training facilities. This makes it vital that ATs be ready to take full advantage of the skill-set they offer to further advance the health of the athletes. As healthcare providers with the highest level of contact with the athletes, it is our responsibility as ATs to advocate for the use of local or "in-house" sports dietitians to help complement the overall care athletes get each day.

— **Kurt Andrews, MS, ATC, PES, CES**

Kurt Andrews is the Director of Sports Medicine, Kansas City Sporting MLS Soccer in Kansas City, Missouri.

Special Considerations

Female Athletes

As more women become involved in organized sports, concerns have been raised regarding special nutritional considerations for female athletes.

In the past, most nutritional information was based on males, thus it is important to recognize the specific dietary needs of female athletes and to formulate individualized nutritional plans. Physiologically, females and males differ in substrate utilization, thermoregulation, body composition, hormones, and bone mineral density. In addition, females respond to training differently than males and tend to have unique behaviors such as underconsuming calories. Therefore, it is important that females consume 20% fat in their diet to support sex-specific needs, increase their protein intake above RDA values, and be aware of their vitamin and mineral needs (e.g., vitamin D, calcium) depending on age, sport/position, menstrual cycle, type of training, body composition, goals, and other variables (Wohlgemuth et al., 2021).

Both males and females are at risk of disordered eating; however, female athletes have a greater risk of acquiring eating disorders, especially for aesthetic sports (Fink & Mikesky, 2021), in an effort to reduce calorie intake. Low body fat percentages in females can lead to hormone abnormalities and possibly menstrual irregularity. The longer a female athlete's menstrual cycles are irregular, the greater the chance of osteoporosis/osteopenia occurring. When these three conditions—eating disorder, menstrual irregularity, and osteoporosis—are present, it is termed the **female athlete triad**. Although not all three conditions need to be present simultaneously, signs and symptoms of any condition should be properly addressed and treated as to prevent the others from surfacing (Fink & Mikesky, 2021). One such prevention method is education such that females should be aware that skipping a period in an already established regular cycle is not a good sign of effective training. In this situation, medical professionals should be alerted so proper investigation can occur.

In other areas of nutrition as mentioned in this chapter, females are susceptible to iron deficiency, which can occur due to their activity (e.g. distance runner), diet choice (e.g. reduced calorie intake or vegetarianism), or related to their menstrual cycle, and can take up to 3–6 months to reverse (Fink & Mikesky, 2021). In particular, young active female athletes require more energy intake to meet demands of growth and their activity, and the same is true of pregnant athletes. In summary, female athletes need to ensure they are acquiring enough energy for activity and growth as well as calcium, vitamin D, iron, and antioxidants during various stages of their life.

Endurance Athletes

Endurance and ultra-endurance athletes have high degrees of muscle and cardiorespiratory endurance to sustain continuous activity for 30 minutes to over 4 hours. Ultra-endurance athletes participate in continuous activity usually lasting over 4 hours. Because of the duration of their activity, endurance athletes expend an enormous amount of calories during training and competition. It is important for them to match energy consumption with energy expenditure as well as replenish energy stores after workouts. Meeting quality calorie requirements may be difficult to achieve depending on their schedule and life demands. These athletes may need to eat smaller meals more frequently and snack throughout the day to consume 3,000–5,000 calories a day. If they need to increase calorie consumption, they can do so by proportionally increasing carbohydrate, protein, and fat so they do not feel full and/or uncomfortable during training or competition.

Endurance athletes should consume the same percentage of macronutrients as other athletes but in much larger quantities. Special attention should be placed on carbohydrate because its stores are limited in the body and it helps to metabolize fat for energy. Furthermore, if the liver and muscle glycogen stores are depleted, extreme fatigue, or **bonking**, will likely occur and decrease performance drastically (Fink & Mikesky, 2021). Carbohydrate should be consumed before endurance exercise because overnight fasting will deplete the liver glycogen stores (Fink & Mikesky, 2021). Between 1 and 4 hours before exercise, 1–4 g of carbohydrate per kilogram of body weight should be consumed in time for adequate digestion without the feeling of hunger. As the activity

---

Female athlete triad Condition when a female athlete has disordered eating (energy deficit), menstrual irregularities, and osteoporosis/osteopenia.

Bonking Extreme fatigue that occurs from depleting carbohydrate stores.

duration increases, glycogen stores decrease, and the body relies on blood glucose for energy; thus, consuming carbohydrate during exercise is beneficial. Typically, ingesting 30–60 g of carbohydrate per hour during endurance exercise is needed (Fink & Mikesky, 2021). This can be accomplished by consuming sports drinks and energy bars and gels. As mentioned previously, replenishing carbohydrate after exercise is very important, and athletes should consume 1–1.5 g of carbohydrate per kilogram of body weight within 15–30 minutes of completing exercise as well as every 2 hours for 6 hours after exercise stops (Fink & Mikesky, 2021).

Endurance athletes should consume adequate amounts of protein daily for the purposes of ensuring protein balance (muscle maintenance and recovery) and providing energy when carbohydrate intake is low. It is suggested that endurance athletes consume 1.2–2 g of protein per kilogram of body weight daily, depending on the intensity of training, weight loss/gain goals, and carbohydrate intake. Likewise, moderate amounts of protein combined with carbohydrate consumed before exercise is recommended. Ultra-endurance athletes will benefit from protein consumption during long training and competitions, however, not too much to cause gastric distress. Last, similar to carbohydrate, 15 g of protein should be consumed within 15–30 minutes after exercise and throughout the day after exercise (Fink & Mikesky, 2021).

Even though endurance training causes the body to rely on fat metabolism for energy during exercise to spare carbohydrate, fat is not of high importance in endurance athletes' diets because decreased performance is usually due to carbohydrate depletion, thus limiting fat metabolism. Additionally, protein and carbohydrate take precedence in an endurance athlete's diet; however, fat consumption should at a minimum meet daily requirements to provide energy, produce hormones, and maintain other essential bodily functions. It is not necessary to consume fat during endurance exercise, but small amounts are reasonable, such as peanut butter and trail mix during ultra-endurance events. Last, it is also not necessary to replace fat immediately after endurance exercise (Fink & Mikesky, 2021).

Another area of focus for endurance athletes is the importance of vitamins B, C, and E, iron, calcium, sodium, and potassium. Vitamin B is involved in energy production, and endurance athletes need high amounts of energy. It is common for endurance athletes to lose iron from hemolysis due to repeated foot impact and sweating. Iron helps to make myoglobin and hemoglobin and transports oxygen. Besides aiding in bone health, calcium is important for fibrin production, which helps with blood clotting, muscle contraction, and nerve function. Vitamins C and E are antioxidants and are needed to counter oxidative damage associated with high-intensity exercise, so intakes of 250–500 mg of vitamin C and 150–400 IU (international units) per day of vitamin E are recommended. Sodium and potassium work together to maintain fluid balance during endurance exercise as well as contribute to nerve function and muscle contraction. Sodium also aids in glucose absorption, but, if levels are too low, it can lead to hyponatremia, which is a life-threatening condition. Needless to say, hydration is critical to the endurance athlete. Please see Table 6.8 for fluid intake recommendations; however, endurance athletes need individualized hydration assessments to determine a hydration plan to better suit their needs during exercise and competition (Fink & Mikesky, 2021).

Strength/Power Athletes

These athletes mainly use the anaerobic system for energy. Carbohydrate is the fuel for short-duration, high-intensity exercise, and these athletes should consume a moderate to high intake of carbohydrate to completely fill glycogen stores before training and competition. Ideally, 6–10 g of carbohydrate per kilogram of body weight per day will replenish glycogen stores, and carbohydrate should be 55–65% of the total calories a day (Fink & Mikesky, 2021). Currently, there are two opposing thoughts on whether to eat carbohydrate 2–4 hours before strength/power exercise. Most research suggests to eat carbohydrate because it will lead to strength gains, whereas other research does not recommend consuming carbohydrate before strength/power exercise, to force the body to use fat as energy. These athletes should experiment with both methods to determine which one is better for them; if athletes choose the latter, they should make certain their diets include adequate carbohydrate the remainder of the day (Fink & Mikesky, 2021).

During training, which can consist of several hours of repeated high-intensity exercise, these athletes may consume 1–1.1 g of carbohydrate per minute in a form of easily digestible sources, such as sports beverages. Conversely, competitions may consist of only a few minutes of exercise; therefore, it is not necessary to consume carbohydrate unless it is a multievent competition, where the athlete is competing several times in one day. In that case, athletes should consume small, easily digestible snacks/meals between events during the day (Fink & Mikesky, 2021).

Regarding recovery, strength/power athletes should consume a source of carbohydrate 15–30 minutes after exercise and 1–1.5 g of carbohydrate per kilogram of body weight every 2 hours for 6 hours after exercise to replenish glycogen stores (Fink & Mikesky, 2021).

As a strength/power athlete, focus is usually on protein versus carbohydrate due to the muscle repair and rebuilding related to this type of exercise. It is true that these athletes have an increased need for protein, but it may not be to the level portrayed by media, retail, and local gyms. There are limits to how much protein can be digested and effectively used at one time (Fink & Mikesky, 2021). Overconsumption of protein can lead to greater urea production, which causes the body to flush it out via the urine and potentially lead to hypohydration, conversion of extra protein to fat, and negative cardiovascular health due to increased saturated fat in animal products (Fink & Mikesky, 2021). Having said that, strength/power athletes should consume 1.4–2.0 g of protein per kilogram of body weight daily or 15–20% of total calories. Eating real food sources of protein at every meal and/or snack and eating a variety of protein sources, such as lean meats, fish, dairy, nuts, seeds, and beans, can achieve this (Fink & Mikesky, 2021). It is recommended that strength/power athletes consume 6 g of easily digestible protein in combination with 35 g of carbohydrate before exercise to gain anabolic effects. It is also recommended to consume 6 g of protein and 35 g of carbohydrate after exercise to benefit protein synthesis (Fink & Mikesky, 2021).

As mentioned previously, strength/power athletes burn very little fat for energy during exercise; however, fat should be consumed on a daily basis for overall health and function. For this purpose, 20–35% of daily total calories should be from fat, depending on the individual's needs, and some suggest 2 g of fat per kilogram of body weight per day. Because fat takes longer to digest, it should be consumed minimally before and during exercise, and it does not need to be replenished immediately after exercise (Fink & Mikesky, 2021).

Team Sport Athletes

Team sport athletes utilize all three energy systems, with the anaerobic system contributing a majority of the energy needed. Depending on the sport and position played, a big difference in calorie requirements exists. However, the underlying principle prevails that these athletes need to match expenditure with calorie intake, and thus energy needs should be calculated. Exercise intensity will determine the number of grams of carbohydrate per kilogram of body weight per day. These amounts range from 5–12 g of carbohydrate per kilogram of body weight per day, with a general recommendation of 6–10 g or 55–65% of daily total calories coming from carbohydrate (Fink & Mikesky, 2021). Similar to endurance athletes, team sport athletes should consume 1.4 g of carbohydrate per kilogram of body weight 1–4 hours before a game. Even though glycogen stores will not be depleted during team sports, time outs and halftime are good opportunities to consume 30–60 g of carbohydrate per hour via sports drinks. To restore carbohydrate after exercise, carbohydrate intake should begin as soon as possible after exercise. It is recommended that 1–1.5 g of carbohydrate per kilogram of body weight be consumed every 2 hours for 6 hours after exercise (Fink & Mikesky, 2021).

Similar to carbohydrate and calorie requirements for team sport athletes, protein requirements depend on an individual's position, sport, training status, and body weight. Athletes who endure more contact during exercise may need more protein intake; generally, 1.2–1.6 g of protein per kilogram of body weight per day is recommended and should be within 15–20% of daily calories. However, some athletes may need 2.5–3 g per kilogram of body weight, depending on their size and exercise goals (Fink & Mikesky, 2021). After exercise, consumption of protein is recommended for tissue healing and muscle rebuilding. This can be accomplished with 6 g of amino acids (15 g of high-quality protein) immediately after exercise (Fink & Mikesky, 2021).

Again, similar to other athletes, fat is not the primary source of fuel for team sports, but it does provide energy, especially during recovery and rest periods.

Fat should be 20–35% of total daily calories to meet bodily needs. Last, like other athletes, fat should be included as part of the diet for taste and satiety during recovery from exercise.

See Table 6.9 for a summary of nutrient requirements before, during, and after exercise for various athletes.

Unfortunately, there are scenarios in which athletes, both males and females, are not consuming enough calories, and this situation presents a new concern that is emerging in athletics called **athletic energy deficit**. Athletic energy deficit or relative energy deficiency in sport (RED-S; Murphy & Koehler, 2022) occurs when an athlete is not matching his or her caloric output by consuming enough calories to properly sustain body function. Typically, athletic energy deficit develops when there is a pressure to change eating habits in an effort to accomplish a sporting goal (Murphy & Koehler, 2022) or when schedules become too hectic and there is not enough time for eating well. Beyond not having enough energy to properly fuel the activity, athletes with athletic energy deficit will be unable to support vital body functions, including bone growth, and may see an increase in fatigue, illnesses, and injuries. In many cases of athletic energy deficit, athletes are at a deficit of 500–1,000 kcal per day. When there is insufficient energy for the natural repair that occurs after exercise, hormones can be negatively affected. In females, estrogen can be significantly lowered, causing amenorrhea and slower bone growth. In males and females, athletic energy deficit may cause shortages of vitamin D and calcium, both essential to bone growth. As a result, poor bone growth may occur, which can lead to stress fractures and early-onset osteoporosis in males and females. Athletic energy deficit can also lead to a series of other adverse health-related consequences, including depression, lethargy, attention deficits, sleep disorders, increases in body fat, chronic fatigue, hypohydration, increased risk for illness and injuries, and muscle wasting (Fink & Mikesky, 2021; Murphy & Koehler, 2022).

Athletic energy deficit Occurs when an athlete does not consume enough calories to properly sustain body function and his or her caloric needs for exercise. Also known as relative energy deficiency in sport (RED-S).

Wrestling

Wrestling is one of only a few sports that match participants on the basis of weight to create an equal level of competition and minimize injury. Yet, in an effort to gain an advantage, many wrestlers attempt to shed pounds rapidly to compete in a lighter weight category. One common form of rapid weight loss is through dehydration. Water weighs approximately 7 lb per gallon; therefore, an athlete can significantly reduce weight by reducing the body's water content. Wrestlers have been known to use a variety of methods to rapidly lose weight, including fluid and calorie restriction, the use of laxatives and diuretics, artificially induced sweating, and overexercising. There is no definitive proof that such tactics actually present an advantage, and there are plenty of reasons not to engage in such behavior. The short-term effects of repeated bouts of extreme, rapid weight loss include dehydration and its associated signs and symptoms of dizziness, vertigo, increased heart rate, altered central nervous system, and decreased performance, strength depletion, other physical and mental health problems, and even death (Lakicevic et al., 2021). The long-term effects are not known at this time; however, there is speculation in the scientific community that these techniques may interfere with normal growth and development in the adolescent athlete.

To reduce the likelihood of unhealthy weight-loss practices ("weight cutting") in high school wrestlers, the state of Wisconsin instituted the Wrestling Minimum Weight Project (WMWP) in 1989. As a result of the WMWP, starting with the 1996–1997 season, the National Federation of State High School Associations (NFHS) modified wrestling rules such that medical professionals would assist in establishing a minimum weight and weight class through the use of checking body fat and hydration. The recommended minimum body fat should not be lower than 7%. The NCAA has a similar approach to managing weight loss for competition in an attempt to keep wrestlers healthy.

In addition, the ACSM (Burke et al., 2021; Thomas et al., 2016) and NATA (Turocy et al., 2011) have published position statements regarding weight loss in competitive wrestling. The ACSM notes that weight cutting can have several physiological effects on performance, including reduced muscle strength,

Table 6.9

Macronutrients Needed Before, During, and After Exercise

Type of Athlete	Nutrient	Daily Recommendations	1–4 Hours Before Exercise	During Exercise	Immediately After Exercise	Hours After Exercise
Endurance athlete	CHO	6–12 g/kg of BW; 55–65% total calories	1–4 g/kg of BW	30–60 g/hr	1–1.5 g/kg of BW within 30 min	1–1.5 g/kg of BW every 2 hr for 6 hr
	Protein	1.2–2 g/kg of BW; 12–18% total calories	Moderate intake with CHO	OK for ultra-endurance	0.25–0.3 g/kg of BW	Continue to consume throughout day
	Fat	20–35% total calories	Not necessary	Small amount during ultra-endurance	—	Part of diet
Strength/power athlete	CHO	6–12 g/kg of BW; 55–65% total calories	Optional	Optional; 1–1.1 g/min	1–1.5 g/kg of BW within 15–30 min	1–1.2 g/kg of BW per hour for 4 hr
	Protein	1.4–2 g/kg of BW; 15–20% total calories	6 g of amino acids and 35 g of CHO	Optional	0.25–0.3 g/kg of BW	6 g of amino acids & 15 g of CHO within 1–3 hr
	Fat	20–25% of total calories	Minimal	Minimal	—	Part of diet; for taste/satiety
Team sport athlete	CHO	6–10 g/kg of BW; 55–65% total calories	1–4 g/kg of BW	30–60 g/hr	1–1.2 g/kg of BW within 15–30 min	1–1.2 g/kg of BW every hour for 6 hr
	Protein	1.2–2 g/kg of BW; 15–20% of total calories	—	—	0.25–0.3 g/kg of BW	6 g of amino acids or 15 g of high quality within 1–2 hr
	Fat	20–35% of total calories	Minimal	Minimal	—	Part of diet

CHO, carbohydrate; BW, body weight.

anaerobic capacity, and endurance capacity; impaired thermoregulatory processes; and lower oxygen consumption. Weight cutting can also deplete fluids, electrolytes, and glycogen, causing increased protein breakdown, impaired coordination, and cardiac arrhythmias. Based on the variety of health risks associated with the practice of weight cutting, ACSM gives the following recommendations regarding the sport of wrestling:

- Education about the adverse consequences of prolonged fasting and dehydration on physical performance and physical health should be provided to coaches and wrestlers.
- Rubber suits, steam rooms, hot boxes, saunas, laxatives, and diuretics should not be used for making weight.
- State or national governing body legislation that schedules weigh-ins immediately before competition should be adopted.
- Daily weigh-ins need to be scheduled before and after practice to monitor weight loss and dehydration. Any weight lost during practice should be regained through adequate food and fluid intake.
- The body composition of each wrestler needs to be assessed before the season using valid methods for this population. Medical clearances will be needed for males younger than 16 years of age with body fat below 7% or those older than 16 years with body fat below 5% and for female wrestlers below 12–14%.
- Caloric intake needs to support the normal developmental needs of the young wrestler. Emphasize the standard percentages of macronutrients along with a minimal caloric intake of 1,700 to 2,500 kcal per day. Remind wrestlers that rigorous training will increase the requirement up to an additional 1,000 calories per day.

Wrestling is a time-honored sport, but techniques used in the past to make weight are not only out of date but also can cause life-threatening consequences. Therefore, these recommendations need to be carefully implemented at all levels of participation and competition. Overall, many of these recommendations can apply to any sport, but they are significantly important for male and female wrestlers.

WHAT IF ❓

You are asked to make a presentation to parents of high school wrestlers on the topic of effective weight-loss techniques. What specific recommendations would you make to parents regarding their children's dietary habits?

Conclusions

Based on the results of research pertaining to the nutritional behavior of athletes, it appears that some important conclusions can be made regarding their dietary practices (Fink & Mikesky, 2021; Thomas et al., 2016):

- Athletes should consume the proper proportions of protein, carbohydrate, fat, and energy needed for their activity and health. Consumption should also be timed appropriately to limit fatigue and account for activity. Athletes should consume diets that provide at least the RDA, AI, or DRI for all micronutrients.
- Significant body composition changes should take place before the competitive season to avoid any potential problems from workout and dietary changes to achieve ideal body weight.
- Carbohydrate consumption should be approximately 3–12 g per kilogram of body weight per day. Targets should be individualized for activity, gender, age, activity schedule, and environmental conditions (see Table 6.2). Also, if the activity is over 60 minutes or there is sustained high-intensity exercise for long durations, carbohydrate intake during activity should be about 30–60 g per hour, and an individualized plan to determine needs would be beneficial.
- Protein recommendations for endurance and strength-trained athletes range from 1.2–2 g per kilogram of body weight per day. These recommended protein intakes can generally be met through diet alone, without the use of protein or amino acid supplements. For example, to compute the recommended 1-day protein intake for an 85-lb female gymnast, make the following calculations:
    - Body weight in kilograms is 38.6.
    - 85 lb divided by 2.2 lb per kg = 38.6 kg

- 38.6 kg × 1.4 g of protein = 54 g daily protein requirement
- A chicken breast (6 oz) will provide the protein requirement.

- Fat intake should range from 20–35% of total energy intake. Consuming less than or equal to 20% of energy from fat does not benefit performance because fat is a source of energy, fat-soluble vitamins, and essential fatty acids. Athletes should avoid junk food and fast food. (Figure 6.4).
- Consuming carbohydrate 1–4 hours before an event should add to the existing carbohydrate stores. Also, ensuring hydration before an event is good practice. An individualized approach to achieving this is ideal.
- Remaining hydrated before, during, and after activity is ideal as is an individualized fluid plan.
- Recovery from activity should include fluids, electrolytes, energy, and carbohydrate. Consuming 1–1.2 g of carbohydrate per kilogram of body weight per hour up to 4–6 hours after activity is recommended along with 0.25–0.3 g per kilogram of body weight of protein.
- Generally, if an athlete consumes a healthy, balanced diet, vitamin and mineral supplements are not necessary. However, in some cases, as with vegetarians, supplementation may be necessary to counter the potentially low intake of energy, protein, fat, creatine, carnosine, iron, calcium, zinc, and vitamin B_{12}.

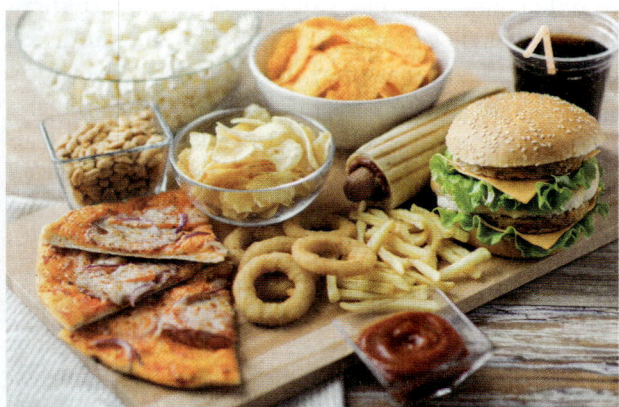

Figure 6.4 Fast foods contain many nutrients but are typically high in fat content.
© Syda Productions/Shutterstock.

Nutritional Knowledge of Athletes and Coaches: What the Research Shows

As presented previously, athletes are largely uneducated regarding proper nutrition, even though they understand the importance of adhering to a quality diet (Torres-McGehee et al., 2012). Therefore, this lack of knowledge might result in damaging nutritional practices because they often fail to incorporate sound principles of nutrition into their training diets. The good news is that they are relying on trained professionals more often, such as registered dieticians, athletic trainers, and strength and conditioning specialists, who demonstrate solid understanding of the importance of athletes adhering to quality diets and the athletes' nutritional needs (Torres-McGehee et al., 2012).

Torres-McGehee et al. (2012) reported that 55% ± 13% of athletes scored above a benchmark of adequate knowledge on a comprehensive test on macronutrients, micronutrients, supplements, weight control, and hydration. In general, the lowest area of knowledge was on weight control and eating disorders, where only 47% ± 22% of athletes scored above the benchmark.

Educating Athletes: What Can the Coach Do?

While not all coaches have basic nutritional education, those planning to coach should incorporate at least one nutrition course into their undergraduate or continuing education. Coaches can attend in-service meetings, professional conferences, community education programs, and online courses on nutrition-related topics. An excellent source of current nutritional information can be obtained via a subscription to a professional journal in the field of coaching or sports science. Furthermore, many excellent books on sports nutrition are now on the market, and hospitals often employ registered dietitians, who are highly trained and may be more than happy to provide information on nutrition for a coach's athletes. For assistance in locating an expert in their area, coaches can contact the Academy of Nutrition and Dietetics (formerly, the American Dietetic Association; http://www.eatright.org/find-an-expert).

Another option for coaches who live near a university is to contact a member of the institution's sports medicine or strength and conditioning staff. Typically, this is a BOC-certified athletic trainer or certified (by the National Strength and Conditioning Association [NSCA]) strength coach. In addition, universities often employ faculty members with graduate degrees in nutrition science, and they may be willing to serve as a resource as well.

Coaches should encourage, perhaps even require, that athletes keep a record of what they eat and drink. This information can be recorded with pencil and paper, or mobile apps can be used for this purpose. Coaches or other professionals (certified athletic trainer, exercise science professor, or registered dietitian) should periodically review what athletes are eating and make recommendations based on sound nutritional principles. Such a record need not be a complex, detailed document. Athletes need only record the content and approximate amount of foods and beverages consumed during each meal. Most food packages provide information regarding the nutritional content of the product. With practice, it is relatively simple to determine whether an athlete is consuming the correct amount of nutrients.

Recently, programs designed to teach athletes nutrition and life skills have been developed. The National Collegiate Athletic Association (NCAA) works in cooperation with the ACSM and Academy of Nutrition and Dietetics to provide athletes with up-to-date information regarding nutrition and performance. The Oregon Health and Science University has developed a program for females, titled Athletes Targeting Healthy Exercise and Nutrition Alternatives (ATHENA). This program is peer led and addresses the connection between young women in sports, disordered eating behaviors, and body-shaping drug use (Elliot et al., 2008). Students learn attitudes and skills that will help them make healthy choices in sports and throughout their lives. Coaches and student team leaders are trained to teach goal setting and self-monitoring of nutritional behaviors. Long-term follow-up studies indicate that females who go through ATHENA training report better nutrition habits and reduced use of diet pills and supplements.

When working with children, coaches should discuss the nutritional needs of athletes with parents. A significant amount of nutritional information is available online from the Sports, Cardiovascular and Wellness Nutrition practice group, a division of the Academy of Nutrition and Dietetics (http://www.scandpg.org); STOP Sports Injuries (http://www.stopsportsinjuries.org); Dietary Guidelines for Americans 2020–2025 (https://www.dietaryguidelines.gov); and the USDA Nutrient Data Laboratory website (https://www.ars.usda.gov/northeast-area/beltsville-md-bhnrc/beltsville-human-nutrition-research-center/nutrient-data-laboratory). The USDA site provides an extensive, searchable listing of the nutrient contents of hundreds of foods. This information can be useful when making decisions about food choices. Another useful site is maintained by the USDA Center for Nutrition Policy and Promotion (http://www.cnpp.usda.gov), which provides online dietary analyses. After registering and entering all necessary dietary information, a detailed nutritional assessment is generated. Because this analysis is completed online, athletes should be encouraged to complete it at home; minors will ideally have parental involvement.

General Dietary Guidelines for Athletes

Daily Diet: Nutritional Maintenance

Although every sport and every athlete has specific nutritional requirements and preferences, some general recommendations can be made based on current knowledge. The basic differences between a nonathlete's and an athlete's diet are that athletes require additional energy to support physical activity and additional fluid to cover sweat losses. It should be noted, however, that, like a conditioning program, the athlete's diet should be tailored to meet individual needs. A gymnast may need to control her body composition within a very narrow set of parameters; a football lineman may wish to gain additional lean body mass. Thus, the nutrition program must be based on the physical characteristics of the athlete and the individual demands of the sport.

All sports nutrition programs should prepare athletes for practice and competition, encourage athletes to consume food and beverages during competition to maintain energy sources, and ensure adequate recovery between training sessions and after competitions (Thomas et al., 2016).

Athletes need to be educated about proper food selections to maintain the correct proportions of carbohydrate, fat, and protein. Scientists recommend the following breakdown for Americans: vegetables, 2.5–4 cups per day; fruit, 1.5–2.5 cups per day; grains, 6–10 cups per day; dairy, 3 cups per day; protein, 5–7 ounces per day; and oil, 24–51 grams per day (https://www.dietaryguidelines.gov/sites/default/files/2021-03/Dietary_Guidelines_for_Americans-2020-2025.pdf). These percentages may change for athletes, depending on their activity and individual needs. For tracking purposes, it may be easiest to adhere to carbohydrate dietary recommendations because most foods contain significant amounts of carbohydrate. It is important that athletes understand that many protein sources contain significant amounts of fat; therefore, these foods should be consumed less frequently than lean sources of protein (i.e., beans, eggs, and dairy). Most experts agree that even highly active athletes need only 1.2–2 g of protein per day for each kilogram of body weight (Thomas et al., 2016). This means that a football player who weighs 195 lb (88.6 kg) needs to consume a maximum of 177 g of protein per day. This amount could be supplied in one big meal (typical of many football players). For example, see the protein provided by this simple meal:

5 hard boiled eggs	32 g
3 cups of cow's milk	25 g
4 ounces (deck of cards size) of lean beef	33 g
8 ounces of chicken	60 g
1 cup of Greek yogurt	25 g
Total =	175 g

Not surprisingly, research shows that professional and collegiate football and international rugby players often consume more than 2 g of protein per day for each kilogram of body weight (Holway & Spriet, 2011). Although, many football coaches may recommend a diet high in carbohydrate and low in fat for optimal performance, they also may recommend beef, chicken, fish, beans, dairy products, and protein supplements to football players who want to gain lean body mass. Unfortunately, these recommendations are contrary to each other because diets high in meat products along with protein supplementation are likely to contain more overall calories and fat. Not only are such diets expensive, but they may be unhealthy as well. As described earlier in this chapter, excess protein produces metabolic waste products, especially nitrogen, which can put stress on the kidneys and liver. Dehydration may also occur because the kidneys increase urine output.

Assuming athletes are sticking to a balanced diet, there is no need to be concerned about their getting enough vitamins and minerals. These compounds are needed in small amounts, and there is little evidence that athletes need to consume extra vitamins and minerals to perform (Fink & Mikesky, 2021). However, dietary supplementation may be warranted in cases of identified deficiencies. As discussed previously, two minerals that may prove to be exceptions are iron and calcium. Athletes who complain of chronic fatigue, repeated stress fractures, loss of fitness, or inability to perform—despite adequate diet and rest—should be referred to a physician for evaluation. A simple blood test can determine whether a true iron or calcium deficiency is the problem. Researchers recommend that high-risk groups be tested periodically for iron deficiency, with subsequent supplementation of iron when deemed appropriate by a physician (Thomas et al., 2016).

Coaches should be conservative when making dietary recommendations, especially to younger athletes. Offering a few well-proven, simple guidelines probably represents the most effective approach. An excellent resource is the interactive Choose My Plate website (http://choosemyplate.gov), which is made available to the public by the USDA (Figure 6.5).

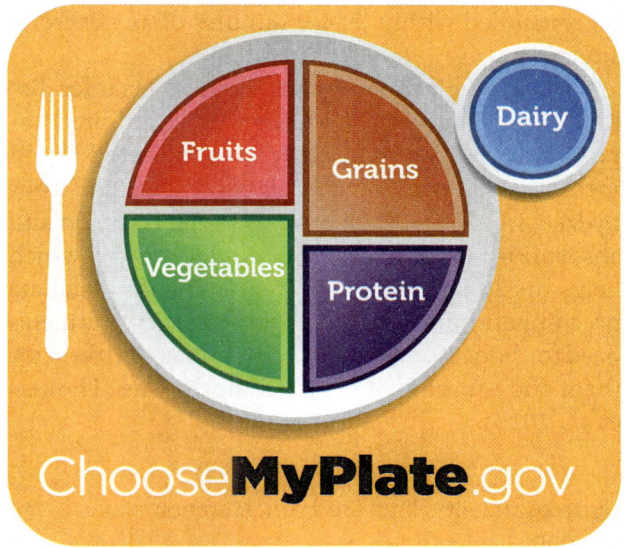

Figure 6.5 ChooseMyPlate.gov.
Courtesy of USDA.

This site enables the user to develop a personalized dietary plan based on factors such as age, gender, and physical activity level; it has replaced the Food Guide Pyramid. However, athletes interested in developing a more sophisticated dietary regimen should consider performing a dietary analysis with a sports dietitian.

Precompetition Diets

Precompetition diets should be determined based on the sport or activity. As a rule, it is advised that athletes, regardless of sport, not consume a meal immediately before an event. The process of digestion takes 2–6 or more hours, depending on the food consumed; thus, foods eaten just before a contest will contribute virtually nothing to performance. It should also be noted that gastrointestinal distress is common if a meal is eaten too close to practice or competition because the body reallocates blood flow to muscles away from the gastrointestinal system once exercise begins. A precompetition meal should provide sufficient fluid to maintain hydration and be relatively high in carbohydrate (low glycemic index), moderate in protein, low in fat, low in fiber, and easy to digest. This facilitates gastric emptying and minimizes gastrointestinal distress while maintaining blood glucose. Experts recommend that the typical pregame meal should be eaten between 1 and 4 hours before the contest (Thomas et al., 2016). However, a very light snack (easy to digest food) and fluid can be consumed within 20–30 minutes of any exercise situation.

If acceptable to the athlete, liquid diets offer distinct advantages over the more traditional precompetition meal. Commercially manufactured liquid meals typically contain a high percentage of carbohydrate in a form that facilitates rapid digestion and absorption. In addition, they contain water, which helps the athlete with respect to achieving adequate precompetition hydration. Remember that athletes need to choose foods and beverages that work best for them and experiment before competitions (Thomas et al., 2016).

Hyperosmolality Increased concentration of a solution.

Nutrition During Competition

Research has shown that consumption of carbohydrate during activity, both aerobic and anaerobic, can be beneficial. It is known that the body has a limited capacity for storing glycogen and that athletes may deplete glycogen supplies in the muscles and liver before completing an event. One hour of highly intense exercise can reduce liver glycogen by 55%, and 2 hours can almost completely deplete both liver and muscle glycogen. Such depletion is commonly referred to as "hitting the wall."

Research supports the premise that consuming carbohydrate during long-duration exercise (1–3 hours at 70–80% maximum aerobic capacity) allows active muscle tissue to rely on blood glucose for energy and not deplete important liver and muscle stores (Thomas et al., 2016). Many commercially made carbohydrate products are available, as well as making one's own preferred beverages. Sports drinks typically provide a 6–8% carbohydrate solution by volume, and approximately 8 oz should be consumed about every 15–20 minutes (between 30 and 60 g per hour). This is especially important in athletes who exercise in the morning after an overnight fast when liver glycogen levels are decreased.

Although the intake of carbohydrate is essential for optimal performance, a relatively high intake of carbohydrate during exercise will likely increase the incidence of upper (e.g., nausea, heartburn, or belching) and lower (e.g., bloating, diarrhea, and abdominal cramps) gastrointestinal symptoms. Two theories are used to explain such gastrointestinal distress, including malabsorption of contents due to limited blood flow to the gut or the attraction of excessive fluid from the blood into the intestines to balance out the excess electrolytes. It is hypothesized that too much carbohydrate or carbohydrate that oxidizes too fast (Table 6.1) can be ingested at rates in excess of 60 g per hour, and this will likely result in **hyperosmolality** of the stomach contents, which then leads to the gastrointestinal discomfort (Fink & Mikesky, 2021).

Postexercise Nutrition

After exercise, dietary goals are to replace muscle glycogen to ensure quick recovery. Composition and timing of the recovery meal or snack depend on the length and intensity of the exercise session

(Thomas et al., 2016). Glycogen depletion can occur after 2–3 hours of exercise at 60–80% VO_2 max. Postexercise meals need to provide adequate fluids, electrolytes, carbohydrate, and protein. A carbohydrate intake of approximately 1.0–1.2 g per kilogram of body weight per hour during the first 4 hours after exercise is adequate to replace glycogen stores (Thomas et al., 2016). The timing of carbohydrate ingestion is important because glycogen levels replenish faster if the food is consumed within 30–60 minutes. The type of food is also significant because consumption of high glycemic index carbohydrate results in higher muscle glycogen levels 24 hours after a glycogen-depleting exercise compared with the same amount of low glycemic index carbohydrate.

Also, there seems to be debate in the literature regarding the rate of muscle protein synthesis for sprint and strength performance when consuming carbohydrate and protein after exercise compared to carbohydrate alone. However, it has been found that consuming carbohydrate and protein (3 g of essential amino acids or 15–25 g of quality protein or 0.25–0.3 g of protein per kilogram) within 2 hours of hard exercise seems to improve net protein balance (Thomas et al., 2016) and muscle protein synthesis as well as glycogen stores (Fink & Mikesky, 2021) compared to carbohydrate alone. Protein consumed after exercise provides amino acids for building and repairing muscle tissue (Thomas et al., 2016) that may have endured microtrauma from contact sports or the long-duration, repetitive, eccentric nature of endurance sports. For certain athletes, it is recommended to consume foods that will provide a ratio of 4 g of carbohydrate to 1 g of protein (e.g., low-fat chocolate milk and sports nutrition bars).

Pamphlets of nutritional information about eating before, during, and after exercise are available online at the Sports, Cardiovascular and Wellness Nutrition practice group (http://www.scandpg.org).

Nutrition and Injury Recovery

A major concern for many injured athletes is weight gain during periods of forced inactivity. During injury rehabilitation, activity may cease, but metabolism often increases because the body is repairing itself and performing other activities, such as utilizing crutches. After trauma or surgery the body may require up to 20% more energy; therefore, athletes should be advised against significantly reducing total caloric intake during rehabilitation out of fear of weight gain. Insufficient energy intake, such as 80% of your normal daily calories, for 10 days can reduce muscle protein synthesis by 20%, thus impacting rate of complete recovery (Knappenberger, 2018).

It is important that an injured athlete be advised about these dietary changes during recovery. It may be possible for some injured athletes to continue exercising with some form of alternate activity. Runners can often ride a stationary bicycle or run in a swimming pool, thereby maintaining aerobic fitness and burning off excess calories. Athletes who are suffering from infectious illnesses may be unable to exercise and should take care to establish a caloric intake based on their BMR until they are healthy.

Unfortunately, direct evidence is still needed to provide solid recommendations for nutrition during injury recovery. However, it is currently recommended that a needs assessment be done throughout the injury recovery process and some simple guidelines followed. Individuals should avoid alcohol and deficiencies in energy, protein, macronutrients, and micronutrients. Simple recommendations regarding macronutrients include maintaining carbohydrate consumption based on healing processes and rehabilitation activity levels; maintaining protein levels as long as they are greater than 1.6–3 g per kilogram per day; and consuming fat, with a concentration on "good" fat (e.g., olive oil, avocados, nuts and seeds, and ground flax or flax oil; Smith-Ryan et al., 2020). Of course, adequate hydration should also be maintained throughout rehabilitation, and increases should occur with fluid loss through sweating.

Carbohydrate is a direct form of energy for cell metabolism. Consuming carbohydrates stimulates insulin and insulin growth factor, both of which help in tissue building. Protein contains the building blocks for connective tissue and muscle. Amino acids in protein are essential, and several, including arginine, ornithine alpha-ketoglutarate, glutamine, and leucine, have been recommended (Knappenberger, 2018); however, caution must be applied when supplementing with amino acids (discussed in more detail later in this chapter). Foods with anti-inflammatory properties are also recommended, but inflammation is a necessary process in healing and should not be stopped.

Finally, free fatty acids, especially omega-3 (anti-inflammatory) and omega-6 (proinflammatory), are known to contain eicosanoids, which can reduce pain as well as cause vasodilation and enhance the immune system. Omega-3 fatty acids can be found in fish oil and cold water fish (e.g., salmon and herring), and omega-6 fatty acids (e.g., linoleic acid) can be found in seeds, nuts, and a variety of vegetable oils. It is important to keep omega-3 and omega-6 fatty acids in balance rather than overconsume one or the other. It is currently recommended to consume 3–9 g per day of each when rehabilitating from an injury (Knappenberger, 2018).

Managing Body Weight

Athletes wishing to gain or lose weight must be educated about the various ways that body weight can be changed. To maintain weight, athletes' caloric intake must equal caloric expenditure (basic metabolic needs plus exercise demands). Unsafe weight management practices can negatively affect athletes' overall health in addition to compromising their athletic performance. Encouraging weight management by limiting calories or specific nutrients, engaging in deadly weight control methods, or simply not eating or drinking much at all are very dangerous practices for anyone but especially for athletes (Turocy et al., 2011). Safe weight loss and management can be accomplished using scientific evidence and credible resources. Foremost, athletes, coaches, and parents are encouraged to visit with a registered dietician when weight management is an issue; however, athletic trainers and strength and conditioning specialists can also be valuable resources. The NATA position statement "Safe Weight Loss and Maintenance Practices in Sport and Exercise" (Turocy et al., 2011) is an excellent resource; it can be downloaded at http://www.nata.org/position-statements.

Body weight can be categorized as three basic forms: water, fat tissue, and lean tissue. Water makes up a substantial portion of nearly all the tissues in the body. From a practical standpoint, skeletal muscles make up the majority of lean-tissue weight. The majority of body fat is found just under the skin and is known as subcutaneous fat. The human body has devised a highly efficient method of storing excess dietary calories. When an athlete consumes more calories per day than the body requires for a given activity level, the excess calories are converted to fat. Conversely, if an athlete fails to consume enough calories to meet the daily requirement, stored fat is metabolized to form energy. Curiously, when athletes severely restrict caloric intake, such as in fasting, the body's energy is not balanced, and at some point they will be in negative nitrogen balance, causing the body to utilize muscle tissue for energy (Fink & Mikesky, 2021). Therefore, an athlete will reduce lean-tissue mass, which in most cases results in loss of performance.

If athletes are striving to maintain a desirable body weight, they should weigh themselves weekly, at about the same time of day, after going to the bathroom. Their body weight should not fluctuate too much from week to week but can fluctuate daily because of sweating from physical activity. It is also important to remember that female athletes may experience weight gains immediately preceding their menstrual period. However, determining body weight by standing on a scale may be of limited value because a given volume of muscle tissue weighs more than the same volume of fat. The ratio of fat to lean body weight is a better measurement; this is commonly referred to as body composition. It is represented as a percentage of body fat; the percentage of essential fat is 2–5% in men, 10–13% in women, 7% for adolescent boys, and 14% for adolescent girls. The range for most active, young females is 14–24% and active, young males, 7–17%; however, obesity is increasing in epidemic proportions across society. From 2011–2014, the prevalence of obesity and extreme obesity in 2- to 19-year-olds was 17% and 5.8%, respectively (Ogden et al., 2016), whereas the prevalence of obesity and extreme obesity in those 20 years and older is 37.9% and 7.7%, respectively, as per body mass index measurements from a 2013–2014 National Health and Nutrition Examination Survey (NHANES; https://www.cdc.gov/nchs/data/hestat/obesity_adult_13_14/obesity_adult_13_14.pdf). And, in a 2015–2016 analysis by the NHANES, the obesity prevalence was 18.5% in youths, which shows an increased upward trend since the previous report (https://www.cdc.gov/nchs/data/databriefs/db288.pdf).

There are athletes who, for a variety of reasons, desire to change their body weight. Those involved in sports that require a specific body weight, such as wrestling, boxing, or lightweight crew, may attempt to lose pounds rapidly to compete in a lighter weight category. These competitors need to understand that rapid weight fluctuations typically involve dehydration and significant water loss can cause a number of undesirable consequences resulting in an overall loss of performance. The sport of wrestling has been very proactive in guarding against short-term weight-loss strategies, such as hypohydration (water deficit), decreased glycogen stores, and pathological methods, and has developed minimum body fat standards for male and female athletes. In the high school setting, male wrestlers cannot have lower than 7% body fat and females, 12%. Currently, all official body fat and body weight measures must be obtained when an athlete is properly hydrated. To determine appropriate hydration, a refractometer and/or urine dipstick assessment can be used to measure urine specific gravity or protein content, respectively. The urine dipstick method is more sensitive to acute dehydration (Turocy et al., 2011). Appropriate hydration is achieved if the urine's specific gravity is less than 1.025. A minimal competitive weight should be established for all weight-class athletes, using the required minimal body fat for the sport or the essential fat guidelines. Wrestlers and other weight-class athletes should determine their healthy body weight and composition during the off-season and then concentrate on preparing for that weight category in the upcoming season. It is important to remember that the current recommendation is to limit weight loss to 1.5% of current body weight per week (Turocy et al., 2011).

Minimal Competitive Weight

Percent body fat is governed by the rules of the sport, minimal essential fat, or personal choice. The minimum percentage of fat for male wrestlers is 7% and 12% for females. The body weight and percentage of fat of the athlete must be determined. Although there are many ways of estimating body fat, the most practical method employs skinfold measurements. However, the technique is only as good as the person administering the test. Hence, testing of body composition should be conducted by a person who has been properly trained, such as an exercise physiologist or BOC-certified athletic trainer.

After the body fat percentage has been determined, **lean body weight (LBW)** can be calculated with the following formula:

$$\text{Fat weight} = \text{Total body weight} \times \text{Body fat \%}$$
$$\text{LBW} = \text{Total body weight} - \text{Fat weight}$$

If a male athlete weighs 135 lb and has 14% body fat, fat weight can be determined by multiplying percentage of fat by total body weight: $0.14 \times 135 = 18.9$ lb. Thus, fat weight is approximately 20 lb. This athlete's LBW is calculated by subtracting fat weight from total body weight: $135 - 20 = 115$ lb. To determine the minimal competitive weight for this athlete, make the following calculation:

$$\text{Minimal competitive weight (MCW)} = \text{Lean body weight} \div (1 - \% \text{ fat desired})$$
$$\text{MCW} = 115 \div 0.93 \, (1 - 0.7) = 124 \text{ lb}$$

Thus, this athlete should not compete if his weight drops below 124 lb. Using the same equation, a 115-lb female wrestler who has 17% body fat should not be allowed to compete if her weight drops below 108 lb:

$$115 \times 0.17 \, (\% \text{ body fat}) = 19.5 \text{ lb of fat}$$
$$115 - 19.5 \text{ lb of fat} = 95.5 \text{ lb LBW}$$
$$\text{MCW} = 95.5 \div 0.88 \, (1 - 0.12) = 108 \text{ lb}$$

Athletes involved in other sports that have aesthetic components, such as gymnastics, dancing, or diving, may also be faced with a dilemma when attempting to alter their appearance. These athletes should never go below a body fat percentage that is essential for maturation. It is important for these athletes to remember that the cost of starvation and other ineffective methods of weight control are likely to affect their muscle mass. Because these activities are considered to be anaerobic (i.e., deriving the required energy from glycogen supplies in working muscles), these athletes may experience more decrements in performance and potential sport injury. Any athlete who demonstrates abnormal eating behaviors or exhibits unusual or unwarranted concerns about excess body fat should be referred to an expert for evaluation and dietary counseling.

Lean body weight (LBW) The amount of weight that is from lean body tissues; also called fat free mass.

Ergogenic Aids

An **ergogenic aid** is a substance that enhances an individual's ability to work or perform. When work output is increased, the person is able to perform at higher intensities and work longer and is capable of putting greater stresses on the body. Based on the overload principle of training, athletes who are using ergogenic aids may be able to increase their capacity to train, thereby increasing their athletic potential (e.g., size or speed). There are different types of ergogenic aids: physiological (i.e., enhancing a body system, e.g., cardiovascular), biomechanical (i.e., external products, e.g., Clap ice skates), psychological (i.e., changing the mental state, e.g., visualization), pharmacological (i.e., drugs or hormones, e.g., anabolic steroids), and nutritional (i.e., supplement or food, e.g., creatine monohydrate). The main focus of this section will be on nutritional or dietary supplements. According to the Dietary Supplement Health and Education Act (DSHEA) of 1994, a supplement contains one or more vitamins, minerals, herbs (i.e., botanical), amino acids, or extracts intended to supplement the diet and not be used as the only food (Fink & Mikesky, 2021). However, this definition does not consider the individual's current diet and the purpose for supplementing because supplements come in various forms, such as functional foods or those enriched with additional nutrients, such as mineral-fortified orange juice; formulated foods or those products that provide energy or nutrients, such as sports drinks and bars; single nutrients; and multi-ingredient products (Maughan et al., 2018).

Sports nutritional supplements have become very popular with athletes of all calibers. The use of supplements, once basically confined to professional or Olympic athletes, has now become a popular technique for gaining an edge for athletes of all ages and categories and has also gained incredible popularity with the general public for various health-related reasons.

Many coaches or parents tell their athletes that, by using nutritional supplements, they can become bigger, stronger, and faster. This message is exactly what the athlete wants to hear, and he or she will often spend significant amounts of money buying a variety of supplements to help reach the goal of becoming the best athlete. For many high school athletes, being a top-tier athlete can mean a college scholarship. Collegiate athletes may want to become better so they can obtain professional contracts. Many supplements are marketed to make athletes think that, by taking a pill or powder or drinking an ergogenic beverage, they will improve their personal performance and reach their goals faster. Typically, the supplement manufacturers claim that these substances are not available in a normal diet, are needed by athletes in greater amounts than the body can acquire through normal dietary habit, are necessary for improved performance via allowing harder training, reduce pain, allow rapid recovery from hard training or injury, or enhance immunity and/or mood (Maughan et al., 2018). These are just a few of the many reasons athletes will take nutritional supplements.

Athletes must remember that not all marketed supplements create bigger, stronger, or faster athletes and that many supplements pose adverse health risks or are illegal and their use will result in disqualification or other penalties. Athletes may assume "more is better" and take megadoses or use supplement protocols inappropriately. Also, supplements may not work the same in all people because an individual's current habitual diet, genes, and microbiota (i.e., gut organisms, such as bacteria) will affect how the supplement does or does not work (Maughan et al., 2018).

Ergogenic aids (Table 6.10) include both illegal and legal substances. In general, the legality of a supplement within a sport is not determined by whether the supplement is considered natural or an athlete can buy it OTC (via retail outlets, catalogs, magazines, and the internet) or have it provided via a physician's prescription. It is important to note that supplements sold in a retail store or online are not guaranteed to be legal in a particular league or sport. Nutritional supplementation can be toxic, resulting in few benefits and many possible negative consequences. Because of these considerations, the NFHS's Dietary Supplement Position Statement states that it strongly opposes supplement use by high school athletes to improve performance because of the lack of scientific research. It also states that coaches and other school personnel should not recommend or encourage the use of dietary supplements for performance enhancement (http://www.nfhs.org/media/1015652/dietary-supplements-position-statement-2015.pdf). The Taylor Hooton

---

Ergogenic aid Anything, however, usually supplements and pharmacological sources, that has the potential to increase the work output of the person consuming or using it.

Table 6.10
Examples of Nutritional and Pharmacological Ergogenic Substances Used by Athletes

Nutritional		
Generic Name	**Perceived Benefits**	**Potential Adverse Effects**
Amino acids (branched chain amino acids [BCAAs])	Development of muscle mass and repair after exhaustive exercise	Fatigue and loss of coordination; various risks associated with liver and kidneys
Creatine	Production of energy at the muscle cell by converting ADP to ATP	Kidney damage, fluid retention, muscle cramps, upset stomach, and diarrhea
Dietary nitrate	Reduces resting blood pressure, lowers the oxygen cost of submaximal exercise (i.e., enhances muscle efficiency), and may enhance overall exercise performance	Health risks associated with the consumption of nitrate salts include cardiovascular collapse, coma, and/or death
Herb (Common Name)	**Perceived Benefits**	**Potential Adverse Effects**
Ephedra (Chinese ephedra, ma huang)	Powerfully stimulates the nervous system and heart	Banned by FDA
	Used for weight loss, increased energy, and enhanced athletic performance	Seizures, anxiety, heart arrhythmias, stroke, heart attack, and death
Arnica (mountain tobacco)	Muscle pain, stiffness, osteoarthritis	May increase effects of anticoagulants
Echinacea (purple coneflower or Indian head)	Weak immune system, colds, infections	May interfere with immunosuppressants
Rhizoma Zingiberis (ginger)	Nausea, vomiting, motion sickness, osteoarthritis	May interact with anticoagulants and antidiabetic drugs
Rhodiola (golden root)	Lethargy, fatigue, poor endurance	May interact with other herbs
Ginseng (Russian root)	Poor endurance performance, low energy, weak immune system	May interfere with anticoagulants
Guarana (zoom cocoa, Brazilian cocoa)	Excess body fat, lethargy	Contains caffeine

(continues)

Table 6.10 (continued)
Examples of Nutritional and Pharmacological Ergogenic Substances Used by Athletes

Pharmacological: Prescription and Over-the-Counter Substances		
Generic Names (Brand Names Vary)	**Perceived Benefits**	**Potential Adverse Effects**
Androstenedione	Development of muscle mass	Reduction of testosterone production Banned by the U.S. government (2005), IOC, and NFL; available by prescription in the United States if medical condition warrants its use
Dehydroepiandrosterone (DHEA complex)	Development of muscle mass, reduction of body fat, and antiaging	Banned by the IOC and NCAA Stomach upset, high blood pressure, changes in menstrual cycle, facial hair in women, deepening of the voice in women, unfavorable cholesterol changes, aggressive behavior
Hydroxymethylbutyrate (HMB, derivative of leucine)	Muscle repair	Undetermined at this point
Estrogen inhibitors	Inhibits estrogen activity to enhance muscle development (typically used in conjunction with androstenedione)	Reduction of estrogen activity in males and females
Gamma-hydroxybutyrate (GHB)	Promotes deep sleep—argued to enhance growth hormone release. Also known as a date rape drug.	ILLEGAL SUBSTANCE—can result in death; available by prescription in the United States if medical condition warrants its use

ADP, adenosine diphosphate; ATP, adenosine triphosphate.

Foundation (http://taylorhooton.org) is also dedicated to educate youth and their adult influencers about the dangers of appearance- and performance-enhancing drugs, including unregulated dietary supplements. The foundation offers a variety of resources, including assemblies designed to discuss the implications of using ergogenic aids.

A supplement usually includes a variety of ingredients. If a supplement contains ingredients that are banned by the FDA, World Anti-Doping Agency (WADA), or U.S. Anti-Doping Agency (USADA), then it should be considered illegal by the athlete or coach. Supplements that contain one or more of the following ingredients typically fall into an illegal category. These ingredients include but are not limited to anabolic steroids, hormones or metabolic modulators, diuretics, and stimulants. For a complete list of illegal (prohibited) ingredients, WADA (http://www.wada-ama.org) and USADA (http://www.usada.org) provide updated lists, as does the NCAA (http://www.ncaa.org).

Unfortunately, even though the DSHEA of 1994 does require manufacturers and distributors of dietary supplements to ensure their products are safe before they are marketed, once the product is marketed, no third-party screening is required to ensure its effectiveness or safety, and it does not require FDA approval. Good manufacturing practice guidelines were developed and continue to evolve to ensure safety, but manufacturers are not required to follow guidelines. To get a product removed from the market, the FDA must show that the supplement is actually unsafe (results in serious health consequences or deaths) before it can be removed from the marketplace (Buell et al., 2013; Kerksick et al., 2018).

It is up to the coach, athlete, and/or parents to be aware of the substances that can be legally purchased but will result in suspensions from teams and events. This process can be challenging because the FDA lacks oversight of the supplement industry. Thus, not all ingredients will be listed on labels, and these hidden ingredients may be banned substances. As mentioned, there is no FDA requirement to prove safety or quality assurance, so even unbanned yet harmful substances can make their way into supplements (Maughan et al., 2018). To help determine the overall safety of nutritional supplements, a tool developed by USADA is now available to the public, called Supplement 411 (http://www.usada.org/supplement411). It presents testimonials from athletes who were banned from sports because of the use of a variety of nutritional supplements and has accurate and official information regarding the safety and efficacy of commonly available supplements. It investigates the athlete's primary dilemma—the risk versus the reward of using various nutritional supplements in light of the fact that their use may result in a positive doping test or serious health consequences, including death. For these reasons and more, it is highly recommended that athletes consult with a nutritional professional for an individual assessment that includes a detailed medical and nutritional history, diet analysis, blood work, and body composition assessment to determine whether supplementation is necessary and, if so, which supplements are safe and legal (Fink & Mikesky, 2021; Maughan et al., 2018). Additional resources for supplement information can be found in Table 6.10.

The popularity of nutritional supplements has increased tremendously since the 1990s, and so has the number of ingredients deemed to be beneficial for athletic performance. As a result, several national organizations have developed position stands regarding supplements in sports. Most recently, NATA released two comprehensive position stands evaluating dietary supplements (Buell et al., 2013) and anabolic-androgenic steroids (Kersey et al., 2012).

Buell and colleagues (2013) emphasized the philosophy of food first to meet nutritional and performance needs because dietary supplement labels do not require third-party verification; purity (i.e., truth in labeling) and noncontamination cannot be assumed. A food-first philosophy indicates that essential nutrients can be obtained naturally from a healthy diet.

Nutritional Ergogenic Aids

Creatine is one of the most common and widely used nutritional ergogenic aids to enhance strength and fat free mass, as well as benefiting high-intensity activities (Cooper, Naclerio, Allgrove, & Jimenez, 2012). Most coaches and athletes are familiar with it because it produces an increase in energy, allowing the athlete to train for longer periods of time. Creatine is a component in the cell that converts adenosine diphosphate (ADP) to ATP and thus produces energy for the cell. By putting more creatine in the system, the cell can produce more energy, and the athlete can train longer. Thus, the athlete can overload the body and produce greater muscle mass. It has been demonstrated that creatine is more helpful to the athlete who uses short bursts of energy (e.g., sprinters and weight lifters) than to endurance athletes (e.g., soccer players and swimmers). Creatine comes in various forms—creatine monohydrate, creatine anhydrous, creatine pyruvate, creatine citrate, creatine malate, and many more. Creatine can be combined with beta-alanine so the athlete can experience a higher-quality workout, which may result in greater strength gains. The addition of beta-alanine as a supplement appears to have a positive effect on lean-tissue accruement and body fat composition.

Creatine is available in many forms, but most athletes use powder combined with some type of fruit juice. It is an expensive supplement and can be purchased OTC without a physician's prescription. Athletes considering the use of creatine should be encouraged to carefully weigh the purpose of using this or any other supplement before they begin its use. Many supplements have additional ingredients found harmful to health; therefore, supplement safety should seriously be considered. Also, long-term effects of creatine supplementation have been determined to be minimal or of no risk (Kreider et al., 2017; Smith-Ryan et al., 2020).

Amino acids (including whey protein) along with beta-hydroxy beta-methylbutyrate (HMB) are marketed for muscle building and repair. A well-balanced diet provides the essential amino acids for most people. Athletes needing extra amino acids are encouraged to eat increased amounts of food during training and conditioning periods to obtain them. Amino acids are water soluble; when excess amounts are taken, they are cleared through the kidneys and eliminated through the urine, which can apply extra stress to the urinary system and result in permanent damage.

Nitric oxide (NO) is a supplement readily available to athletes in a variety of products, particularly multi-ingredient preworkout supplements. NO is readily available in green leafy vegetables and beets; however, the amount of nitrate necessary to produce beneficial changes for the athlete is undetermined; therefore, there are a variety of regimens that are being recommended. Although NO does seem to have a benefit, such as increasing blood flow to active muscles, its unregulated dosing concerns the medical community and dosages found in multi-ingredient preworkout supplements may not be enough to produce ergogenic effects (Harty et al., 2018). At this time, a food-first philosophy (leafy greens and beet root juice) is the best way to get extra amounts of NO into an athlete's diet.

Athletes can also readily purchase and take herbal supplements as ergogenic aids. The standardization of herbs is not required, and there is little consistency among different batches of herbs from different manufacturers (Buell et al., 2013). Some herbs produce a stimulatory effect (e.g., ginseng, guarana and ephedra), and others produce relaxation to reduce musculoskeletal stress in the athlete (e.g., chamomile and arnica). Some athletes do not understand that using herbs in combination with OTC or prescription drugs can result in either reduced effectiveness of both the drug and the herb or increased action of both the herb and the drug in the body, which can have detrimental health effects (Williams, 2021).

Coaches, athletes, and parents should be reminded that there is very poor regulatory control over nutritional and ergogenic supplements, despite attempts by government agencies to improve regulation. Therefore, it is important for the consumer to evaluate the marketing claims, research studies, and safety issues associated with nutritional ergogenic aids (Buell et al., 2013; Kersey et al., 2012). Several studies have identified unrecognized risks of supplementation, so consumers should be aware of deceptive marketing techniques, including outstanding claims, patents, testimonials, and media campaigns. Research studies that are presented outside of peer-reviewed journals should not be trusted. If presented with research, evaluate whether the authors report subject demographics, methods, and study limitations.

Finally, always be aware of safety issues associated with supplement use. Do not attempt to compensate for poor nutrient or energy intake by taking supplements, and be very careful about toxicity effects. Whole-food products provide the essential macro- and micronutrients needed by physically active individuals, and using illegal substances or doses of single supplements in higher quantities than recommended levels may have detrimental effects on healthy tissue and normal absorption of nutrients (Buell et al., 2013). Athletes and coaches should remember that the most promising area of positive health outcomes related to nutrition is with dietary patterns and not nutrient supplementation, unless nutrient deficiencies exist (Burke et al., 2019; Fink & Mikesky, 2021).

Pharmacological Ergogenic Aids: Stimulants and Anabolic-Androgenic Substances

Stimulants are often the most popular legal substances for ergogenic purposes. In many cases, a variety of stimulants are combined in products. Three common products include caffeine, guarana, and ephedra. They all affect the way the brain recognizes exhaustion during exercise. These supplements, in separate ways, override the brain's recognition of exhaustion during exercise and permit the athlete to continue training when the brain is telling the body to stop. Caffeine is the world's most commonly used psychoactive substance. It is natural to tea, coffee, and cocoa and is typically touted to be a safe aid when providing a boost of energy for the athlete. It is purported to aid endurance activities by assisting substrate metabolism and delaying fatigue. However, there have been large ranges of reported performance increases across research studies, and further research should identify the individual factors that make caffeine an ergogenic aid (Guest et al., 2021). Currently, the NCAA is the only organization that restricts the amount of caffeine consumption by athletes because caffeine is metabolized at different rates and in different ways (McCarthy, 2021). To receive a violation, an athlete would have to consume 6–8 cups of coffee within 2–3 hours of an event to reach around 500 mg of caffeine. Therefore, it is highly unlikely that an athlete will receive a NCAA violation for caffeine consumption. On the other hand, guarana and ephedra are very controversial ergogenic aids. Ephedra has been banned as a supplement; however, ephedra continues to be available in foreign countries and can be purchased over the internet or by other illegal means. It is important for the coach or athletic trainer to discourage the use of guarana or ephedra during exercise situations. The use of these mixtures is most prevalent during two-a-day practices to boost energy levels and has been suspected in the deaths of several athletes. Their use is dangerous and even deadly when environmental factors, such as excessive heat and humidity plus excessive training regimens, are coupled with the athlete's unwillingness to stop exercising at the appropriate time.

Stimulants, including amphetamines, can also be obtained by athletes and are used to increase their energy. Athletes can legally and illegally obtain prescription stimulants, such as Dexedrine (dextroamphetamine), Adderall (amphetamine and dextroamphetamine), and Ritalin (methylphenidate) in an effort to boost energy and focus. In general, amphetamines are commonly used during two-a-day practices or before intense competitions. These prescription stimulants affect the brain and body much the same way as do the OTC stimulants (i.e., caffeine and guarana) do because they block the fatigue messages to the brain and increase focus so athletes can exercise beyond their usual capability. However, like other stimulants, these drugs can make the body more sensitive to heat or cardiac problems. Major League Baseball (MLB) is taking an aggressive approach to the overuse of attention deficit hyperactivity disorder (ADHD) stimulants (i.e., Ritalin and Adderall) by requiring players who have ADHD diagnoses to seek approval by a three-expert panel for a therapeutic use exemption in order to take ADHD medication (Thurm, 2012).

The use and abuse of anabolic-androgenic steroids goes well beyond nutritional supplements and borders on illicit drug use. The most notable supplements in this category are anabolic steroids, growth hormone, and erythropoietin (EPO). These products cannot be purchased in a retail store; thus, they are typically purchased through an underground source. Athletes will go to extreme measures to obtain and use these supplements. They will also go to extreme lengths to hide the use of these illegal supplements. Unfortunately, many can be legal substances when prescribed by a medical professional for the proper reasons. Kersey and colleagues (2012) indicated that anabolic-androgenic products can be used safely in therapeutic doses; however, it is the nontherapeutic and unregulated use by athletes that can pose serious health risks.

Anabolic steroids are legal products, used by many medical doctors and veterinarians in therapeutic dosages to help heal muscle damage and treat other medical conditions, but they are used by athletes illegally in much higher dosages to build muscles. Because the athlete is obtaining these supplements through an illegal source, the dosages used are sometimes as high as 100 times or more than the therapeutic dose. Athletes can use oral or injectable steroids, and, many times, they use both types in a "stacking" routine, or taking multiple doses. (Kersey et al., 2012). Steroids injected directly into the muscle are more effective than those taken by mouth because a higher percentage is delivered directly to the muscle after injection. Oral intake allows the drug to metabolize and degrade in the digestive and hepatic (i.e., liver) systems. Unfortunately, many times, the athlete injecting steroids does not have the proper equipment for injections and must share needles and syringes, which is very dangerous. By using anabolic steroids in large amounts, athletes can contract bloodborne diseases, damage internal organs, increase risk of heart attack, develop unwanted aggression and secondary sex characteristics, and cause changes to their body composition that may not help them in their preferred sport. The NSCA rejects the use of anabolic steroids on the basis of fair play and concerns for the athlete's health. It also encourages that research and funding be dedicated to educational programs and documentation of both short- and long-term effects of anabolic steroid abuse (Bhasin et al., 2021; Hoffman et al., 2009). The Taylor Hooton Foundation also offers educational material on steroids and other supplements (http://taylorhooton.org).

Other commonly known substances the athlete may be tempted to use are testosterone precursors. Androstenedione is a testosterone precursor taken by athletes with the intent to build muscle tissue. Androstenedione (andro) was made famous by professional baseball player Mark McGwire. OTC sales of andro were banned by the U.S. government in January 2005; however, an athlete may be able to purchase this drug over the internet, and it is also available by prescription; thus, an athlete may be able to obtain it legally. Another testosterone precursor currently popular with athletes is dehydroepiandrosterone (DHEA), a hormone found in the blood that is converted to androstenedione and then to testosterone. Testosterone increases protein synthesis and slows protein breakdown, which can generate increased muscle bulk with proper training. The adverse effect of using testosterone or testosterone precursors is the reduction of natural androgen hormone production by the body. Andro is banned by the International Olympic Committee (IOC), NFL, and MLB; DHEA is banned by the IOC, NFL, National Basketball Association (NBA), MLB, and NCAA. Many of the athletes using testosterone precursors also use estrogen inhibitors, which increase the effectiveness of the andro. Using an estrogen inhibitor reduces the estrogen in the body. In female athletes, this reduction of estrogen combined with the increase in overall testosterone over a long period of time leads to an increase in male characteristics.

EPO is a natural substance produced by the kidneys that stimulates red blood cell proliferation. EPO can now be synthesized in the laboratory and is used for cancer patients undergoing chemotherapy and other individuals with chronic illnesses who need to augment their red blood cell levels. Athletes who compete in endurance activities can benefit from an increase in the number of circulating red blood cells. The red blood cells carry oxygen; the more oxygen the bloodstream can carry to the cells, the longer the cells can function. The longer the cells function, the longer the athlete can compete at a higher level. Endurance athletes, such as swimmers, marathon runners, and cyclists, have been known to use this drug. The adverse effect of using EPO is that the athlete may take too much and get too many red blood cells circulating. This situation increases the viscosity of the blood and makes the heart work much harder to pump this thick blood through the body. If the heart has to work too hard for too long, the athlete can experience heart failure and die (Salamin et al., 2018).

Gamma-hydroxybutyrate (GHB) is an illegal substance (it is also known as a date rape drug) but can be obtained by some athletes. Those who sell GHB to athletes claim it helps the athlete get into the deepest phase of sleep and stay in that sleep phase longer. Deep sleep is suggested to be the cycle during which human growth hormone is released, making longer deep sleep potentially valuable for increased muscle growth (Chennaoui et al., 2015). The use of GHB can be lethal to an athlete. It is an illegal substance, and all athletes should be discouraged from its use.

Review Questions

1. Describe the similarities and differences between the basic molecular structure of carbohydrate, fat, and protein.

2. Describe the major problems associated with excessive consumption of dietary protein.

3. According to the chapter, a survey of coaches, athletes, and BOC-certified athletic trainers revealed that athletes depended on which sources for their information about nutrition?

4. What is the recommended level of dietary protein for adolescent athletes?

5. How much water does the body need under conditions of heavy exercise in high ambient temperatures?

6. Calculate the BMR for an 18-year-old male athlete who weighs 200 lb, is 6 ft tall, and has 18% body fat.

7. Calculate the MCW for the athlete from question 6 if he would like to have 16% body fat.

8. Discuss briefly the short-term effects of repeated episodes of extreme, rapid weight loss.
9. What should be the three goals of any sports nutrition program?
10. What are the recommended percentages of protein, fat, and carbohydrate in an ideal training diet?
11. Using the equation provided in the chapter, compute the protein requirement (in grams) for a football player who weighs 94 kg.
12. Briefly list the general guidelines regarding the composition of a precompetition meal.
13. True or false: During times of heavy exertion, it is not possible to lose more than 0.5–1 L of water for each hour of exercise.
14. Compute the fluid deficiency (% dehydration and amount of fluid [ounces] necessary for proper replacement) of an athlete (175 lb) who weighs 5.5 lb less after practice than he did before practice.
15. What are the effects of dietary fasting on muscle tissue?
16. True or false: Sports scientists recommend a training diet in which 30–40% of daily calories consumed are in the form of protein.
17. What are the nutritional concerns of an injured athlete who is recovering from an injury?
18. Name the risks associated with nutritional supplementation.
19. What drugs are typically used illegally in sports to obtain an advantage?
20. What resources should an athlete use to obtain credible information about ergogenic aids?

References

American Diabetes Association. (2014). Glycemic index and diabetes. Retrieved from http://www.diabetes.org/food-and-fitness/food/what-can-i-eat/understanding-carbohydrates/glycemic-index-and-diabetes.html?loc=ff-slabnav

Aragon, A. A., Schoenfeld, B. J., Wildman, R., Kleiner, S., VanDusseldorp, T., Taylor, L., Earnest, C. P., Arciero, P. J., Wilborn, C., Kalman, D. S., Stout, J. R., Willoughby, D. S., Campbell, B., Arent, S. M., Bannock, L., Smith-Ryan, A. E., & Antonio, J. (2017). International Society of Sports Nutrition position stand: Diets and body composition. *Journal of the International Society of Sports Nutrition, 14*, 16.

Bhasin, S., Hatfield, D., Hoffman, J., Kraemer, W., Labotz, M., Phillips, S., & Ratamess, N. (2021). Anabolic-androgenic steroid use in sports, health, and society. *Medicine & Science in Sports & Exercise, 53*(8), 1778–1794.

Buell, J., Franks, R., Ransone, J., Powers, M. E., Laquale, K. M., & Carlson-Phillips, A. (2013). National Athletic Trainers' Association position statement: Evaluation of dietary supplements for performance nutrition. *Journal of Athletic Training, 48*(1), 124–136.

Burke, L. M., Castell, L. M., Casa, D. J., Close, G. L., Costa, R. J. S., Desbrow, B., Halson, S. L., Lis, D. M., Melin, A. K., Peeling, P., Saunders, P. U., Slater, G. J., Sygo, J., Witard, O. C., Bermon, S., & Stellingwerff, T. (2019). International Association of Athletics Federations consensus statement 2019: Nutrition for athletics. *International Journal of Sport Nutrition and Exercise Metabolism, 29*(2), 73–84.

Burke, L. M., Slater, G. J., Matthews, J. J., Langan-Evans, C., & Horswill, C. A. (2021). ACSM expert consensus statement on weight loss in weight-category sports. *Current Sports Medicine Reports, 20*(4), 199–217.

Chennaoui, M., Arnal, P. J., Sauvet, F., & Leger, D. (2015). Sleep and exercise: A reciprocal issue? *Sleep Medicine Reviews, 20*, 59–72.

Cooper, R., Naclerio, F., Allgrove, J., & Jimenez, A. (2012). Creatine supplementation with specific view to exercise/sports performance: An update. *Journal of the International Society of Sports Nutrition, 9*(33).

de la Puente Yagüe, M., Collado Yurrita, L., Ciudad Cabañas, M. J., & Cuadrado Cenzual, M. A. (2020). Role of vitamin D in athletes and their performance: Current concepts and new trends. *Nutrients, 12*(2), 579.

Dietary Guidelines Advisory Committee. (2015). *Dietary guidelines for Americans 2015–2020*. Government Printing Office. Retrieved from https://health.gov/dietaryguidelines/2015/guidelines/

Elliot, D. L., Goldberg, L., Moe, E. L., DeFrancesco, C. A., Durham, M. B., McGinnis, W., & Lockwood, C. (2008). Long-term outcomes of the ATHENA (Athletes Targeting Healthy Exercise and Nutrition Alternatives) program for female high school athletes. *Journal of Alcohol & Drug Education, 52*(2), 73–92.

Fink, H. H., & Mikesky, A. E. (2021). *Practical applications in sports nutrition* (6th ed.). Burlington, MA: Jones & Bartlett Learning.

Fishman, M. P., Lombardo, S. J., & Kharrazi, F. D. (2016). Vitamin D deficiency among professional basketball players. *Orthopedic Journal of Sports Medicine, 4*(7), 1–5.

Glycemic Index. (2017). Retrieved from http://www.glycemicindex.com/index.php

Guest, N. S., VanDusseldorp, T. A., Nelson, M. T., Grgic, J., Schoenfeld, B. J., Jenkins, N. D., Arent, S. M., Antonio, J., Stout, J. R., Trexler, E. T., Smith-Ryan, A. E., Goldstein, E. R., Kalman, D. S., & Campbell, B. I. (2021). International Society of Sports Nutrition position stand: Caffeine and exercise performance. *Journal of the International Society of Sports Nutrition, 18*(1), 1–37.

Harty, P. S., Zabriskie, H. A., Erickson, J. L., Molling, P. E., Kerksick, C. M., & Jagim, A. R. (2018). Multi-ingredient pre-workout supplements, safety implications, and performance outcomes: A brief review. *Journal of the International Society of Sports Nutrition, 15*(1), 1–28.

Hector, A. J., & Phillips, S. M. (2018). Protein recommendations for weight loss in elite athletes: A focus on body composition and performance. *International Journal of Sport Nutrition and Exercise Metabolism, 28*(2), 170–177.

Hildebrand, R. A., Miller, B., Warren, A., Hildebrand, D., & Smith, B. J. Compromised vitamin D status negatively affects muscular strength and power of collegiate athletes. *International Journal of Sport Nutrition and Exercise Metabolism, 26*(6), 558–564. doi:10.1123/ijsnem.2016-0052

Hoffman, J. R., Kraemer, W. J., Bhasin, S., Storer, T., Ratamess, N. A., Haff, G. G., . . . Rogol, A. D. (2009). Position stand on androgen and human growth hormone use. *Journal of Strength and Conditioning Research, 23*(5), S1–S59.

Holway, F. E., & Spriet, L. L. (2011). Sport-specific nutrition: Practical strategies for team sports. *Journal of Sports Sciences, 29*(Supp. 1), S115–S125.

Jenkins, D. J., Dehghan, M., Mente, A., Bangdiwala, S. I., Rangarajan, S., Srichaikul, K., ... & Yusuf, S. (2021). Glycemic index, glycemic load, and cardiovascular disease and mortality. *New England Journal of Medicine, 384*(14), 1312–1322.

Kerksick, C. M., Wilborn, C. D., Roberts, M. D., Smith-Ryan, A., Kleiner, S. M., Jäger, R., Collins, R., Cooke, M., Davis, J. N., Galvan, E., Greenwood, M., Lowery, L. M., Wildman, R., Antonio, J., & Kreider, R. B. (2018). ISSN exercise & sports nutrition review update: Research & recommendations. *Journal of the International Society of Sports Nutrition, 15*(1), 1–57.

Kersey, R., Elliot, D. L., Goldberg, L., Kanayama, G., Leone, J. E., Pavlovich, M., Pope, H. G. Jr. (2012). National Athletic Trainers' Association position statement: Anabolic-androgenic steroids. *Journal of Athletic Training, 47*(5), 567–588.

Knappenberger, K. (2018, July). Nutrition for injury recovery and rehabilitation. *NATA News*, 14–17.

Kreider, R. B., Kalman, D. S., Antonio, J., Ziegenfuss, T. N., Wildman, R., Collins, R., Candow, D. G., Kleiner, S. M., Almada, A. L., & Lopez, H. L. (2017). International Society of Sports Nutrition position stand: Safety and efficacy of creatine supplementation in exercise, sport, and medicine. *Journal of the International Society of Sports Nutrition, 14*(1), 1–18.

Lakicevic, N., Mani, D., Paoli, A., Roklicer, R., Bianco, A., & Drid, P. (2021). Weight cycling in combat sports: Revisiting 25 years of scientific evidence. *BMC Sports Science, Medicine and Rehabilitation, 13*(1), 1–6.

Maroon, J. C., Mathyssek, C. M., Bost, J. W., Amos, A., Winkelman, R., Yates, A. P., Duca, M. A., Norwig, J. A. (2015). Vitamin D profile in National Football League players. *American Journal of Sports Medicine, 43*(5), 1241–1245.

Maughan, R. J., Burke, L. M., Dvorak, J., Enette Larson-Meyer, D., Peeling, P., Phillips, S. M., . . . Engebretsen, L. (2018). IOC consensus statement: Dietary supplements and the high-performance athlete. *International Journal of Sport Nutrition and Exercise Metabolism, 28*(2), 104–125.

McCarthy, C. (2021). Caffeine can affect student-athlete health, performance. *College Athletics and the Law, 18*(5), 1–5.

McDermott, B. P., Anderson, S. A., Armstrong, L. E., Casa, D. J., Cheuvront, S. N., Cooper, L., ... Roberts, W. O. (2017). National Athletic Trainers' Association position statement: Fluid replacement for the physically active, 52(9), 877–895.

Murphy, C., & Koehler, K. (2022). Energy deficiency impairs resistance training gains in lean mass but not strength: A meta-analysis and meta-regression. *Scandinavian Journal of Medicine & Science in Sports, 32*(1), 125–137.

National Institutes of Health (NIH). (n.d.). Nutrient Recommendations: Dietary Reference Intakes (DRI). Retrieved from https://ods.od.nih.gov/Health_Information/Dietary_Reference_Intakes.aspx

Ogden, C. L., Carroll, M. D., Lawman, H. G., Fryar, C. D., Kruszon-Moran, D., Kit, B. K., & Flegal, K. M. (2016). Trends in obesity prevalence among children and adolescents in the United States, 1988–1994 through 2013–2014. *JAMA, 315*(21), 2292–2299.

Riviere, A. J., Leach, R., Mann, H., Robinson, S., Burnett, D. C., Babu, J. R., & Frugé, A. D. (2021). Nutrition knowledge of collegiate athletes in the United States and the impact of sports dietitians on related outcomes: A narrative review. *Nutrients, 13*(6), 1772.

Salamin, O., Kuuranne, T., Saugy, M., & Leuenberger, N. (2018). Erythropoietin as a performance-enhancing drug: Its mechanistic basis, detection, and potential adverse effects. *Molecular and Cellular Endocrinology, 464*, 75–87.

Smith-Ryan, A. E., Hirsch, K. R., Saylor, H. E., Gould, L. M., & Blue, M. N. (2020). Nutritional considerations and strategies to facilitate injury recovery and rehabilitation. *Journal of Athletic Training, 55*(9), 918–930.

Thomas, D. T., Erdman, K. A., & Burke, L. M. (2016). American College of Sports Medicine joint position statement: Nutrition and athletic performance. *Medicine & Science in Sports & Exercise, 48*(3), 543–568.

Thurm, W. (2012). Is there an ADHD epidemic in major league baseball? Retrieved from http://www.baseballnation.com/2012/6/29/3104332/is-there-an-adhd-epidemic-in-major-league-baseball

Torres-McGehee, T., Pritchett, K., Zippel, D., Minton, D., Cellamare, A., & Sibilia, M. (2012). Sports nutrition knowledge among collegiate athletes, coaches, athletic trainers, and strength and conditioning specialists. *Journal of Athletic Training, 47*(2), 205–211.

Turocy, P. S., DePalma, B. F., Horswill, C. A., Laquale, K. M., Martin, T. J., Perry, A. C., . . . & Utter, A. C. (2011). National athletic trainers' association position statement: Safe weight loss and maintenance practices in sport and exercise. *Journal of athletic training, 46*(3), 322–336.

Williams, C. T. (2021). Herbal supplements: Precautions and safe use. *Nursing Clinics, 56*(1), 1–21.

Wohlgemuth, K. J., Arieta, L. R., Brewer, G. J., Hoselton, A. L., Gould, L. M., & Smith-Ryan, A. E. (2021). Sex differences and considerations for female specific nutritional strategies: A narrative review. *Journal of the International Society of Sports Nutrition, 18*(1), 1–20.

CHAPTER 7
Emergency Plan and Initial Injury Evaluation

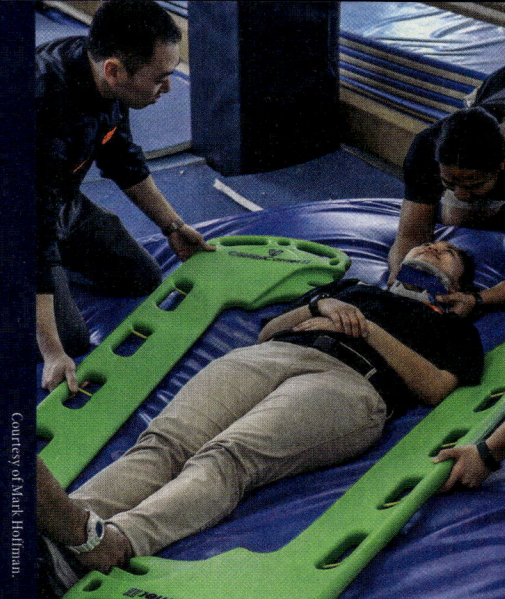

MAJOR CONCEPTS

Coaching and other athletic personnel have a legal duty to develop and implement an emergency action plan to be followed if an athlete is injured while participating in sports. To be effective, the emergency plan must be carefully planned by all the principal parties involved, including all members of the athletic healthcare team in conjunction with emergency medical services (EMS) providers in the community. In the primary and secondary school settings, the appropriate institutional representatives, such as the athletic trainer (AT; if one is employed by the school district), athletic director, and school principal, should be involved as well, whereas in the collegiate/university setting the AT, athletic director, medical director, police department, vice president, and board of regents are the ones most often involved in emergency planning. Youth leagues, sports complexes, and other venues that host events should also have an emergency action plan, which would involve the league commissioner, facilities administrator for the venue, and any other sports or event director with influence over the league or facilities in the development and implementation of the plan. The plan must be flexible to allow for changes in personnel or facilities and venues and should be revisited annually. In addition, the plan must incorporate an education component that includes annual rehearsal to ensure it will work effectively if and when an emergency arises. Skills of available personnel must be recognized, and roles and responsibilities should be carefully documented. Details such as emergency equipment inventory, communications, and transportation must be carefully considered. Moreover, the emergency plan must extend beyond the traditional game-day and practice paradigm to include off-season components, such as summer conditioning camps and the strength and conditioning room if it is a separate facility. As well, the plan must address the potential issue of an injured or ill fan, sideline participant, or official. This chapter provides a step-by-step outline of the vital components in the development of an effective emergency plan and discusses the process of injury evaluation in the unique situations presented in the sports environment.

Sports injuries are an inevitable outcome of participation for millions of high school athletes and hundreds of thousands of collegiate athletes each year. The lack of emergency planning, policies, medical staff, and proper emergency equipment is often the major safety concern that faces youth sports and secondary school athletics (Adams et al., 2018; Casa et al., 2013). A recent assessment

(Adams et al., 2018) of evidence-based polices related to health and safety of secondary school athletes produced sobering results. Although all 50 states and the District of Columbia have regulations that mandate concussion referral plans and will not allow return to play without written release from a qualified healthcare provider, only 24 states require that every school or organization sponsoring athletics develop an emergency plan for managing any serious or life-threatening sport-related injuries (Adams et al., 2018). However, a recent national survey of secondary school ATs revealed that 89% of respondents reported having a written EAP at their schools (Scarneo et al., 2019). On another positive note, most (50–90%) of the respondents indicated that their EAPs list emergency equipment, provide venue specific directions, and are updated, reviewed, rehearsed, and distributed by relevant athletic staff members annually (Scarneo et al., 2019). Proper planning is essential to ensure appropriate initial first aid management of limb and life-threatening injuries because many of these injuries occur without warning (Andersen et al., 2002; Parsons et al., 2019). Developing a formal emergency action plan for sports injuries is important for two primary reasons. First, anything that can be done ahead of time to improve the health care of injured athletes, coaches, officials, or fans should be a priority. Second, from a legal standpoint, failure to have an emergency plan in place has been found to constitute negligence in litigation resulting from a sports injury (Quandt et al., 2009). According to Mirsafian (2016), although coaches often do not have satisfactory knowledge to manage all emergency situations, they owe their athletes various legal duties regardless of the type and level of sport they are involved in, and a breach of those duties can lead to their civil or criminal liability. Moreover, causing unnecessary aggravation or complications by failing to identify and properly deal with injuries presents a legal liability (McCaskey & Biedzynski, 1996). Therefore, planning ahead for potential emergencies is essential.

Emergency action plans (EAPs) are written blueprints for handling emergencies; such plans should be easily understood and clearly establish accountability for the management of emergencies (Andersen et al., 2002). First and foremost, each entity sponsoring or hosting athletic events must have a written EAP that is comprehensive, practical, and flexible to adapt. A summary of the key elements identified by the National Athletic Trainers' Association (NATA; Andersen et al., 2002) for the development of EAPs follows; these elements can be found on NATA's website at https://www.nata.org/sites/default/files/emergencyplanninginathletics.pdf:

1. An EAP for athletics identifies the personnel (i.e., emergency team) involved in carrying it out and outlines the qualifications. All personnel should be trained in automatic external defibrillator (AED) use, cardiopulmonary resuscitation (CPR), first aid, and prevention of disease transmission.
2. The EAP should specify the equipment needed to carry out the tasks required in the event of an emergency and the location of the emergency equipment. The level of training of the personnel involved determines the type of equipment made available.
3. Arrangements need to be made to have EMS personnel present at all athletic events whenever possible (Figure 7.1). However, if EMS personnel

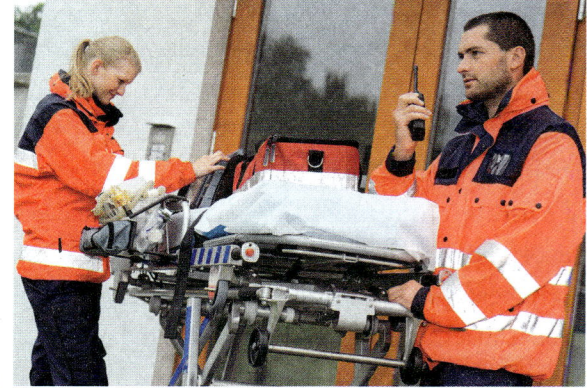
(a)

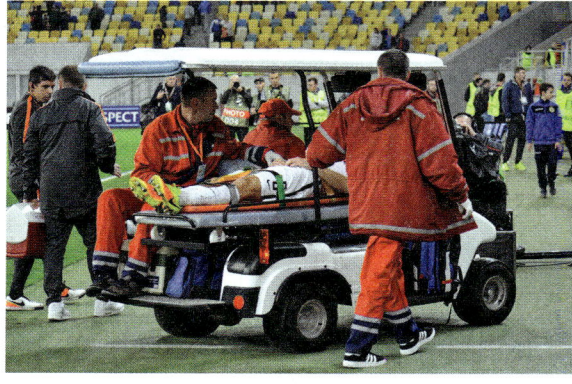
(b)

Figure 7.1 Arrangements must be made to have EMS personnel present at athletic events whenever possible.
(a) © CandyBox Images/Shutterstock; (b) © Vlad1988/Shutterstock.

are not present at the event, then all staff members should know the mechanisms for communication to summon the appropriate emergency care service providers. Situations are different from community to community, so all key members of the staff must know the emergency access numbers and have access to either a cellular phone or a landline. In many cases, an emergency call box may be available to summon EMS directly. In addition to notifying EMS, EAPs must identify the mode of transportation for the injured participant to the emergency vehicle if the EMS cannot directly access the field or court of play.

4. The EAP should be specific to the activity venue. In particular, specific addresses to each venue, access routes to playing areas from roads, and the location of keys to any gates or doors that may present barriers to emergency personnel should be delineated in the EAP.

5. The EAP should also have specific checklists for the care of injuries when the timing and accuracy of care can be the difference between life and death. The recommendation is that checklists should be developed for moderate to severe brain trauma, massive hemorrhaging, cervical spine injury, asthma, exertional heat illness, exertional sickling, rhabdomyolysis, diabetes, and cardiac arrest (Drezner et al., 2007; Parsons et al., 2019).

6. EAPs should incorporate the emergency care facilities to which the injured individual will be taken. Emergency receiving facilities should be notified in advance of large scheduled events and contests. If possible, personnel from the emergency receiving facilities should be included in the development of the EAP for the institution or organization.

7. The EAP specifies the necessary documentation supporting its implementation and evaluation. This documentation should identify responsibility for documenting the actions taken during the emergency, evaluation of the emergency response, and institutional personnel training.

8. The EAP should be reviewed and rehearsed annually, although more frequent review and rehearsal may be necessary if there are staff changes. Changes in staff, facilities, playing schedules, EMS personnel, and playing seasons can affect the EAP's effectiveness. The results of these reviews and rehearsals should be documented and should indicate whether the EAP was modified, with further documentation reflecting how it was changed.

9. The administration and legal counsel of the sponsoring organization or institution should review the EAP.

Emergency Team

In any school setting or facility, the recommendation is that all personnel directly involved with the interscholastic sports program take part in the development and implementation of the EAP. These personnel should include coaches, directors and administrators, the team physician and AT (if available), school nurses, local EMS personnel, **athletic training student aides** (if present), and other staff members (e.g., managers and administrative assistants) involved with the program. Typically, the ATs and athletic training student aides, team physician, coaches, and managers associated directly with the interscholastic sports program are the personnel who comprise what is known as the emergency team at an event. They provide four functions regarding the EAP: (1) immediate care of the athlete, (2) emergency equipment retrieval, (3) activation of EMS (when the situation is deemed of sufficient magnitude), and (4) signaling the EMS to the field if they are already present or directing EMS to the scene of the injury if they were not originally present. A decision should be made ahead of time as to who will remain with the injured athlete, who will call or signal emergency personnel, and who will retrieve equipment and/or unlock/open access points for arriving emergency services. The emergency team should stipulate ahead of time what type of signals will be used to (1) alert on-site EMS personnel to come onto the field and render care if necessary, (2) alert the team physician to come to the field, and (3) indicate the specific equipment that is needed on-site (Andersen et al., 2002). In particular, emergency signals and equipment retrieval instructions or locations are also best reviewed and disseminated before the start of each athletic event

Athletic training student aides Students who observe and experience the field of athletic training under the direct supervision of a certified or licensed athletic trainer.

in a "time-out" meeting (NATA, 2012). The time out gathers together the athletic healthcare professionals who comprise the emergency response team to go through pre–athletic-event checklists to review the venue's EAP. Time outs allow for all healthcare providers to become familiar with each other, the roles of the team, the equipment available and its location, and any signals, thereby allowing for a coordinated and decisive emergency response and outcome (NATA, 2012). Because of the serious nature of many injuries, time outs should also review any specific checklists established for the immediate care and disposition of these injuries to avoid conflict or confusion at the time of the injury (Parsons et al., 2019).

Best Practices for Emergency Planning for Athletics

The general agreement is that the most effective way to prevent fatalities and manage nonfatal events is through a sound and well-rehearsed EAP. As a result, several best practices related to the construction and implementation of EAPs within institutional athletic settings have been developed to guide secondary schools and colleges in the removal of barriers that jeopardize the delivery of optimal safety and preventive measures to the athletic community (Casa et al., 2012a; Casa et al., 2013; Cooper et al., 2019; Parsons et al., 2019). Best practices have also been established for youth sports that can be used as a road map for youth leagues and associations (Huggins et al., 2017).

Institution-Based Athletics

These best practices contain standards that address many areas associated with institution-based athletics, including standards aligned with readiness for participation; access to healthcare teams; safe participation relative to the environment; hydration and nutrition; and equipment choice, fitting, and maintenance. The inclusion of comprehensive athletic EAPs integrated with local EMS per athletic venue are also included in the best practices. Regarding standards that facilitate emergency planning and the creation of a safe environment for sports participation, the following areas are considered as essential best-practice actions for institutions that sponsor athletics.

1. The sponsoring organization should have a comprehensive athletic EAP to ensure that appropriate care can be provided in a timely manner, even in the absence of on-site medical providers (Cooper et al., 2019).
2. No scheduled athletic activity, including conditioning sessions, should occur until the appropriate administrators have confirmed that coaches and all support staff are fully familiar with the EAP and the EAP is posted at each venue (Casa et al., 2013; Cooper et al., 2019; Parsons et al., 2019).
3. All athletics staff who have contact with student-athletes should possess current certification in first aid and CPR/AED, be educated about factors contributing to sudden death and how to recognize life-threatening situations, and be responsible for documenting competencies and continuing education specific to preventing sudden death in sports (Casa et al., 2012a; Casa et al., 2013).
4. Establish an efficient internal and external communication system to activate on- and off-site emergency team members.
5. Post the specific location of all emergency equipment and assign team members responsibility for specific equipment retrieval and readiness checks before the event. For example, AEDs and other CPR equipment should be placed for immediate retrieval (no more than 1 to 3 minutes is ideal) after recognizing an emergency (Casa et al., 2013; Parsons et al., 2019).
6. Train members of emergency team in proper use and maintenance of all equipment, including battery replacement and documentation of maintenance records.
7. Provide guidelines on who will advocate for a minor in the event of an emergency incident when the parent or guardian is absent (Cooper et al., 2019).

Youth Sports–Based Athletics

In the United States, youth sports and fitness participation has grown significantly over the years as evidenced by the numbers: over 28 million youth (ages 6–17 years) participate in a team sport (Endres et al., 2019) and over 60 million participate in some form of organized sports (McKay et al., 2019).

Around 56.6% of Generation Z (i.e., those born after 2000) indicate that they participate in a team sport as compared to 30.4% of Millennials (i.e., those born between 1980 and 1999); however, recent data from 2020 indicates that inactivity is consistent between both generations at about 20–27% (Physical Activity Council, 2021). Unfortunately, sports are a leading cause of injury, with an estimation that around 59 of every 1,000 individuals aged 5–24 will sustain a sports- or recreation-related injury each year in the United States (McKay et al., 2019). Therefore, the need is great to have education and best practices designed to protect youth sports participants.

While most youth sports have a national governing board (NGB) to give instruction to the lower levels, not all NGBs provide directives to those levels regarding best practices for the health and safety of the participants. Because of the variety of sports and NGBs involved with youth participation, determining injury rates for the participants is difficult. From 2007 to 2015, 45 deaths were reported in youth sports (Endres et al., 2019). In general, sudden deaths occur more often in males, with basketball having the highest incidence, and they occur more often in practices than in competitions (Endres et al., 2019). As is the case with other research regarding deaths within this age group, the highest percentage of the deaths were attributed to cardiac issues (Endres et al., 2019). As is the case with secondary schools and colleges, youth sports leagues should utilize best practices to ensure the health and safety of their participants and staff (Huggins et al., 2017).

1. Each youth sports league should have an EAP for each venue that the league uses. This EAP should be designed by local personnel and approved by the league commissioner or director.
2. Each league should devote financial resources for the purchase and maintenance of emergency equipment, such as AEDs, medical kits, splints, and venue-specific emergency items. For example, a large soccer complex may want to have some type of motorized vehicle to help transport injured participants. Emergency equipment should be at each venue that the youth sports league utilizes for competitions and practices.
3. All league officials and coaches should be required to have CPR/AED certification and be educated in the prevention of sudden death.
4. League officials, coaches, and parents should have access to training modules regarding emergency situations, including exertional heatstroke, concussion, and sudden cardiac arrest.
5. Participants' parents should be required to report to the league any past or current medical conditions, allergies, and medications for their children.
6. Coaches in youth sports leagues should be trained in best coaching practices to minimize injury risk to the participants.

Emergency Care Training

All personnel involved with organized sports programs must be trained in basic first aid and CPR (Figure 7.2). Recent developments in AEDs (Figure 7.3) have made these devices available to schools and recreational facilities. As such, members of the athletic healthcare team should be trained in the use of AEDs and bag valve masks (Figures 7.4 and 7.5). First aid, CPR, and AED training is available through several agencies nationwide, including the National Safety Council, the American Heart Association, the Red Cross, and the Emergency Care and Safety Institute. All personnel are strongly encouraged to upgrade their training according to recommendations by each agency; however, annual practice and periodic mock emergency drills should be done to verify the effectiveness of the emergency plan. Emergency care skills deteriorate quickly and should be reviewed regularly. In addition to completing

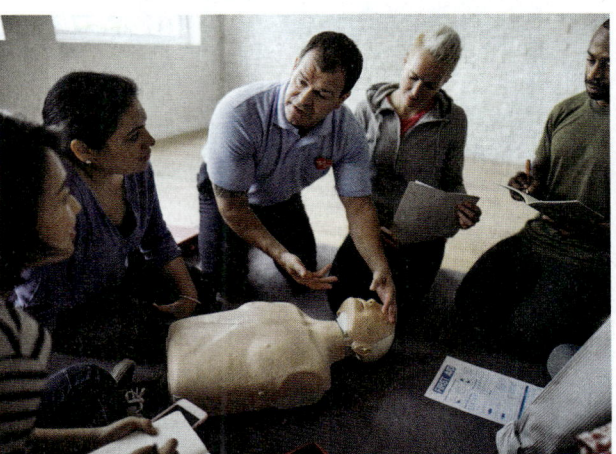

Figure 7.2 Instructor leading CPR training.
© Rawpixel.com/Shutterstock.

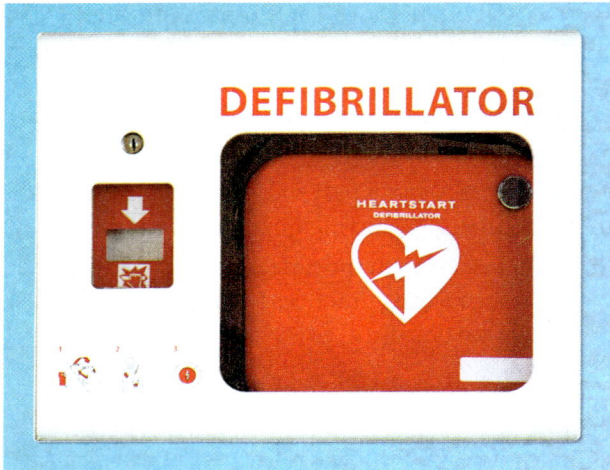

Figure 7.3 Automated external defibrillator (AED) hanging on wall.
© Flowersandtravelin/Shutterstock.

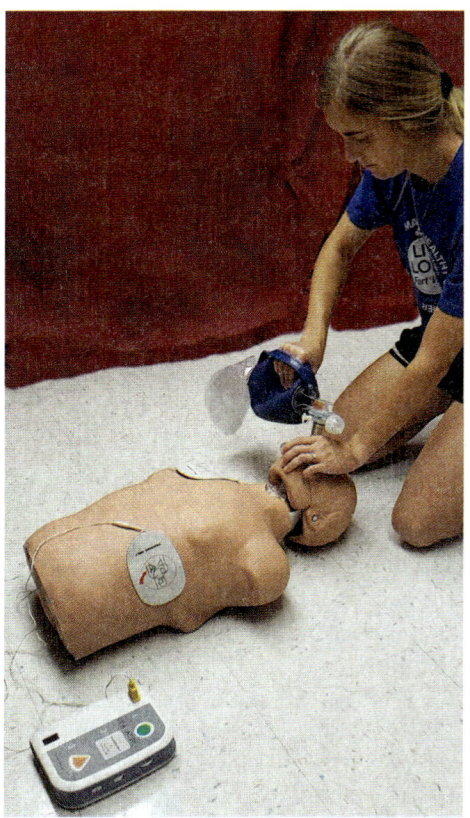

Figure 7.5 Rescuer giving rescue breaths to a training mannequin using a bag valve mask.
Courtesy of Cindy Trowbridge.

emergency skills training, coaches should be trained to recognize life-threatening situations and educated about factors contributing to sudden death (Casa et al., 2012a; Casa et al., 2013).

Injury Evaluation Procedures

To be effective in the initial process of injury management, the person rendering first aid must have a prepared protocol to follow. The emergency treatment protocol must be generic enough to be effective regardless of the type of injury. By following a preplanned format, the coach or physical educator is assured of first evaluating all vital life functions and following up with a step-by-step examination to determine any serious injuries that the athlete may have sustained. In this way, tragedy can be avoided. For example, not recognizing exertional sickling and treating it as heat illness or treating an unconscious athlete's head wound without first assessing the airway and determining whether the athlete is breathing could result in sudden death.

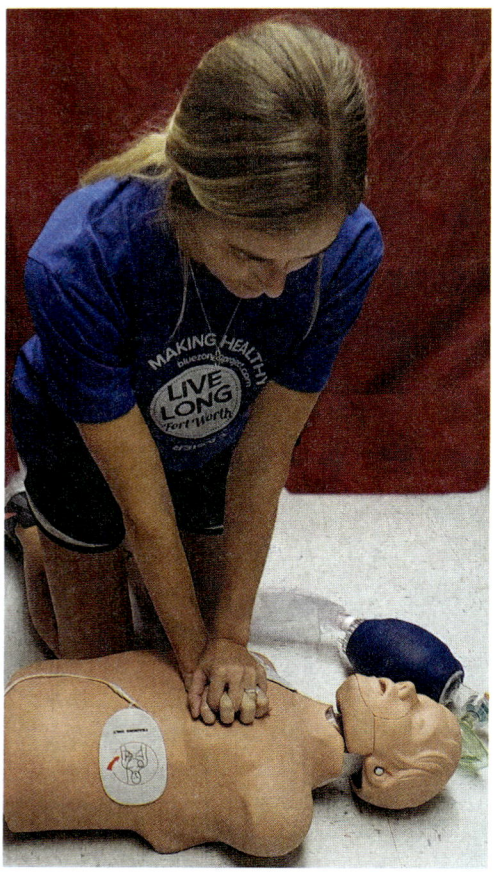

Figure 7.4 Rescuer performing chest compressions on a training mannequin after AED analyzed heart rhythm and provided shock.
Courtesy of Cindy Trowbridge.

> ### WHAT IF ❓
>
> You are a football coach in Tucson, Arizona. You are trained in CPR, first aid, and AED use, and all of your athletes have been cleared to participate and have a preparticipation physical examination on file. What equipment and student-athlete information would you request from your athletic director or AT to prevent sudden death from occurring at practices that often take place when the temperature is above 100°F?

Each injury presents initial responders with a unique set of circumstances; however, their responsibilities remain the same. They must have a basic knowledge of sports injuries and, more important, the ability to differentiate between life-threatening, major, and minor injuries, which requires the development of initial assessment skills necessary to determine which injuries should be referred to medical personnel and which can be treated with simple first aid. Such determinations represent a major dilemma for many in the coaching or physical education profession and is especially true when no AT is immediately available, as is often the case. Secondary school survey findings reveal that 67% of the schools ($n = 10,553$) had access to AT services; however, only 35% had full-time access, 30% had part-time access, and 3% had per diem contracts, but the remaining 32% of respondents reported no access to AT services (Huggins et al., 2018). Because almost one-third of secondary schools do not have an AT, the importance of other people within the athletic department being familiar with the preexisting emergency plan and able to function effectively as "first responders" on the athletic healthcare team is clear.

Initial Responders' Limitations

In the absence of a Board of Certification (BOC)–certified or state-licensed AT, medical doctor, or other designated healthcare provider, initial responders may be responsible for the earliest management of injuries sustained by an athlete. Initial responders must take special care not to overstep the bounds of their training, experience, and expertise. In short, they should avoid the urge to provide care beyond their first aid training. All the procedures described so far can be classified as appropriate first aid care that should be rendered by coaching personnel at the time of an injury. The critical point to remember, however, is that initial responders should not perform procedures that are clearly in the domain of medical doctors or allied health personnel, such as ATs. For example, performing special tests on joints to determine injury to ligaments; reducing (i.e., putting back into place) a dislocated joint; and removing stitches, a splint, or a cast are clearly procedures that fall in the domain of trained medical professionals and not initially responding staff members.

Immediate management of an acute emergent sports injury presents initial responders with a challenge unlike their normal day-to-day activities. The primary objective of immediate management by the personnel who are initially responding is for them to provide appropriate initial care, including sustaining the injured athlete's life if necessary. In a best-case scenario, the initial responders would be BOC-certified ATs, state-licensed ATs, or qualified medical personnel (QMP), such as a physician, physician assistant, emergency medical technician, paramedic, or advance practice nurse. However, if the initial responders are a coach, an administrator, or another layperson, they have no less of a responsibility to ensure the health and safety of the sick or injured person. Initial responders are in charge of the immediate care of the sick or injured person to determine the severity of the injury and sustain life. Because sports injuries generally occur amid the confusion of a contest or practice, initial responders must maintain a clear head and remain objective in the earliest assessment of any injury.

In the absence of an AT or other QMP, coaches or other individuals should be seen as first responders to an injured athlete and should focus on providing emergency first aid care to the extent of their training and expertise. These individuals must avoid going beyond their level of training when assessing and treating an injured athlete. For example, performing clinical tests for the integrity of the ligaments of a joint is something that an AT or a QMP has training and background in but goes beyond the training of most initial responders. These skills should be performed only by those personnel who have advanced training and are qualified. However, initial responders can be trained in the recognition of life-threatening conditions, such as exertional heatstroke, head and neck injuries, exertional sickling, rhabdomyolysis, sudden cardiac arrest, or airway obstructions and respiratory arrest. If left unattended, any of these conditions can result in sudden death. By law, initial responders are the persons most often held accountable for proper injury management when no AT or QMP is present. Therefore, even though every situation is unique, initial responders must clearly convey to everyone in the immediate vicinity of the injured athlete that they are in charge until someone more qualified arrives. Typically, athletes (i.e., victims) should not be moved unless they are in imminent danger, such as being struck by lightning or needing immediate cooling.

First, cervical spine injury should be assumed in unconscious patients and ruled out for all traumatically injured but conscious patients before moving them. Reports of neck pain, altered sensation and/or motor function, or tenderness/deformity on the vertebrae of the neck are key signs and symptoms (see Chapter 9 for more details). Second, in cases where athletes may be suffering from exertional heat stress, immediate cooling should be implemented before transport by EMS (Casa et al., 2012b). Immediate cold-water immersion is preferred, but any cooling modality can be used until immersion is ready (see Chapter 18 for more details). Third, all individuals who work with a specific group of athletes need to be aware of which athletes have the sickle cell trait and recognize that lower extremity or low back pain/spasm, weakness, difficulty recovering, or shortness of breath may indicate exertional sickling (Casa et al., 2012b). Such symptoms require that the athlete stop participating immediately and be attended to using advanced care, including oxygen supplementation. Finally, coaches must be trained to deal effectively with cardiac arrest or respiratory problems, so CPR and the use of an AED or removing obstructions and performing rescue breathing (with pocket or bag valve masks) must be practiced periodically. Most states have recommendations in place that require all coaches to be CPR and AED

certified before beginning coaching; however, no national and only a few state mandates are in place for coaches to maintain adequate knowledge regarding emergency care for youth athletes (Strand et al., 2019). However, recent research has found that even coaches who possessed certifications in first aid and resuscitation still had knowledge gaps in areas related to youth CPR and AED as well as asthma (Strand et al., 2019).

Assessment of the Injured Athlete: Scene Safety

Scene safety or sizing up the scene refers to the action of a coach or physical educator to be aware of issues that can range from minor difficulties to major dangers at the scene of an injury. Even though typical athletic scenes may appear relatively safe (i.e., athletic practice or game), they can turn unsafe with very little notice. In particular, weather conditions can change in a manner of minutes and threaten not only the victim but also the rescuers. Trained emergency medical professionals refer to this as the concept of situational awareness, or the need to pay attention to the environment and people around them at all times, so they can react to or prevent any actions that might add further risk to the situation (Pollak, 2021). Sizing up the scene is also helpful so that the individual who is tasked with calling on emergency services can also provide information that might be valuable to the responding emergency personnel.

Assessment of the Injured Athlete: Initial Check and Physical Exam

The assessment of the injured athlete consists of two general phases known as the initial check (i.e., primary assessment) and the physical exam (i.e., secondary assessment). The purpose of the initial check is to determine whether the athlete's life is in immediate jeopardy caused by excessive bleeding, a compromised airway, or lack of breathing or circulation. The purpose of the physical exam is to focus on the specific area or region that is reported as being injured because information from this assessment can provide important guidance in the continued care and eventual transportation of the athlete to the

---

Rhabdomyolysis As a result of overexertion or traumatic injury, muscle fibers are damaged and die, which, in turn, causes a release of their contents into the bloodstream; this condition can lead to serious complications, such as renal (i.e., kidney) failure.

sidelines or a medical care center. To be effective, the physical exam must be conducted in a preplanned, sequential fashion. In cases in which injuries are obvious (e.g., fracture), skipping certain portions of the physical exam may be possible to render appropriate first aid sooner. However, even after attending to the obvious injury, initial responders should complete the remaining portions of the survey to rule out other conditions. A good example is a basketball player who falls to the floor immediately after having attempted to get a rebound. If initial responders see the incident—and notice that the athlete grabbed his or her ankle and was in obvious pain—they would be correct in performing a quick check followed by a visual assessment of the ankle to determine whether the athlete has any obvious fractures or open wounds. Then, assuming no serious injuries are present, the application of ice and compression as well as elevation of the injured ankle would be appropriate. This entire process should take no more than a few minutes, after which initial responders should perform a more thorough physical exam if other medical personnel have not arrived.

Generally, an athlete should not be moved unless a good reason exists to do so, such as further risk of injury because the scene is not safe. Therefore, during the initial check, first responders should make every effort to perform the assessment without moving or allowing others to move the athlete. In some cases, this may not be possible; for example, rolling athletes onto their back may be necessary to deliver life-saving CPR or to immediately cool athletes because of exertional heat illness. First responders must remember that following appropriate first aid procedures whenever moving an athlete is important and moving an athlete is often not necessary until advance care has arrived, especially if the athlete is breathing. If the athlete needs no life-saving measures, then the secondary assessment, which includes a physical exam, can be conducted. Again, initial responders are reminded not to diagnose injuries and to perform only essential stabilization of bones or joints, stop severe bleeding, or provide appropriate first aid for obvious closed (i.e., sprains or strains) or open (i.e., cuts or abrasions) wounds. If the athlete is bleeding, wearing medical exam gloves is important because doing so is included as a protective measure called **standard precautions** (universal precautions). Hand hygiene should also be emphasized before and after the care of an injured athlete (Pollak, 2021).

Initial Check (Primary Assessment)

According to the American Academy of Orthopaedic Surgeons (AAOS; Pollak, 2021), the initial check must include assessments of the following (in order of importance) with the general purpose of identifying and treating life threats:

- Scan for signs of uncontrolled bleeding (hemorrhage).
- Assess responsiveness or level of consciousness.
- Assess the airway.
- Assess breathing.
- Assess circulation.
- Identify life threats.
- Determine priority of patient care and transport.

Hemorrhage Assessment

Uncontrolled bleeding takes priority over all other assessments. Extensive external bleeding is extremely rare in athletics but can occur if a major artery is severed. Arterial bleeding is bright red and spurts along with the pulse; venous bleeding is darker and will flow either slowly or rapidly, depending on the size of the vein; and capillary bleeding is red and oozes from the wound. Most external bleeding is obvious and can be controlled by the appropriate first aid procedures—use of direct pressure, pressure bandage, or tourniquet (Pollak, 2021). In major injuries to extremities where bleeding cannot be stopped with pressure and elevation, the application of tourniquets is recommended (Kragh et al., 2008) to save limbs and lives. Understandably, initial responders may not feel comfortable applying a tourniquet, but new first aid training includes instruction in application techniques. As a reminder, any time blood or other bodily fluids are exposed, initial responders should, whenever possible, take standard precautions to protect against the transmission of blood-borne pathogens. Initial responders are encouraged to wear medical exam gloves and consider eye protection (i.e., glasses or sunglasses) to help prevent exposure.

> **Standard precautions** Protective measures that have been recommended by the Centers for Disease Control and Prevention (CDC) for use in dealing with blood and body fluids or other potentially hazardous materials.

Internal hemorrhaging is difficult if not impossible to detect during the initial assessment. One of the earliest signs of severe internal bleeding is **hypovolemic shock**, which is caused by too little blood in the vascular system. Two important signs of this condition are rapid, weak pulse and rapid, shallow breathing. Changes in the condition of the skin surface may also provide clues to this condition. Moist, clammy-feeling skin and a blue color inside the lips and under the nail beds indicate shock. Dizziness, confusion, thirst, and weakness can also be observed. Such cases represent true medical emergencies, and the primary objective must be to treat for shock by improving blood flow to the heart, lungs, and brain and arrange for transport to a medical facility. Treatment of shock is discussed later in this chapter.

Determining Responsiveness

Before making any decisions about rendering care to injured athletes, first responders must determine the athletes' level of responsiveness or consciousness. Assessment of the neurological status of an injured person can be a daunting task, even for the experienced medical professional. The complexity of the central nervous system (CNS) cannot be disputed; however, from an assessment standpoint, dividing the CNS into the brain and spinal cord is helpful. As recommended by AAOS (Pollak, 2021), this can be accomplished quickly and consistently by using the AVPU scale: A = *a*lert and *a*ware, V = responds to *v*erbal stimulus, P = responds to *p*ainful stimulus, and U = *u*nresponsive to any stimulus.

When assessing alertness, initial responders should note whether the athletes' eyes are open and, further, whether they can accurately identify person (name), place (location), and time (date or day of week). If athletes can successfully accomplish these simple tasks, they are said to be alert. If they do not appear to be alert, then initial responders must verify the athletes' ability to respond to verbal stimulus. If verbal communication can be established, regardless of the accuracy of the communication, they are said to be "responsive to verbal stimulus." In the event athletes do not appear to be able to communicate verbally at any level, initial responders must verify a response to painful stimuli by pinching the skin overlying a bone, such as the clavicle or skin on the inside of the upper arm or thigh. If initial responders observe a response to these stimuli either verbally, through facial gestures, or by attempts to move a limb to avoid being pinched, the athletes are said to be "responsive only to painful stimuli." If the athletes fail to show any form of response, that is, opening of the eyes, verbal communication, or response to painful stimuli, they are said to be "unresponsive to any stimuli." If spinal or head injury is suspected, steps must be taken immediately to immobilize the head and neck to prevent aggravation of the injury (Pollak, 2021). However, the concepts and processes of spinal immobilization depend on local emergency protocols. In this case, immobilization refers to preventing any excessive motions that could aggravate the current situation and does not refer to the actual technique used to accomplish the protection of the spinal column (e.g., stretcher vs. long spine board).

Respiratory System

Assessment of the respiratory system is the next priority when rendering first aid to injured athletes. This portion of the initial check should require only a few seconds (no more than 5–10 seconds) and can be started as the initial responders are approaching the injured athletes if they are within visual proximity. If the athletes are obviously responsive (easily talking or crying), then the initial responders can assume that the airway is open and respiration is occurring. When level of responsiveness is in question or the athletes are unresponsive, other means of airway and respiration assessment may be necessary.

Airway Assessment

Initial assessment can be facilitated by asking the athletes a simple question. A verbal response implies the airway is open but does not mean that they can breathe appropriately to sustain life. If victims are unresponsive, the initial responders should assess for breathing first by looking for chest rise in the position in which they were found. If the victims are on their stomach or side and appear not to have chest rise, then life takes priority over the spine. Initial responders must carefully roll the athletes as a unit onto their back to continue the assessment.

Hypovolemic shock Inability of the cardiovascular system to maintain adequate circulation to all parts of the body.

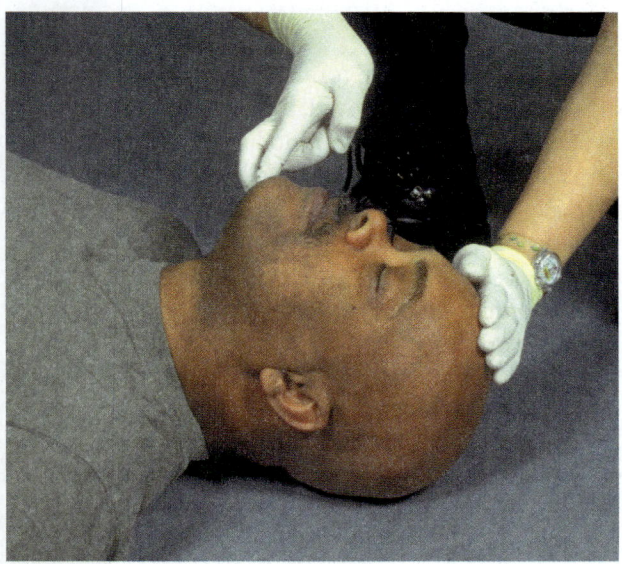

Figure 7.6 Head-tilt/chin-lift method.

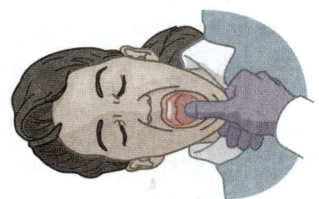 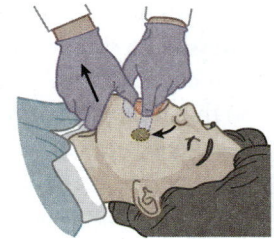

Finger-sweep method
- With index finger of your hand, slide finger down along the inside of one cheek deeply into mouth and use a hooking action across to other cheek to dislodge foreign object.
- If foreign body comes within reach, grab and remove it. Do not force object deeper.

Figure 7.8 Finger-sweep method.

If serious head or spinal injury is not indicated, initial responders should use the head-tilt/chin-lift technique (Figure 7.6). The procedure is as follows: Place one hand on the athlete's forehead while gently lifting the chin with the other hand. In the case of a helmeted athlete, such as a football player, a coach or physical educator should not remove the helmet or face mask to open the airway. Opening an airway and checking for breathing can be accomplished with the helmet in place. Removing the helmet can easily aggravate an existing spinal injury and should be done by trained QMPs.

When initial responders suspect a spinal injury may have occurred, the preferred method of opening the airway is the jaw-thrust technique (Figure 7.7).

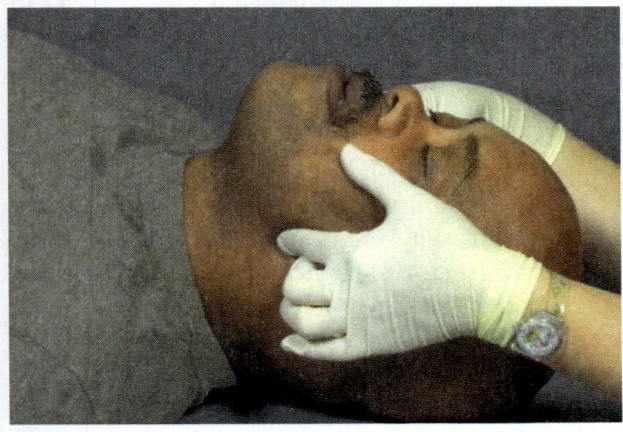

Figure 7.7 Jaw-thrust maneuver.

The procedure is as follows: While at the athlete's side, place fingers below the ear lobes and gently push the jaw upward while not moving the head; this should open the airway.

Initial responders should remember to check for any foreign objects in the airway, such as gum, a mouthpiece, chewing tobacco, a dental appliance, or other material. If they see an object, it should be removed using the finger-sweep method (Figure 7.8).

Breathing Assessment

If the airway, had to be opened using the head-tilt/chin-lift method or jaw-thrust method, then the initial responders need to look for chest rise, listen for breathing sounds, or feel for chest rise from airflow. If the athletes are responsive, simply watching and listening to them speak, cry, or breathe may provide important information regarding the adequacy of their airway (Pollak, 2021). Wheezing; gasping; labored speaking; or short, rapid breaths can be problematic and result in a poor supply of oxygen to key organs. Unresponsive athletes may not be breathing; however, initial responders must assess the circulation, and if no signs of circulation are present, then they need to immediately start CPR chest compressions and request an AED.

Circulation Assessment

Determining the status of the circulatory system is a critical component of the initial assessment and is intended to verify the integrity of the heart and blood vessels. Besides excessive external or internal hemorrhage, the major concern is the presence or absence of the signs of circulation (e.g., heart rate). The circulation assessment should be executed quickly by looking at skin color and feeling for a pulse at the carotid artery on the neck. Skin color is best assessed at areas of good perfusion, such as the lips, inside the mouth, fingernail beds, palms, and soles of feet. Pale, gray, or blue skin indicates either lack of circulation or poor perfusion of the blood (Pollak, 2021). The carotid pulse should be readily identifiable and strong if circulation is sufficient.

A responsive athlete who is breathing and communicating will have the signs of circulation, including pulse and blood flow. In an unresponsive victim, initial responders should determine whether the signs of circulation are present after opening the airway and quickly checking for breathing. If the initial responders see no signs of circulation (no pulse or altered skin color), they must immediately begin chest compressions associated with CPR. Several years ago, updates to the American Heart Association guidelines (Neumar et al., 2015) emphasized a change in the order of emergency treatment of unresponsiveness and identified important characteristics of successful resuscitation efforts, including compressions and breathing. Although an open airway and breathing are essential, circulation is of prime importance because blood flow is what allows the body to function. Delay in providing circulation and perfusion of blood may cause further complications. Therefore, the airway should be carefully opened, and breathing should be quickly assessed along with pulse (5–10 seconds), but if there are signs of decreased circulation, then chest compressions should be started before providing ventilation to the unresponsive athlete. The sequence is circulation, airway, and breathing (C-A-B), and airway maintenance and breaths follow compressions if circulation is compromised. However, if after the assessment, the initial responders determine that circulation is intact but airway and breathing are compromised, then they must be treated first.

Physical exam The process of evaluating an individual for signs and symptoms associated with injury or illness.

Sign Objective evidence of an abnormal situation within the body.

Symptom Subjective evidence of an abnormal situation within the body.

Summary

All rescue methods are continued until advanced care arrives, the athlete is revived, the scene becomes unsafe, or the rescuer tires and can no longer continue. In an unresponsive athlete situation, the initial responder's primary responsibility is to keep the athlete alive and to ensure that advanced care help is summoned. The athlete does not need to be moved from the playing field or practice area because delaying a game or practice does not justify moving someone.

Physical Exam (Secondary Assessment)

The **physical exam** should include specific components that enable the initial responders to collect as much information about the injury as possible under the circumstances and within their training. The essential parts of the survey are as follows:

- **History.** Discuss the mechanism of injury with the athletes and/or onlookers. Ask the athletes about their current signs and symptoms.
- **Observation.** Observe for obvious signs and/or symptoms related to the injury.
- **Palpation.** Feel the injured area to collect more information.

Overall, the purpose of the physical exam is for initial responders to note signs and symptoms related to the injury. While administering the physical exam, initial responders must continually monitor the injured athletes' signs of breathing and circulation (responsiveness). Although the purpose of the initial assessment is to verify circulation and respiration, both of these vital functions may change quickly related to the body's response to the injury. For example, athletes who have sustained a significant head injury may initially have normal circulation and respiration, both of which rather quickly decline as bleeding in the skull continues. As such, initial responders must remain ever vigilant during the physical exam for changes in the condition of the athletes that may be life threatening. Initial responders must also be observant for signs and symptoms of hypovolemic shock, which can also escalate into a life-threatening phenomenon. Critical to this is a basic understanding that a **sign** involves objective findings, such as bleeding, swelling, discoloration, and deformity. **Symptoms** are subjective in nature and may not be as reliable in determining the nature of the injury. Symptoms include findings such as headache, nausea, pain, and **point tenderness**. Initial responders begin observing for signs and symptoms related to the athletes even before they are near enough to render any aid. As initial responders approach the injured athletes, they must note the body position and look for signs of possible significance, such as odd behavior or actions. If they saw the injury occur, the forces involved and the mechanism of injury will be clearer. This information can be related to possible types of injury (e.g., fracture vs. sprain).

Medical History

Whether the athletes are responsive or unresponsive, collecting a history is considered the third part of victim assessment. Obviously, if the athletes are unresponsive, initial responders need to collect information from bystanders, typically teammates or other coaching personnel. Regardless of the circumstances, when rendering care to unresponsive athletes, initial responders must always assume that serious head and spinal injuries are present, which require the stabilization of the athletes' head and neck. The priorities must be basic life support—cardiac function, airway, and breathing—followed by contacting EMS. In the case of conscious athletes, the history process begins as soon as initial responders arrive on the scene (Figure 7.9). Its purpose is to collect information critical to identifying the body areas involved as well as the severity and mechanisms of injury (Prentice, 2017). Traumatic injuries usually present a more obvious set of complaints and possible causes than do chronic injuries.

Although each injury is unique, coaches' questions to athletes should be phrased in simple, easy-to-understand terms that can elicit the desired information without leading athletes to giving a preferred answer. Initial responders should avoid using terminology too advanced for athletes and always take care not to increase athletes' anxiety level by losing their composure. Questions should require only brief responses—preferably a yes or no. Initially, initial responders can gain the confidence of the athletes by letting them know what they are doing and that they are there to ensure the athletes' welfare. In the case of rendering care to persons unknown to initial responders, they should always identify themselves and indicate that they are there to render first aid care. They should ask the athletes to explain what happened and to describe perceptions of the injury; whether they are in pain and, if so, where; and whether they heard any strange sounds during the injury or felt anything abnormal. Regarding injuries of the extremities, initial responders should ask whether the athletes heard a pop or felt a snap, as if something "let go" within the joint or elsewhere within the extremity. If possible, initial responders should compare the injured side with the uninjured area on the opposite side of the body. The athletes' answers provide essential information to assist the initial responders in the evaluation of both the location and magnitude of the injury. Initial responders should not forget to inquire about the injury history (both long and short term) of the involved area. A good example of how such information could be useful is the case of a suspected shoulder subluxation (partial dislocation). Such an injury may be very difficult to evaluate. However, if during the history taking, the athletes admit that their shoulder has been dislocated several times in the past year, the initial responders may then focus on determining the integrity of that specific joint because that injury tends to have a high rate of recurrence. Information regarding the injury history of the athletes should always be passed on to the medical personnel who evaluate the athletes later.

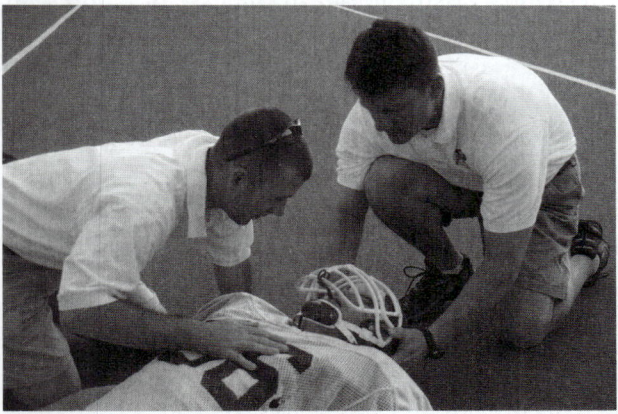

Figure 7.9 A coach obtains a history of injury from an injured athlete while the AT stabilizes head and neck.

Point tenderness Pain produced when an injury site is palpated.

In some cases, the medical emergency may be difficult to ascertain, as is the case with certain conditions, such as diabetes, exercise-induced asthma (EIA), and head injury. Clues to the problem may be given during the history process if done correctly. In the case of metabolic emergencies, the questions are obvious ("Do you have diabetes—and if so, did you take your insulin today?" "Do you have epilepsy—and if so, are you on any sort of medication?"). In the case of EIA, the athletes are usually having trouble catching their breath, have chest tightness, and are wheezing (see Chapter 19). They might also feel dizzy or have bluish gray lips, which indicate poor oxygen delivery. In the case of conscious athletes with a possible head injury, behavior may be incongruent with the circumstances. The initial responders' questions should assist in determining the level of consciousness as well as the integrity of higher thought processes by assessing orientation, concentration, and short-term memory (see Chapter 9).

Observation and Palpation

Essentially, the goal of the physical exam is to identify all injuries, regardless of severity; treat them appropriately; and refer the athletes for medical care if it is deemed necessary. With responsive athletes, initial responders can ask them to point out the site of injury. They can then look and feel for the signs of injury, including deformity, open wounds, tenderness, and swelling. With unresponsive athletes, if breathing and circulation are maintained, the physical exam should be thought of as a head-to-toe assessment of the athletes. Initial responders should look and feel (i.e., palpate) for abnormalities or open wounds by starting at the head and progressing through the neck, chest, abdomen, pelvis, and extremities. Palpation is the process of feeling or touching with the fingertips to determine any abnormalities (Pollak, 2021). With good palpation skills, any noticeable irregularities could indicate fractures, dislocations, or other types of tissue damage. With practice, palpation skills can be refined to the point where identification of injury-related problems, such as swelling, muscle spasm, localized fever, abdominal rigidity (i.e., sign of internal bleeding in abdominal cavity), deformity, crepitus (i.e., grating feeling beneath the skin surface), and skin tension can be easily detected.

Palpation is a learned skill and does involve some amount of contact with the injured athlete (Figure 7.10). Consequently, great care must be taken to avoid aggravation of existing injuries. Also, when evaluating a conscious athlete, an explanation of the purposes of the evaluation can be helpful in relieving anxiety. The recommendation is that whenever possible the palpation process should begin in a body area away from where there are obvious injuries (Prentice, 2017). This allows the athlete to develop confidence in the initial responder's palpation skill before the initial responder evaluates the injury (or injuries). As well, in the case of injury to an extremity, the recommendation is to evaluate the uninjured limb first. This provides an immediate basis for comparison when the actual injury is evaluated.

In cases of possible significant injury in which much of the body is covered with equipment and clothing, equipment or garments should be removed from the suspected area of injury by cutting away the equipment or clothing with scissors rather than removing it in a normal fashion. In this way, unnecessary movement of athletes can be avoided. Obviously, care must be taken not to cause athletes embarrassment, but in the case of a potential

---

Exercise-induced asthma (EIA) A constriction of the airway resulting from participation in exercise. Also known as exercise-induced bronchoconstriction (EIB), the term preferred by the American College of Allergy, Asthma, and Immunology.

Palpation The act of feeling with the hands for the purpose of determining the structural integrity of the tissue beneath.

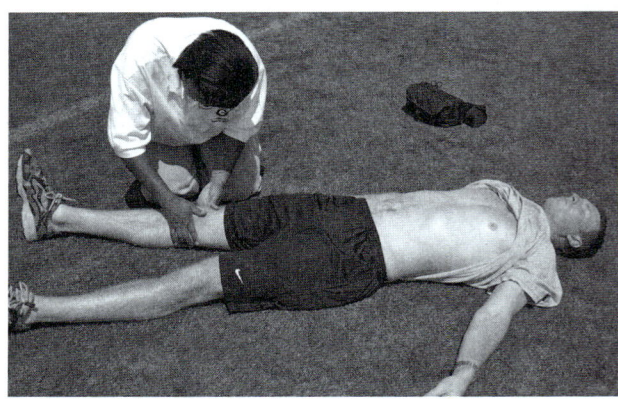

Figure 7.10 Palpation of a knee injury.

life-or-death situation, saving their life must always take priority over modesty.

Shock

Shock is an acute, life-threatening condition that involves the body's failure to maintain adequate circulation to the vital organs. As previously described, hypovolemic shock may result from severe hemorrhage; however, shock can be caused by several other conditions, including cardiogenic (i.e., heart failure), neurogenic (i.e., dilated blood vessels), and simple psychogenic (i.e., fainting) conditions. The signs and symptoms of shock can include any combination of the following: profuse sweating; cool, clammy-feeling skin; dilated pupils; elevated pulse and respiration rate; irritable behavior; complaints of extreme thirst; and nausea and/or vomiting.

Treatment for shock includes having athletes in a supine position with the legs elevated approximately 8 to 12 inches. Initial responders should calm athletes with reassuring comments. To avoid further loss of body heat, they can cover athletes with blankets. In the case of a suspected spinal injury, initial responders should not move athletes from the position they are in. Rather, they should monitor athletes' vital signs and cover them with blankets if environmental conditions are such that loss of body heat is possible.

Removal from Field or Court

During all phases of the athlete examination process, significant findings should be noted and recalled for later use. Normally, the entire evaluation process should be completed in a matter of minutes, after which the appropriate first aid treatment should be initiated. If further evaluation is deemed necessary, the decision must be made to move athletes from the playing field or practice area. Athletes who are conscious and responsive and have no obvious lower extremity injuries that preclude walking may be able to leave the area under their own power or with assistance. If a lower extremity injury exists, some form of transport device should be used, such as a stretcher, spine board, or even a two-person carry, to remove athletes from the site of injury. In the case of unconscious athletes or those who may have sustained a head or neck injury, the best policy is for initial responders to stay with them, monitor vital signs, treat for shock, and summon EMS personnel. Unless athletes are in immediate danger of being injured further, movement before the arrival of EMS personnel is not justified.

Return to Play

In the absence of any QMP, such as a physician or BOC-certified or state-licensed AT, initial responders must decide whether athletes should be allowed to return to play. In some cases, making this decision is easy, such as when a head or neck injury or a fractured bone is suspected, in which case the answer is no. In other cases, initial responders are often presented with ethical dilemmas that arise whenever athletes' best medical interests conflict with the performance expectations of the athletes, team, or parents. In such cases, initial responders must understand their legal liability in relationship to negligent treatment of a suspected injury. For example, all athletes who must leave a practice or game because of a neurological injury (e.g., concussion) should not be allowed to return until they are evaluated by a trained medical professional. Returning to play after a suspected concussion can lead to serious and even life-threatening complications if athletes are allowed to return to participation without medical evaluation. Likewise, athletes who appear to be suffering from heat-related problems should be removed from participation and cleared for return only by QMP.

Without question, the most difficult decisions for initial responders involve injuries to athletes' musculoskeletal system, such as joint injuries, muscle strains, and contusions. In general, if the injury results in any degree of functional loss, athletes should not be allowed to return to participation. Initial responders can verify functional loss in the lower extremities by asking athletes to perform simple drills, such as hopping up and down on one leg or running a figure eight. In the case of upper extremity injury in the shoulder region, for example, asking athletes to place their hand on the center of their upper back as if to scratch their back will verify normal range of motion. To test muscle strength and joint integrity, initial responders should ask athletes to perform a push-up. Failure to execute any simple functional test should result in removal from participation that day and medical referral. Such athletes should be allowed to return to participation only after having received

WHAT IF ❓

You are coaching junior varsity football, specifically the linebackers, when suddenly someone yells that an athlete has been hurt on the other end of the practice field. When you arrive on the scene, the athlete is lying face down on the field and not moving. What should your initial actions be in this situation?

medical clearance from a physician or BOC-certified or state-licensed AT.

Initial responders must always remember that signs such as swelling, discoloration, limping, and facial expressions related to pain and symptoms such as pain, popping, clicking in a joint, or uncontrolled muscle spasm potentially indicate a more serious injury. When in doubt, initial responders should always err on the conservative side and remove athletes from participation until QMP can perform a more complete evaluation.

Athletic Trainers SPEAK OUT

How important is an emergency action plan, and is there a situation you can describe where it worked really well?

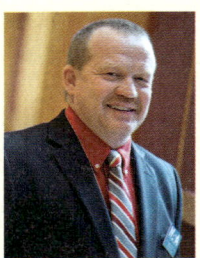

Courtesy of Larry Cooper, MS, LAT, ATC.

The single most important safety procedure that you can have in place for your student-athletes is an EAP. The EAP should be a detailed, venue-specific plan that is practiced annually with all emergency personnel. The EAP is the single best way that you can prepare for a positive outcome in the event of a catastrophic or life-threatening athletic injury. The two critical components are venue specific and rehearsed with all first responders.

While working a holiday wrestling tournament at a local high school, we had a suspected neck injury with loss of sensation and movement in the lower extremities. I was the AT who was on the mat first, so I went to stabilize the head. Because we were not at my school, I got to see up close and personally the EAP go into action and work flawlessly. Every cog of the wheel (i.e., AT, security, EMS, athletic director, tournament director, and referees) worked together, and the athlete was loaded, strapped, and transported within minutes of the injury. There was time for reflection and review during a break in the tournament, and everyone had an opportunity to voice concerns or praise. The athlete ended up being okay. To see the EAP work as it was planned and rehearsed was a great experience and reinforced the importance of every school having a venue-specific EAP.

—**Larry Cooper, MS, LAT, ATC**

Larry Cooper is an AT and a retired teacher at Penn Trafford High School, Harrison City, Pennsylvania.

Review Questions

1. What are the key elements to an EAP?
2. List several best practices for an EAP that help eliminate barriers to optimal health and safety.
3. Regarding emergency planning, what are the four items the emergency team should stipulate before a game or other competition?
4. What is the order of assessment and performance of life-saving skills when a participant appears not to be breathing or not to have a pulse?
5. Briefly describe the initial check and the physical exam as they relate to the initial assessment of an injured athlete.

6. When performing an initial check of an injured athlete, what is the recommended procedure for opening an airway when a neck injury is suspected?

7. True or false? Removing a helmet from an injured, unresponsive football player as soon as possible to establish an open airway is imperative.

8. What is one of the earliest clues that internal bleeding may be occurring?

9. List the essential components of the physical exam.

10. Differentiate between a sign and a symptom.

11. True or false? When collecting a history from an injured athlete, questions should be brief and using complicated terminology should be kept to a minimum.

12. True or false? An initial responder should put the team's priorities over the health of an athlete.

13. What differences if any should there be between an EAP for a high school, a college, and a youth league?

References

Adams, W. M., Scarneo, S. E., & Casa, D. J. (2018). Assessment of evidence-based health and safety policies on sudden death and concussion management in secondary school athletics: A benchmark study. *Journal of Athletic Training, 53*(8), 756–767.

Andersen, J. C., Courson, R. W., Kleiner, D. M., & McLoda, T. A. (2002). National Athletic Trainers' Association position statement: Emergency planning in athletics. *Journal of Athletic Training, 37*(1), 99.

Casa, D. J., Anderson, S. A., Baker, L., Bennett, S., Bergeron, M. F., Connolly, D., . . . Thompson, C. (2012b). The inter-association task force for preventing sudden death in collegiate conditioning sessions: Best-practices recommendations. *Journal of Athletic Training, 47*(4), 477–480.

Casa, D. J., Guskiewicz, K. M., Anderson, S. A., Courson, R. W., Heck, J. F., Jimenez, C. C., . . . Walsh, K. M. (2012a). National Athletic Trainers' Association position statement: Preventing sudden death in sports. *Journal of Athletic Training, 47*(1), 96–118.

Casa, D. J., Almquist, J., Anderson, S. A., Baker, L., Bergeron, M. F., Biagioli, B., . . . Valentine, V. (2013). The Inter-Association Task Force for Preventing Sudden Death in Secondary School Athletics Programs: Best-practices recommendations. *Journal of Athletic Training, 48*(4), 546–553.

Cooper, L., Harper, R., Wham, G. S., Jr., Cates, J., Chafin, S. J., Jr., Cohen, R. P., . . . Valovich-McLeod, T. C. (2019). Appropriate medical care standards for organizations sponsoring athletic activity for the secondary school–aged athlete: A summary statement. *Journal of Athletic Training, 54*(7), 741–748.

Drezner, J. A., Courson, R. W., Roberts, W. O., Mosesso, V. N., Jr., Link, M. S., & Maron, B. J. (2007). Inter-Association Task Force recommendations on emergency preparedness and management of sudden cardiac arrest in high school and college athletic programs: A consensus statement. *Prehospital Emergency Care, 11*(3), 253–271.

Endres, B. D., Kerr, Z. Y., Stearns, R. L., Adams, W. M., Hosokawa, Y., Huggins, R. A., . . . Casa, D. J. (2019). Epidemiology of sudden death in organized youth sports in the United States, 2007–2015. *Journal of Athletic Training, 54*(4), 349–355.

Huggins, R. A., Scarneo, S. E., Casa, D. J., Belval, L. N., Carr, K. S., Chiampas, G., . . . Westin, T. (2017). The Inter-Association Task Force document on emergency health and safety: Best-practice recommendations for youth sports leagues. *Journal of Athletic Training, 52*(4), 384–400.

Huggins, R. A., Attanasio, S. M., Endres, B. D., Coleman, K. A., & Casa, D. J. (2018). *Athletic training locations and services (ATLAS) project: 1st Annual report.* Retrieved from https://ksi.uconn.edu/wp-content/uploads/sites/1222/2018/09/ATLAS-2018-Report-Final.pdf

Kragh, J. F., Walters, T. J., Baer, D. G., Fox, C. J., Wade, C. E., Salinas, J., & Holcomb, J. B. (2008). Practical use of emergency tourniquets to stop bleeding in major limb trauma. *Journal of Trauma, 64*(Suppl 2), S38–S50.

McCaskey, A. S., & Biedzynski, K. W. (1996). A guide to the legal liability of coaches for a sports participant's injuries. *Seton Hall Journal of Sports and Entertainment Law, 6*(1), 8–97.

McKay, C. D., Cumming, S. P., & Blake, T. (2019). Youth sport: Friend or foe? *Best Practice & Research Clinical Rheumatology, 33*, 141–157.

Mirsafian, H. (2016). Legal duties and legal liabilities of coaches toward athletes. *Physical Culture and Sport Studies and Research, 69*(1), 5–14.

National Athletic Trainers' Association (NATA). (2012, August). *National Athletic Trainers' Association official statement on athletic health care provider "time outs" before athletic events.* Retrieved from https://www.nata.org/sites/default/files/timeout.pdf

Neumar, R. W., Shuster, M., Callaway, C. W., Gent, L. M., Atkins, D. L., Bhanji, F., . . . Hazinski, M. F. (2015). Part 1: Executive summary: 2015 American Heart Association guidelines update for cardiopulmonary resuscitation and emergency cardiovascular care. *Circulation, 132*(18 Suppl 2), S315–S367.

Parsons, J. T., Anderson, S. A., Casa, D. J., & Hainline, B. (2019). Preventing catastrophic injury and death in collegiate athletes: Interassociation recommendations endorsed by 13 medical and sports medicine organisations. *Journal of Athletic Training, 54*(8), 843–851.

Physical Activity Council. (2021). *2021 Physical Activity Council's overview report on U.S. participation.* Retrieved from https://eb6d91a4-d249-47b8-a5cb-933f7971db54.filesusr.com/ugd/286de6_610088e5e73d497185ac181a240833a9.pdf

Pollak, A. N. (2021). *Emergency care and transport of the sick and injured [AAOS]* (12th ed.). Burlington, MA: Jones & Bartlett Learning.

Prentice, W. E. (2017). *Principles of athletic training: A guide to evidence-based practice* (16th ed.). New York, NY: McGraw-Hill.

Quandt, E. F., Mitton, M. J., & Black, J. S. (2009). *Legal liability in covering athletic events. Sports Health, 1*(1), 84–90.

Scarneo, S. E., DiStefano, L. J., Stearns, R. L., Register-Mihalik, J. K., Denegar, C. R., & Casa, D. J. (2019). Emergency action planning in secondary school athletics: A comprehensive evaluation of current adoption of best practice standards. *Journal of Athletic Training, 54*(1), 99–105.

Strand, B., Lyman, K. J., David, S., Landin, K., Albrecht, J., & Deutsch, J. (2019). High school coaches' knowledge of emergency care. *International Council for Health, Physical Education, Recreation, Sport and Dance Journal of Research, 10*(2), 33–39.

CHAPTER 8
The Injury and Healing Processes

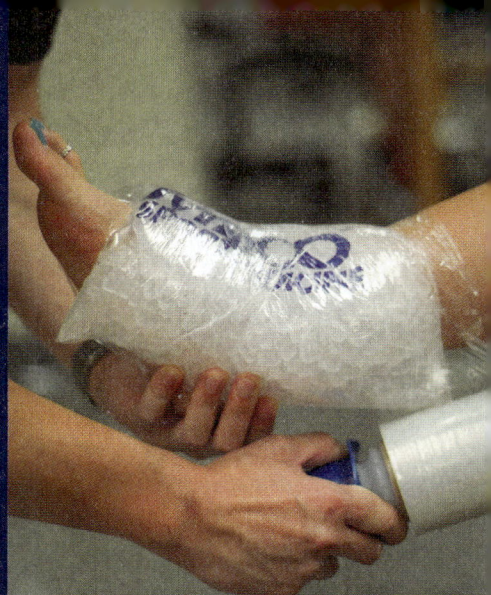

Courtesy of Mark Hoffman

MAJOR CONCEPTS

This chapter examines the complex topic of the tissue healing process in reaction to physical trauma associated with physical activity. It begins with an overview of the types of tissues and the forces involved in sports injuries, followed by a detailed, phase-by-phase description of the healing process, which includes the inflammatory response, fibroblastic repair, and maturation and remodeling phases. The inflammatory response phase is often the most limiting phase to physical activity or exercise; therefore, coaches and physical educators must grasp the basic physiology of this process to better understand the recommended procedures for assisting the necessary processes of inflammation as well as limiting the negative consequences. Successful management depends on whether the inflammatory response phase is acute or chronic, so correctly recognizing the signs and symptoms associated with these phases can guide management. Depending on the signs and symptoms, treatment can include application of therapeutic cold (e.g., crushed ice or commercial cold packs), compression, and elevation or the administration of therapeutic heat (e.g., hot packs or warm whirlpool). Pharmacological agents, such as anti-inflammatories or pain relievers, should be recommended by a physician or another allied healthcare provider. Even though many pharmacological agents are available over the counter, recent evidence suggests that dosage mistakes are common and can result in serious side effects, including death. This chapter concludes with a discussion of the role of exercise in the overall rehabilitation process.

The Physics of Sports Injury

The human body consists of many types of tissue, each serving a specific purpose. Some tissues are highly specialized (e.g., the retina of the eye contains tissue that is sensitive to light and is not found anywhere else in the body), whereas other types of tissue are distributed throughout the body. The most common type of tissue in the body is **connective tissue** (Moini, 2020). Areolar (i.e., loosely woven and irregularly arranged) and dense (i.e., tightly packed and

> **Connective tissue** The most common tissue in the body; includes ligaments, bones, retinaculum, joint capsules, cartilage, fascia, and tendons.

organized) connective tissues help form ligaments, retinaculum, joint capsules, bone, cartilage, fascia, and tendons (Houglum, 2016). Moini (2020) classified other general categories of tissue as epithelial (for protection, secretion, and absorption), muscular (for contraction), and nervous (for sensation and conductivity). Connective tissues are the primary components that create the musculoskeletal system, so not surprisingly they are commonly involved in both acute and chronic sports injuries. Collegiate athletes experience a variety of injuries, and recent research has established that the musculoskeletal system is involved in a significant portion of those injuries (Yang et al., 2012). For example, the most common acute injuries over three seasons of data were sprains and strains (62% of total), and one of most common chronic injuries was tendonitis (15% of total). High school athletes also experience a variety of injuries, including strains, sprains, fractures, and other injuries to the musculoskeletal system. These types of injuries to the lower and upper extremity account for 7 of the top 10 injuries experienced in both competition and practice and rank just behind concussions as the most common (Comstock & Pierpoint, 2020).

Three basic types of forces can affect connective tissues: tensile, compressive, and shear (Figure 8.1). Tendons are designed to resist tensile forces but are less effective when subjected to shear forces and are poorly designed to deal with compressive forces. Conversely, bone tissue is designed to absorb compressive forces, but it is less effective against tensile and shear forces (Prentice, 2017; Starkey & Brown, 2015). Ligament tissue, like that of tendons, is best suited to resist tensile forces while being more vulnerable to shear and compressive mechanisms.

Tendons act as mechanical bridges and allow muscle force to pass to bones and joints (Sözen, 2019). Shorter compared to longer tendons exhibit greater tensile strength because they typically have a larger diameter, but a longer tendon may be able to undergo a greater overall deformation before it tears (Sözen, 2019). Tendons are extremely strong structures able to withstand significant compressive and tensile stresses. Yet activities such as running and jumping may generate forces in excess of these physiological limits because tissue stress is often two to 3.5 times body weight during running (Keller et al., 1996) but can exceed nine times with high-speed downhill running. In addition, running is a highly repetitive movement, and forces can be applied through the lower limbs approximately 90 times per minute (Lorimer & Hume, 2014).

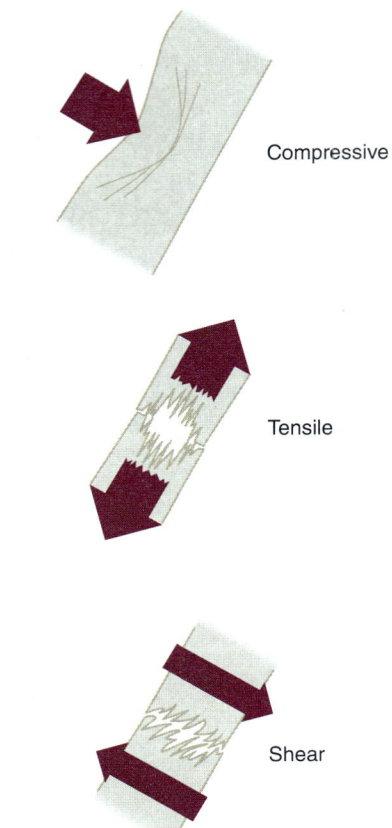

Figure 8.1 Mechanical forces of injury: compression (application of inward pushing force), tensile (application of outward pulling force), and shear (application of forces to displace layers parallel to one another).

Muscle tissue and its surrounding connective tissue (i.e., fascia) are most commonly injured when excess tension is applied while contraction (i.e., shortening) is occurring. Furthermore, the common belief is that more injuries to muscles and fascia occur during eccentric contractions when the musculotendinous unit is lengthening at the same time a force is being applied (LaStayo et al., 2003). When strains occur, the damage is typically found at the proximal musculotendinous junction (Ingersoll & Mistry, 2006).

Each tissue type (e.g., muscle, tendon, bone, or skin) has a limit to how much force it can withstand. This limit has been referred to as the critical force or ultimate failure point (Prentice, 2017; Starkey & Brown, 2015). The critical force value varies for each type of tissue in the body. Even within the same type of tissue, the critical force value may vary owing to changes in the tissue structure, including length, diameter, and fiber organization. Factors such as age, temperature, skeletal maturity, gender, and body weight can also affect the mechanical properties of ligaments (Prentice, 2017; Starkey & Brown, 2015). More research into the specific causes of musculoskeletal injuries is warranted because soft-tissue injuries being very common in sports is well documented (Yang et al., 2012).

The Physiology of Sports Injury

Whenever tissues are damaged as a result of **trauma**, the body reacts quickly with a predictable sequence of physiological actions designed to ultimately lead to the resolution, regeneration, or repair of the involved tissues. **Resolution** is complete healing in which dead cells and cellular debris are removed and the tissue is left functionally the same. **Regeneration** occurs when damaged tissue is replaced by cells of the same type along with scar tissue and retains most of its original structure. **Repair** occurs when the original tissue is replaced by scar tissue and the original structure and function are lost. Using the skin as an example, if individuals suffer a laceration but then heal completely and cannot find any marks that indicate where the injury occurred, then they have experienced resolution; if they can see a small scar that is not as large as the original injury, then they have experienced regeneration; and if they end up with a significant scar that replaced the original skin, then they have experienced repair.

The physiological process of healing includes three phases that are unique but fall along a continuum where they overlap; to fully enter the subsequent phase, the preceding phase must be finished (Houglum, 2016; Ingersoll & Mistry, 2006). Each phase serves a specific purpose, and all are essential to proper repair of the structures involved. The three phases are commonly referred to as the **inflammation phase**, **fibroblastic phase**, and **maturation and remodeling phase** (Figure 8.2). The amount of time necessary to finish the healing depends primarily on the severity of the injury and the type of tissue; therefore, laying out an exact timeline for completion is impossible. For example, a mild ligament sprain (i.e., first-degree injury) can take weeks to fully heal, whereas a mild muscle strain can take only a few days, and a complete ligament tear (i.e., third-degree injury) can take up to 12 months, whereas a complete muscle tear can take as little as 6 weeks to fully heal. Each phase overlaps

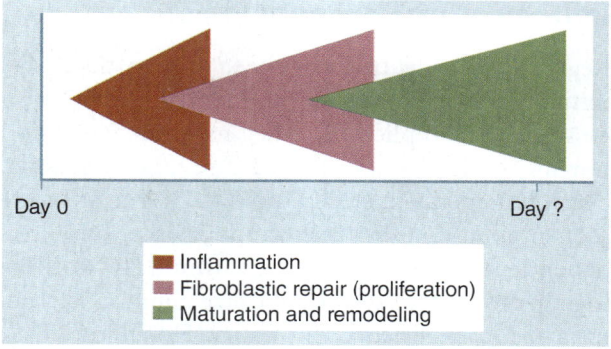

Figure 8.2 The healing process is typically separated into three overlapping and continuous phases: inflammatory, fibroblastic (proliferation), and maturation and remodeling. Courtesy of Cindy Trowbridge.

and shares some of the same duties, but each phase has its own specific goals. Unfortunately, several factors can impede healing, including the extent of the injury; poor tissue vascularization; uncontrolled muscle spasm; amount of hemorrhage, swelling, and edema; infection; age; overall health; nutrition; and the climate (i.e., humidity and oxygen tension) (Houglum, 2016; Prentice, 2017), but the good news is that the human body has an amazing ability to heal and restore itself after injury.

Trauma Wound or injury.

Resolution Complete healing whereby dead cells and cellular debris are removed, and the tissue is left functionally the same.

Regeneration Damaged tissue is replaced by cells of the same type along with scar tissue, but the tissue retains most of its original structure.

Repair Original tissue is replaced by scar tissue or repaired tissue.

Inflammation phase The first of the healing phases in which the body is responding to the threat of infection while trying to assess and contain the original injury.

Fibroblastic phase The second of the healing phases in which the body is beginning to build the infrastructure necessary for the injured site to recover.

Maturation and remodeling phase The third of the healing phases in which the body is completing the process of recovery and tissue is beginning to be formed according to how it will be used.

Inflammatory Response Phase

Regardless of what tissue has been injured, the body's initial response to trauma is inflammation. This process is very complicated; it begins immediately following the injury and includes several sequential and interdependent steps (Table 8.1). The steps are sequential in that they follow one another but interdependent in that they are continuously working together to protect, destroy, localize, dilute, and clean the area that experienced the injury (Houglum, 2016). The normal immediate signs and symptoms of inflammation include swelling, pain, reddening of the skin (i.e., **erythema**), increases in the temperature of the area involved, and loss of function (Ingersoll & Mistry, 2006; Scott et al., 2004; Figure 8.3).

When tissues are damaged as a result of trauma, millions of cells are destroyed. However, the destruction is what actually triggers the body's healing response. This phase is characterized by several steps, which are designed to minimize the initial (i.e., primary) injury and begin the development of new tissue. These steps include vascular, cellular, and metabolic changes that are mediated by a variety of chemicals, including **histamine**, **bradykinin**, and **prostaglandins** (Table 8.1). A good analogy for understanding this process is the construction of a new building. The first step is the implosion or removal of the old and damaged structure so a new building can be started. After the implosion, the site is fenced in, and crews begin to clean up the debris. The new foundation can be laid only when the debris has been cleared. Basically, the inflammatory response phase is meant to destroy injured tissue, contain the area, localize the actual site of injury, protect the injured tissue, and defend against infection (Houglum, 2016). In essence, the entire acute inflammatory phase results in a walling off of the damaged area from the rest of the body along with forming a mass of cellular debris, enzymes, and chemicals that serve to clean up the destroyed structures and protect the area against infection while also providing the necessary components for tissue repair. The acute inflammatory phase of injury lasts until new tissue material can arrive (approximately 2 to 4 days; Prentice, 2017). However, if athletes return to participation too soon and the area is disturbed by additional trauma, the inflammatory response phase would last much longer. Therefore, protection (i.e., splinting or crutches) and rest are often the prescribed treatment. For example, with the majority of fractures, some type of immobilization is required, usually in the form of a splint or a plaster or synthetic cast. In severely displaced fractures, surgical placement of appliances, such as plates and screws, may be necessary to stabilize the bony fragments to facilitate healing.

The mechanical force of the injury usually results in damage to a variety of soft tissues, including the blood vessels. As a result, blood flow into the interstitial (i.e., between the cells) spaces suddenly increases, which results in the formation of a hematoma (i.e., blood and plasma pooling within tissue, which can

Table 8.1
Sequential and Interdependent Steps of the Inflammatory Process

1	Tissue injury and ultrastructural change
2	Chemical mediation (chemotaxis)
3	Hemodynamic alteration (i.e., vasoconstriction, vasodilation, and clotting)
4	Increase in tissue metabolism
5	Increase in vascular permeability
6	Leukocyte migration (i.e., neutrophils, macrophages, and monocytes—ordered from early to late arrival)
7	Phagocytosis

Erythema Red discoloration of the skin.

Histamine Powerful inflammatory chemical that causes an increase in vascular permeability and vasodilation.

Bradykinin Inflammatory chemical released when tissues are damaged; it causes increased pain in the area and may play a role in the production of other inflammatory chemicals, such as prostaglandins.

Prostaglandins Perhaps some of the most powerful chemicals produced in the body; related to the inflammatory process, they cause a variety of effects, including vasodilation, increased vascular permeability, pain, fever, and clotting.

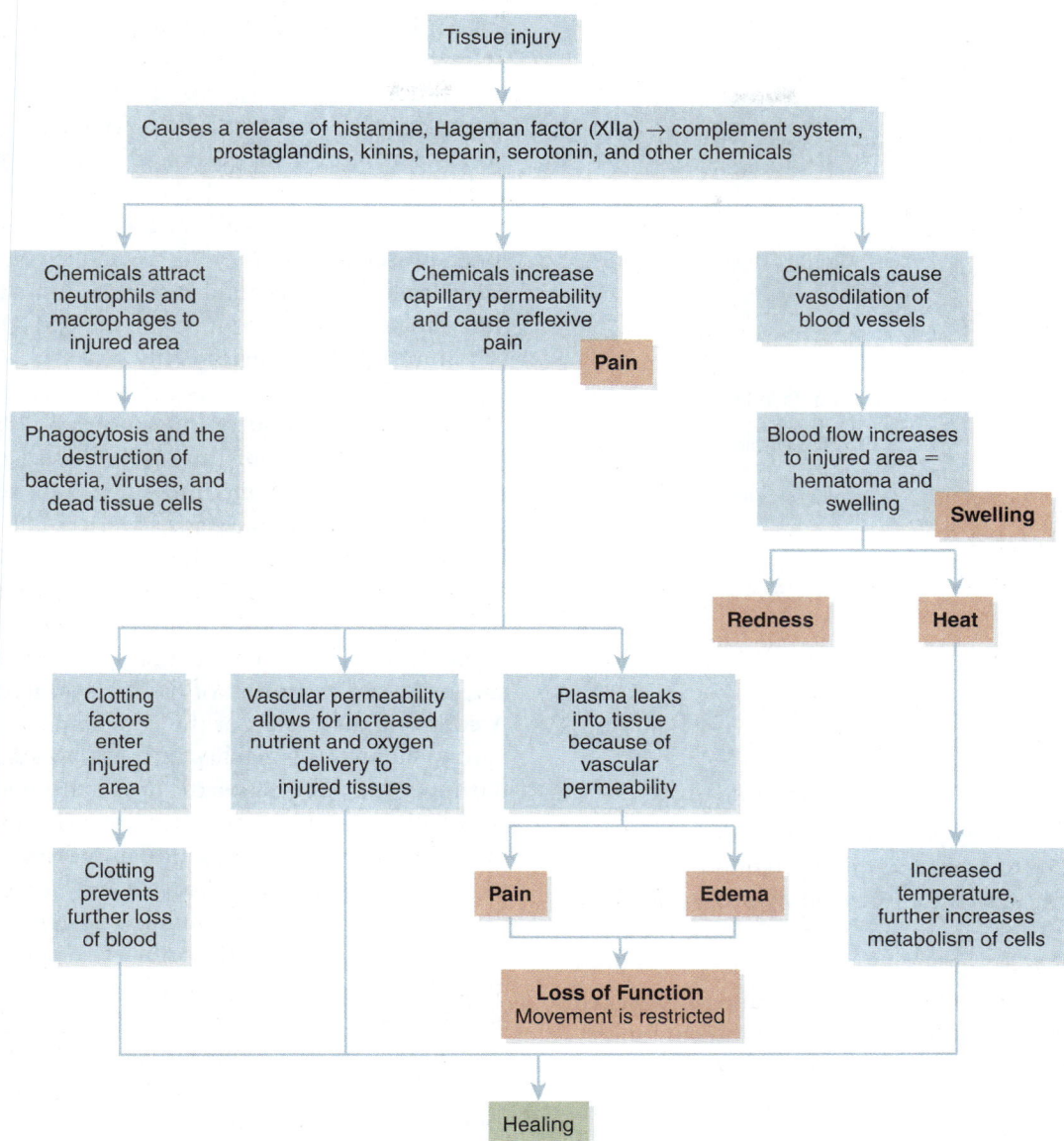

Figure 8.3 Inflammatory process.
Data from Chiras, D. D. (1999). *Human biology: Health, homeostasis, and the environment* (3rd ed.). Sudbury, MA: Jones and Bartlett Publishers.

cause damage). To prevent a hematoma from forming, a process known as **hemostasis** is initiated, which is an important step within the inflammatory process that helps prevent significant tissue damage (Houglum, 2016; Scott et al., 2004). A hematoma can develop quickly, so **vasoconstriction** is initiated to reduce blood flow and assist the cellular mechanisms of clotting in the damaged vessels. However, after only a few minutes, vasoconstriction is followed by **vasodilation** of blood vessels. The increased diameter of the blood vessels also increases vessel permeability,

Hemostasis Platelets and clotting factors in the bloodstream move to the site of injury to prevent excessive blood pooling; the mechanism that leads to the end of bleeding. This step helps attract other chemicals and cells to fully begin the inflammation phase.

Vasoconstriction Decrease in the diameter of a blood vessel resulting in decreased blood flow.

Vasodilation Increase in the diameter of a blood vessel resulting in increased blood flow.

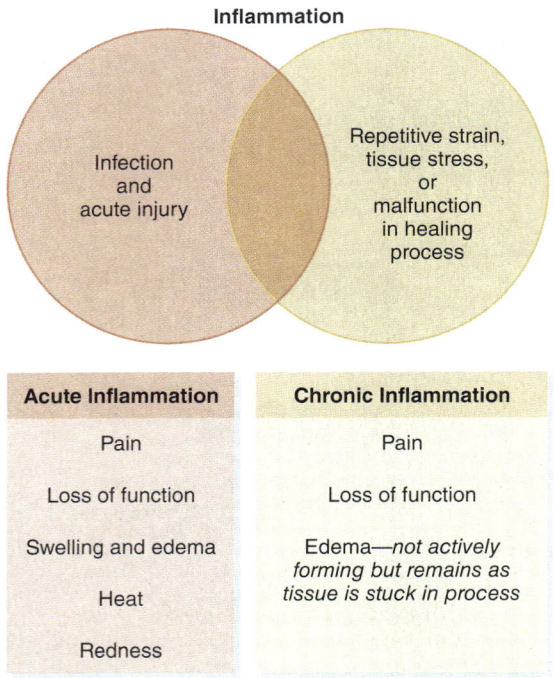

Figure 8.4 Acute versus chronic inflammation.
Courtesy of Cindy Trowbridge.

which will bring essential cells and chemicals to the site of injury to assist the inflammation phase. This phase is critical to the entire healing process because normal healing cannot happen if the inflammatory phase does not accomplish its goals, or it does not subside (Prentice, 2017). That differences exist between inflammation associated with acute injury and infection (i.e., acute inflammation) and inflammation associated with repetitive stress or incomplete healing (i.e., chronic inflammation) is important to understand (Figure 8.4). Although the two types of inflammation share common characteristics, they are more different than alike, and therefore must be treated differently. The section on intervention procedures presented later in the chapter will discuss these differences.

Complement system Refers to the part of the immune system that involves the complement proteins which assist host defense and inflammation.

Leukocyte White blood cell.

Lysosome Cellular organelle that contains enzymes that break down waste materials and cellular debris.

Three groups of chemicals have been identified as being active during the acute phase of the inflammatory response: vasoactive substances, which cause vasodilation; chemotactic factors, which mediate function and attract other types of cells; and degenerative enzymes, which cause cellular breakdown (Scott et al., 2004). These chemical mediators are responsible for the vascular, cellular, and metabolic changes that precede all the other cellular changes initiated in the inflammatory response phase (Figure 8.3). Histamine is a powerful inflammatory chemical and is released from several types of cells, resulting in short-term vasodilation and increased vascular permeability. Histamine is also known for causing redness around the site of trauma and sometimes an itching sensation, especially when the trauma is an insect bite or sting. In addition to histamine, when tissue damage occurs, an enzyme known as Hageman factor (XIIa) becomes active within the bloodstream. The Hageman factor induces several localized changes in the region of damage, including activation of the **complement system**. A complete discussion of the complement system is beyond the scope of this chapter, but for this discussion, the important information to know is that it includes a variety of chemically similar structures (i.e., cytokines) that play major roles in the inflammatory response, including activation of **leukocytes** and **lysosomes** and the attraction of cellular building material into the area. The leukocytes are the primary response team to injury; they are essential to healing and transported via blood vessels to the injury site (Chazaud, 2020; Scott et al., 2004). Through a complex process, which includes vasodilation, these leukocytes (e.g., neutrophils, macrophages, and monocytes) adhere to blood vessel walls and then fall off into the tissue space owing to the gaps created by vasodilation and permeability (Chazaud, 2020; Scott et al., 2004). Lysosomes contain powerful enzymes that, when released, hasten the breakdown of cellular structure (i.e., degradation effect). The process of attracting lysosomes, leukocytes, and other cellular building material is known as chemotaxis (Table 8.1) and is essential to the process of inflammation. The Hageman factor is also responsible for the manufacture of another powerful inflammatory chemical called bradykinin. It affects the vasculature by increasing vascular permeability and causes a pain response (Houglum, 2016). In addition, bradykinin triggers the release of prostaglandins, which are among the most powerful chemicals in the human body (Scott et al., 2004). Prostaglandins produce several effects in the damaged area, including vasodilation, increased vascular permeability, increased pain, and stimulation of the clotting mechanism (Scott et al., 2004). Another important chemical mediator of the acute inflammatory process is **arachidonic acid**, which is the product of the interaction between enzymes supplied by leukocytes and phospholipids derived from the membranes of destroyed cells (Scott et al., 2004). Arachidonic acid serves as the catalyst for a series of reactions that yield a variety of substances, including leukotrienes, which play a role in the inflammatory phase by attracting leukocytes to the damaged area. In the end, the combination of these chemical mediators and hemodynamic (vasoconstriction and vasodilation) and metabolic changes is what allows for the necessary cleanup of damaged tissue and the initiation of cellular building (Table 8.1).

The hemodynamic changes initiated by the chemical mediators are essential because the tissue cleanup process is made possible owing to an increase in vascular permeability, which allows large structures, such as plasma proteins, platelets, and leukocytes (primarily neutrophils), to pass out of capillaries and into the damaged tissue (Scott et al., 2004). By way of **phagocytosis** (i.e., cell eating), leukocytes and lysosomes dispose of damaged cells and tissue debris. The number of neutrophils in the damaged area can increase greatly in the first few hours of acute inflammation, to as high as four to five times the normal levels (Chazaud, 2020). Neutrophils arrive quickly at the site of injury; however, they live for only a short time (approximately 7 hours) and have no means of reproduction (Chazaud, 2020). When neutrophils expire, they release chemicals that attract a second type of leukocyte known as a macrophage. Macrophages also consume cellular debris via the process of phagocytosis. However, unlike neutrophils, macrophages can live for months and do have the ability to reproduce (Chazaud, 2020; Knight, 1995).

Unfortunately, the inflammatory response phase can last longer or be of a larger magnitude than optimally needed for all types of trauma. As a result, previously healthy tissue can be damaged as part of the repair process, which is called secondary injury. Secondary injury (Figure 8.5) adds to the total trauma area. An example of secondary injury is after a lateral ankle sprain, the hemorrhage (i.e., swelling) and subsequent **edema** (i.e., fluid accumulation) can often affect the lower leg and toes. When edema and the associated chemicals, lysosomes, and leukocytes start to invade areas of healthy tissue, they cause tissue destruction. The fluid accumulation along with the previously damaged blood vessels may cause further obstruction of blood flow to the area surrounding the tissue damage. In turn, the lack of blood flow prevents the arrival of oxygen and other energy sources to not only the injured tissue but also the surrounding undamaged tissue, which may result in a specific type of secondary injury called **secondary metabolic injury** (Figure 8.5a). This type of secondary injury results from the energy needs of tissue being greater than the energy available, which causes healthy tissue to die because of a lack of appropriate metabolic provisions (Knight, 1976; Merrick, 2002). Furthermore, during extended phagocytosis, the neutrophils and some macrophages cause another type of secondary injury called **secondary enzymatic injury** (Figure 8.5b). Basically, the cell membranes of healthy cells are compromised by the chemical waste products produced by the necessary phagocytosis of real tissue debris (Merrick, 2002). When a cell membrane is compromised, it can no longer maintain homeostasis and will likely experience **apoptosis** (i.e., programmed cell death). In addition

---

Arachidonic acid Chemical released when cells are damaged that serves as a precursor to the formation of other inflammatory chemicals, including leukotrienes and prostaglandins.

Phagocytosis The uptake of large particles from the extracellular matrix into the cell for the purpose of cleaning up debris and assisting with immune system function.

Edema Abnormal accumulation of fluid in the interstitial tissue; disruption of homeostatic fluid balance in the tissues.

Secondary metabolic injury Indirect result of tissue trauma. Healthy tissues surrounding primary injury die from lack of blood flow and metabolic supplies. The energy needed exceeds that of the energy available.

Secondary enzymatic injury Indirect result of tissue trauma. Healthy tissues surrounding primary injury die as a result of aggressive eating of healthy tissue within the area of the original injury. Waste products also damage cell membranes of healthy cells, causing cell death.

Apoptosis Process of programmed cell death. Biochemical events can lead to changes in cell characteristics, thereby causing cell death.

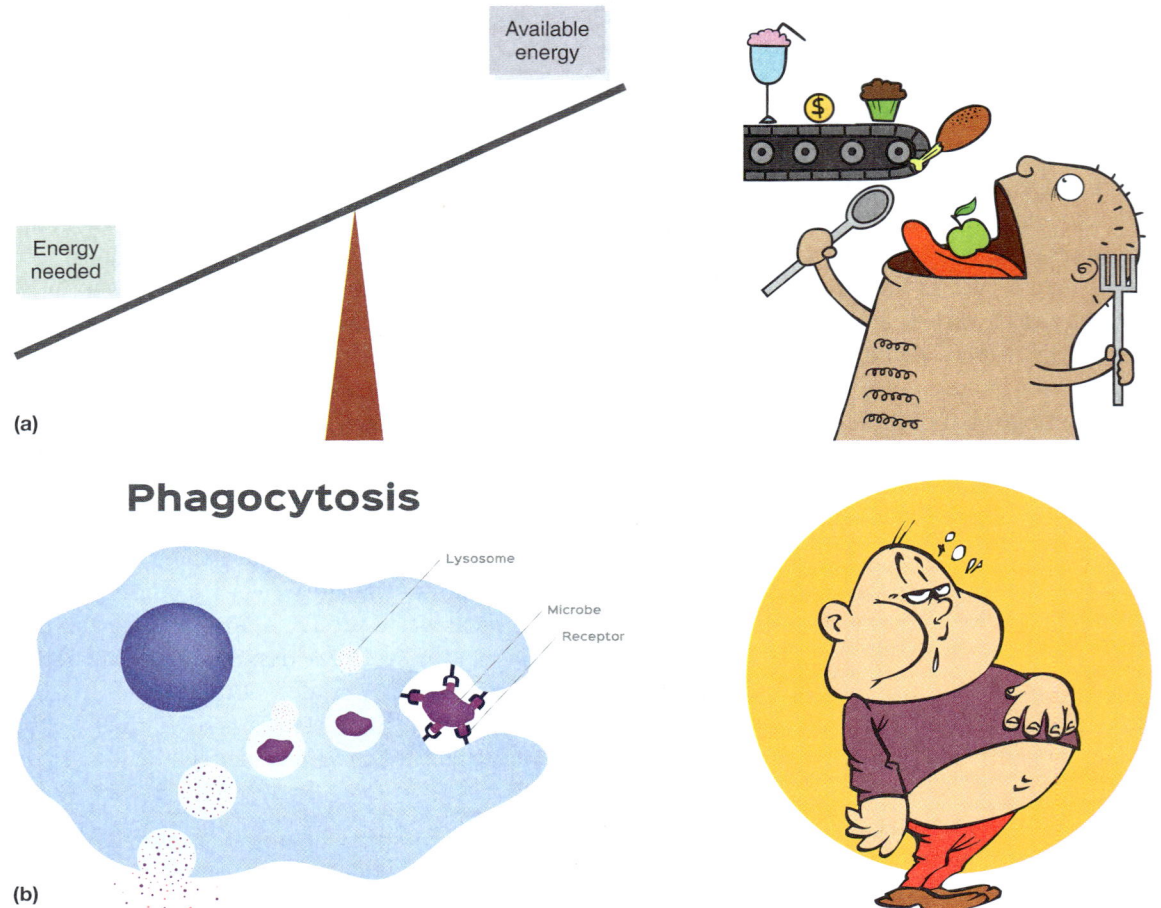

Figure 8.5 Secondary injury is associated with **(a)** secondary metabolic tissue death (injury) that occurs because the energy needs of tissue are greater than the energy available, which causes healthy tissue to die because of a lack of appropriate metabolic provisions, and **(b)** secondary enzymatic tissue death (injury), whereby the phagocytes devour everything in sight and eat way too much tissue, including originally healthy tissue, thus creating even more destruction.
(Top Left) Courtesy of Cindy Trowbridge; (Bottom Left) © gritsalak karalak/Shutterstock; (Top Right) © zetwe/Shutterstock; (Bottom Right) © humphrey/Shutterstock.

to apoptosis, some healthy cells are even consumed by overly aggressive neutrophils and macrophages because they are unable to distinguish between the tissue debris and surrounding healthy tissue and therefore an "overeating" syndrome occurs that results in general dysfunction or death of the originally healthy tissue (Merrick, 2002).

As previously stated, in the absence of further irritation or trauma, the inflammatory phase usually ends 2 to 4 days after the initial injury (Prentice, 2017). At this time, the earliest steps in tissue repair can begin to occur, with the migration into the area of specialized cells, including polymorphs and monocytes (both specialized forms of leukocytes) and histiocytes (a type of macrophage). These cells continue the process of breaking down the cellular debris to prepare for generation of new tissue. Building of new tissue is always a two-step process of tissue breakdown (i.e., lysis) and tissue buildup (i.e., synthesis). The balance between these two processes allows for the appropriate growth of new tissue, which then begins the fibroblastic repair phase.

Fibroblastic Repair Phase

With the exception of bones, connective tissues of the body heal themselves by replacing damaged cells with like cells (i.e., resolution and regeneration) or forming scar tissue (i.e., regeneration and repair). New connective tissue begins to form as soon as the inflammatory response phase nears its end. If we continue with the analogy of building a new structure, this phase is where the scaffolding (walls) is secured to the foundation to form the overall structure of the new building. At this point, the tissue now has some form and can withstand some pressure; therefore, early mobilization of joints and muscles is often favored at this time (Kannus et al., 2003). The fibroblastic repair phase begins with the damaged capillaries repairing themselves in just a few days after the initial injury. This process, known technically as **angiogenesis**, involves the actual formation of new capillaries, which interconnect to form new vessels (Houglum, 2016). With the formation of a new vascular supply, the new tissue is able to receive valuable nutrients and proteins to assist in the rebuilding process. Then, the process continues with the migration of fibroblasts into the area (Figure 8.6). **Fibroblasts** are immature, fiber-producing cells located in healthy connective tissue; they are responsible for producing **collagen** and other structures as part of tissue healing (Ingersoll & Mistry, 2006; Watson, 2016). Because of chemical mediation (complement system), fibroblasts become active at this time and produce collagen fibers and proteoglycans (i.e., protein macromolecules) also become active and help retain water in the tissues (Houglum, 2016). The retention of water is particularly important in tissues such as articular cartilage, which acts much like a sponge when exposed to fluids in joints. Bone injuries heal in a fashion similar to how soft tissue injuries heal; however, specialized cells known as **osteoclasts** migrate to the region of injury and remove destroyed cells and other debris, and then specialized fibroblasts known as **osteoblasts** migrate to the injured area from adjacent periosteum and bone. Moreover, new osteoblasts are manufactured on a large scale in the same region (Watson, 2016). The function of the osteoblasts is to develop a vascularized zone of collagen and cartilage, which is known as a callus. A callus fills the space between the fractured bone ends and can be seen quite clearly on a standard X-ray photograph (Figure 8.7). As in the building analogy, the callus is

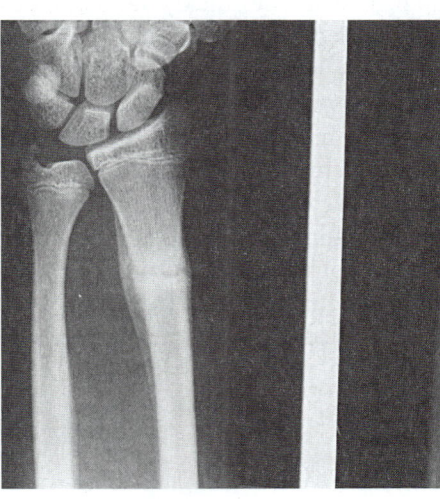
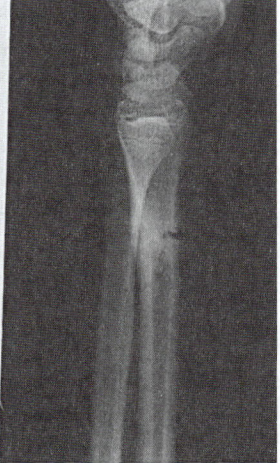

Figure 8.7 Callus forming around a fracture of the distal radius.
Courtesy of Ron Pfeiffer.

Angiogenesis Formation of capillaries that interconnect, resulting in the formation of new vessels.

Fibroblast Immature, fiber-producing cell of connective tissue that can mature into one of several cell types.

Collagen The major protein of connective tissue.

Osteoclast Bone cell that breaks down bone tissue for the purposes of maintaining, repairing, and remodeling bony tissue.

Osteoblast Bone cell that synthesizes bone.

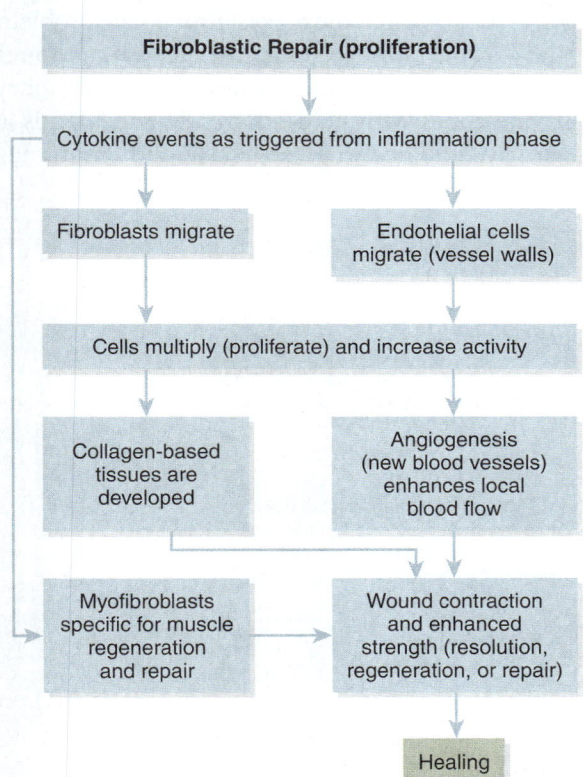

Figure 8.6 Fibroblastic repair (proliferation) phase.
Data from Watson, T. (2016). *Soft tissue repair and healing review*. Retrieved from http://www.electrotherapy.org/downloads

only the scaffolding and is not of sufficient strength to substitute for the original bone; it is just the beginning phase, which, through a process of maturation, will become fully functional bone.

Maturation and Remodeling Phase

Continuing the analogy of building a new structure, this phase is when the finishing touches are put on the structure (Figure 8.8). For example, with a building, walls are fortified (matured) and landscaping (remodeling) is done so the property is functional. Maturation and remodeling are the processes of the final phase of healing and may last up to 12 months, depending on the type of tissue injured (Houglum, 2016). Tendons and ligaments often take the longest because they are required to be strong and elastic and their blood supply can be limited (Cantu & Steffe, 2013). In contrast, muscle tissue can heal relatively quickly because it has a very extensive network of capillaries and specialized cells that trigger muscle growth. In cases where scar tissue (collagen based) is necessary to heal the injured area, it also undergoes maturation and remodeling. Although scar tissue demonstrates stiffness characteristics similar to those of uninjured tissue, it has reduced resistance to failure and a lower load compliance in addition to not always being aligned directionally according to common tissue stresses (Corr & Hart, 2013). Under ideal conditions, scar tissue can be 90–95% as strong as the original tissue; it may, however, achieve considerably less strength, perhaps up to 30% less (Cantu & Steffe, 2013).

Stress from exercises is essential in this phase; the new tissue will adapt its new collagen and tissue-specific fibers along the stress lines to form a much stronger configuration. Appropriate rehabilitative exercises are critical to this process, guided by two principles: the overload principle and the specific adaptations to imposed demands (SAID) principle. Tissue must be overloaded above normal demands to adapt and grow. Also, tissue will adapt according to the type of stresses placed on it (SAID principle; Houglum, 2016). For example, rehabilitation exercises must be prescribed to challenge the individual and must be done in directions or modes (i.e., strength, endurance, and power) that are specific to the required needs (Houglum, 2016).

Pain and Acute Injury

Although swelling, or edema, is often the most visible aspect of an acute injury, from the athlete's perspective, pain is often the biggest immediate problem. An important point to remember is that, although everyone has experienced pain associated with injury, everyone copes with pain differently and pain is as much psychological (i.e., cognitive and emotional)

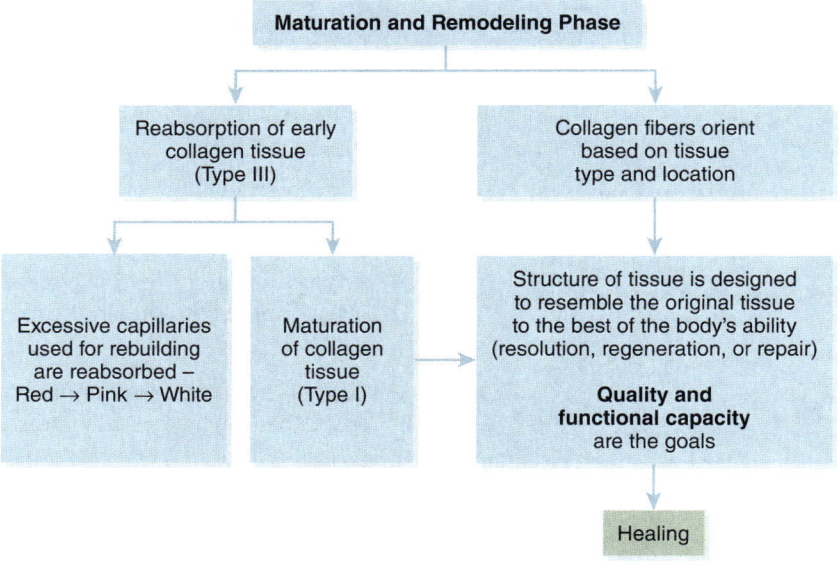

Figure 8.8 Maturation and remodeling phase.
Data from Watson, T. (2016). *Soft tissue repair and healing review*. Retrieved from http://www.electrotherapy.org/downloads

as it is physiological (Denegar, 2016; Moseley & Butler, 2015). Therefore, pain must be considered to be multimodal, or a biopsychosocial, phenomenon (i.e., biological, psychological, and sociological). As a physiological (i.e., biological) phenomenon, pain is essentially the result of sensory input received through the nervous system that indicates the location of the tissue damage or potential tissue damage.

Pain is typically defined as the perception of an unpleasant sensation associated with tissue damage or the emotional experience associated with the potential for tissue damage (Denegar, 2016). As such, knowing that each individual responds to pain differently is an important concept (Moseley & Butler, 2015). Therefore, during the initial evaluation of an injury, coaches must be familiar with the athletes' typical response to pain. Athletes with an extremely high pain tolerance may underestimate the severity of an injury, whereas athletes with low pain tolerance may grossly exaggerate the severity of an injury. Injured athletes may also downplay the level of pain out of fear of losing a starting position on the team. Pain is typically measured subjectively using different scales to rank the severity and quality of pain. One common scale is the numeric rating scale, for which no pain receives a 0 and the most severe pain receives a 10 (Houglum, 2016). However, recent evidence is providing scientists with an objective way to measure pain using functional magnetic resonance imaging of the brain (Wager et al., 2013), but this technology is a long way from being used clinically. In short, because pain is largely subjective, it may not be a useful indicator of the severity of an injury, but it must be addressed. When coaches must decide the significance of an injury, they are cautioned to err on the conservative side and, when in doubt, to refer athletes to medical personnel. Pain may also be thought of as athletes' friend in that it serves as a mechanism to reduce their activity level until adequate tissue healing has occurred (Denegar, 2016). The treatment of pain must be the domain of qualified medical

Athletic Trainers SPEAK OUT

Why is understanding the injury process essential when treating athletes of all ages and skill levels?

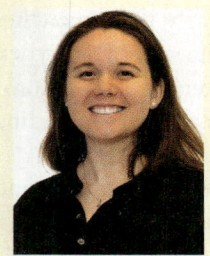

Courtesy of Breanna Hamilton, MEd, LAT, ATC.

By understanding the unique needs of each patient in conjunction with the intrinsic and extrinsic factors that affect the healing process, such as age and skill level, we, as clinicians, gain a clearer picture of how we can have the greatest beneficial impact on an injury. In addition, it is important to recognize that the specific therapeutic techniques selected will vary depending on what we, as clinicians, have been exposed to and are comfortable with. This is important to remember because, while the specifics of each injury process will differ, the foundations and techniques used will largely remain the same.

Looking closer at how both age and skill level affect the injury process, it is important to keep several key concepts in mind. Most importantly, as an individual ages, the rate at which tissue heals slows. Thus, what may take a 16-year-old soccer player a week to heal, may take 3 or more weeks for a 75-year-old recreational athlete. Additionally, parental consent is mandatory in the United States when treating individuals under the age of 18, and for older individuals, some therapies may be contraindicated due to medical conditions such as a pacemaker, arthritis, or osteoporosis. With skill level, the degree to which they are performing at and the frequency of said performance are largely the determining factors of what techniques will be used. A balance has to be struck between allowing the tissue to heal and stressing it in a manner that benefits the body's natural healing process. This can be a challenge at any level, but particularly at higher levels of competition, where individuals have a harder time resting an injury. Having a thorough understanding of the factors that affect the injury process allows us as clinicians to augment treatments to provide the maximum benefit to our patients.

—Breanna Hamilton, MEd, LAT, ATC

Breanna Hamilton athletic trainer for the United States Marine Corps, Camp Hansen, Okinawa, Japan.

Table 8.2
Common Modalities Used to Treat Pain

Modality	Afferent Nerve Stimulated
Ice	Temperature receptors
Heat	Temperature receptors
Electrical stimulation	Touch receptors
Massage	Touch receptors
Prophylactic wrapping or compression	Touch and proprioceptive receptors

personnel (QMP), including athletic trainers (ATs). Even though the main goal is for athletes to return to play, coaches, athletes, and parents should not treat the pain associated with an injury by using prescription medications or unproven techniques. Sports medicine personnel can use a variety of **modalities** to treat pain associated with injury (Table 8.2).

Intervention Procedures

Although the acute inflammatory process is clearly a necessary component of healing, athletes, coaches, and even many sports medicine personnel typically think of inflammation as something to be avoided at all costs. This sentiment is so common in the sports community that the variety of suggested first aid treatments for acute injuries can be overwhelming. Suggested treatments for inflammation include the application of **cryotherapy** (i.e., therapeutic use of cold), such as crushed ice packs, ice cups applied

Modality Therapeutic agent or technique that helps create an optimal healing environment.

Cryotherapy Therapeutic use of cold.

Thermotherapy Therapeutic use of heat.

Anti-inflammatory drug Drug designed to prevent swelling. Two basic categories are currently in use: steroidal and nonsteroidal.

Analgesic Agent that relieves pain without causing a complete loss of sensation.

via massage, ice-water baths, commercially available chemical cold packs, intermittent compression and cold, and aerosol coolants (i.e., ethyl chloride; Denegar, 2016). After the acute inflammatory phase has passed (i.e., no redness or heat is present) and ice is no longer bringing significant change (Denegar, 2016), **thermotherapy** (i.e., therapeutic use of heat)—including commercially available hydrocollator packs, warm and moist towels, ultrasound, and diathermy (i.e., radio-frequency energy)—may be appropriate, but cryotherapy is still appropriate based on clinical goals. The use of modalities such as ultrasound and diathermy should always be done under the direct supervision of trained QMP, such as Board of Certification (BOC)–certified ATs, physical therapists, or physicians.

In addition to cold and heat therapy, pharmacological agents—drugs designed to prevent swelling (**anti-inflammatories**) or drugs designed to prevent pain (**analgesics**)—are often used to treat the signs and symptoms of the inflammatory phase. Many of these drugs must be prescribed by a medical doctor and represent treatment beyond the training of coaching personnel or an AT. However, some anti-inflammatory drugs, such as aspirin, ibuprofen, and naproxen, and some analgesics, such as acetaminophen, are available over the counter (OTC) and are often effective for minor acute injuries. However, caution should be exercised, particularly when coaches are dealing with athletes under the age of 18 years; they should always consult with parents before recommending any sort of pharmacological agent, including OTC medications.

Experts agree that some sort of treatment beyond simple rest be applied during both the inflammatory phase as well as in the later stages of healing. Available research supports the use of modalities such as ice, compression, and elevation in addition to some pharmacological agents during the inflammatory phase to help control the likely overwhelming response of the body's innate immune system. Likewise, clinical evidence strongly supports the use of modalities such as ice and therapeutic heat (e.g., moist hot packs, whirlpool, and paraffin) and more sophisticated modalities such as ultrasound, diathermy, and electrotherapies (e.g., transcutaneous electrical nerve stimulation [TENS], neuromuscular electrical stimulation [NMES], and interferential stimulation [IFS]) during the fibroblastic repair and maturation and remodeling phases. Application of any of these modalities is typically regulated by medical practice acts in each state; therefore, they should be applied only by QMP under the direct supervision of physicians and in the parameters stipulated by the state's allied healthcare practice act.

Cryotherapy and Thermotherapy

Using cold or hot therapies to change the temperature of injured tissues can have dramatic effects on the physiological activities of healing and may affect the mechanical properties and range of motion of tissue after injury (Bleakley & Costello, 2013; Bleakley & Davison, 2010). Inflammation is a fundamental part of the healing process and should not be considered a negative effect; however, excessive vasodilation and vessel permeability can cause the swelling or edema to be too much or to last too long and thus cause pain (Bleakley & Davison, 2010). Therefore, during the first few minutes of the inflammatory phase, direct application of cold (generally in the form of crushed ice) may reduce vasodilation and pain, thereby reducing the amount of initial swelling, or edema, and dysfunction (Denegar, 2016). In classic research by Knight (1985), the immediate application of ice to an injury (i.e., during the early inflammatory response phase) helped to decrease the overall recovery time. Knight (1985) hypothesized that this occurred for two reasons. First, the tissue cooling slows aggressive neutrophils and macrophages and helps prevent excessive waste products and unnecessary destruction of healthy cells (i.e., secondary enzymatic injury). Second, the tissue cooling reduces the metabolic activity of the healthy cells in the injured area, thereby reducing their need for oxygen (i.e., secondary metabolic injury; Merrick, 2002). Consequently, the healthy cells are better able to survive the initial period of inflammation when oxygen may be in short supply. This sparing of cells contributes to a smaller collection of debris in the region of the initial (i.e., primary) injury, thereby promoting an earlier onset of the fibroblastic repair phase. In essence, the immediate application of ice helps reduce the signs and symptoms of acute inflammation and the overall severity of the secondary injury, as described earlier in this chapter. The application of ice immediately following an injury mitigates the metabolic changes associated with inflammation, thereby preventing an overresponse and subsequent secondary injury (Bleakley & Hopkins, 2010). Finally, ice provides an analgesic effect that can reduce muscle spasm and promote early mobilization. In the end, these two effects allow athletes to engage in other techniques, including therapeutic exercise.

A combination of techniques, known as PRICE (i.e., protection, rest, ice, compression, and elevation), has often been the mainstay of caring for an injury to an extremity. The application of PRICE is a standard first aid procedure for injuries such as sprains, strains, dislocations, contusions, tendonitis, and fractures. However, controversy has developed regarding the use of cryotherapy, and recent evidence has demonstrated that rest should not be complete and early mobilization of the joint or muscle will assist in the healing process (Bleakley et al., 2012; Dubois & Esculier, 2020).

One set of clinical researchers (Bleakley et al., 2006; Bleakley et al., 2012) continues to believe that the application of cold can provide significant pain relief and thereby promote motion and the body's natural responses related to healing, so they have recommended a removal of the *R* from PRICE and have developed a new combination of techniques whose acronym is POLICE (i.e., protection, optimal loading, ice compression, and elevation) for the treatment of acute musculoskeletal injuries. The emphasis of the POLICE model is to use ice with the goal of restoring protected and optimal loading so the tissue will not be delayed in healing because of weakness resulting from rest. Another set of clinical researchers, Dubois and Esculier (2020), insist that ice delays the inflammatory process and can result in negative consequences and rest delays tissue healing. They recommend protection, elevation, avoiding anti-inflammatories, compression, and education (i.e., PEACE) and load, optimism, vascularization, and exercise (LOVE) to manage acute musculoskeletal injuries. These two opinions are not as divergent as they may originally seem because they both focus on protecting the injured area, reducing edema, and promoting mobility. The main difference is the use of cryotherapy; therefore, the following paragraph is a discussion of the physiology surrounding tissue cooling and its myths and misconceptions (Long & Jutte, 2020). Ultimately, a one-size-fits-all formula is not the solution. The following discussion surrounding this topic is a reminder to athletes, coaches, and allied healthcare professionals to think differently and seek out new and innovative strategies for safe and effective pain relief and loading of tissues after the injury so healing is promoted and not delayed.

The use of cryotherapy was once a mainstay in the treatment of musculoskeletal injury, and the differences seen in clinical practice were more related to the type of cryotherapy (e.g., crushed ice, cubed ice, and cold whirlpool). But over the past 15 years, a vigorous discussion has ensued regarding when and if cryotherapy should be used to manage musculoskeletal injuries (Bleakley et al., 2006; Bleakley et al., 2012; Dubois & Esculier, 2020). The advent of whole body cryotherapy (WBC) cooling chambers has also muddied the waters related to the evidence for using cryotherapy in the management of musculoskeletal injuries, especially muscle soreness, and the mechanics of recovery after workouts (Costello et al., 2015; Patel et al., 2019). Unfortunately, limited evidence exists regarding a definite clinical benefit to WBC, with weak evidence regarding a positive effect on functional recovery following exercise (Patel et al., 2019). Therefore, more high-quality clinical research is required to determine whether WBC can reduce the negative consequences of inflammation, improve performance, and promote functional recovery (Costello et al., 2015; Patel et al., 2019).

Though many variations on application of cryotherapy exist, experts recommend that the most effective way of applying cold to the body is a plastic bag filled with crushed ice (de Estéfani et al., 2020; Figure 8.9). Nothing exotic need be used—a plastic sandwich bag with some type of closure is most effective. Crushed ice is made relatively inexpensively by ice machines, which are a good investment for a school athletic department. Crushed ice can even be purchased before a game or practice session and stored in a cooler for later use. Commercially available chemical cold packs and aerosol sprays (i.e., ethyl chloride) are less effective than crushed ice and can even be dangerous in some situations (Denegar, 2016). Research has shown that the risk of frostbite during the application of a bag of crushed ice is minimal. Human tissue freezes at around 25°F (−3°C), and a bag of crushed ice reaches a low temperature of only 32°F and is gradually warmed by the heat from the body. The traditional recommendation is that an ice bag be left in place for 20–30 minutes and then removed owing to the fact that metabolism may be slowed to levels that hinder normal physiology or the cold produces no further benefit. Because we do not have high-quality evidence on the efficacy of ice for treating musculoskeletal injuries (Vuurberg et al., 2018), many clinicians who are against the use of ice for musculoskeletal injuries often cite that no evidence exists for its use and that it can possibly disrupt the inflammatory process, especially angiogenesis and initial proliferation (Dubois & Esculier, 2020; Vuurberg et al., 2018). However, the only studies that have shown significant reductions in cellular metabolism were done on animals, and the ice was applied continuously for five to six hours (Bleakley, 2009; Bleakley & Hopkins, 2010; Long & Jutte, 2020). On the other side of the argument, studies are available that demonstrate successful reduction in skeletal muscle damage and markers of inflammation, which indicates a benefit of cryotherapy in controlling excessive inflammation from both acute injury (Puntel et al., 2013) and excessive exercise (Santos et al., 2012). Therefore, we do not really have any evidence that icing disrupts the inflammatory process in a negative way, nor do we have a defined duration or type of application that is best for cryotherapy. However, research comparing an intermittent application of ice (i.e., 10 minutes on, 10 minutes off, 10 minutes on) to 20 minutes of continuous application of ice on acute ankle injuries demonstrated a greater reduction in pain during the first week of treatments for athletes who used the intermittent technique (Bleakley et al., 2006), even though both groups improved overall. Therefore, the current recommendation for pain relief is to cool the skin enough to provide for analgesia and to promote early mobilization (5–15 minutes), and the recommendation for the clinical goal of

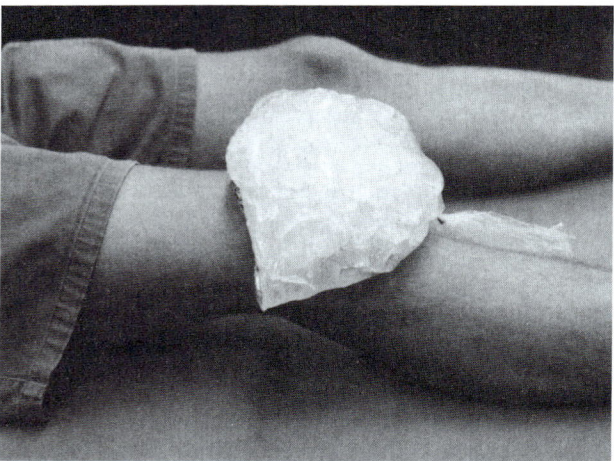

Figure 8.9 Bags filled with crushed ice are the most convenient way to apply cold to an injury.
Courtesy of Ron Pfeiffer.

preventing secondary injury is to cool the skin for 20–50 minutes, depending on the type of cryotherapy (Kwiecien & McHugh, 2021; Merrick et al., 2003) used and the subcutaneous adipose thickness over the targeted musculoskeletal injury (Otte et al., 2002). However, more controlled research needs to be performed regarding the use of cryotherapy during the inflammatory response phase and the amount of time required to achieve decreases in tissue temperature necessary for slowing the onset of secondary injury (Bleakley & Hopkins, 2010; Long & Jutte, 2020).

Compression is best achieved by using a commercially available elastic wrap (Tomchuk, 2010; Figure 8.10a). Wraps come in a variety of sizes and widths that can accommodate almost any anatomic site and body size. Placing the ice bag directly against the skin with the elastic wrap secured over the bag is the best way. The wrap should be wound in a closed spiral fashion, starting distally and finishing proximally. Care must be taken not to make the wrap excessively tight because doing so could compromise circulation. A rule of thumb is that two fingers should be able to easily be slipped under the elastic after it has been secured. After the wrap is in place, the pulse distal to the wrap should always be checked. Leave the wrap in place until the injury is seen by medical personnel. Newer forms of compression are also available. Systems that deliver intermittent pneumatic compression and cold via sleeves are gaining popularity in the sports medicine setting (Figure 8.10b). In essence, the air-based compression enhances the cooling capabilities of the cold modality because it increases skin surface contact.

Elevation of the injury is self-explanatory; however, some precautions are necessary. When an injury to the lower extremity is elevated, adjacent joints should be supported with padding. Elevation during sleep can be accomplished simply by raising the foot end of the bed a few inches off the floor. The purpose of elevation is to promote venous and lymph return to main circulation and limit edema in distal extremities. However, it is best combined with active movement, which allows the muscles to act as a pump on the venous and lymphatic system.

Thermotherapeutic agents, such as moist heat packs, diathermy, or ultrasound, may also have a beneficial effect on soft-tissue injury. However, available research is unanimous that such treatments should never be applied during the acute inflammatory phase

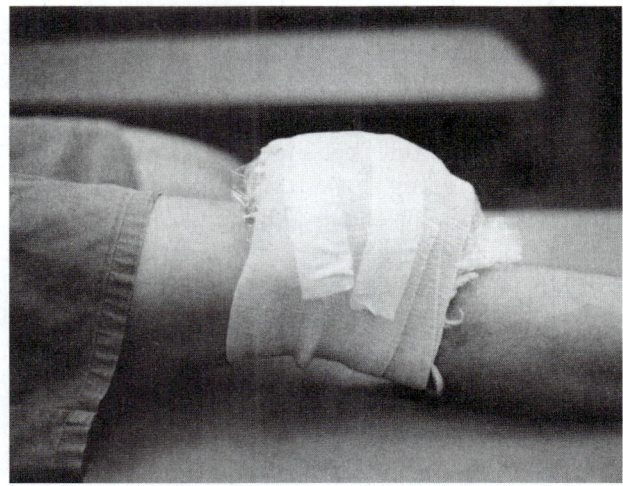

(a)

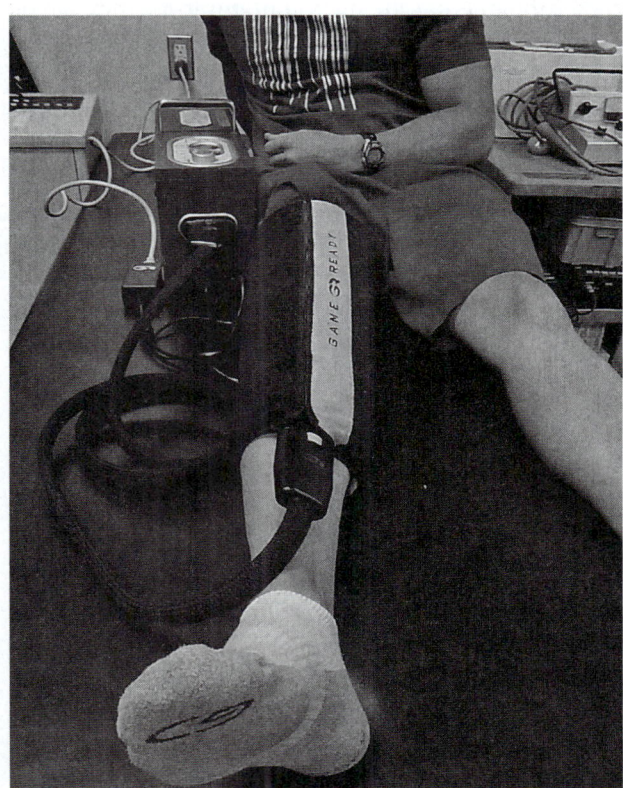

(b)

Figure 8.10 (a) Elastic wrap provides a convenient method of compression. (b) A common continuous cooling and intermittent compression device.
(a) Courtesy of Ron Pfeiffer; (b) Courtesy of Cindy Trowbridge.

when redness and heat are present (Denegar, 2016). By heating the tissue during the early phases of the injury, the metabolic activity of the inflammatory agents is increased, thereby resulting in an increase in inflammation (Denegar, 2016). However, thermotherapies may be useful during the final phases of injury repair by increasing available oxygen and stimulating vasodilation in the region of the injured tissues. In addition, heat increases local metabolic activities, including those resulting in regeneration of tissues, and relieves pain that might be preventing therapeutic exercises. Therefore, coaches can recommend heat-based thermotherapies to their athletes if they are confident the acute signs of inflammation (i.e., redness, heat, and active edema) are not present.

Pharmacological Agents

A wide variety of pharmacological agents are currently available for the treatment of inflammation. Based on their fundamental chemical configuration, they can be classified into two groups: steroidal and nonsteroidal anti-inflammatory drugs (NSAIDs). Both groups seem to interfere with some aspect of the inflammatory process, thereby reducing either the amount of swelling (i.e., anti-inflammatory) or pain (i.e., analgesic).

Steroidal Anti-Inflammatory Drugs

Steroidal drugs (i.e., corticosteroids) are manufactured in such a way as to resemble a group of naturally occurring chemicals in the body known collectively as glucocorticoids, which are active in the body relative to the metabolism of carbohydrates, fats, and proteins. Curiously, the exact mechanism of action of steroidal drugs on the inflammatory process is not clearly understood (Scott et al., 2004). Evidence is available that steroids suppress cytokines, block the release of arachidonic acid, lower the amount of chemicals released from intracellular lysosomes, decrease the permeability of capillaries, diminish the ability of white blood cells to phagocytize tissues, and reduce local fever (Scott et al., 2004). Probably the best known of the steroidal preparations is cortisone; however, others commonly used include hydrocortisone, prednisone, prednisolone, triamcinolone, and dexamethasone.

Steroidal preparations are generally either orally ingested or injected. They may even be introduced through the skin via **phonophoresis** (using ultrasound energy) or **iontophoresis** (using electrical current; Denegar, 2016). Problems with steroidal chemicals involve the negative effects they have on the process of collagen formation. In essence, steroids can decrease the overall strength of the connective tissue structures in an injured region (Scott et al., 2004). Great care must be taken when using these powerful drugs. The medications should be prescribed only by a physician, and the risks and benefits should be discussed with the athlete and parents (if the athlete is a minor) before treatment.

Nonsteroidal Anti-Inflammatory Drugs

Nonsteroidal anti-inflammatory drugs (NSAIDs) block specific reactions in the inflammatory process; however, they do not seem to significantly delay collagen formation. As a group, these drugs appear to block the breakdown of arachidonic acid to prostaglandin, which in turn decreases the inflammatory response to injury (Hatt et al., 2018). Aspirin, known chemically as acetylsalicylic acid, produces several effects—anti-inflammatory, analgesic, and **antipyretic** (i.e., reduces fever). These drugs have become extremely popular in the medical community, but they do have side effects and may not be the most appropriate first choice for treating musculoskeletal injuries (Stovitz & Johnson, 2003). Coexisting renal, cerebrovascular, cardiovascular, and gastrointestinal diseases can be adversely affected by the intake of NSAIDs owing to the side effects that are common in these organ systems (Hatt et al., 2018).

Though the physiological effects of NSAIDs on inflammation are quite clear, what remains to be clarified is their effect if any on the rate and completeness of the healing process. Each phase of injury repair is necessary for the subsequent phase to occur, and if the inflammatory phase is significantly blocked, then theoretically NSAIDs may delay the healing of musculoskeletal injuries. Scientists and physicians have concerns that the consumption of NSAIDs during the acute stages of injury may slow or even stop the very important inflammatory response phase. Recall that, for new tissue to rebuild, the damaged

---

Phonophoresis The use of ultrasound to assist with the topical or transdermal delivery of drugs or possibly other substances into the tissues of the body.

Iontophoresis Using an electrical current to drive a chemical/medication directly through the skin.

Nonsteroidal anti-inflammatory drugs (NSAIDs) Class of agents that block specific reactions in the inflammatory process.

Antipyretic Agent that relieves or reduces fever.

tissue must first go through a complete inflammatory response phase. When healing tissue does not complete the early inflammatory phase, the tissue strength of the regenerated tissue is in question (Hertel, 1997; Scott et al., 2004). Even though NSAIDs are widely used to treat acute soft-tissue injury, their efficacy is not in the scientific literature. In fact, their side effects on a variety of organ systems often garner more attention (Hatt et al., 2018; Hertel, 1997). Also, little evidence exists to support the claim that NSAIDs hasten the return of injured athletes to competition (Hertel, 1997). Important factors regarding NSAIDs are to be realistic about their capabilities and to help athletes understand that they are very rarely a substitute for rehabilitation and activity modification (Stovitz & Johnson, 2003). The commonly used NSAIDs are listed in Table 8.3.

Acetaminophen (i.e., Tylenol) is not an NSAID and is strictly an analgesic and antipyretic that is used to relieve pain and fever. However, concerns are increasing over the safety of Tylenol and the current recommended dosages, and new warnings by the FDA have been posted regarding liver damage and death (Harvard Health Publishing, 2020).

Until more conclusive research is available, the best approach to treating the majority of soft-tissue injuries appears to be the application of ice during the acute inflammatory phase; followed by a combination of protected optimal loading exercises designed to meet the patient's needs and prescribed pharmacological agents or monitored OTC medications; followed by advanced rehabilitative exercises that are properly supervised by QMP. From a legal and ethical standpoint, the coach or other nonmedical personnel should provide only initial first aid to any soft-tissue injury (i.e., ice and protection) and then refer the athlete to the appropriate medical authority. Nonmedical personnel should avoid recommending any type of medication, even an OTC drug, such as aspirin or acetaminophen. The best approach is to have any injury seen by QMP before further treatment (in any form) is given.

Table 8.3
Examples of Nonsteroidal Anti-Inflammatory Drugs

Category	Examples
Salicylic acid derivates	Acetylsalicylic acid (aspirin)
	Sodium salicylate
	Diflunisal
	Salicylsalicylic acid
	Sulfasalazine
	Olsalazine
Para-aminophenol derivatives	Acetaminophen
Indole and indene acetic acid	Indomethacin
	Sulindac
	Etodolac
Heteroaryl acetic acid	Ibuprofen
	Naproxen
	Flurbiprofen
	Ketoprofen
	Fenoprofen
	Oxaprozin
Anthranilic acid (fenemates)	Mefenamic acid
	Meclofenamic acid
Enolic acid derivatives (oxicams)	Piroxicam
	Tenoxicam
	Meloxicam
Napthylalkanones	Nabumetone
Pyrenecarboxylic acids	Etodolac
Pyrroles	Ketorolac
COX-2 inhibitors	Celecoxib
	Etoricoxib

Data from Kowalski, M. L., & Makowska, J. S. (2015). Seven steps to the diagnosis of NSAIDs hypersensitivity: How to apply a new classification in real practice? *Allergy, Asthma, & Immunology Research, 7*(4), 313; Conaghan, P. G. (2012). A turbulent decade for NSAIDs: Update on current concepts of classification, epidemiology, comparative efficacy, and toxicity. *Rheumatology International, 32*(6), 1492; and Hatt, K. M., Vijapura, A., Maitin, I. B., & Cruz, E. (2018). Safety considerations in prescription of NSAIDs for musculoskeletal pain: A narrative review. *PM & R, 10*(12), 1406.

WHAT IF ?

A parent asks you for advice on what OTC drug would be best to give his daughter to help her recover from a second-degree ankle sprain. What would you suggest?

Role of Exercise Rehabilitation

What may seem paradoxical is that the most effective treatment for many sports injuries, especially those involving soft tissues, is physical activity. Obviously, asking an athlete to run on a sprained ankle is incorrect, but a properly constructed and supervised exercise regimen can have a dramatic effect on the healing process when the overload and SAID principles are followed (Figure 8.11). Research indicates that rehabilitative exercise can exert a variety of positive effects on collagen formation (Houglum, 2016). Because collagen is a major constituent of tendon and ligament tissues, exercise is a logical form of treatment. According to Knight (1995), exercise is essential during the healing process for two reasons. First, exercise results in increased circulation with a concomitant increase in oxygen supply to the healing tissue. Second, exercise stresses the healing tissue and in essence "guides" the proper structuring of collagen. Although exercise is essential to proper tissue healing, the old saying "too much too soon" is worth remembering during the rehabilitation process (Houglum, 2016). At the very least, the process of collagen formation and tissue regeneration requires 2–3 weeks and full functional healing can take 12–15 months for severe injuries (Houglum, 2016). Further, after the final phase of healing, when appropriate the athlete should have the area properly protected with adhesive taping, wrapping, or bracing.

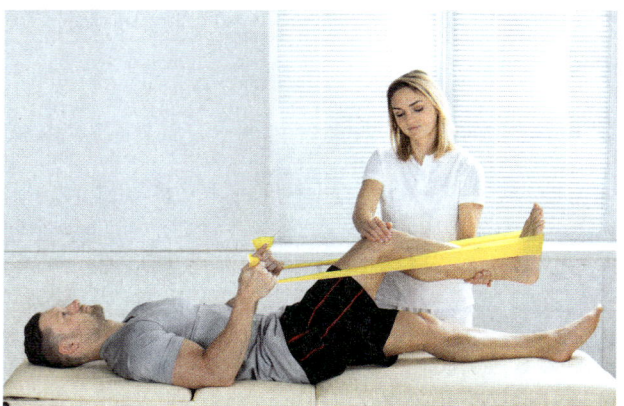

Figure 8.11 Exercise can be the most effective treatment for many athletes who have sustained sports injuries.
© Andrey_Popov/Shutterstock.

Decisions concerning returning to play should be made by a medical professional with experience in sports injuries and return-to-play assessment techniques or screening. Coaches should avoid returning athletes to participation too early just because they may be critical to the team's success.

Any injury severe enough to warrant a medical diagnosis should be treated with a comprehensive program of exercise rehabilitation. Such a program must consist of essential components and be planned by professionals with the appropriate training, either a BOC-certified AT or a physical therapist who has sports medicine training. Responsibility for implementation and supervision of the out-of-clinic exercise program (e.g., home exercise programs) may fall on the parent, coach, or physical educator. Thus, communication among the athlete, coach, parent, and medical personnel is essential for any program to be effective.

Rehabilitative exercise, often called therapeutic exercise, is a four-phase process consisting of categories of exercise based on a continuum of severity and recovery (Houglum, 2016). If the athlete's injury is severe, the initial exercise protocol may make the athlete a passive participant; a therapist actually moves the injured extremity through a series of passive exercises. The benefits are the reestablishment of a normal range of motion (ROM) and reduction of swelling and muscle spasm. As the injury improves, the next phase of exercise is active assisted. During this phase, the athlete becomes a working partner in the exercise process, making a voluntary effort to move the injured joint while being assisted by a therapist. The benefits of this phase are improved ROM and increased muscle strength. The next phase in the rehabilitation process is active exercise. At this point, the athlete continues moving the joint through a full ROM, using gravity as resistance to stimulate development of muscle strength. The important aspect of this phase is that the therapist merely supervises the activity; no physical assistance is given to the athlete. The final phase of the recovery program is known as resistive: External resistance is applied to the joint movements. This can be done via manual resistance provided by the therapist or the use of resistive exercise machines or even free weights. The primary objective of this phase is to improve the strength of the muscles surrounding the injured area to protect the injured area from future injury. This last phase must incorporate exercises known as "functional" activities, which include movements identical to those typically exhibited in the athlete's sport, for example, running and cutting drills for those athletes in sports such as basketball, football, and soccer. Published experts within the sports medicine community concur that such a protocol is necessary for adequate healing of damaged soft-tissue structures, especially in the lower extremities (Herring et al., 2012; Houglum, 2016; Prentice, 2017).

Injury rehabilitation should be considered an ongoing process. Injury-specific exercise should be a permanent component in the total training and conditioning program of the athlete. Without such an approach, the likelihood of reinjury is high in many cases. The coach must communicate with the appropriate members of the athletic healthcare team—AT, physical therapist, and/or physician—to plan and implement an effective program of therapeutic exercise.

Review Questions

1. During which type of muscular contraction does the majority of muscle or fascia injuries occur?
2. True or false? The proximal musculotendinous junction has been found to be the most common site for injuries.
3. List the three types of mechanical forces that can cause soft-tissue injury.
4. Define *critical force* or *failure point* of tissue.
5. Describe the major steps that occur during the healing process of an injury, with particular emphasis on vasoconstriction, vasodilation, and subsequent hematoma formation.
6. Define *chemotaxis*.
7. Briefly describe two of the chemical mediators and their physiological effects during the acute phase of an injury.
8. Briefly describe the overall purpose of the inflammatory phase of an injury.
9. List the types of cells that migrate to the injured area during the early part of the resolution phase.
10. What are the five clinical signs of inflammation?
11. What are fibroblasts?
12. What is angiogenesis?
13. What is the relationship between a bony formation known as a callus and the healing of a fracture?
14. Describe the mechanism for secondary injury as described by Knight (1976) and Merrick (2002).
15. What is the effect of ice application on a secondary injury?
16. Briefly explain the physiological effects of the application of ice, compression, and elevation on acute inflammation.
17. What do the POLICE, PEACE, and LOVE acronyms stand for regarding the treatment of musculoskeletal injuries?
18. What is an easy and effective way of applying cold and compression simultaneously to an injury?
19. What is the recommended duration of ice application for the treatment of pain during acute inflammation?
20. At what temperature does human tissue typically freeze?
21. At what point during the process of injury repair can thermotherapies be useful?
22. Differentiate between steroidal and nonsteroidal anti-inflammatory pharmacological agents.
23. What is the mode of action of NSAIDs regarding the acute inflammatory phase of an injury?
24. What does the acronym OTC stand for?
25. What are the concerns about the administration of NSAIDs over a period of time?
26. Give a brief explanation of the four types of therapeutic exercise outlined in the chapter—passive, active assisted, active, and resistive.

References

Bleakley, C. (2009). Current concepts in the use of PRICE for soft tissue injury management. *Physiotherapy Ireland, 30*(2), 19–20.

Bleakley, C. M., & Costello, J. T. (2013). Do thermal agents affect range of movement and mechanical properties in soft tissues? A systematic review. *Archives of Physical Medicine and Rehabilitation, 94*(1), 149–163.

Bleakley, C. M., & Davison, G. W. (2010). Cryotherapy and inflammation: Evidence beyond the cardinal signs. *Physical Therapy Reviews, 15*(6), 430–435.

Bleakley, C. M., Glasgow, P., & MacAuley, D. C. (2012). PRICE needs updating, should we call the POLICE? *British Journal of Sports Medicine, 46*, 220–221.

Bleakley, C., & Hopkins, J. (2010). Is it possible to achieve optimal levels of tissue cooling in cryotherapy? *Physical Therapy Reviews, 15*(4), 344–350.

Bleakley, C., McDonough, S., & MacAuley, D. (2006). Cryotherapy for acute ankle sprains: A randomized controlled study of two different icing protocols. *British Journal of Sports Medicine, 40*, 700–705.

Cantu, R., & Steffe, J. A. (2013). Soft tissue healing and considerations after surgery. In L. Maxey & J. Magnusson (Eds.), *Rehabilitation for the postsurgical orthopedic patient* (pp. 15–25). Elsevier. https://doi.org/10.1016/B978-0-323-07747-7.00002-2

Chazaud, B. (2020). Inflammation and skeletal muscle regeneration: Leave it to the macrophages! *Trends in Immunology, 41*(6), 481–492.

Comstock, R. D., & Pierpoint, L. A. (2020). *Summary report: National High School Sports-Related Injury Surveillance Survey (2018–2019)*. Retrieved from https://coloradosph.cuanschutz.edu/docs/librariesprovider204/default-document-library/2018-19.pdf?sfvrsn=d26400b9_2

Corr, D. T., & Hart, D. A. (2013). Biomechanics of scar tissue and uninjured skin. *Advanced Wound Care, 2*(2), 37–43.

Costello, J. T., Baker, P. R., Minett, G. M., Bieuzen, F., Stewart, I. B., & Bleakley, C. (2015). Whole-body cryotherapy (extreme cold air exposure) for preventing and treating muscle soreness after exercise in adults. *Cochrane Database of Systematic Reviews*. doi:10.1002/14651858.CD010789.pub2

de Estéfani, D., Ruschel, C., Benincá, I. L., dos Santos Haupenthal, D. P., de Avelar, N. C. P., & Haupenthal, A. (2020). Volume of water added to crushed ice affects the efficacy of cryotherapy: A randomised, single-blind, crossover trial. *Physiotherapy, 107*, 81–87.

Denegar, C. R. (2016). *Therapeutic modalities for musculoskeletal injuries* (4th ed.). Champaign, IL: Human Kinetics.

Dubois, B., & Esculier, J-F. (2020). Soft tissue injuries simply need PEACE & LOVE. *British Journal of Sports Medicine, 54*(2), 3–5.

Harvard Health Publishing. *Acetaminophen safety: Be cautious but not afraid*. (2020, April 15). Retrieved from https://www.health.harvard.edu/pain/acetaminophen-safety-be-cautious-but-not-afraid

Hatt, K. M., Vijapura, A., Maitin, I. B., & Cruz, E. (2018). Safety considerations in prescription of NSAIDs for musculoskeletal pain: A narrative review. *PM & R, 10*(12), 1404–1411.

Herring, S. A., Kibler, W. B., & Putukian, M. (2012). The team physician and the return-to-play decision: A consensus statement 2012 update. *Medicine & Science in Sports & Exercise, 44*(12), 2446–2448.

Hertel, J. (1997). The role of nonsteroidal anti-inflammatory drugs in the treatment of acute soft tissue injuries. *Journal of Athletic Training, 32*(4), 350–358.

Houglum, P. (2016). *Therapeutic exercise for musculoskeletal injuries* (4th ed.). Champaign, IL: Human Kinetics.

Ingersoll, C. D., & Mistry, D. J. (2006). Soft tissue injury management. In C. Starkey & G. Johnson (Eds.), *Athletic training and sports medicine* (p. 24). Sudbury, MA: Jones and Bartlett Publishers.

Kannus, P., Parkkari, J., Järvinen, T. L. N., Järvinen, T. A. H., & Järvinen, M. (2003). Basic science and clinical studies coincide: Active treatment approach is needed after a sports injury: A short review. *Scandinavian Journal of Medicine & Science in Sports, 13*(3), 150–154.

Keller, T. S., Weisberger, A. M., Ray, J. L., Hasan, S. S., Shiavi, R. G., & Spengler, D. M. (1996). Relationship between vertical ground reaction force and speed during walking, slow jogging, and running. *Clinical Biomechanics, 11*(5), 253–259.

Knight, K. L. (1976). Effects of hypothermia on inflammation and swelling. *Athletic Training, 11*, 7–10.

Knight, K. L. (1985). *Cryotherapy: Theory, technique and physiology*. Chattanooga, TN: Chattanooga Corp.

Knight, K. L. (1995). *Cryotherapy in sport injury management*. Champaign, IL: Human Kinetics.

Kwiecien, S. Y., & McHugh, M. P. (2021). The cold truth: The role of cryotherapy in the treatment of injury and recovery from exercise. *European Journal of Applied Physiology, 121*(8), 2125–2142.

LaStayo, P. C., Woolf, J. M., Lewek, M. D., Snyder-Mackler, L., Reich, T., & Lindstedt, S. L. (2003). Eccentric muscle contractions: Their contribution to injury, prevention, rehabilitation, and sport. *Journal of Orthopaedic & Sports Physical Therapy, 33*(10), 557–571.

Long, B. C., & Jutte, L. S. (2020). 21st Century attacks on cryotherapy in sports health care—Clinician beware. *Athletic Training & Sports Health Care, 12*(3), 99–101.

Lorimer, A. V., & Hume, P. A. (2014). Achilles tendon injury: Risk factors associated with running. *Sports Medicine, 44*(10), 1459–1472.

Merrick, M. A. (2002). Secondary injury after musculoskeletal trauma: A review and update. *Journal of Athletic Training, 37*(2), 209–217.

Merrick, M. A., Jutte, L. S., & Smith, M. E. (2003). Cold modalities with different thermodynamic properties produce different surface and intramuscular temperatures. *Journal of Athletic Training, 38*(1), 28–33.

Moini, J. (2020). *Anatomy and physiology for health professionals* (3rd ed.). Burlington, MA: Jones & Bartlett Learning.

Moseley, G. L., & Butler, D. S. (2015). Fifteen years of explaining pain: The past, present, and future. *Journal of Pain, 16*(9), 807–813.

Otte, J. W., Merrick, M. A., Ingersoll, C. D., & Cordova, M. L. (2002). Subcutaneous adipose tissue thickness alters cooling time during cryotherapy. *Archives of Physical Medicine and Rehabilitation, 83*(11), 1501–1505.

Patel, K., Bakshi, N., Freehill, M. T., & Awan, T. M. (2019). Whole-body cryotherapy in sports medicine. *Current Sports Medicine Reports, 18*(4), 136–140.

Prentice, W. E. (2017). *Principles of athletic training: A guide to evidence-based practice* (16th ed.). New York, NY: McGraw-Hill.

Puntel, G. O., Carvalho, N. R., Dobrachinski, F., Salgueiro, A. C. F., Puntel, R. L., Folmer, V., . . . Soares, F. A. A. (2013). Cryotherapy reduces skeletal muscle damage after ischemia/reperfusion in rats. *Journal of Anatomy, 222*(2), 223–230.

Santos, W. O. C., Brito, C. J., Júnior, E. A. P., Valido, C. N., Mendes, E. L., Nunes, M. A. P., & Franchini, E. (2012). Cryotherapy post-training reduces muscle damage markers in jiu-jitsu fighters. *Journal of Human Sport and Exercise, 7*(3), 629–638.

Scott, A., Khan, K. M., Roberts, C. R., Cook, J. L., & Duronio, V. (2004). What do we mean by the term "inflammation"? A contemporary basic science update for sports medicine. *British Journal of Sports Medicine, 38*(3), 372–380.

Sözen, H., (Ed.). (2019). Introductory chapter: Tendons. In *Tendons*. IntechOpen. doi:10.5772/intechopen.88995

Starkey, C., & Brown, S. D. (2015). *Examination of orthopedic and athletic injuries* (4th ed.). Philadelphia, PA: F.A. Davis.

Stovitz, S. D., & Johnson, R. J. (2003). NSAIDs and musculoskeletal treatment: What is the clinical evidence? *Physician and Sportsmedicine, 31*(1), 35–52.

Tomchuk D. (2010). The magnitude of tissue cooling during cryotherapy with varied types of compression. *Journal of Athletic Training, 45*(3), 230–237.

Vuurberg, G., Hoorntje, A., Wink, L. M., van der Doelen, B. F. W., van den Bekerom, M. P., Dekker, R., . . . Kerkhoffs, G. M. M. J. (2018). Diagnosis, treatment and prevention of ankle sprains: Update of an evidence-based clinical guideline. *British Journal of Sports Medicine, 52*(15), 956.

Wager, T., Atlas, L., Lindquist, M., Roy, M., Woo, C., & Kross, E. (2013). An fMRI-based neurologic signature of physical pain. *New England Journal of Medicine, 368*, 1388–1397.

Watson, T. (2016). *Soft tissue repair and healing review.* Retrieved from http://www.electrotherapy.org/modality/soft-tissue-repair-and-healing-review

Yang, J., Tibbetts, A. S., Covassin, T., Cheng, G., Nayar, S., & Heiden, E. (2012). Epidemiology of overuse and acute injuries among competitive collegiate athletes. *Journal of Athletic Training, 47*(2), 198–204.

CHAPTER 9
Injuries to the Head, Neck, and Face

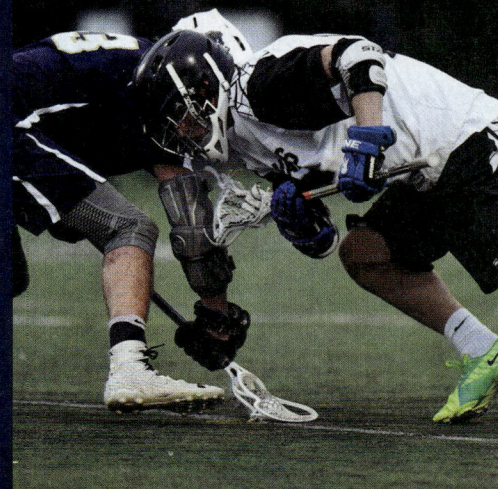

Courtesy of Mark Hoffman.

MAJOR CONCEPTS

Injuries to the head, neck, and face present some of the most perplexing problems associated with sports injuries. The current state of knowledge regarding these injuries is constantly being updated, and the reader is encouraged to always seek the most current peer-reviewed research regarding prevention, recognition, treatment, and disposition of these injuries. The chapter begins with a review of the gross anatomy of the head, neck, and face and goes on to describe the central nervous system, giving special attention to the structures often involved in head and neck injuries, along with data on the incidence and severity of such injuries in a variety of sports. It provides new evidence-based material regarding prevention, recognition, treatment, and return-to-play (RTP) progression after a concussion. Severe forms of head injury, including intracranial injuries and second impact syndrome (SIS), are presented, along with recommendations on how best to avoid these potentially lethal problems. In addition, the chapter contains a special section on the helmeted tackle football player, which includes guidelines on the initial treatment of suspected head and neck injuries.

Next, the chapter outlines major mechanisms of cervical spine injuries, followed by a discussion of the various types of injuries that can occur, including simple sprains and strains as well as more severe forms, such as disk herniations and vertebral dislocations and fractures. In addition, it presents information regarding the mechanisms and signs and symptoms of brachial plexus injuries. As with head injuries, it features guidelines for the initial treatment of suspected injuries to the cervical spine.

The remainder of the chapter deals with recognition and care of injuries to the maxillofacial region (face, teeth, eyes, nose, and ears).

Anatomy Review

The head is technically a housing structure. It encloses the delicate brain; provides sockets for the eyes and openings for the ears, nose, and mouth; and provides sites of attachment for the soft connective tissue and vertebral column (spine). The head is connected to the body via the neck vertebrae, but because of its structure, it provides a significant potential for a multitude of injuries. The anatomy works well for the day-to-day functions of our species, but in the context of sports, this anatomic arrangement provides a significant potential for a multitude of injuries. The potential forces involved in many sports and activities can seriously affect the structure and function of the structures housed in the head and neck.

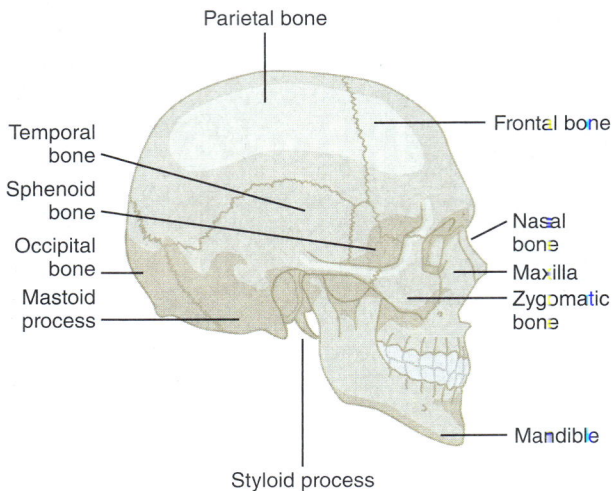

Figure 9.1 The bones of the human cranium.

Skull

Consisting of 8 cranial bones and 14 facial bones, the skull is a complex structure. The brain (encephalon) is housed in the cranium and is afforded considerable protection via an ingenious system of bony and soft-tissue structures. The brain consists of neural tissues that are easily damaged, and it must be protected, especially when one considers the potential forces involved in many sports and activities (i.e., car racing, skiing, and sledding sports) owing to contact and acceleration forces of gravity.

The bones of the cranium (Figure 9.1) form a rigid housing for the brain and are held together by specialized articulations known as suture joints. The suture joints of the cranium have much more space between them at birth to allow for growth, and as an individual ages the suture joints come closer together and ossify (i.e., harden; Moini, 2020). Not all suture joints look the same because some have more toothlike projections, such as the sagittal suture, than others. These joints are surrounded by connective tissue and allow a tiny amount of movement, which accommodates compliance and elasticity of the skull, but the anatomic arrangement of the cranial bones and their respective joints provides a protective outer structure for the brain.

The soft-tissue structures also serve a protective function; they include the five layers of the tissues of the scalp: the skin, a layer of dense connective tissue, the galea aponeurotica (essentially a broad, flat tendon), loose connective tissue, and the periosteum of the cranial bone (Figures 9.2 and 9.3).

The Meninges

Found below the cranial bones are soft-tissue structures that protect the brain and spinal cord. These are collectively referred to as the *cerebral meninges* (Figures 9.2 and 9.3); they consist of three distinct layers of tissues between the underside of the cranium and the surface of the brain. The outermost layer is known as the *dura mater*. It consists of tough, fibrous connective tissue that is fused to the inside surfaces of the cranial bones and continues to form vertical and horizontal sheets within the brain that separate the hemispheres and the cerebrum from the cerebellum, respectively. The dura also serves as a protective membrane to the brain and spinal cord, houses the **cerebrospinal fluid (CSF)**, and contains arteries and veins that transport blood to and from the cranial bones (Figure 9.2; Moini, 2020). The middle meningeal layer is the delicate *arachnoid membrane*; compared with the dura mater, it has significantly less strength and contains no blood supply. The arachnoid membrane is also separated from the layer below it by the subarachnoid space, which also contains CSF. The purposes of space and CSF are to allow motion between layers and to protect the brain from acute blood pressure changes, transport chemicals, and cushion the brain and spinal cord from external forces

Cerebrospinal fluid (CSF) Clear fluid that surrounds the spinal cord and brain.

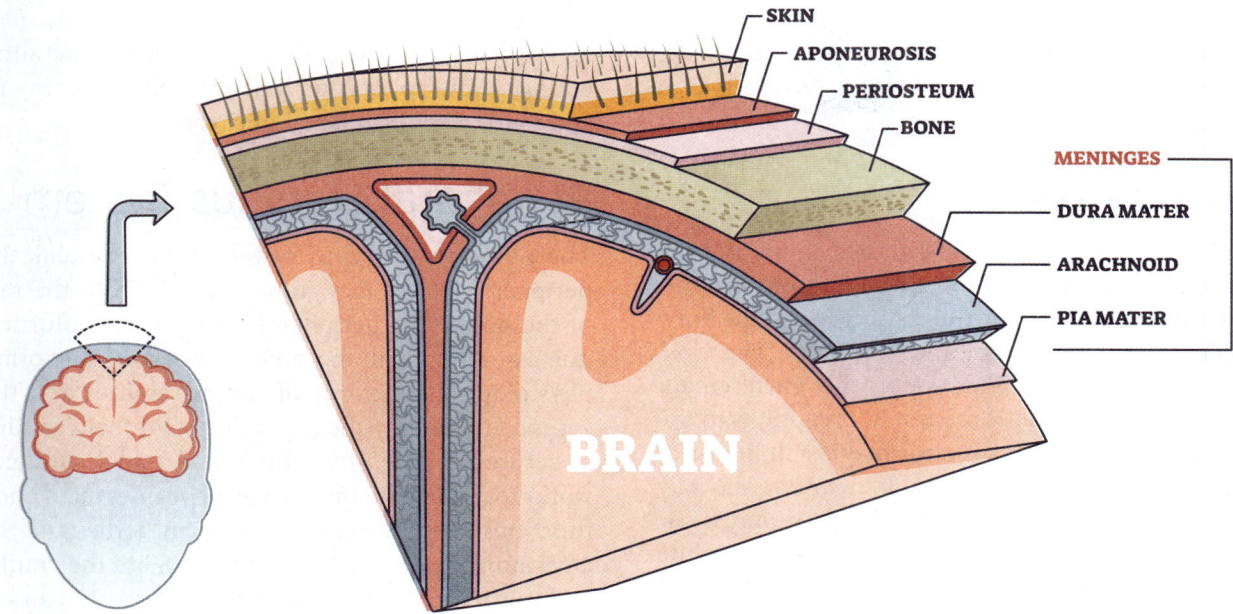

Figure 9.2 A cross-section of the human scalp.
© VectorMine/Shutterstock.

such as those encountered in collision and contact sports. CSF gives the brain natural buoyancy, so its density of neurons does not impair its own blood supply because of the weight of the brain. The CSF suspends the mass of the brain so that even though a brain can weigh as much as 1,400 grams, it feels like 25 grams (Saladin, 2007). Children's brains typically have less CSF during certain stages of development, which might create extra brain weight. Therefore, any blow to the head might result in more impairment of blood supply because the brain was not able to absorb the impact (Chatelin et al., 2012). The innermost meningeal layer is the *pia mater*, which is physically attached to the brain tissue and serves to provide a framework

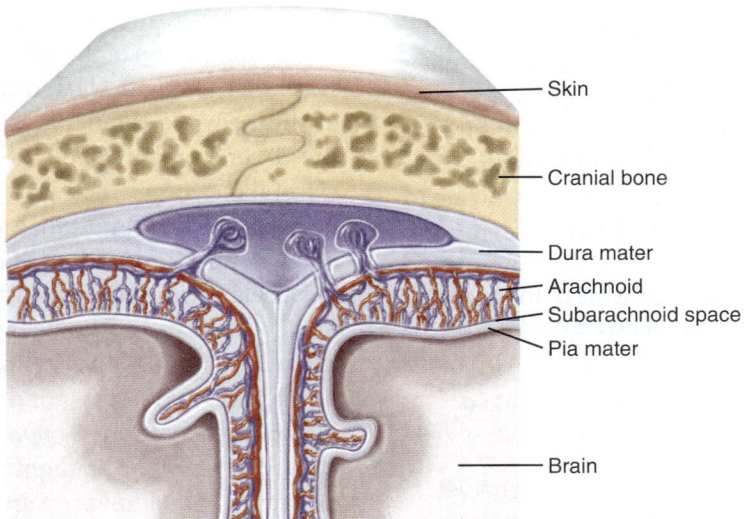

Figure 9.3 The cerebral meninges.

for an extensive vasculature that supplies the brain. The pia mater is a very thin, delicate membrane; like the arachnoid membrane, it is more susceptible to trauma than the dura mater is.

Central Nervous System

The brain, along with the spinal cord, composes the **central nervous system (CNS)**. Both the brain and spinal cord are protected by the meninges and the bony structure of the cranium and vertebrae. The CNS receives an extensive blood supply that must remain constant for it to function. Even interruptions to the blood flow lasting only seconds may result in loss of consciousness (LOC). As a result, neural tissue may be destroyed when deprived of blood for only a few minutes. The CNS tissue consists of gray and white matter that represents two distinct types of neural tissues. The brain of an adult weighs 3 to 3.5 pounds and contains approximately 100 billion neurons (Van De Graaff, 1998). The brain basically consists of three parts: cerebrum, cerebellum, and brain stem. The *cerebrum* is the largest of the three and is involved in complex functions, such as cognition, reasoning, and intellectual functioning. The *cerebellum*, which is in the lower posterior portion of the cranial area, performs functions related to complex motor skills and potentially other functions as our understanding of the brain progresses. The *brain stem* is at the base of the brain and serves to connect the brain to the spinal cord.

The young child's brain appears to be three to four times less stiff than the adult brain; therefore, children's brains are far more plastic or impressionable than the adult brain (Chatelin et al., 2012). This plasticity clearly has positive effects during maturation but can have negative effects associated with brain injury because the child's brain is less resistant to trauma. The child's brain may also have a slower recovery owing to lower quantities of **myelin** (fatty cells that cover nerves)

Central nervous system (CNS) Consists of the brain and spinal cord and is the processing center for bodily functions.

Myelin A structure, composed of fats and proteins, that insulates the axon of a nerve.

Peripheral nervous system (PNS) Consists of nerves that reside outside of the spinal cord and brain that relay information from brain to body.

and metabolic sensitivities (Field et al., 2003). Because myelin is much more highly concentrated in the adult brain, it allows for quicker repair to nerves after injury and more controlled metabolic responses.

Peripheral Nervous System

The **peripheral nervous system (PNS)** contains the peripheral nerves that connect the CNS to the rest of the body. The peripheral nerves carry information associated with movement, sensation, and other physiological functions of the extremities and the organs. It is simply the nervous system that contains structures outside of the brain and spinal cord and works together with the CNS to allow integrated body functions internally and between our bodies and the environment. The nerves in the PNS are the cranial and spinal nerves. The cranial nerves have 12 pairs of nerves that are labeled with Roman numerals (I–XII). The cranial nerves originate at the midbrain (cranial nerve I [optic] and cranial nerve II [olfactory]) or the base of the brain (cranial nerves III–XII) and make their way to other structures in the brain and lower in the body via the foramen magnum (opening in the base of skull). Some of the cranial nerves go to the face and eyes, and others go to the heart, lungs, and digestive organs and enable our senses of sight, smell, taste, hearing, and touch (on the face). Cranial nerves also have motor functions, such as chewing, facial expressions, tongue movement, and swallowing. The spinal nerves comprise 31 pairs (8 cervical, 12 thoracic, 5 lumbar, 5 sacral, and 1 coccygeal) that originate from the spinal cord and exit through the vertebrae.

A subdivision of the PNS is the *autonomic nervous system (ANS)*, which handles unconscious activities of the body via the nerves that connect the CNS to the visceral organs. The ANS monitors and regulates visceral (i.e., organ) activity; responds to the environment, including emotional stress; and prepares the body for physical activity. When a person feels safe and has a healthy functioning body, the physiological state often reflects one of social engagement, self-soothing behaviors, and positive feelings. When a person feels unsafe, the ANS will respond in various ways depending on the situation. *Sympathetic nerves* are associated with the fight-or-flight response (i.e., increased heart rate and blood pressure) or the freeze response (i.e., extreme sleepiness), and *parasympathetic nerves* are associated with the rest and digest functions (i.e., decreased heart and respiration rate, relaxation, and digestion).

Another subdivision of the PNS is the *somatic nervous system (SNS)*, which is involved in conscious skeletal muscle activity as well as some unconscious neuromuscular reflexes.

Face

The human face is composed of an outer layer of skin placed loosely over underlying bones. It also includes subcutaneous muscles, cartilage, and fat deposits, which offer minimal protection from trauma. The facial bones consist of the maxilla, the right and left palatine, the right and left zygomatic, the right and left lacrimal, the right and left nasal, the right and left inferior nasal concha, the vomer, the mandible, and the hyoid (Moini, 2020).

Several areas around the face are especially prominent and thus prone to injury. The orbits for the eyes, particularly the supraorbital regions, are vulnerable to contusions. The nasal bones are located centrally on the face and can also receive direct blows, often resulting in fractures. The mandible is subject to excessive external forces as well.

Neck (Cervical Spine)

The bones of the neck are the seven cervical vertebrae (Figure 9.4), which provide support for the head and protection for the upper portion of the spinal cord. The first cervical (C-1) vertebra (i.e., atlas) articulates directly with the occipital bone to form the right and left atlanto-occipital joints. The skull and C-1 articulate as a unit with the second cervical (C-2) vertebra (i.e., axis) to form the atlantoaxial joint, which allows for rotation of the head on the neck. The remaining five cervical vertebrae become progressively larger as they approach the thoracic spine.

Head Injuries in Sports

Background Information

Although the majority of injuries to most parts of the body are without serious consequence and are self-correcting, even relatively minor trauma to the head can result in severe injury. If the injury is severe enough, death can result. The possible mechanisms, types, and severity of head injuries in sports are nearly infinite, especially as the exposure to contact sports at younger ages continues. However, significant advances in our understanding regarding head injuries in sports have been made in recent years, and many organizations have published position statements and jurisdictions have passed legislation mandating education about head injuries. As a result, with appropriate education, healthcare providers, coaches, physical educators, and parents can learn to recognize head injuries and render effective first aid when necessary.

Head injuries can occur in almost any sport or activity. Currently, many definitions exist for head injuries, such as sports-related concussion (SRC) and mild traumatic brain injury (mTBI). Scientific surveys have provided additional insight into which sports appear to carry a higher risk, but as definitions of head injury, reporting standards, and public awareness have changed, including the often underreporting of head injuries by athletes, comparing survey data over multiple decades is challenging. Epidemiological research on the incidence of head, brain, and neck injuries is ongoing and improving, and accurate data from relatively recent playing seasons are available at multiple sports participation levels and can provide a macro view of these injuries.

According to the Centers for Disease Control and Prevention (CDC), traumatic brain injuries are a serious public health concern as evidenced by the

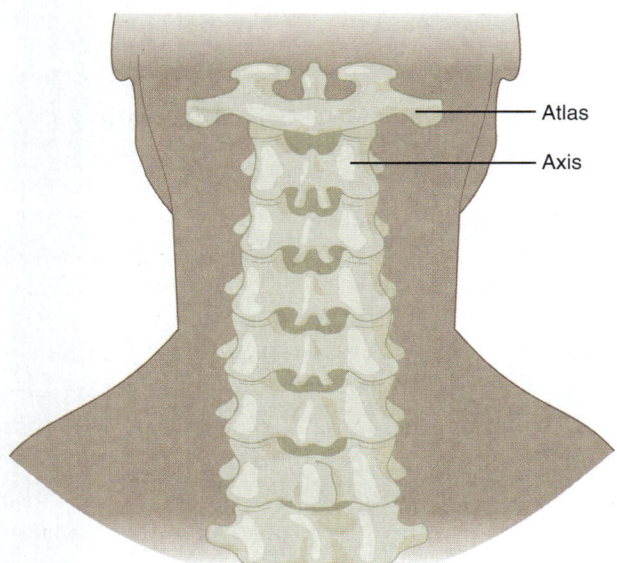

Figure 9.4 Posterior view of the cervical spine.

fact that in 2013 almost 2.8 million of the 26 million emergency department visits, hospitalizations, and deaths were associated with them (Peterson et al., 2014). Because reporting standards and awareness have changed over time, wide variability exists in the literature regarding the occurrence of concussions in sports since the 1990s. Recent data from the High School Sports-Related Injury Surveillance Study catalogued injuries (males: $n = 804,828$; females: $n = 400,346$) during the 2018–2019 boys' and girls' high school sports seasons (175 high schools surveyed) and reported that the head and face were the locations of the highest percentage of injuries across competitions (26.8%) and the second highest percentage across practices (14.1%), whereas neck injuries were one of the most uncommon areas with the percentage of injuries across competitions (1.6%) and practice (1.2%; Comstock & Pierpoint, 2020). Ankle injuries were second most common in competitions (19.6%) and the most common in practices (16.5%), and knee injuries were third most common for both competitions and practices (13.8%; Comstock & Pierpoint, 2020). See Table 9.1 for the percentage of concussions in each sport surveyed.

For collegiate sports, including Division I, II, and III institutions (2011–2012 to 2014–2015 seasons), 1,485 concussions were sustained by 1,410 student-athletes across 13 sports (Kerr et al., 2017). Men's football (80.6%) had the highest proportion of team seasons (competitions and practice) with at least one reported concussion across all schools and sports, followed by men's ice hockey (70.8%), men's wrestling (58.6%), women's ice hockey (55.2%), women's soccer (50.5%), men's lacrosse (45.5%), women's lacrosse (44.4%), and women's basketball (42.7%; Kerr et al., 2017). The overall rate of exposure was highest for men's wrestling (4.31 per 1,000 athlete exposures [AEs]), followed by men's football (3.25 per 1,000 AEs), and highest for women's ice hockey (2.11 per 1,000 AEs), followed by women's soccer (1.65 per 1,000 AEs; Kerr et al., 2017).

According to the CDC, athletes are not the only population at risk for head and spine injuries as evidenced by the number of emergency room visits for traumatic brain injury increasing by 53% from 2006 to 2014 and on average 155 people dying each day from injuries associated with a traumatic brain injury in the United States (CDC, 2021). The leading

Table 9.1

Concussion Statistics at High School Sports Level

High School Sports Season (2018–2019)	% Concussions of Total Injuries	Rank (Top 10 Injuries)	Most Common Sports Situation
Boys' football	21.7%	1	Being tackled
Boys' soccer	16.8%	1	Heading ball
Girls' soccer	21.2%	1	Defending/general play
Boys' and girls' volleyball	15.3%	2	Digging
Boys' basketball	10.5%	2	Defending
Girls' basketball	20.9%	2	Defending
Wrestling	19.5%	1	Takedown
Baseball	9.2%	2	Fielding a batted ball
Softball	14.2%	1	Fielding a batted ball

Data from Comstock, R. D., & Pierpoint, L. A. (2020). *National High School Sports-Related Injury Surveillance Survey (2018-2019)*. Retrieved from https://coloradosph.cuanschutz.edu/research-and-practice/centers-programs/piper/research-practice/research-projects cause of traumatic brain injury is falls, and the second leading cause is being struck by or against an object (CDC, 2021). The Traumatic Brain Injury Program Reauthorization Act of 2018 directs the CDC (2019) to implement a National Concussion Surveillance System (https://www.cdc.gov/traumaticbraininjury/ncss/). This system will eventually estimate the number of people with a disability caused by brain injury and provide estimates for SRCs in and outside of organized sports at all levels. Having this database will also provide information about the common cause of concussion, monitor trends, and give insight to medical personnel.

Clearly, concussions are a high-volume injury in high school and collegiate sports. More importantly, players sustaining one concussion had a threefold increased risk of sustaining an additional concussion when compared with their nonconcussed teammates (Guskiewicz et al., 2000), and one in 11 SRCs are recurrent across 25 National Collegiate Athletic Association (NCAA) sports (Zuckerman et al., 2015). Previously concussed children and adolescents have four times the risk of sustaining a concussion compared with those with no previous concussion history (Van Ierssel et al., 2020). Thus, this information confirms that concussions are very common and subsequent concussions are more likely to occur after a first concussion, so immediate recognition and referral for treatment can make a big difference in the care of these injuries.

The most recent research available from the National Center for Catastrophic Sport Injury Research (NCCSIR; https://nccsir.unc.edu/) indicates that fatal and nonfatal (incomplete recovery) and serious head and neck injuries continue to occur in many sports (Kucera & Cantu, 2020). During the 2018–2019 collection year (high school, college, and junior college), 80 sports-related catastrophic events occurred, with 78% at the high school level mostly among males (91%). Overall, 31.3% of cases were fatal, 8.8% were nonfatal but permanently disabling, 53.8% were serious with a recovery, and 6.3% had unknown outcomes. Of these 80 catastrophic injuries, the spine experienced 22.5% (spine fractures over 55%), and head and brain experienced 16.3% (brain trauma over 76%; Kucera & Cantu, 2020).

Unfortunately, cheerleading was the second most common cause of nonfatal and serious catastrophic injuries behind football at both the collegiate and high school levels, and most of these were attributed to head and neck trauma (Kucera & Cantu, 2020). From 1983 to 2011, cheerleading led to 3 fatal injuries, 45 nonfatal injuries, and 71 serious injuries among high school and collegiate participants (Mueller & Cantu, 2011).

Data related directly to brain injury in football (professional, semiprofessional, high school, and college) have provided some interesting numbers. As a whole, the number of fatalities in football that can be attributed to brain injuries has decreased since 1961; however, the number of disabilities associated with brain injury has increased (Mueller & Cantu, 2012). Fewer fatal injuries demonstrate significant strides in rules, tackling techniques, and injury management; however, the fact that more injuries occur that result in disability is still very disturbing (Mueller & Cantu, 2012). Fatal injuries related to football are also related to concerns regarding repeated head contacts and the occurrence of chronic traumatic encephalopathy (CTE); however, these data are not included in the NCCSIR reports because the deaths tend to happen years after competition ceases. CTE is a neurodegenerative disease associated with head trauma, but the literature on neurobehavioral sequelae and long-term consequences of exposure to recurrent head trauma is inconsistent (Maroon et al., 2015; McCrory et al., 2017). Only speculation can be drawn from the current CTE research regarding a cause-and-effect relationship between sports concussion and CTE (Maroon et al., 2015; McCrory et al., 2017). Therefore, the communities of healthcare providers, coaches, physical educators, and parents need to better understand brain injury and the importance of proper management.

Mechanism of Injury and Type

A multitude of descriptive classifications exist for head injuries. However, all head injuries can be placed into three general categories: concussion, intercranial hemorrhage, and skull fracture (Newman, 2020). Injuries to the head can happen via direct or indirect contact or be a result of other medical factors (e.g., stroke). Direct mechanisms involve a blow to the head resulting in brain injury at the site of impact, known as a *coup* type of injury. When injury also happens on the opposite side of the skull from the site of impact, the injury is known as a *contrecoup* type. The contrecoup-associated injury occurs when the head is moving and stops abruptly. For example, when a tackle is made in football, the brain keeps moving in the skull and is subsequently compressed on the side opposite the initial impact. Indirect mechanisms of injury involve damaging forces traveling from other areas of the body, such as blows to the face or jaw. Rapid and violent movement of the cervical spine, especially when the blow is not expected, such as seen in whiplash injury (automobile accidents), results in indirect injuries to the brain. An understanding of these mechanisms of injury highlights the validity of the often-used cliché in sports medicine circles, "Treat every head injury as if there is also a neck injury and every neck injury as if there is also a head injury."

Concussion

Concussions can happen from forces applied directly (e.g., direct contact) or indirectly (e.g., whiplash) to the skull, causing the brain to move rapidly within the skull. When the brain rapidly moves within the skull, metabolic and ionic changes occur that affect the complex physiological processes of the brain (Broglio et al., 2014; McCrory et al., 2017). Concussions usually result in immediate and often short-lived impairment of neurological functions (**Time Out 9.1**), but many times signs and symptoms can evolve over several minutes to even hours (McCrory et al., 2017). Recent evidence suggests that in most cases of concussion the injury occurs owing to a complex metabolic crisis in the brain often related to restrictions in blood flow; however, in other cases structural damage may occur (Giza & Hovda, 2014; Harmon et al., 2019; MacFarlane & Glenn, 2015). Nerve cells (i.e., axons) suffer from a metabolic and ionic disruption that causes energy

Coup Brain contusion injury to the same side as the site of the impact.

Contrecoup Brain contusion injury to the opposite side of the site of impact.

TIME OUT 9.1

Signs and Symptoms of Sports-Related Concussion

PHYSICAL (SIGNS OR SYMPTOMS)
- Headache from the impact
- Dizziness and balance problems
- Fatigue
- Visual problems (tracking, depth, and double vision)
- Diminished pupil reaction or unequal pupils
- Dazed or stunned
- Ringing of ears (tinnitus)
- Sensitivity to light and noise
- Vomiting
- Nausea
- Loss of consciousness
- Unstable gate

COGNITIVE
- Confusion or feeling "foggy" or "slowed down"
- Inability to quickly answer questions or repeats questions
- Poor concentration
- Forgetful of recent information or conversations
- Memory lapses

SLEEP DISTURBANCES
- Drowsiness
- Trouble falling asleep
- Sleep more or less than usual

EMOTIONAL
- Irritability
- Actions uncharacteristic of the individual
- Anxiousness
- Sadness
- Depression

Adapted from Harmon, K. G., Clugston, J. R., Dec, K., Hainline, B. Herring, S., Kane, S. F., Kontos, A. P., Leddy, J. J., McCrea, M., Poddar, S. K., Putukian, M., Wilson, J. C., & Roberts, W. O. (2019). American Medical Society for Sports Medicine position statement on concussion in sport. *British Journal of Sports Medicine, 53*(4), 213–225.

deficits and neural transmission problems; as a result, the axons cannot transmit signals with the efficiency or effectiveness they had before injury (Giza & Hovda, 2014; MacFarlane & Glenn, 2015). Researchers now understand that brain tissue not destroyed remains extremely vulnerable to subsequent trauma or other stresses (physical, cognitive, or emotional), which may result in phenomena such as minor changes in brain blood flow, intracranial pressure, or oxygen delivery (Giza & Hovda, 2014; MacFarlane & Glenn, 2015).

Current science has moved away from classification systems for cerebral concussion. Any trauma that causes one or more signs and symptoms (Time Out 9.1) is considered a concussion. No one concussion is like another, so grading systems have been abandoned and serial monitoring of signs and symptoms, including duration and intensity, is currently the best way to determine the severity and the required medical treatment (Broglio et al., 2014; McCrory et al., 2017). Recent evidence has indicated that LOC and posttraumatic amnesia (PTA) were not appropriate designates of concussion severity because LOC occurs in only 9% and PTA in only 27% of concussions (Guskiewicz et al., 2000). Even though their presence does not indicate severity, any LOC or extended PTA is a significant sign and symptom and should be respected. The intent of moving away from a grading system was to simplify the decision-making process of the athletic healthcare team members when evaluating the status of athletes suspected of having sustained a head injury. Given the potential implications of a bad decision in such situations, *the current recommendation states that any athlete who exhibits signs and symptoms of a concussion should be removed from play or practice and not return that day* (Broglio et al., 2014; Harmon et al., 2019; McCrory et al., 2017). Any RTP decisions should be made by a qualified healthcare provider, thereby helping the coaching staff avoid errors in judgment (Broglio et al., 2014; Harmon et al., 2019; McCrory et al., 2017).

The majority of concussions (80–90%) typically resolve in 10–14 days in adults and within 4 weeks in children without medical intervention (McCrea et al., 2013; McCrory et al., 2017). Youths are more susceptible to concussions owing to their maturing brains and skulls and weaker neck musculature and may need a longer time to recover from concussions and RTP to reduce the risk of **second impact syndrome** (Broglio et al., 2014).

Postconcussive syndrome (PCS; discussed in more detail in the section that follows), or persistent symptoms, is not uncommon after concussions; it does not reflect a single pathophysiological entity but typically involves long-lasting posttraumatic signs and symptoms, such as headaches and balance disturbance, memory problems, poor concentration, fatigue and sleep problems, and emotional changes (McCrory et al., 2017). Memory problems that occur after concussions are referred to as PTA (Russo et al., 2022). Two types of PTA have been identified as resulting from head injury: anterograde and retrograde. **Anterograde amnesia** involves an inability to recall events that have transpired since the time of the injury. **Retrograde amnesia** is present when the athlete is unable to recall events that occurred just before the injury. Now, however, the general thought is that retrograde amnesia is hard to measure and poorly reflective of the severity of head injury (Russo et al., 2022). Recent evidence suggests that the *duration* of all postconcussive symptoms, rather than the presence, type, or duration of amnesia, is what suggests persistent neurological problems (Broglio et al., 2014; McCrory et al., 2017). All cases of concussions that have prolonged symptoms (more than 14 days in adults and 4 weeks in children) should be managed in a multidisciplinary way (i.e., involving physicians, neuropsychologists, psychiatrists, and counselors; McCrory et al., 2017). The multidisciplinary management should minimally include symptom-limited aerobic exercise, a targeted physical therapy program, and cognitive behavioral therapy (McCrory et al., 2017).

Second impact syndrome Significant brain swelling that can occur rapidly if a person suffers a second concussion before symptoms from an earlier concussion have subsided.

Anterograde amnesia Inability to recall events that have occurred after an amnesia-inducing injury.

Retrograde amnesia Inability to recall events that occurred just before an injury.

Postconcussive Syndrome

PCS involves cases in which the signs and symptoms of a concussion last weeks, months, and even years beyond the initial injury (Harmon et al., 2019). Unfortunately, PCS is ill defined and poorly understood because signs and symptoms are both subjective and objective and are often vague (Ellis et al., 2016; Harmon et al., 2019; Leddy et al., 2016). Several common signs and symptoms include headaches, anxiety, depression, sensitivity to light and noise, memory loss, poor concentration and problem solving, and insomnia (Harmon et al., 2019; Leddy et al., 2016). Two recent studies have emphasized that postconcussion symptoms can last for years. In investigations of retired NFL football players, those who experienced concussions were more likely to demonstrate cognitive deficits and depression (Guskiewicz et al., 2005; Hart et al., 2013) and changes in cerebral blood flow and some white matter abnormalities when compared to controls matched by age, IQ, and education (Hart et al., 2013). Although significant research has been conducted regarding PCS, no proven or accepted correlations have been made between the severity of the concussion and initial symptoms and the likelihood of developing physical, cognitive, or emotional PCS (Harmon et al., 2019). However, some risk factors are gaining attention but need more scientific investigation. These risk factors include being female and younger; having a history of learning disabilities, migraines, and depression; and having a dangerous style of athletic play and weak cervical muscles (Broshek et al., 2005; Eckersley, Nightingale, Luck, & Bass, 2019; Harmon et al., 2019; Scorza et al., 2012).

As mentioned in the previous section, a multidisciplinary healthcare team should manage the treatment of persistent symptoms of head injury (McCrory et al., 2017; Reynolds et al., 2014). Poor evidence exists for the use of medications for PCS because some medications can mask any worsening effects (Scorza et al., 2012). Recovery can be very frustrating because it is a long, slow process that may remove athletes from their normal activities, such as work and school. However, evidence exists to suggest that following a concussion clinical trajectory model that includes assessment and therapy for a sequelae of symptoms, including vestibular (balance), cognitive and fatigue, ocular motor, anxiety and mood, cervical pain, and posttraumatic migraine, may provide recovery guidance (Reynolds et al., 2014). Research continues in these areas, and evidence is being gathered on a variety of therapeutic interventions (Ellis et al., 2016).

Because of recent media coverage and the outcome of a major lawsuit filed by former players against the NFL, the condition of **chronic traumatic encephalopathy (CTE)** should be discussed. CTE is diagnosed only postmortem and was long associated with boxers. Its recent discovery in the brains of several deceased football players alerted the medical community to investigate it further. Qualified scientists are engaging in seminal research to better understand CTE and its relationship to concussions and contact sports. First and foremost, though, is that research science has yet to establish a cause-and-effect relationship between CTE and concussions or exposure to contact sports (Carson, 2017; Maroon et al., 2015; McCrory et al., 2017; Stein et al., 2015). The conclusions are that the clinical findings that relate to CTE overlap with many neurodegenerative diseases and significant limitations exist connecting CTE to contact sports (Maroon et al., 2015). Therefore, any fears caused by media pressure should be mitigated by rational behaviors until there is clear evidence of the exact relationship.

Second Impact Syndrome

SIS primarily affects children and adolescents and occurs when a second concussion happens before symptoms of an initial concussion have resolved, thereby causing diffuse and often catastrophic cerebral edema (McLendon et al., 2016). The cerebral edema is believed to be caused by a failure of cerebral autoregulation of blood pressure and a surge in adrenaline (catecholamine) when a second impact is received before full recovery from an original concussive injury (Wetjen et al., 2010). Essentially, SIS involves the rapid development of catastrophic swelling of the brain, specifically to a region known as the uncus of the temporal lobes, which puts pressure directly against the brain

---

Chronic traumatic encephalopathy (CTE) Condition that can be identified only after death with a brain autopsy. It is a degenerative disease characterized by a distinct collection of tau proteins in several areas of the brain that affect function.

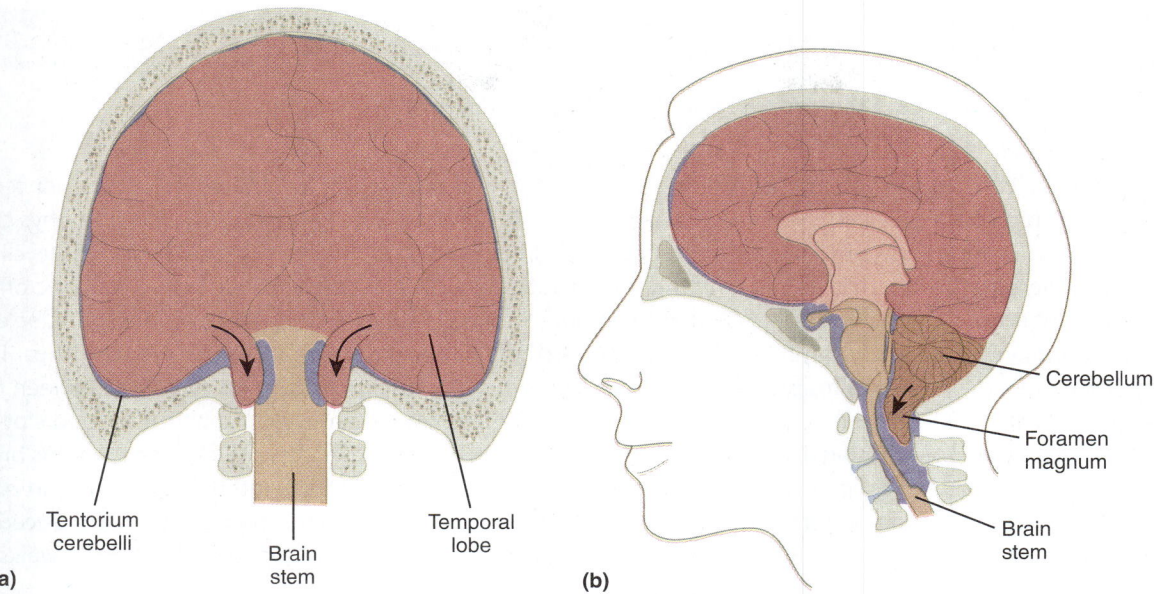

Figure 9.5 In second impact syndrome, vascular engorgement in the cranium increases intracranial pressure, leading to **(a)** herniation of the uncus of the temporal lobes (arrows) below the tentorium in this frontal section or to **(b)** herniation of the cerebellar tonsils (arrows) through the foramen magnum in this midsagittal section. These changes compromise the brain stem, and coma and respiratory failure rapidly develop. The shaded areas of the brain stem represent the areas of compression.
Robert Cantu, MD, FACSM, Neurological Surgery, Inc., Concord, Massachusetts. Reprinted with permission.

stem (Figure 9.5). Ultimately, SIS can cause coma or death. Researchers disagree about how far apart the two hits can be when considering SIS because they believe that ongoing metabolic abnormalities after a concussion may leave the brain more susceptible to a second impact (McLendon et al., 2016). Even though a limited number of cases of SIS have been reported in the research literature, it is more common in adolescents under the age of 18 (Harmon et al., 2019; Wetjen et al., 2010), and the sports medicine community needs to be concerned and adopt a more cautious approach to the care and management of athletes who sustain concussions.

A typical scenario for SIS might involve an athlete receiving a concussion with associated symptoms that include headache, nausea, poor concentration, and excessive drowsiness. Unfortunately, because of not being honest with their symptoms (i.e., the athlete did not report the symptoms to the athletic trainer [AT]), they return to play before the resolution of symptoms, such as the headache and poor concentration. Upon return to the sport, the same athlete, while engaging in the same activity, receives another relatively minor blow to the head. Shortly thereafter, the athlete collapses, becomes unresponsive, and is taken to a healthcare facility. While there, the athlete lies in a deep coma, and brain scans reveal significant brain edema. If death results, on autopsy, the cause of death is confirmed as massive cerebral edema resulting from uncontrolled vascular engorgement of brain tissue. Any athlete who sustains what appears to be even a minor concussion must be examined carefully by a healthcare provider and cleared by a physician before being allowed to return to participation (see **Time Out 9.2**). This concern is especially acute in the case of athletes with a history of concussions. An important point to remember is that symptoms related to a concussion may take days or even weeks to be resolved. As such, medical personnel, athletes, coaches, and parents should apply extreme caution when making decisions regarding RTP for athletes with a history of head injuries.

Intracranial Injury

Strong evidence exists that intracranial injury in sports also represents a potentially life-threatening situation. These injuries can be the result of a variety of mechanisms, including direct blows, rapid deceleration, and even rapid rotational motions of

> ### TIME OUT 9.2
>
> **Two Cases of Second Impact Syndrome That Changed Lives Forever**
>
> **PRESTON PLEVRETES**
>
> On November 5, 2005, at the age of 19, Preston's life was irreversibly changed. On October 4, he experienced a helmet-to-helmet hit at a LaSalle University football practice and was diagnosed with a concussion by a physician in his hometown in New Jersey. However, he eventually went back to school and was cleared by a campus clinic nurse and AT despite the fact that he still had throbbing headaches. Unfortunately, he did not tell anyone other than a few close friends about how he felt. On that November Saturday, while Preston was covering a punt, he collided with a Duquesne University player at the visitors' 37-yard line. He never got up and was rushed to the hospital. The collision tore a major vein in his brain, which resulted in three strokes and lapsing into a coma between the football field and hospital next door. Emergency surgery lasted more than 2 hours, during which a blood clot on the surface of his brain was removed. In addition, the right side of his skull was so severely swollen that his brain could not heal, and he needed reconstructive surgery after 5 months. He underwent another brain surgery in 2009 because of frequent grand mal seizures. As a result, Preston has no peripheral vision, and his speech is reduced to fits and spurts of breathy words. His right arm is difficult to move, and he has balance problems when he walks.
>
> TheBalrog. (2011, March 3). *Preston Plevretes story* [Video]. YouTube. https://www.youtube.com/watch?v=F4foY1EtmKo
>
> **ZACKERY LYSTEDT**
>
> In October 2006, Zackery, a 13-year-old middle school athlete, experienced an initial concussion in the second quarter of a football game but was allowed to return to play even though he had a headache and was confused and having difficulty remembering plays. Unfortunately, throughout the rest of the game, he experienced many more blows to his head and eventually collapsed in his father's arms at the end of the game. Emergency brain surgery followed, and he was on life support for 7 days owing to excessive cerebral edema. For him to speak and move his left arm took almost a year, and to be free of a feeding tube, over 2 years. It took more than 5 years before he could stand and walk a few steps and then return to his wheelchair.
>
> UW Medicine. (2013, May 13). *Zackery Lystedt: Then and now* [Video]. YouTube. https://www.youtube.com/watch?v=v-KUUW02VXg

the head. By far, the majority of intracranial injuries result from blunt trauma to the head. The injury is characterized by disruption of the blood flow in either veins or arteries, resulting in the development of a hematoma or swelling in the confines of the cranium. Such a condition places the brain tissues in jeopardy because these structures are extremely sensitive to pressure.

Jordan (1989) identified the major forms of **intracranial injury** as **epidural (extradural) hematoma** (bleeding between the dura and the cranial bones), **subdural hematoma** (bleeding below the dura mater), **intracerebral hematoma** (bleeding within the brain tissues), and **cerebral contusion** (bruising of the brain tissue). Because an epidural hematoma involves arterial bleeding, the signs and symptoms of injury will usually develop rather quickly, and because of the vascular anatomy of the dura mater, a subdural hematoma (i.e., under the dura) can involve rapid arterial bleeding with symptoms developing in minutes or venous bleeding with pooling and clotting developing over many hours. In some cases, symptoms don't appear for hours or even days after the initial injury. Although no particular signs and symptoms exist that

Intracranial injury Head injury characterized by disruption of blood vessels, either veins or arteries, resulting in the development of a hematoma or swelling within the confines of the cranium.

Epidural (extradural) hematoma Bleeding between the dura and the cranial bones.

Subdural hematoma Bleeding below the dura mater.

Intracerebral hematoma Bleeding within the brain tissues.

Cerebral contusion Bruising of the brain tissue.

may worsen, any changes in visual functioning and pupil reaction or increases in disorientation or equilibrium are of extreme concern. If these changes are not recognized immediately and the injured athlete is not transported immediately to the hospital, any of these conditions can result in some degree of permanent neurological damage and even death. Therefore, serially monitoring the signs and symptoms of concussed athletes is extremely important (Time Out 9.1). Any worsening of signs and symptoms indicates the need for immediate follow-up with a physician, possibly including an emergency room visit. If athletes are taken to the emergency room and advanced scanning techniques (magnetic resonance imaging or computed tomography scan) are performed, coaches and parents need to be aware that negative findings of bleeding or structural damage to the brain *do not* clear the athletes from complications of a concussion and extended recovery. Imaging is often overused and contributes little to management of concussion other than ruling out more serious traumatic brain injuries or skull fractures (Scorza et al., 2012). These negative findings indicate only that the damage was not structural and likely is metabolic.

Cranial Injury

Cranial injuries involve the bones of the skull. In the majority of cases, the force injuring the bones is of sufficient magnitude to also cause damage to the tissues of the scalp. Thus, some bleeding and soft-tissue damage, along with cranial injury, may also be present. Skull fractures can be simple, linear fractures with no damage to underlying tissue. In many cases, these injuries produce few neurological problems. The more severe forms of cranial injuries involve what are known as **depressed skull fractures**, which are potentially much more serious because bone fragments have been pushed into the cranial region. Obviously, this type of injury is more likely to produce serious and possibly life-threatening neurological damage. Fractures to the cranial base can also be very serious and involve tearing of internal carotid artery and the pooling of blood in the ophthalmic veins of the eyes, thereby causing **exophthalmos** (eyeball protrusion; Agur & Dalley, 2018). A variety of signs and symptoms of cranial bone injuries may also be present depending on the site of injury. These are discussed in some detail later in the chapter.

Initial Treatment of a Suspected Head Injury, Including Sports-Related Concussion: Guidelines

As mentioned previously, as a general rule, any athletes who sustain an apparent head injury should be treated as if a neck injury is also present; conversely, any athletes sustaining a neck injury should be treated as if a head injury is also present. The mechanism of injury for both is similar; consequently, they could occur simultaneously.

The following guidelines for the emergency care of athletes suspected of having sustained a head injury are divided into procedures while the athletes are at the site of injury, followed by guidelines for injured athletes after they have been removed to a secondary site (e.g., sideline or courtside). If any significant signs and/or symptoms of head or neck injury (i.e., numbness, tingling, LOC, deformity, or tenderness directly on spine) are present when evaluating athletes at the site of initial injury, they must be stabilized (Figure 9.6) and not moved until emergency medical services (EMS) personnel have arrived on the scene. By default, any athletes who, based on the initial evaluation, have sustained

WHAT IF ?

You are coaching soccer practice when suddenly a wing player collides with the goalie while attempting to kick a goal. On your arrival at the scene, the goalie appears to be okay; however, the other player is conscious but confused and unable to remember the current score or the team she is playing against. What type of injury has probably occurred given this history and these symptoms?

Depressed skull fracture A fracture of the skull where it is sunken in from a trauma; can occur with or without a cut in the scalp.

Exophthalmos A bulging of the eye anteriorly out of the orbit.

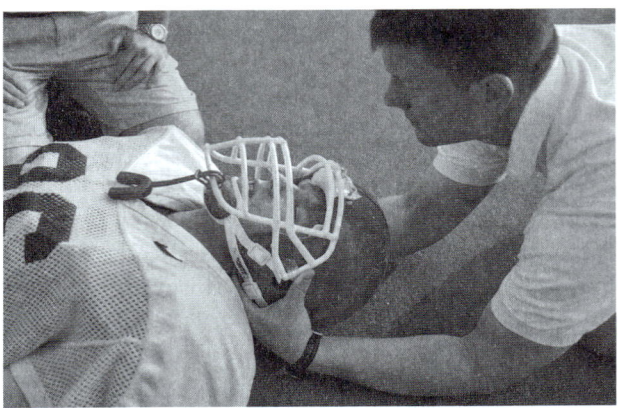

Figure 9.6 Stabilizing an athlete's head and neck.

a concussion must be removed from play and not allowed to return until examined by a qualified member of the athletic healthcare team (Broglio et al., 2014; Harmon et al., 2019; McCrory et al., 2017; Scorza et al., 2012).

Concussions are one of the most complex sports-related injuries to evaluate and manage because of the complexity of the concussive injury. Despite the urge, often encouraged by overzealous athletes, teammates, parents, and even coaches, to return players to participation, this must not be allowed in cases when athletes sustain any form of head trauma, including a concussion. The best policy is to remove athletes who sustain what appears to be a head injury, regardless of how minor it seems, from further participation; administer the appropriate sideline assessment; and refer them to an allied healthcare provider or physician for further evaluation to obtain follow-up care and directions regarding RTP (Broglio et al., 2014; Harmon et al., 2019; McCrory et al., 2017; Scorza et al., 2012). The potential consequences associated with SRC make the decision to remove injured athletes from play an essential step in their care. Although strict enforcement of a removal-from-play policy may not be popular with all athletes, fans, and even some coaches, the reality is that not taking the time to evaluate the injury and the potential occurrence of signs and symptoms may result in more serious and in some cases irreversible injury. A point worth noting is that management of athletes suspected of having suffered a head injury is becoming a major legal issue at the state level. In May 2009, the state of Washington was the first state to pass a law ("Zackery Lystedt Law") that required removal and clearance for RTP among youth athletes. In fact, by 2014, all 50 states and the District of Columbia had enacted some form of legislation regarding youth sports and SRC. All entities have an RTP law that involves removal from the field or court after an injury; however, two states allow athletes to return the same day if they are cleared by an allied healthcare provider (Potteiger et al., 2018). Many of the laws (more than 80%) require parents to sign an information sheet regarding concussions (Tomei et al., 2012), but the type of information given to parents is usually left up to schools or state high school federations (Harvey, 2013). The state legislation also varies in what policies are applied to different school settings (public vs. private or K–6 vs. K–12) and different age groups of children (Harvey, 2013; Potteiger et al., 2018; Tomei et al., 2012). Most state policies also leave out club and recreational sports, but all states require that coaches complete some type of concussion education program on a regular basis (Potteiger et al., 2018).

Consensus Statements Regarding Concussion Management

Starting in 2001, allied healthcare professionals started meeting internationally to develop consensus statements regarding SRC. These statements are numbered and identified according to the city where the meeting was held (first, Vienna in 2001; second, Prague in 2004; third and fourth, Zurich in 2008 and 2012; and fifth, Berlin in 2017). Each successive statement is designed to present conceptual understanding of SRC using an expert consensus-based approach (McCrory et al., 2017). The statements are meant for healthcare providers who are involved in athlete care at any level, but parents, coaches, and physical educators should be aware that the policies are based on clinical science and centered on protection of the injured athlete. Another important point is that the authors of the consensus statements acknowledge that the science related to SRC prevention, recognition, treatment, and rehabilitation is evolving and that the individual management of each suspected concussion will always remain in the realm of clinical judgment (McCrory et al., 2017). The most recent statement from Berlin (McCrory et al., 2017) provides a list of 11 guidelines to govern the logical flow of the clinical management of SRC:

recognize, remove, reevaluate, rest, rehabilitation, refer, recover, return to sport, reconsider, residual effects and sequelae, and risk reduction. They are presented in detail in **Time Out 9.3**.

The NCAA and the Department of Defense (DOD) have collaborated to form the Concussion Assessment, Research and Education (CARE) Consortium to provide scientific expertise to study concussion with the goal of improving the safety and health of student-athletes, service members, and youth sports participants (http://www.careconsortium.net/). The consortium supports research, education, presentations, and publications regarding concussion and is a reliable and trusted source of information for healthcare providers and the broader public.

Baseline Concussion Screening

Baseline testing is widely used at both the secondary school and collegiate levels, but controversy still exists among the healthcare community regarding its validity and reliability (Fallows et al., 2020; Kirkwood et al., 2009). Kirkwood and colleagues

---

TIME OUT 9.3

The 11 Rs for the Clinical Management of Sports-Related Concussion

1. **Recognize (the injury)**
   - Understand the pathology of the injury and its complex presentations.
   - Use organized multidimensional testing that assesses the following:
     - Symptoms:
       - Somatic (e.g., headache)
       - Cognitive (e.g., feeling as if in a fog)
       - Emotional (e.g., rapid emotion changes)
     - Physical signs (e.g., LOC, amnesia, neurological deficit)
     - Balance impairment (e.g., gait unsteadiness)
     - Behavioral changes (e.g., anxiety or depression)
     - Cognitive impairment (e.g., slowed reaction times)
     - Sleep and wake disturbance (e.g., somnolence or drowsiness)
2. **Remove (from play)**
   - Cautious of cervical or other emergent conditions
   - No RTP on that day
3. **Reevaluate (must be a follow-up exam)**
   - Needs to include medical and neurocognitive assessment; may or may not include advanced testing
4. **Rest (complete rest is *not* supported)**
   - Relative rest staying below cognitive or physical symptom exacerbation
5. **Rehabilitation**
   - Needs to be multimodal and to address the patient's signs and symptoms, especially neuromuscular responsiveness (perception and action)
6. **Refer**
   - Persistent symptoms need to be addressed by appropriate medical personnel.
   - More than 10–14 days in adults and 4 weeks in children is considered prolonged or persistent.

(continues)

TIME OUT 9.3 (continued)

7. **Recovery**
   - Clinical recovery is defined as a return to normal activities (school, work, and sport).
   - The strongest and most consistent predictor of a slower recovery is the severity of the initial symptoms in the first few days after the injury.
   - Risk factors for prolonged recovery: children (adolescents); females; a history of migraine headaches, depression, ADHD, or learning disabilities; and a history of previous concussions
   - Not possible to define a single physiological time window for SRC recovery, nor is a tool available that could provide this definitive evidence

8. **Return to sport (and return to learn)**
   - Both should be a graduated stepwise process with success at a preliminary step before progressing.

9. **Reconsider**
   - Pay attention to evolving evidence, especially regarding different populations.
   - Children and adolescents should not return to full sports until they have returned to school and learning.

10. **Residual effects and sequelae**
    - Clinicians need to be aware of potential long-term problems (i.e., postconcussive syndrome) and permanent brain damage with repetitive head impacts.
    - A cause-and-effect relationship has not yet been demonstrated between CTE and SRC or exposure to contact sports.

11. **Risk reduction**
    - Preparticipation SRC history is very important, as is the quality of protective equipment.
    - Prevention areas that need more investigation include sports technique (head-up tackling and helmetless practices), helmet mandates and manufacturing, officiating (calling bad hits), neck strength, and video and sensor equipment.

Data from McCrory, P., Meeuwisse, W., Dvorak, J., Aubry, M., Bailes, J., Broglio, S., ... Davis, G. A. (2017). Consensus statement on concussion in sport: The 5th International Conference on Concussion in Sport held in Berlin, October 2016. *British Journal of Sports Medicine, 51*(11), 838–847.

(2009) indicated that undoubtedly baseline testing may minimize the negative effects of concussions in young athletes. They noted, though, that young athletes' brains are in a state of active and rapid maturation, and the validity and reliability of different baseline tests remains in question because limited evidence exists to show that they truly lower risk or improve outcomes. These authors also noted that normative data were not inclusive of race, previous concussion history, mental disorders, and learning disabilities (Kirkwood et al., 2009). However, much has been accomplished regarding normative data for a variety of baseline tests (Asken et al., 2012; Fallows et al., 2020). Normal variability is now recognized (Fallows et al., 2020), and basic demographics (sex and race), medical history (concussions and learning disabilities [e.g., ADHD]), and psychiatric disorders are incorporated (Asken et al., 2012).

Therefore, we (authors of this text) recommend that athletes in collision and contact sports undergo a baseline concussion screening test before the start of the season. Adolescents should be tested annually thereafter owing to their developing brain, and both adolescents and collegiate athletes should establish new baselines at least 6 months after a previous concussion (NCAA, n.d.). The baseline test should involve history of concussion or brain injury; neurological disorders; and mental health symptoms and disorders, symptom evaluation, cognitive assessment, and balance evaluation (NCAA, n.d.).

An important point is that the concussion screening test is used for both preinjury and postinjury assessment and management of concussions. The tool used should be validated and appropriate for use based on the age of the individual. The recommendation is that this concussion assessment should be done outside of the normal preparticipation physical exam so that full attention of the athlete and administrator can be devoted to the exam. Several screening tests are available for use and cover the systems most often effected by SRC (Table 9.2). Some tests, such as the Sport Concussion Assessment Tool 5 (SCAT5; Echemendia et al., 2017), Military Acute Concussion Evaluation (MACE 2), Vestibular/Ocular Motor Screening (VOMS), King-Devick Test, and Balance Error Scoring System (BESS), are typically used for acute assessment and follow-up but can also be used as baseline tests; they are available for free and largely easy to administer. The Sensory Organization Test (SOT) is done on equipment typically not available outside of a clinical research laboratory. The computer neurocognitive tests are the most common baseline and follow-up tests used across secondary and collegiate athletic programs and are covered in detail following. Ultimately, the purpose of a baseline test is to have individual performance data for comparison after a concussion and during recovery. Any retesting of the athlete should be done using the same concussion screening test in the same environment at approximately the same time of day as the initial testing was done to determine a potential area of brain disruption (visual, vestibular, or cognitive)

Table 9.2
Concussion Baseline Assessment Tools

Name of Test	Web Access
Paper or App Assessment Tools	
Sport Concussion Assessment Tool 5 (SCAT5)	https://bjsm.bmj.com/content/bjsports/early/2017/04/26/bjsports-2017-097506SCAT5.full.pdf
Military Acute Concussion Evaluation (MACE)	https://www.health.mil/Reference-Center/Publications/2020/07/30/Military-Acute-Concussion-Evaluation-MACE-2
Computerized Neurocognitive Tests	
Immediate Post-Concussion Assessment and Cognitive Testing (ImPACT)	https://impactconcussion.com/
CogSport/Axon	http://headsafe.com.au/wp-content/uploads/Axon-Cogstate-Guide.pdf
Automated Neuropsychological Assessment Metrics (ANAM)	https://armymedicine.health.mil/~/media/Files/ArmyMedicine/Documents/R2DANAM_Info_Brochure.ashx
Balance Tests	
Balance Error Scoring System (BESS)	https://www.physio-pedia.com/Balance_Error_Scoring_System
Sensory Organization Test (SOT)	https://www.sralab.org/rehabilitation-measures/sensory-organization-test
Eye Function Tests	
Vestibular/Ocular Motor Screening (VOMS)	https://www.physio-pedia.com/Vestibular/Oculomotor_Motor_Screening_(VOMS)_Assessment
King-Devik Test	https://kingdevicktest.com

Data from Cleveland Clinic. (2022). Concussion test. Retrieved from https://my.clevelandclinic.org/health/diagnostics/22267-concussion-test

and thus guide rehabilitation and potentially provide valuable progression information.

Computerized Neurocognitive Assessment

Paper-and-pencil neuropsychological testing has been identified as the cornerstone of concussion management and is still widely used by neuropsychologists in clinical settings. However, since the early 2000s the use of computerized platforms for neurocognitive testing has emerged (Lovell, 2002). Even though they are no substitute for formal neurocognitive evaluation, these brief cognitive evaluation tools have become the mainstay of many collegiate and high school sports programs. Currently, a variety of platforms are available for use under the guidance of an AT, team physician, or neuropsychologist. Each platform contains a variety of assessments that typically include verbal and visual memory, visual motor speed, reaction time, impulse control, and symptom scales. Added value has been demonstrated of having a personal neurocognitive baseline test (Roebuck-Spencer et al., 2013; Van Kampen et al., 2006), but as discussed earlier the neuroscience community believes some issues still exist regarding validity and reliability, though they are progressively being addressed (Asken et al., 2012; Fallows et al., 2020; Kirkwood et al., 2009). Ultimately, recent research has highlighted the false positives (i.e., software says athletes have a concussion and they do not) and false negatives (i.e., software says athletes are fine, but they do have a concussion; Resch et al., 2013; Resch et al., 2016). However, previous research indicates that the ability to correctly and accurately diagnose a concussion goes up significantly when computerized testing is included as a part of a test battery that includes a thorough severity- and duration-graded symptom scale and a balance assessment (Broglio et al., 2007). Therefore, computerized testing can be included with other tests but should not be used as a stand-alone diagnostic tool. Although some controversy exists regarding their usefulness (O'Neill et al., 2017), neurocognitive computerized tests may be helpful for school-related issues (e.g., attention or memory retention) and may serve as a guide for determining learning accommodations (e.g., shorter assignments or extended time for tests; Broglio et al., 2014). In the end, the clinician, not a computer, needs to make the return-to-physical-training and return-to-learn decisions.

Initial Assessment for Head Injury

For athletes who remain on the ground after the injury, which indicates a head injury could have been sustained, the first step in their management incorporates basic first aid procedures after reaching them. This is accomplished by executing the initial check. The first few seconds of the initial check should provide important information about the injured players. On reaching the athlete, body position; movement; unusual limb positions; and the position of the helmet, face mask, and/or mouth guard should be noted. All athletic and healthcare staff must be trained and well-rehearsed in dealing with such situations because immobilization of the head and neck should also take place at this time until severe injury has been ruled out (Courson et al., 2020; Mills et al., 2020). The head and neck should be stabilized (Figure 9.6) before arousing the injured athlete by placing hands on the shoulders, chest, or upper back and speaking loudly and directly toward the athlete's head. If the athlete is conscious, the airway in all probability is open. If the athlete appears to be unconscious, a designated person should make a mental note of the time; this will be of great value when the athlete arrives later at an emergency healthcare facility. Now, a determination needs to be whether the athlete is in either respiratory or cardiac arrest. Any problems, such as an obstructed airway or cardiac arrest, must be attended to before continuing with any further evaluation of injuries.

Circulation and Breathing Assessment

Assessing circulation and breathing can be done simultaneously because they are associated with each another. A responsive and talking athlete is a sign of good circulation because both talking and responsiveness require blood flow, whereas with an unresponsive athlete circulation must be determined by looking for other signs, including pulse, skin color, and movement of extremities. Breathing can usually be detected by observing the chest cavity or abdomen for the rise and fall associated with breathing or by placing an ear near the athlete's face and listening for the typical sounds of respiration. By doing this, sounds can also be detected that indicate airway obstruction, such as gagging, wheezing, or choking. In the case of a helmeted football player, the helmet does not need to be removed to determine whether the athlete is breathing.

If no signs of circulation are present, the emergency plan should be activated and cardiopulmonary resuscitation (CPR) initiated; if circulation is present but the athlete is not breathing, then rescue breathing should begin. If the athlete is prone, the athlete should carefully be rolled to a supine position following accepted first aid guidelines, which include vital steps such as stabilizing the head and maintaining an airway while rolling the athlete. If the athlete has football or other protective equipment on, the equipment should be removed so the chest and airway can be accessed (refer to the guidelines later in this section regarding removing a helmet and face mask from a football player with a head or neck injury). In a situation where circulation and/or breathing is lacking, the primary responsibility of the first responder is to keep the athlete alive and ensure that advanced help is summoned. The possibility of delaying a game or practice does not justify moving someone in this situation.

Physical Examination

At no time should staff attempt to revive an unconscious athlete by using a commercially made inhalant such as ammonia capsules. Athletes may reflexively jerk their head away from the inhalant, which could result in aggravation of an existing neck injury. Obviously, athletes who are conscious and alert represent a less complicated case than do athletes who appear to be unconscious and not breathing. Once the initial check has been completed, which can be accomplished in around 10–30 seconds, and the athlete's vital signs have been ascertained to be stable at the moment, then the physical exam can proceed, whereby as much information about the suspected head injury can be collected. At this point, retaining stabilization of the head and neck is prudent until specific signs and symptoms have been ruled out, including focal spine tenderness, numbness or tingling, or deformity (Mills et al., 2020). The physical exam (using the mnemonic CEMEPS) must include assessments of the following (see detailed descriptions later in the chapter):

C—Consciousness (Is it altered or changing?)

E—Extremity sensation and strength ("Can you feel where I am touching you?" "Squeeze my hand." "Pull your foot up." Perform these tests without moving the athlete's neck.)

M—Mental function ("What is your name?" "Who are we playing?" "Can you tell me what half or quarter it is?")

E—Eye signs (pupil equality and reactivity) and movements

P—Pain specific to the neck or on palpation to neck structures

S—Spasm of neck musculature (palpation reveals)

The staff must know the following information when evaluating a helmeted athlete with a suspected head injury:

- Don't remove the helmet of a football player. Remove other helmets only if they are impeding stabilization and evaluation efforts.
- Don't move the athlete until you are sure the cervical spine is not involved.
- Don't rush through the physical exam.

For athletes who are conscious, a series of quick, simple tests can be conducted to determine whether any significant neurological damage has occurred. First, if the athlete's consciousness is diminishing, assessors should note whether they are no longer opening their eyes or following verbal commands with answers or movements. To test extremity sensation, assessors can check the athlete's sensation on both sides by lightly touching or pinching their arm, torso, and leg and asking them to identify the general location of the sensation. To test strength, assessors should place two fingers in one of the athlete's hands and ask them to squeeze as hard as possible, then perform the test on the opposite hand to compare grip strength. Assessors can also place their hands on the tops of the athlete's feet and ask them to dorsiflex (i.e., move the top of their feet toward their legs) to compare bilateral strength. To determine orientation, assessors can ask a number of quick, easy-to-answer questions that help to establish the athlete's mental awareness of self and location (person, place, and time). Because the eyes are often the great revealers of neurological damage, assessors can determine possible brain injury by monitoring the athlete's eyes for size and equality of the pupils. To determine reactivity of the pupils, assessors can place one hand over one of the athlete's eyes and remove it quickly to determine whether the pupil reacts to light. Assessors should perform the tests on both eyes. Pupils are generally the same size; however, in rare cases, some people normally have pupils of unequal size, which is technically known as **anisocoria**. To test peripheral vision, assessors can hold a finger or pen directly in front of the athlete's face and slowly move it from side to side while asking them to indicate when it is no longer visible. Assessors should also have the athletes follow a finger or pen with their eyes only (no head movement) as it is slowly moved side to side and up and down and note any difference in peripheral vision by comparing right and left as well as any jerking movements of the eyeballs, which is called **nystagmus**. Loss of peripheral vision or jerking of the eyes is indicative of possible brain injury. Finally, assessors should ask about neck pain and spasm and gently palpate the athlete's neck, beginning at the base of the skull, then working slowly down to the bottom of the neck. Assessors should note any deformity, such as cervical protrusions or muscle spasms, and ask the athlete whether pain occurs at any specific bony area during the evaluation.

Based on the results of this portion of the injury evaluation, assessors should be able to determine whether athletes need immediate transportation to a hospital and the amount of neck stabilization that is necessary. Any concussion represents a potentially serious medical emergency. Continued LOC or deterioration of physical condition during the on-field evaluation also indicates that the injury is a medical emergency. If athletes experience signs and symptoms of a concussion (Time Out 9.1), regardless of whether they were rendered unconscious (even if only for a few seconds), they are not to return to the activity. Athletes should remain near the site of initial injury if they continue to suffer severe symptoms or altered consciousness, their vital signs should continue to be monitored, and EMS should be summoned. Before EMS arrive, even if the athlete's condition improves, no attempt should be made to move the athlete away from the site of initial injury because doing so may aggravate the injury.

In all probability, athletes who suffer a concussion will be able, with assistance, to walk to the sideline or courtside. At that point, they should be monitored, and an allied healthcare provider or physician should perform a complete medical evaluation. Of course, the process of referral and medical evaluation should be predetermined by way of the emergency action plan (EAP). Removal from the site of injury should be done with great care and without haste. Assuming the athlete does not have a cervical spine injury and is in a laying-down position, the first step in moving them is to raise them to a sitting position. With assistance from two members of the emergency team on both of their sides, the athlete should be raised into a sitting position by applying some force under their armpits while providing support in the event they lose balance. After the athlete is in a sitting position, their vital signs and overall behavior should be monitored for 1 to 2 minutes. If they appear to be normal, the next step is to assist them to a standing position, again with support on both of their sides from members of the emergency team. After the athlete is in a standing position, again their vital signs and sense of balance should be monitored for 1 to 2 minutes. If they appear to be normal, they should be asked to begin walking slowly toward the area, away from the site of the initial injury, where they can be examined more carefully. Again, members of the emergency team must provide continuous physical support on both sides of the athlete as they walk in case they lose their balance and begin to fall. After the athlete arrives at the site for further evaluation, they need to be assisted to a seated position and the next phase of the examination begun.

Finally, important points to remember are that concussion symptoms may be similar in nature to those observed in athletes who have been exercising intensely and are hypohydrated, and athletes may intentionally avoid reporting or being completely forthcoming about their symptoms to an AT or coach for fear of not playing (Broglio et al., 2014). Athletes who have sustained a concussion may willingly pull themselves from activity to take a break but not know exactly what is happening or what they are feeling; as a result, they may not seek medical care. For an AT to watch every athlete at every activity for subtle nuisances is difficult, so an important point is educating athletes and coaches before injury that athletes need to seek help in such situations. For athletes who

Anisocoria Unequal size pupils that may be related to an acute condition such as head injury or occur naturally. It is important to perform a thorough clinical evaluation to determine the appropriate management.

Nystagmus Vision condition where the eyes make repetitive, uncontrolled movements when tracking.

have removed themselves from activity, the initial assessment can begin with the sideline assessment, as described below.

Sideline Assessment

Once the athlete is seated away from the playing area and can be assessed without interference from fellow athletes, a more detailed assessment of their condition must be conducted. The objective of this phase of the evaluation is to determine the presence of any signs or symptoms of head injury that may have developed since the time of the initial injury. This information is of vital importance to making decisions regarding appropriate medical referral. No longer acceptable is the practice of simply sitting athletes out for a few minutes and then returning them to participation based on an apparent return to preinjury status because doing so is against the law in all 50 states and the District of Columbia.

Clinical research and discussions (McCrory et al., 2017) examining best practices in dealing with athletes who may have sustained a concussion indicate that even in the absence of trained medical professionals follow-up assessments that include a standardized list of typical symptoms should be used to help determine the status of someone suspected of having sustained a concussion. Although the ideal situation would employ the skills and training of a medical professional, such as a Board of Certification (BOC)–certified AT, nurse practitioner, physician assistant, or physician, options are available to programs that do not have trained medical professionals directly on staff (McCrory et al., 2017). With very little training, a tool called the Pocket Concussion Recognition Tool (http://bjsm.bmj.com/content/47/5/267.full.pdf) can be used to identify a suspected concussion (McCrory et al., 2017). It is a very simple tool that instructs the evaluator to look for visible signs of a concussion (e.g., dazed or stunned look), identify any signs and symptoms the athlete may be experiencing (Time Out 9.1), and briefly assess the athlete's memory (e.g., "Where are we?" "What team did we play last week?"). It also identifies several red flags (e.g., seizures and deterioration of mental status) that indicate the athlete needs immediate medical attention and EMS should be called. But this is a basic tool that is used for recognition only. The pocket guide clearly states, "Any athlete with a suspected concussion should be *immediately removed from play*, and should not be returned to activity until they are assessed medically. Athletes with a suspected concussion should not be left alone and should not drive a motor vehicle" (McCrory et al., 2017).

Currently, ATs and other medical professionals are using the SCAT5, which was developed as a part of the Fifth International Conference on Concussion (Echemendia et al., 2017; McCrory et al., 2017). The tool's authors encourage distribution in printed form, but with the advent of easy-to-use handheld devices, it is also available as an app. The SCAT5 is intended for anyone age 13 or older, and it can be downloaded for free here: https://bjsm.bmj.com/content/bjsports/early/2017/04/26/bjsports-2017-097506SCAT5.full.pdf. For children 12 years and younger, the Child SCAT5 can be downloaded for free here: https://bjsm.bmj.com/content/51/11/862.

Both the SCAT5 and the Child SCAT5 assessment tools include six major areas: on-field assessment, symptom evaluation, cognitive screening, neurological screening, delayed recall, and clinical decision. The differences between the Child SCAT5 (Davis et al., 2017) and the SCAT5 (Echemendia et al., 2017) are subtle, but the Child SCAT5 involves parents and more relevant memory and cognitive questions for those younger than 12 years of age. Both tools begin with an assessment of red flags, observable signs for consciousness and general appearance (blank stare or vacant look), quick cervical spine assessment, and the Glasgow Coma Scale (GCS) for responsiveness because any of these conditions warrant emergency referral. The GCS gives a score on a scale of 15 points for eye movement, verbal response, and motor response to commands and pain. A score of less than 8 indicates a severe condition that needs immediate emergency medical treatment. The SCAT5 also includes the Maddocks Score for immediate orientation and memory to person place and time. Once evaluators have established that a head injury is not in need of emergency treatment, they can complete the remainder of the tool questions on the sidelines or in a clinical setting.

The second section is a graded symptom-scale checklist with duration and severity assessments as well as simple history questions regarding previous concussive injuries, history of headaches, hospitalizations, mental disorders, and learning disabilities. The Child SCAT5 is slightly different than the SCAT5 in that it has a symptom scale for the child and a symptom scale for the parent. The third section is a cognitive assessment for concentration and short-term memory. This assessment is accomplished by evaluators asking the injured athlete to answer a series of questions as well as perform some cognitive skills, such as knowing the correct month, date, year, and time of day. Memory tests include testing the ability to recall five words in the correct order plus reciting lists of numbers and months of the year in reverse order. The fourth section is a neurological screening with an eyes closed balance examination (modified balance error scoring system [mBESS]), a coordination test (finger to nose), neck range of motion, visual accuracy with reading, and a tandem gait walk. If children are not of reading age, they are asked to describe the scene in a picture on the form. The mBESS assesses athletes' ability to hold an eyes closed hands on hips position on two different surfaces (flat and foam) using three different positions: double-leg, tandem (one foot in front of the other), and single-leg stances without shoes. The goal is to complete 20 seconds without many errors (more than 10), such as opening eyes, lifting hands, or stumbling. The foam surface and the single-leg stance are removed for the mBESS for children younger than 10 years old. The fifth section is a delayed recall for the five words used on the immediate memory test.

The sixth and final section involves a recording of scores from the other sections and an area to diagnose the athlete with a concussion or an area to indicate that the test is a follow-up and whether an improvement or a decline in health is indicated.

Additional sign and symptom assessment options for follow-up testing of athletes by an allied healthcare provider are listed in Table 9.3; they are the Graded Symptom Scale Checklist (GSSC), Post Concussion Symptoms Scale (PCSS), Post-Concussion Symptom Inventory (PCSI), Acute Concussion Evaluation (ACE), Concussion Symptom Inventory (CSI), and the Rivermead Post-Concussion Symptoms Questionnaire (RPCSQ; Committee on Sports-Related Concussions in Youth; Board on Children, Youth, and Families; Institute of Medicine; & National Research Council, 2014). Each tool has only subtle differences, but any follow-up assessment should be validated for use with the appropriate age group (Lumba-Brown et al., 2018) and not be used as a stand-alone measure for recovery from concussion. Coaches or parents can use these assessment tools to obtain critical information while at or near the site of injury (courtside or sideline) if they are the only supervising personnel available, after which the information can be relayed

Table 9.3
Self-Reported Symptom Scales

Scale Name	Access
Graded Symptom Scale Checklist (GSSC)	https://sjschools.org/images/Athletics_HS/graded_symptom_checklist.pdf
Acute Concussion Evaluation (ACE)	https://www.cdc.gov/headsup/pdfs/providers/ace-a.pdf
Concussion Symptom Inventory (CSI)	https://bsbproduction.s3.amazonaws.com/portals/2969/docs/concussions_csi-12_-_nscn-form1.pdf
Post Concussion Symptom Scale (PCSS)	https://hawaiiconcussion.com/downloads/Post-Concussion-Symptom-Scale.pdf
Post-Concussion Symptom Inventory (PCSI)	https://www.nhmi.net/media/pdf-files/Parent-Symptom-Scale.pdf
Rivermead Post-Concussion Symptoms Questionnaire (RPCSQ)	http://www.tbi-impact.org/cde/mod_templates/12_F_06_Rivermead.pdf

Data from Committee on Sports-Related Concussions in Youth; Board on Children, Youth, and Families; Institute of Medicine; & National Research Council. (2014). *Sports-related concussions in youth: Improving the science, changing the culture.* Washington, DC: National Academies Press.

to medical personnel. However, administration by a coach or parent *does not* provide a diagnosis. Qualified medical professionals make diagnoses because determination of a concussion is a clinical judgment (McCrory et al., 2017). In the absence of qualified medical professionals, coaches and parents must receive proper training on the use of these assessment tools. Further, they must understand that their main role is to protect the health and safety of athletes and that "if in doubt, sit them out" is the rule and not the exception. Athletes may have a concussion even if their SCAT5 or other symptom scale appears "normal" (McCrory et al., 2017), so the rule of *no RTP* should be strictly followed for all athletes if they experience even one sign or symptom after having experienced a direct or indirect blow (McCrory et al., 2017).

Home Instructions and Postconcussion Care

Because most young athletes will be released to the care of a parent or guardian and college-age athletes will be released to roommates or friends, instructions must be provided for immediate follow-up care and the concussion management plan, which outlines the treatment and resources during concussion management (Broglio et al., 2014). The plan should be included in the institution's policies and clearly communicate the care, resources (e.g., physicians and school nurses), and accommodations offered to the concussed athletes.

For home care instructions, a paper with a list of symptoms should be given to the caregivers with instructions indicating that the appearance of any severe symptoms or a significant increase in the intensity of common symptoms (e.g., headache) indicates immediate referral to an emergency department. The general changes that are considered serious are repeated vomiting, seizures, slurred speech, inability to speak, worsening headache, increased confusion or irritability, decreasing consciousness or LOC, and numbness in arms or legs. In addition, a follow-up evaluation is scheduled and written on the paper, along with additional instructions such as only sparingly taking acetaminophen for headaches, eating a carbohydrate-rich diet, avoiding exercise that induces any increase in symptoms, resting the mind's activity by limiting activities that require heavy levels of concentration or multisensory events (e.g., video games), sleeping as needed, and avoiding alcohol and driving (Broglio et al., 2014). Instructions should stress avoiding taking nonsteroidal anti-inflammatory drugs (e.g., ibuprofen) during concussion management, because they might prevent awareness of a worsening condition involving brain swelling, and consulting a physician for any other medication concerns. The notion that concussed athletes should not be allowed to sleep uninterrupted is outdated, as is the recommendation of complete physical and mental rest (Strelzik & Langdon, 2017).

Each concussion is unique based on many factors (e.g., physical, cognitive, emotional, and sleep related); therefore, predicting how someone will recover is difficult. Typically, recovery will be delayed if the individual is a female and has lower cognitive abilities, neurological or psychological diseases or conditions (e.g., migraines or depression), learning disabilities, and a history of concussion. However, a point that is comforting to share with parents, coaches, and athletes is that 70–80% of concussed athletes do not show any physical or mental differences 1 to 3 months after a concussion (Broglio et al., 2015; Collins et al., 2016; Lumba-Brown et al., 2018).

As mentioned previously, the understanding of the role of physical and mental rest within concussion recovery has changed over the years based on gathered patient-centered evidence. Athletes should be encouraged to participate in activities of daily living as long as those activities do not increase symptoms (Collins et al., 2016; Lumba-Brown et al., 2018; Strelzik & Langdon, 2017). "Cocooning" athletes or prescribing strict brain rest (e.g., sitting in a dark room, taking naps, and no reading or computers) is not recommended (Collins et al., 2016). However, temporary accommodations (e.g., excused from physical education and school) should be granted when deemed necessary (i.e., the physical or academic activity increases symptoms). Other activities, such as text messaging, video games, and loud social activities, may need to be limited during concussion recovery only if they are aggravating symptoms (Harmon et al., 2019; Strelzik & Langdon, 2017) because during recovery injured athletes need to maintain social and emotional support (Lumba-Brown et al., 2018).

Concussion Rehabilitation

Many different types of clinicians (e.g., ATs, pediatricians, emergency room physicians, concussion specialists, and school nurses) may see athletes with a concussion, and their background information may vary greatly. For example, recent research (Collins et al., 2016; Lumba-Brown et al., 2018) recommends that athletes *do not* stop exercising, reading, or engaging socially like once recommended; however, some healthcare practitioners (e.g., nurses and internists) may still suggest doing so because they may not have kept up on the latest concussion recovery research. Therefore, a concussion care program must always include a healthcare provider with current training in concussion recovery who will include a multidisciplinary approach (Collins et al., 2016; Reynolds et al., 2014). Targeting active treatments to each individual's clinical situation may improve recovery and the rate of returning to school or work (Collins et al., 2016).

Although the recommendations for physical and cognitive rest during concussion recovery exist, an important point is that rest continuing beyond the acute stage may be the reason athletes develop symptoms (e.g., anxiety and sleep disorders) that are unrelated to the actual concussion but may be confused for concussion symptoms (Broglio et al., 2015; Schneider, 2019). Recent research has provided significant evidence that subthreshold aerobic activity may be effective for concussion recovery (Leddy et al., 2016; Leddy et al., 2019), which now is the standard recommendation in concussion recovery programs. The program is called the Buffalo Concussion Protocol. To begin the subthreshold activity portion, athletes are fitted with a heart rate monitor and assessed with the question "If 100% is feeling perfectly normal, what percentage of normal do you feel now?" When the assessment is greater than 70%, the athlete is cleared to begin a light aerobic program based on their rating of perceived exertion (Borg scale 6–20) and any aggravation of signs or symptoms. A bike or treadmill can be used with increasing the incline or resistance, followed by the speed, until the athlete reports a Borg scale of greater than 19.5, have exacerbation of current symptoms by more than 3 points on a 10-point Likert scale, or have an occurrence of several new symptoms not reported before exercise (Leddy et al., 2016; Leddy et al., 2019). When one of more of these conditions is met, then the test is concluded, and the exertional heart rate recorded. Future aerobic exercise is based on this heart rate to remain below symptom aggravation but to take advantage of the benefits of aerobic exercise on brain blood flow. A typical exercise progression based on the Buffalo Concussion Protocol begins with 20 minutes of daily aerobic exercise (free of symptom exacerbation) at 80% of the recorded exertional heart rate as determined from the test. Each week, the target exercise heart rate can be raised by 10–15 beats/minute, and this protocol can be continued until no symptoms are present and the athlete has reached their predicted maximum heart rate during exercise (Leddy et al., 2016; Leddy et al., 2019). Once the athlete is able to complete exercise at their predicted maximal heart rate without the onset of new or increasing symptoms, they are then cleared for the later stages of RTP (see additional information below).

Beyond aerobic conditioning and before beginning more aggressive sport-specific RTP activities, the visual and vestibular systems, as well as any psychological or cognitive sequelae, must be rehabilitated (Broglio et al., 2015; Schneider, 2019). Choosing where to concentrate athletes' rehabilitation can be aligned with the identified profiles based on presentation of symptoms. Kontos, Sufrinko, Sandel, Emami, and Collins (2019) identified these profiles as cognitive/fatigue, vestibular, ocular, migraine, and mood/anxiety, with vestibular and ocular disturbance being the most common. This study also found that some individuals shared two or more profiles, such as vestibular/ocular and migraine (Kontos et al., 2019). Therefore, VOMS screening and rehabilitation exercises must be included in rehabilitation programs (Broglio et al., 2015). Mucha and colleagues (2014) developed a simple screening tool called the VOMS (Table 9.2) to assess the vestibular and oculomotor profile. It has several visual tests involving eye movements and head movements and assesses any increases in nausea, headache, dizziness, and fogginess. Exercises focused on improving vestibular and ocular function can enhance concussion recovery (Broglio et al., 2015; Kontos et al., 2018; Murray et al., 2017). Detailed information regarding targeted vision and vestibular rehabilitation methods for concussions is beyond the scope of the chapter; however, parents, coaches, and medical personnel should be aware of this option for concussion recovery.

Another new approach in the rehabilitation of concussions is based on increasing evidence that athletes with a concussion history have a significant increased risk of lower extremity musculoskeletal injury (Eagle et al., 2020; Herman et al., 2017) as a result of diffuse neuron injury and a delay in neuromechanical responsiveness resulting from postconcussion changes in brain function (Eagle et al., 2020; Herman et al., 2015; Wilkerson et al., 2017; Wilkerson et al., 2020). The odds of experiencing a lower extremity injury are 1.5 to 4 times higher in athletes with a concussion history (Wilkerson et al., 2020) than in those without. The injuries are hypothesized to result from the initial metabolic energy crisis experienced in the brain at the time of the concussive injury, which damages a key connection between perception and motor action (Eagle et al., 2020; Wilkerson et al., 2020). Exercises that involve perception–action coupling or exercises with dual tasks are recommended in concussion rehabilitation (Eagle et al., 2020; Wilkerson et al., 2017; Wilkerson et al., 2020). A dual-task exercise involves an athlete performing two motor tasks (e.g., ball toss while standing on one leg) or a motor and cognitive task (e.g., jumping jacks while counting backward from 100 by sevens [serial sevens]). Rehabilitation that is focused on perception–action coupling can be accomplished in a variety of ways. Simple tools are available, such as colored balls and verbal math or memory games that can be combined, and high-tech computer-driven light action array scenarios that require the completion of tasks with both motor and cognitive components (e.g., stand on balance board and hit board when and where a red blinking light appears). Detailed information regarding targeted perception–action coupling rehabilitation methods for concussions is beyond the scope of the chapter, but the reader is encouraged to follow the ever-developing evidence regarding the ability to rehabilitate concussions as well as preventing subsequent concussions and lower extremity injuries.

Return to Play and Return to Learn

Gradual RTP and return-to-learn (RTL) plans are recommended by physicians for athletes who have experienced a concussion and are symptom-exacerbation free with activities of daily living and have normal objective (i.e., physical) tests and subjective (i.e., neurocognitive) tests (Broglio et al., 2014; Harmon et al., 2019; McCrory et al., 2017; Schneider, 2019; Scorza et al., 2012). All RTP and RTL protocols need to begin with healthcare provider clearance. Each state has different rules as to the credentials and training of the healthcare provider, but most require either a physician, nurse practitioner, physician assistant, or AT to provide clearance (Potteiger et al., 2018). The general steps are listed in Table 9.4. All RTP protocols begin with a resolution of all signs and symptoms during activities of daily living. After the no-activity intense activity period ends, each step should be performed in no less than a 24-hour period. Successful completion of a step is performance of exercise tasks without an aggravation or reoccurrence of any signs and symptoms that day or the following day. If any signs and symptoms are experienced during one of the exercise steps, then the athlete is to stop all activity and rest until the next day. Assuming the athlete is symptom free the following day, they then drop back to the previously asymptomatic level (Broglio, 2014; McCrory et al., 2017), and the progression begins again. The minimum time for a gradual RTP is typically 7 days; however, a period of months may be necessary to successfully return an athlete to play, depending on the individual responses and any modifying circumstances (Harmon et al., 2019; Schneider, 2019). For example, for athletes with multiple concussions, concussions occurring with less force involved, and/or concussions with increased severity, the concussion management RTP plan should be very conservative.

RTL (school setting; Table 9.5) also has a graduated progression into full cognitive activities and long days. Halstead and colleagues (2013) emphasized the importance of a progressive and guided increase in school activities because of the effects concussions can have on cognitive faculties. Aggressive and early return to high-level cognitive tasks or an environment with excessive lights and noise may cause an exacerbation of signs and symptoms and delay recovery. RTL protocols should be multidisciplinary (Halstead et al., 2013) with an emphasis on communication between the treating medical provider and the school nurse, principal, and/or social worker so the teacher and parents can be aware of restrictions on in-class and out-of-class work. As a rule of thumb, athletes should return to classroom activities (stage 2 or 3; Table 9.5) before beginning stage 3 of the RTP protocol (Table 9.4). Unfortunately, the public has been slower to accept the need for RTL strategies as evidenced by the fact that only a very few states have laws that mandate a written protocol and accommodations for the classroom, whereas all 50 states and the District of Columbia have RTP criteria and clearance protocols (Potteiger et al., 2018).

Table 9.4
Return-to-Play Progression

Instructions: Follow a stepwise progression typically with 24 hours between each step. Progression through steps is delayed if postconcussive signs or symptoms develop at any point. Before progression begins again, all signs and symptoms need to have cleared.

Stage	Aim	Activity and Goals
1	Symptom-limited activity	Activities of daily living; no strenuous activity and limited cognitive and physical activity; general rest; gradual reintroduction of tasks.
2	Light aerobic exercises	Walking or stationary cycling at slow to medium pace; no resistance training (70% maximum heart rate or 80% of Buffalo concussion threshold); increasing heart rate under controlled circumstances.
3	Sport-specific exercises	Sport-specific exercises and drills; no head impact activity; movement techniques without risk of contact.
4	Noncontact training drills	Noncontact training drills and resistance training; harder training drills (e.g., passing drills); may start progressive resistance training and add cognitive challenging tasks.
5	Full-contact practice	Normal training activities; restore confidence and assess readiness to return.
6	Return to play	Normal game play.

Data from McCrory, P., Meeuwisse, W., Dvorak, J., Aubry, M., Bailes, J., Broglio, S., . . . Vos, P. E. (2017). Consensus statement on concussion in sport: The 5th International Conference on Concussion in Sport held in Berlin, October 2016. *British Journal of Sports Medicine, 51*(11), 838–847.

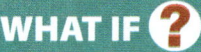

WHAT IF

You are confronted with a situation during a tackle football game in which a player is apparently knocked unconscious during a play. When you arrive at the scene, the player is lying face down and is not moving. What would you do to ascertain the athlete's level of injury? What would you not do, and why?

Concussion Education

Athletes, parents, and coaches need to seek out continuing education on concussions because the understanding and general treatment of these injuries changes all the time. The good news is that all states require some type of concussion awareness (Glasgow, 2017; Potteiger et al., 2018). However, the requirements are not always specific to a type of healthcare provider and these policies cover some or all student-athletes, coaches, parents, and officials. Healthcare providers typically need to complete training yearly or every 2 years; however, most states are just assuming that all healthcare providers, no matter their specialty, will "just know about concussions," so the bad news is that there are no specific education sessions required (Glasgow, 2017). But despite some of these limitations, most states often allow schools to choose their concussion management teams, so the hope is that the healthcare providers on this team would be up to date on the latest concussion evidence. To demonstrate concerns over concussion education and state laws, a recent research paper reported that club coaches for recreation sports, where many children and adolescents engage in physical activity, were less likely to have mandates that require leagues or organizing bodies to provide concussion education materials or proof of training, and a group of club coaches also scored

Table 9.5
Return-to-Learn Progression

Instructions: Schools need to have an SRC policy that includes education on prevention and management for teachers, staff, students, and parents. Appropriate academic accommodations and support to students recovering from an SRC need to be established and followed. In general, if athletes cannot concentrate or tolerate academic stimulation for at least 30 minutes, they should stay at home and continue with activities of daily living. Children and adolescents should not return to sport until they have successfully returned to school. However, early introduction of symptom-limited physical activity is appropriate.

Stage	Aim	Activity and Goals
1	Daily activities at home that do not give the child symptoms	Normal activities of daily living that children can do if they do not increase symptoms (e.g., reading, texting, and screen time). Start with 5–15 minutes at a time and gradually build up the time to increase tolerance.
2	School activities	Homework, reading, or other cognitive activities outside of the classroom that take more than 30 minutes to complete.
3	Return to school part-time	Gradual introduction to school attendance. May need to start with a partial school day or increased breaks during the day, be allowed longer time for tests, and have their activities altered to protect against light and noise sensitivity.
4	Return to school full-time	Gradually progress school activities until a full day can be tolerated and all activities have returned to normal. May need to catch up on missed work.

Data from McCrory, P., Meeuwisse, W., Dvorak, J., Aubry, M., Bailes, J., Broglio, S., . . . Vos, P. E. (2017). Consensus statement on concussion in sport: The 5th International Conference on Concussion in Sport held in Berlin, October 2016. *British Journal of Sports Medicine, 51*(11), 838–847; and Halstead, M. E., McAvoy, K., Devore, C. D., Carl, R., Lee, M., & Logan, K. (2013). Returning to learning following a concussion. *Pediatrics, 132*(5), 948–957.

lower on a concussion knowledge quiz when compared to secondary school coaches working within school districts (Stamm et al., 2020).

A variety of programs offer information to coaches and athletes, and some high school federations have made concussion training mandatory for all participants. The Sports Legacy Institute Concussion Education (SLICE) campaign for youth athletes (http://staging.sportslegacy.org/sports-legacy-institute-concussion-education-programs/slice/; Bagley et al., 2012), the Centers for Disease Control and Prevention's HEADS UP to Youth Sports campaign for coaches and medical providers (https://www.cdc.gov/headsup/youthsports/training/index.html; Sarmiento et al., 2010), and the coach training program for coaches from BrainLine (https://www.brainline.org/article/active-free-concussion-training-sports-coaches; Glang et al., 2010) have been able to increase knowledge of concussions in these populations. Many other entities, such as local hospitals, have also developed training modules that can be completed online to satisfy any training requirements.

The AT is responsible at the school for educating athletes, parents, coaches, and administrators before the season begins on the importance of reporting concussion symptoms and completing any requested testing protocols (both baseline and follow-up) and explaining that collision and contact sports inherently have more risk of concussion than other noncontact sports. ATs can never place too much emphasis on explaining to athletes why they should report symptoms of a concussion immediately.

ATs should also be involved with protective equipment decisions and conditioning exercises as they relate to concussion prevention and safety as well as educating those involved with equipment management. For example, well maintained helmets can reduce the incidence of concussions but do not significantly prevent concussions in sports (Rowson et al., 2014) and neck musculature strengthening with short-latency ballistic contractions may reduce the risk of concussions (Gilchrist et al., 2015). Another important point to note is that evidence is growing that over a collegiate football season, athletes who participated in helmet-less football practices that emphasize rugby-type tackling techniques demonstrated a lower head-impact frequency per athlete exposure during the season compared to a control group (normal helmeted practices; Swartz et al., 2019). Unfortunately, this behavioral intervention produced only short-term changes and were lost by the end of the season, so more research needs to be completed (Swartz et al., 2019).

ATs should also be in charge of developing the written concussion plan that details procedures for baseline testing, the steps for the recognition and treatment of concussion, follow-up testing, and RTP and RTL protocols. After a concussion, proper care and education about the recovery process should be conveyed to all parties involved. Specifically, ATs should communicate that severity and an exact time to recover cannot be accurately predicted because each concussion is unique depending on age, gender, mental health, symptoms, past concussions, and medications, but that most concussions resolve within 2 weeks (Broglio et al., 2015; Collins et al., 2016; Lumba-Brown et al., 2018).

Cervical Spine Injuries

Background Information

Injuries involving the cervical spine occur in almost any athletic event but most often in tackle football, lacrosse, rugby, ice hockey, soccer, diving, cheerleading, and gymnastics. Neck (cervical) injuries can involve a variety of tissues in the region, including bones, ligaments, intervertebral disks, spinal cord, spinal nerve roots, and the spinal nerves themselves (Schroeder & Vaccaro, 2016). Any injury to this region of the body is potentially serious; therefore, those personnel charged with providing emergency care must be as prepared as possible for such injuries. Although a single catastrophic (nonfatal) cervical spine injury (CSI) is devastating, the overall incidence in athletics should be viewed in perspective: 17,810 new CSI cases are reported each year (54 cases for every 1 million people) in the United States, and only 7.8% of those CSIs are linked to sports (National Spinal Cord Injury Statistical Center [NSCISC], 2021). Vehicle accidents (38.6%), falls (32.2%), and violence (14%) account for two to five times more injuries (NSCISC, 2021). According to high school and collegiate data collected by the NCCSIR, during the 2018–2019 season, 80 sports-related catastrophic injuries and conditions were captured, with 18 injuries to the spinal cord and/or vertebrae out of 37 catastrophic injuries (Kucera & Cantu, 2020). Unfortunately, the number of spinal injuries has stayed relatively the same over the past 3 years, but both increases and decreases have been demonstrated over the past decade (Kucera & Cantu, 2020).

Spinal cord injuries are very serious but represent a fairly small number of total injuries. If the assumption is made that statistics of overall direct catastrophic injuries provide some representation of the incidence of spinal cord injuries in sports, then tackle football produced the highest number of traumatic injuries in the catastrophic category (Kucera & Cantu, 2020). Another point that is also important to note is that football has a very large number of participants (almost 2 million). As such, the relative incidence of all catastrophic injuries in tackle football is quite low on an athlete exposure basis. For example, for the years from 1982–2019, the rate of all direct catastrophic injuries in high school sports indicated that football had 2.64 per 100,000 AEs, whereas the rates were 3.21 for male cheerleading, 2.62 for female cheerleading, 3.31 for male gymnastics, 1.3 for female gymnastics, 2.6 for male ice hockey, and 1.73 for female ice hockey (Kucera & Cantu, 2020). For collegiate sports (1982–2019), the rate of all direct catastrophic injuries indicated that football had 0.78 per 100,000 AEs, whereas the rate for male skiing was 4.53; female skiing, 4.48; and female equestrian, 3.68 (Kucera & Cantu, 2020). Data presented in the 2020 annual football injury report (Kucera et al., 2020) are shown in Table 9.6. These data represent the incidence of CSIs in football that resulted in some level of disability at the time of the injury and incomplete recovery. The data in Table 9.6 have been reduced to represent groups of years together. Overall, the total number of injuries across all levels has generally declined, despite an uptick in incidences during the 2000–2009 seasons, and this can be considered good

Table 9.6

Annual Survey of Catastrophic Cervical Cord Football Injuries

Years	Organized Youth	Pro and Semipro	Middle and High School	Collegiate	Total
1977–1989	2	2	113	18	135
1990–1999	3	3	60	9	75
2000–2009	2	8	76	8	94
2010–2019	4	2	52	14	72
Total	11	15	301	49	376

Data from Kucera, K. L., Klossner, D., & Cantu, R. C. (2020). *Annual survey of catastrophic football injuries, 1977–2019*. Retrieved from https://nccsir.unc.edu/reports/

news. Since the period from 1977–1989, very recent numbers (2010–2019) demonstrate a reduction in the occurrence of catastrophic cervical injuries at the high school level but a return to higher numbers of injuries at the college level over this same period (Table 9.6). Therefore, the number of catastrophic neck injuries in high school football may be decreasing over time because of the many rules that have been established to reduce their number; the education of athletes, coaches, and parents on appropriate tackling and falling techniques; and the increasing presence of emergency medical care on the sidelines and the accuracy of the medical response. However, the slight increase at the collegiate level might be a result of more opportunities for playing time at the college level and more aggressive play related to national coverage and exposure on television as the rules, education, and medical care have improved at this level, too.

The extent and severity of neurological damage that occurs in a neck injury depend on the magnitude of the mechanism of injury, the resulting movement of the neck, and the extent of tissue damage (Schroeder & Vaccaro, 2016). In the case of simple neck muscle strains, neurological involvement is extremely rare. Cervical injuries are expressly more serious when displacement of an intact vertebra occurs; fragments of a vertebral fracture are displaced; or an intervertebral disk ruptures, which places pressure directly on the spinal cord or nerve roots. In these situations, the potential for permanent neurological damage is high. Curiously, even when considerable damage has occurred to tissues surrounding the spinal cord, significant neurological symptoms may be totally absent at the time of the injury. Therefore, the certified AT, coach, or other first responder must be objective and complete an initial assessment process and immobilization of the head and neck (Figure 9.6) to avoid converting a treatable into a permanent injury. Although a coach is not expected to conduct as complete a neurological evaluation as would be expected of an AT or a physician, the simple field tests including assessment of consciousness, extremity strength and sensation, mental function, eye signs, pain specific to neck area, and neck musculature spasm (CEMEPS) described earlier in the chapter can often yield sufficient information to make an informed decision regarding initial management of the athlete. See **Time Out 9.4**, which shares Tommy Mallon's story and the creation of the organization Advocates for Injured Athletes, whose mission is to promote sports safety and provide essential support, education, and resources to help keep student-athletes safe (http://injuredathletes.org/about-us/).

Mechanisms of Injury

Historically, the mechanism of injury considered to be potentially the most common and serious was excessive forced flexion (hyperflexion) of the cervical spine. However, extensive film analysis and objective research have disputed this long-held belief. Most experts now agree that the mechanism known technically as *axial load* produces the majority of serious

> ### TIME OUT 9.4
>
> **Tommy Mallon Story**
>
> In the spring of 2009, Tommy Mallon was playing lacrosse when he collided with another player as they both went for a ball on the ground. Tommy wanted to get up and "shake it off," but Riki Kirchoff, the responding certified AT, insisted he stay down because her CEMEPS initial evaluation revealed that he had slight numbness at the back of his head. Tommy was spine boarded and transported to a trauma hospital, where doctors discovered that he had a neck fracture and had severed one of his vertebral arteries, which had caused a dangerous clot to form. Attending physicians all agreed that Tommy's life was saved by not allowing him to get up and to the care he received by all the emergency responders present.
>
> Advocates for Injured Athletes (A4IA). (n.d.). *A4IA story*. Retrieved from http://injuredathletes.org/about-us/

CSIs, which is especially true in tackle football. Before the mid-1970s, tackling with the crown of the helmet (spearing) was a common practice. Axial loading of the cervical spine occurs when the head is lowered with slight flexion just before impact—the net effect being a straightening of the normal vertebral curve (Boden et al., 2006; Schroeder & Vaccaro, 2016). In this position, forces applied to the top of the head are absorbed directly by the bones of the vertebral column without the protective assistance of surrounding ligaments and muscles. In 1976, the NCAA enacted a rule change that prohibited spearing, or leading with the head, for contact. The results seemed impressive because the number of CSIs significantly dropped the following year. However, the data in Table 9.6 seem to show that despite ongoing efforts to reduce the incidence of these injuries, they are still a problem. Classic research by Heck (1996), designed to see whether 15 years of the spearing rule implementation decreased its incidence rate, determined that the overall rate of spearing differed very little in two seasons of New Jersey high school football games: spearing was present one in 2.5 plays in 1975 compared with one in 2.4 plays in 1990. More current research on football that catalogued cervical injuries resulting in quadriplegia (paralysis) from 1989–2002 demonstrated that making a tackle (classic mechanism of spearing) caused 79.7% of injuries resulting in quadriplegia, whereas only 10.1% were a result of being tackled (Boden et al., 2006). On the contrary, general cervical cord **neurapraxia** (temporary loss of motor and sensory function) was quite similar between making a tackle (44.7%) and being tackled (36.8%; Boden et al., 2006). Therefore, the football community likely needs to continue to emphasize the importance of teaching young athletes not to practice this extremely dangerous maneuver. All coaches, officials, parents, and sports medicine personnel share some responsibility in monitoring young athletes during games and practice as well as providing them with education, such as HEADS UP to Youth Sports training (https://www.cdc.gov/headsup/youthsports/training/index.html). To address spearing and dangerous tackling, in 2005 the NCAA updated its tackle football rules by eliminating the problem of determining whether the maneuver was performed *intentionally* by the athlete to discourage athletes from contacting any opponent with the top or crown of the helmet or the face mask (Boden et al., 2006). Over the past 10 years, Pop Warner (U.S. youth football league) has consistently updated practice and game rules to prohibit full-speed head-on straight blocking or tackling with players more than 3 yards apart; eliminate kickoffs for Pee-Wee football (9- to 11-year-olds); eliminate three-point stances and head-down positioning; require coaches take the USA Football's Heads Up Football training; and implement a transition game called "Rookie Tackle," which helps kids go from flag football to tackle football (Pop Warner Little Scholars, 2019). The National Athletic Trainers' Association (NATA), National Football League (NFL), Pop Warner Youth Football, and NCAA are committed to educating football participants regarding the dangers of these high-risk maneuvers. A classic video from 2009 is still relevant for the education of players, coaches, and parents regarding proper tackling (https://vimeo.com/6398919), and USA Football has several videos and courses designed for education and presented in this video (https://www.youtube.com/watch?v=FgsU3bOvTZ0).

Neurapraxia A temporary loss of motor and sensory function owing to blockage of nerve conduction.

Although spearing (axial loading) has been identified as a continuing problem and an extremely hazardous practice among football players, also true is that any forced movement of the cervical spine, including hyperflexion, hyperextension, rotation, and lateral flexion, can result in injury. Whiplash, or a rapid, forceful back-and-forth motion of the neck, is also not uncommon because athletes falling off equipment or hitting the ground quickly can cause this motion. The types and severity of injury to the cervical spine are extensive; however, they can be classified according to the tissues involved and the extent of the damage. In order of severity, these injuries range from a simple compression or stretch of the brachial plexus nerve complex, which is self-correcting within minutes of the injury, to more severe problems involving ruptures of the intervertebral disks, fractures of the vertebrae, or damage to the spinal cord.

Brachial Plexus Injuries

Known commonly as "burners" or "stingers," brachial plexus (cervical nerve root 8 and thoracic nerve root 1 [C8-T1]) injuries are a frequent occurrence in sports such as football and rugby, where the athlete's body may be forced in one direction while an arm may be pulled in the opposite direction, causing a contralateral neck flexion and same-side shoulder depression (Schroeder & Vaccaro, 2016). An injury to the brachial plexus typically results in significant but transient symptoms ranging from an intense burning sensation in the shoulder, arm, and hand to loss of sensation or some motor function in the shoulder, arm, wrist, and hand. As shown in Figure 9.7, injury to the brachial plexus typically involves one of two mechanisms—an abnormal traction or abnormal compression of one or more of the large nerves that comprise the entire brachial plexus (C8-T1; Schroeder & Vaccaro, 2016).

Signs and symptoms of brachial plexus injury include the following:

- Immediate neurological symptoms radiate into the affected arm, often described as an intense burning or stinging sensation.
- Voluntary use of the arm significantly decreases (often the arm appears limp).
- Symptoms should be self-correcting, and the involved extremity should return to normal sensation in a few minutes.
- In repeat cases, symptoms as described may persist for days or even weeks. Muscle atrophy, especially of the deltoid muscle, may be apparent. In such cases, medical evaluation is essential before athletes are allowed to return to participation.

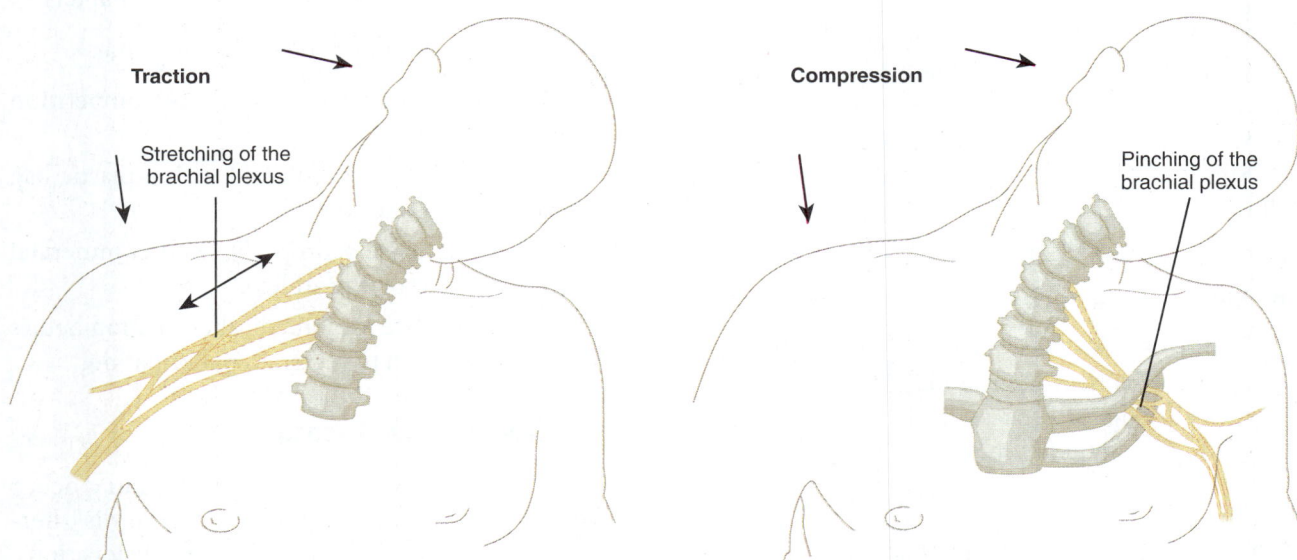

Figure 9.7 Common mechanisms of injury to the brachial plexus.

First aid care of brachial plexus injury involves the following:

1. Because of the nature of brachial plexus injuries, little can be done regarding first aid other than to remove athletes from participation until the symptoms subside.
2. Once on the sideline, continue to monitor the athlete's recovery and do not allow them to return to participation until the symptoms have abated and grip strength in the affected extremity is normal compared to the opposite arm. An ice bag applied to the side of the suspected injury (compressed or distracted side) can often help alleviate symptoms.
3. If symptoms as described do not abate after 10 minutes, refer the athlete for a medical evaluation, after which medical clearance is required before return to participation.

Sprains

Sprains of the cervical spine are common in some sports and generally involve portions of the major ligaments that serve to stabilize the vertebrae. The common mechanisms for these injuries are hyperflexion, hyperextension, lateral flexion, and rotation. These injuries generally involve a significant amount of force, as is seen in contact/collision sports, such as football, ice hockey, rugby, NASCAR racing, and wrestling. Such injuries are usually self-correcting and resolve themselves over a period of days. Occasionally, however, the mechanism of a sprain is severe enough to result in an actual displacement of vertebrae, which can result in more serious neurological problems.

Signs and symptoms of sprains include the following:

- Localized pain in the region of the cervical spine
- Point tenderness over the site of the injury
- Limited range of motion in neck movements
- No obvious neurological deficits (as verified by the neurological test described in the section titled "Physical Examination" earlier in the chapter)

First aid care of sprains involves the following:

1. Remove the athlete from practice/competition that day.
2. Apply ice (best accomplished with a plastic bag filled with crushed ice).
3. If available, place a properly sized commercial cervical collar on the athlete.
4. Refer the athlete for a medical evaluation before they are allowed to return to participation.

Strains

Strains involve the muscles and tendons of the neck region and are normally more painful than serious. Exceptions to this are injuries such as a whiplash, which consists of a combination of joint sprain and musculotendinous strain to the region because of the rapid and forceful back-and-forth movement of the neck. Another point that is important to remember is that indirect head injury is also possible with whiplash because the brain will accelerate in the skull. The mechanism of injury for strains is virtually the same as that described previously for sprains.

Signs and symptoms of strains include the following:

- Localized pain in the region of the cervical spine
- Muscle spasm
- Limited range of motion in neck movements
- No obvious neurological deficits (as verified by the neurological test described in the section titled "Physical Examination" earlier in the chapter)

First aid care of strains involves the following:

1. Remove the athlete from practice/competition that day.
2. Apply ice (best accomplished with a plastic bag filled with crushed ice).
3. If available, place a properly sized commercial cervical collar on the athlete.
4. Refer the athlete for a medical evaluation before they are allowed to return to participation.

Fractures and Dislocations

The most extreme forms of cervical injury occur when the damage involves intervertebral disk herniation, cervical stenosis, fractures, and dislocations, all of which result in pressure being placed directly on the spinal cord. The spinal cord is extremely sensitive to such trauma, and permanent neurological damage and even death can occur depending on the specific location of the injury. Any of the forceful ranges of motion described earlier can result in either a fracture or dislocation; however, axial loading is associated with many of the more severe forms of injury (Boden et al., 2006). The effect of a vertebral fracture or dislocation on the spinal cord is fairly obvious because the movement of bones or bone fragments can impinge or damage the spinal cord; however, discussing cervical disk herniation and cervical stenosis is important. Cervical disk herniation is quite common in tackle football and rugby players and may result in transient sensation and strength loss (Schroeder & Vaccaro, 2016). Cervical stenosis, which involves the spinal canal being too small for the spinal cord and nerve roots, can be congenital or can occur as a result of repeated poor tackling techniques, which ultimately change the curvature of the cervical spine and narrow the spinal canal width (called **spear tackler's spine**; Schroeder & Vaccaro, 2016). The spinal cord may also suffer damage secondary to the initial trauma as a result of circulatory problems caused by severed or impinged arteries and swelling of the spinal cord. When bleeding and swelling happen, neurological problems will likely be present (Brigham & Capo, 2013). Therefore, these injuries represent true medical emergencies and require the best care possible.

Signs and symptoms of factures and dislocations include the following (in the case of unconscious athletes, the primary objectives are to stabilize the head and neck, summon EMS, and provide basic life support by gaining access to the airway and/or chest):

- Report from athlete of having felt or heard something pop or snap in their neck at the time of injury
- Severe pain localized in the region of the cervical spine associated with muscle spasm
- Difficulty swallowing
- Deformity in the vertebrae, as detected by palpation
- Burning, numbness, or tingling sensations in the neck, extremities, and/or trunk
- Weakness in either bilateral or unilateral grip strength and/or ankle dorsiflexion
- Complete absence of or altered sensation in the neck, extremities, and/or trunk
- Complete absence of or altered motor function in the extremities and/or trunk
- Loss of bowel/bladder control

First aid care of fractures and dislocations involves the following:

1. Complete the initial check (by using the CEMEPS mnemonic) and ascertain status of vital signs.
2. After initial check is complete, proceed to the physical examination. If any of the previously listed signs and symptoms are present, proceed to the following steps.
3. Stabilize the head and neck immediately. The emergency plan should designate a team leader who will immediately apply manual spinal stabilization (Figure 9.6 and Figure 9.9); in the case of helmeted football players, do not immediately remove the helmet to gain stabilization; rather, use the helmet to assist in stabilization of the head and neck.
4. If CPR is necessary, both the helmet and shoulder pads should be removed to maintain proper spinal alignment (Courson et al., 2020).
5. Summon EMS.
6. Do not attempt to move the athlete without a full medical team present; rather, when other trained personnel arrive, work as a team to ensure the neck is stabilized with a cervical collar (or other device) and place the athlete onto the spine board or other spinal immobilization device.
7. Continue to monitor vital signs until EMS arrives.

Spear tackler's spine Diagnosed via X-ray, the cervical spine shows changes, including a narrowing of the spine at the neck or loss of the normal curvature of the spine, and/or changes resulting from trauma to the spine; a strict contraindication for further participation in tackle sports.

Athletic Trainers SPEAK OUT

What Is the Role of the AT When a Concussion Is Suspected?

A concussion is a complex traumatic brain injury that if undetected can put athletes at risk for catastrophic injury. Evidenced-based research suggests that the best course of action when a concussion is suspected is immediate removal from participation. ATs play a vital role following a concussive incident because they are often the only healthcare professional on-site with the knowledge and skills to properly assess the injury. The AT becomes even more crucial when you consider the possibility that an athlete may also be suffering from a severe neurological, cranial, or cervical spine injury due to their sharing a common mechanism with concussion. Additionally, concussions are highly individualized, and no two will have the same presentation, further complicating the situation and making the AT's role more challenging. Therefore, ATs are responsible for being vigilant and continually monitoring athletes throughout athletic practices and competitions for a concussion.

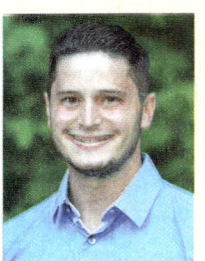

Courtesy of Christopher P. Tomczyk, MS, ATC.

Recognition of a concussion is key to activating the acute assessment process. An AT needs to be equipped with the most up-to-date knowledge surrounding the injury to be effective. Concussions can be the result of a direct blow to the head, face, or neck or a blow to the body that transmits biomechanical forces up to the brain. It should be on an ATs list of differential diagnoses following any collision and/or rotational-based mechanism involving the head. Early recognition of a concussion is critical to maximizing favorable postinjury outcomes.

Evaluation is vital to the acute assessment process to identify the present state of the athlete. Current literature suggests that a multifaceted approach be used to assess a concussive injury that includes a physical exam, a symptom checklist, postural-stability and vestibular/ocular assessments, and neurocognitive testing. The role of the AT is to be proficient in the administration and interpretation of multiple sideline tools that address these areas. An important point to remember is that concussion signs and symptoms do not always present immediately after injury and may take up to 24–48 hours to develop. Therefore, the recommendation is for an AT to perform a follow-up assessment the following day. If at any point a concussion is suspected, the ATs job is to remove the athlete from participation immediately!

Management of a concussed athlete through the stepwise RTP progression should begin within 24–48 hours after a concussion diagnosis. The AT will facilitate the athlete's reintegration into sports participation, which aims to gradually introduce daily physical activity, exercise, and sports-related activities. This process will be individualized, and the AT will need to understand the goals of each stage accurately to safely progress the athlete through participation.

Overall, the ATs role when a concussion occurs is complex. It requires extensive knowledge of injury specifics in combination with proficient evaluation and management skills. ATs are equipped for the challenge if they can **recognize**, **evaluate**, and **manage** athletes who have incurred a concussion.

—Christopher P. Tomczyk, MS, ATC

Christopher P. Tomczyk is a doctoral student in the Sport Injury Research Lab at Michigan State University in Lansing, Michigan.

Initial Management of a Suspected Cervical Spine Injury: Guidelines

When considering specific actions in treating an athlete with a suspected CSI, an immediate distinction must be made. Is the athlete conscious or unconscious? With the unconscious athlete, the assumption must be that both head and neck injuries are present; therefore, spinal motion restriction with head and neck stabilization will be necessary (Figure 9.6) throughout. Next, the primary objective is to determine whether the athlete's life is in immediate jeopardy. Does the athlete have a pulse? Does the athlete have an open airway? Is the athlete breathing? These questions are answered during the initial check discussed earlier in the chapter. If the answer to any of these questions is no, EMS must be summoned, and basic life support must be initiated and continued until EMS personnel arrive. With the conscious athlete, the level of spinal motion restriction necessary can be determined by asking questions and performing the short CEMEPS evaluation. Blunt trauma and altered level of consciousness, spinal pain or tenderness, loss of cervical range of motion, neurological complaint or findings (e.g., numbness or motor weakness in more than one limb), and/or anatomic deformity of the spine are reasons to proceed with in-line head and neck stabilization (Figure 9.6) and spinal motion restriction with a spine board (Figure 9.8), scoop stretcher (Figure 9.9a), or vacuum body immobilizer (Figure 9.9b; Courson et al., 2020). In general, when dealing with a suspected CSI (unconscious or conscious), the most important criterion should be prevention of further injury by ensuring the best method of spinal motion restriction and mode of transfer (Courson et al., 2020; Mills et al., 2020). The appropriate prehospital treatment of a suspected CSI may mitigate long-lasting health and financial effects on the injured athlete and/or family members (Courson et al., 2020).

Regarding CSI, athletes are either equipment laden (e.g., tackle football, lacrosse, and ice hockey) or nonequipment laden (e.g., soccer, gymnastics, and track and field). To effectively access the chest and airway with equipment-laden athletes, the face mask and/or helmet will need to be removed

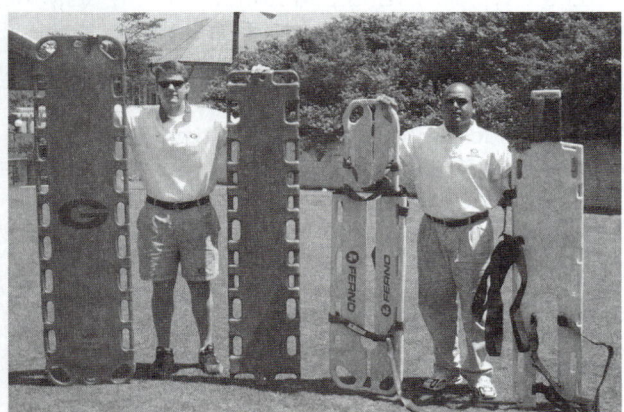

Figure 9.8 Examples of spine boards used to immobilize injured athletes.

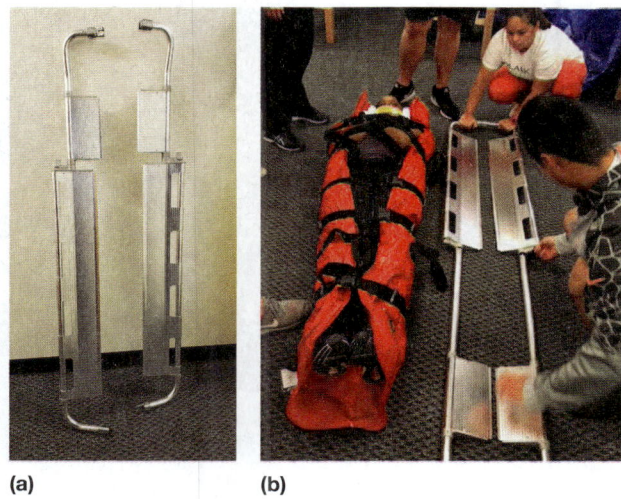

Figure 9.9 (a) Scoop stretcher. **(b)** Vacuum immobilizer and scoop stretcher.
Courtesy of Cindy Trowbridge.

(Courson et al., 2020). If the helmet must be removed and the athlete is wearing shoulder pads, then the shoulder pads and helmet should be removed as one unit to maintain spinal motion restriction (Courson et al., 2020). For nonequipment-laden athletes, no special instructions apply regarding spinal motion restriction.

Though head and neck injuries carry the potential of catastrophic results regardless of the sport, equipment-laden athletes who sustain such injuries do present special problems because of their equipment. The standard equipment protecting the player's head and neck is a helmet with an attached face mask and chin strap (Figure 9.10). Mouth guards for protection of teeth and shoulder pads for chest protection are also used. Dealing with a compromised airway or circulation problems (i.e., lack of pulse or arrhythmia) can be made very difficult by helmets and face masks and shoulder pads, respectively. Management procedures for equipment-laden athletes have become a major issue in the sports medicine community; however, medical organizations are relying on evidence-based recommendations, and management protocols are updated regularly to reflect the understanding of CSIs and appropriate immediate management related to different equipment types (Courson et al., 2020; Mills et al., 2020). Ultimately, the proper planning of an event will optimize care, and all protocols should be developed specific to the sports venue, sports equipment, and the available medical resources, with

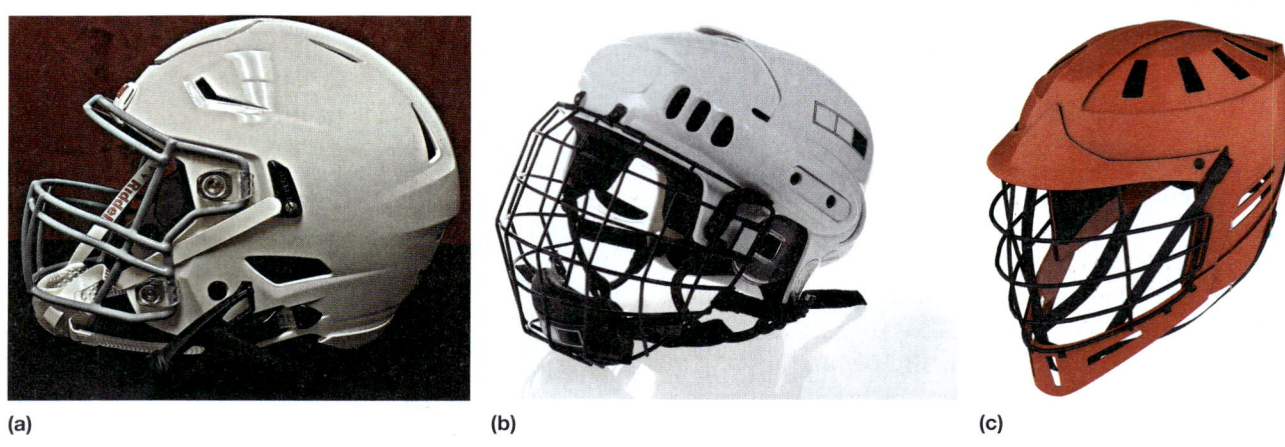

Figure 9.10 Examples of helmets used in football, ice hockey, and lacrosse. **(a)** Football helmets can come in a variety of designs; pictured is the quick-release Riddell helmet, which has a small tool available to release the face mask. **(b)** Ice hockey and **(c)** lacrosse helmets often fit differently than football helmets and have more rigid face-mask and jaw-protection attachments.
(a) Courtesy of Cindy Trowbridge; (b) © Flashon Studio/Shutterstock; (c) © VitaminCo/Shutterstock.

guidelines that focus on controlling scene safety, activating the EMS system, directing EMS to the scene, and initiating and directing care of injured athletes based on their presentation (Courson et al., 2020).

The sponsoring organization of the sport should have an EAP for handling athletes with head and neck injuries (see Chapter 7). One staff member, typically a qualified medical professional (QMP), must be designated as the emergency team leader, whose primary responsibility is the supervision of the entire management process. In addition, the team leader must monitor the position of the athlete's head and neck, making sure that they are not moved unnecessarily (Figure 9.11). Special consideration must be given to the care and handling of equipment-laden football players (**Time Out 9.5**). If no QMP is present, then a coach or physical educator must assume the emergency team leader position and ensure that the injured athlete is not moved and the EAP is implemented. The techniques of how to effectively and safely transport athletes with head and neck injuries must be practiced on an annual basis so that if and when an injury happens all personnel will be ready for their role (Courson et al., 2020). Training does not mandate correct implementation, so practice of these techniques is essential. This is especially true when the potential for catastrophic injury if a head or neck injury is improperly handled is considered. Fortunately, in the vast majority of school sports situations, EMS should be readily available. Even in rural or remote settings, EMS are typically within 30 minutes. If any delay of EMS is anticipated in excess of 30 minutes, having multiple people trained in effective head and neck in-line stabilization is prudent so the transfer of care can continue until a larger medical team arrives with equipment (Courson et al., 2020).

Prehospital Care for the Treatment of Head and Neck Injuries in Football

An interagency task force with several medical societies, including the NATA, was convened in 1998 to develop standardized medical guidelines for the

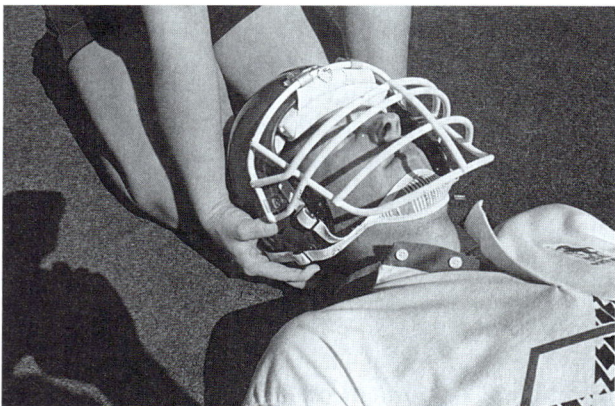

Figure 9.11 In the event of a neck injury, the helmet provides an excellent means of cervical immobilization, along with the steady hands of a rescuer.
Courtesy of Ron Pfeiffer.

TIME OUT 9.5

Guidelines for Appropriate Care of the Spine-Injured Athlete

EMERGENCY PREPAREDNESS

- The EAP is an essential component of care for CSI injuries. Development of the EAP should be a collaborative effort of the sports medicine team, local EMS personnel, coaches, administrators, officials, and others who might be involved in helping to provide emergency care.
- Medical time-outs need to be performed before each event to avoid miscommunications that can lead to serious errors. During the medical time-out, members of the care team and others should review who the QMP are on-site and their roles, what equipment is available, the management protocols for patients with suspected CSI, and information on transport protocols and signals and communication used to summon advanced emergency care.

INITIAL CARE

The initial care of athletes with a suspected CSI may involve a variety of techniques to ensure the maintenance of breathing and circulation and the stabilization of the spinal column so no further damage occurs. Key areas to consider are scene control and equipment removal.

- Scene control
  - Ensuring a calm and orderly environment with a buffer zone around injured patients will facilitate optimal medical care. Usually, nonmedical personnel, including coaches and officials, can assist in scene control.
- Equipment removal for airway and chest access
  - The top focus when considering helmet, face mask, and shoulder pad removal is maintaining circulation, airway, and breathing. Important considerations when deciding to remove equipment are the athlete's weight, equipment make and model, and types of immobilization devices available.
  - If transport is essential, then the face mask must be removed regardless of airway status so that if there is compromise in breathing, the airway can be accessed. Individuals with the highest level of training, comfort, familiarity, and experience in managing patients with a suspected CSI should remove equipment. Following are evidence-based recommendations:
    - Trained personnel and appropriate tools need to be available, and discretion of how to remove equipment should be dependent on the situation and the personnel at the scene. The highest priority is maintaining cervical alignment throughout the process of equipment removal. Care providers should have more than one method available for removing a face mask because the type of construction and hardware can vary among equipment even on the same team.
    - A variety of techniques can be employed to appropriately and safely remove equipment. Current evidence-based recommendations follow:
      - Removing face mask only: Two people should be involved in removing the face mask (one maintains in-line stabilization and the other uses tools to remove the face mask).
      - Removing helmet and shoulder pads: At least two people should be involved in removing the helmet and two to four people for optimally removing shoulder pads. Both depend, though, on the equipment, athlete's size, and technique being used.

SPINAL MOTION RESTRICTION AND SAFE TRANSFER

A procedure should be developed to ensure that athletes with a suspected spinal column injury be appropriately restricted and transported to a designated Level I or II trauma center as quickly and safely as possible. However, the use of a long spine board and complete immobilization for any suspected CSI has declined as evidence has emerged regarding its effectiveness (Morrissey, 2013; NATA, 2014). Being aware of any local or state EMS protocols

(continues)

> **TIME OUT 9.5** *(continued)*
>
> regarding these changes is also important. Spinal motion restriction in some form is essential if any of the following conditions are present:
>
> - Blunt trauma or an altered level of consciousness
> - Spinal pain or tenderness
> - Anatomic deformity of the spine
> - Loss of cervical range of motion
> - Neurological complaints or findings, such as numbness or motor weakness
>
> In-line stabilization is the first step when a CSI is suspected and can be accomplished in a variety of ways, including head squeeze or trapezius muscle squeeze. The rescuer's thumbs should always be pointing toward the face of the patient. Evidence regarding the use of neutral alignment and distraction or leaving the head and neck in the position they are found has not been determined. Regardless, neck position should ensure an open airway, and a neutral spine alignment seems to reduce spinal cord morbidity caused by compromised circulation. However, realigning should not be attempted if it is difficult to do or increases the patient's pain or other symptoms.
>
> All emergencies and patients are different, so rescuers should practice a variety of transfer techniques with different types of equipment (rigid spine board, vacuum immobilizer, scoop stretcher, and cervical collar). The rescuer at the head is the one in charge and should deliver clear and direct commands during the spinal motion restriction and transfer of patients. Evidence from data regarding nonathletes with spinal injuries indicates that any equipment used to immobilize should be left in place for transport and if a long, rigid spine board is used, then the time on the board should be minimized. Two general techniques are recommended for transfer to an immobilization device, such as a long spine board, scoop stretcher, vacuum immobilizer, or padded stretcher. Each technique requires a different number of personnel to accomplish the transfer, but both require rescuers at the head, shoulders/chest, hips, and lower extremities.
>
> - The logroll is used for both prone and supine athletes. Athletes are rolled either away or toward rescuers so the spinal immobilization device can be placed appropriately. When using the push technique, athletes are rolled away from rescuers, and when using the pull technique, athletes are rolled toward rescuers. If athletes are prone, the logroll push techniques are superior to the pull technique:
>   - The supine logroll requires at least five rescuers, prone logroll push requires at least five rescuers, and prone logroll pull requires at least four rescuers.
> - The multiperson lift is used for supine athletes and requires at least eight rescuers. Studies on cadavers have demonstrated that this technique seems to result in the least amount of spinal motion.
>
> Use of a cervical motion restriction device (cervical collar) is important if equipment is removed, but placement can be difficult if equipment remains in place. However, even if a device is used, the recommendation is that manual in-line stabilization be continued throughout the transfer until the head is secured. A variety of techniques can be used to secure the head and provide additional stabilization, including head blocks, rolls, blankets, and tape; however, securing the head occurs after the torso and lower extremities are secured. Tape can be applied to the chin and at the eyebrow level on the forehead for optimal stabilization.
>
> A variety of strap types are available to effectively secure a patient: hook and loop, clip, pin, and Velcro. When strapping patients to an immobilization device, the recommendation is to use an X-strap approach whereby the straps come across the shoulders and chest like a seat belt. Other straps at the hips and along the lower extremities are essential as well. The torso needs to be secured first, with the arms free, so that EMS can access veins for intravenous injections or neurovascular assessment, but the wrists can be taped to restrain movement. Restriction of spinal motion should be maintained at all times during transport, but if extra equipment (i.e., long spine board or scoop stretcher) can be removed safely, then do so.
>
> Data from Mills, B. M., Conrick, K. M., Anderson, S., Bailes, J., Boden, B. P., Conway, D., . . . Courson, R. (2020). Consensus recommendations on the prehospital care of the injured athlete with a suspected catastrophic cervical spine injury. *Journal of Athletic Training, 55*(6), 563–572; and Courson, R., Ellis, J., Herring, S. A., Boden, B. P., Henry, G., Conway, D., . . . Walpert, K. P. (2020). Best practices and current care concepts in prehospital care of the spine-injured athlete in American tackle football March 2–3, 2019, Atlanta, GA. *Journal of Athletic Training, 55*(6), 545–562.

proper prehospital care of spine-injured athletes. The intent was to eliminate the confusion that existed at that time among medical providers as to what constituted the proper care for athletes with a suspected CSI. The task force published a position statement that was subsequently updated two times in 2009 with a new position statement (Swartz et al., 2009) and in 2014-2015 with an official statement and executive committee statements (NATA, 2014; NATA, 2015). The most recent update is within a consensus statement (Mills et al., 2020) and a best practices and current care concepts document (Courson et al., 2020). Overall, the updates have reflected a better understanding of equipment removal from equipment-laden athletes and provided evidence-based information regarding the type and technique of spinal motion restriction to use in different situations (Courson et al., 2020; Mills et al., 2020; Morrissey, 2013; NATA, 2014; NATA, 2015; Swartz et al., 2009). Time Out 9.5 briefly outlines several of the guidelines from the two most recent publications by Mills and colleagues (2020) and Courson and colleagues (2020). The purpose of the consensus statement (Mills et al., 2020) was to identify several important prehospital care questions and provide evidence-based responses to these questions from collected and reviewed literature. The purpose of the best practices document (Courson et al., 2020) was to outline details regarding practical treatments based on the consensus recommendations. Figures 9.12 to 9.15 provide examples of proper stabilization and teamwork for placing a spine-injured equipment-laden athlete on a rigid spine board. Exact details regarding the practical management of the spine-injured athlete are not provided because that is beyond the scope of the chapter; however, readers are encouraged to explore this information based on their future career interests.

Coaching and physical education personnel are advised to exercise extreme caution when making decisions about immediate care of equipment-laden athletes with possible head and/or neck injury. Removal of the helmet and other equipment, unless executed by a physician or other emergency care provider, such as an AT or a paramedic, should be avoided unless it is absolutely necessary.

In situations where an airway must be established and breathing assistance must be given by a coach or physical educator, then the carefully and properly executed removal of only the face mask is the most prudent approach. Depending

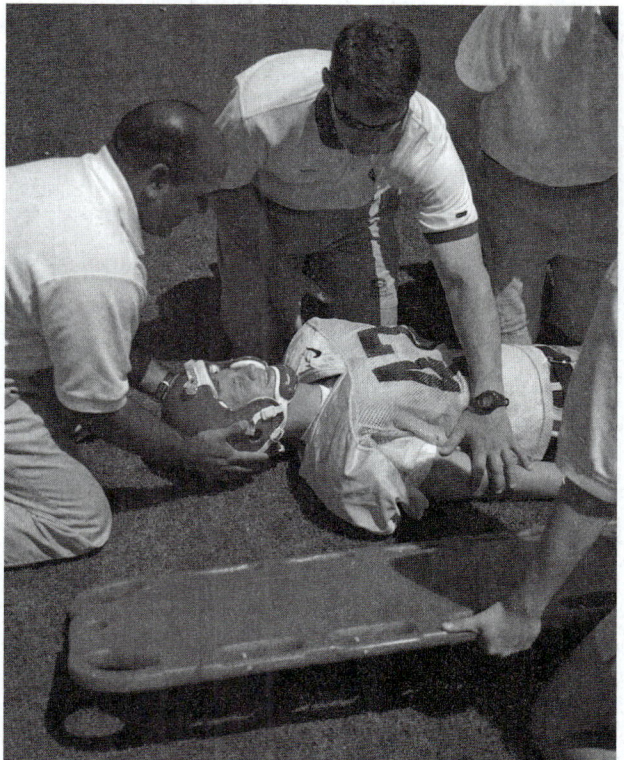

Figure 9.12 Members of the rescue team are stationed at the legs, hips, and shoulders, with the team leader providing stabilization to the head and neck.

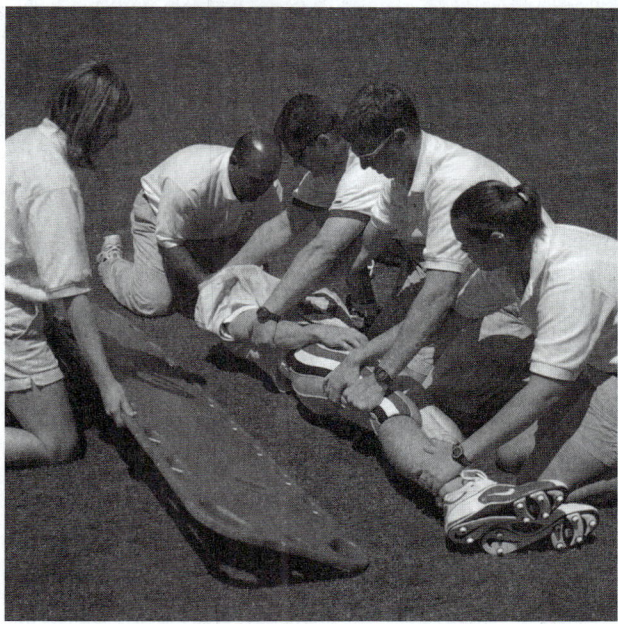

Figure 9.13 At the command of the team leader, the team rotates the athlete, as a unit, to enable movement of the spine board.

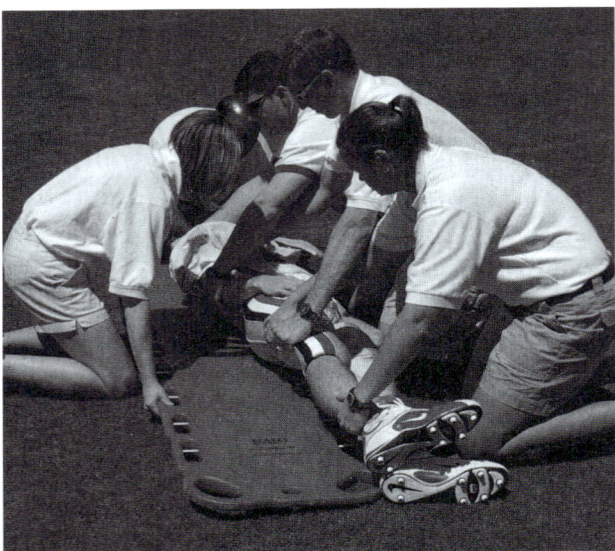

Figure 9.14 A fifth team member slides the spine board under the athlete. Note how the straps are placed to facilitate ease of securing the athlete to the board.

on the age and design of the helmet, removal of the face mask can be accomplished in a variety of ways. Because a variety of types of face masks exist for the various athletic helmets available, their attachments to the helmets are different (Figure 9.10), making the removal of face masks different based on the helmet. Many football face masks are attached by a hard plastic loop-and-strap system with a screw attachment (Figure 9.16). The majority of current designs secure the face mask to the helmet with small plastic clips (loop straps) attached to the helmet with screws, and the loops or straps can be cut off with a cutting tool (Figure 9.17a and b) or removed with a handheld screwdriver or cordless electric screwdriver (Figure 9.17c). However, recent advancements in football helmets have introduced quick-release buttons that require only a plastic tool or any small-tipped device to disengage the connection point (Figure 9.10). Removal of the plastic straps on the top and each side of the face mask—using devices such as a cordless screwdriver, handheld pruner, wire cutters, or tin snips (Figure 9.17)—while the head and neck are stabilized will allow the mask to be removed completely (Figure 9.18). Lifting the face mask from the helmet as opposed to rotating it is important because rotating it causes more motion. Coaching personnel must be aware of the specific types of equipment their athletes are wearing in the event that such an emergency arises. Research on the most effective method of face mask removal has produced varying results, depending on the type of

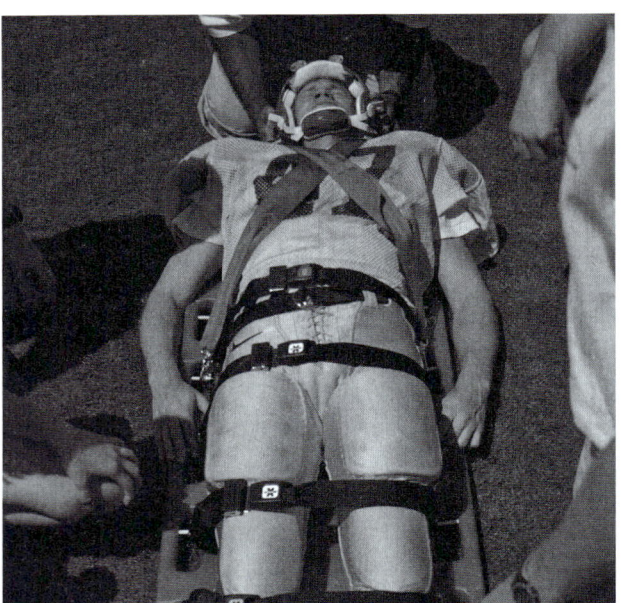

Figure 9.15 The athlete is firmly secured to the board with straps holding the ankles/feet, thigh/pelvis/arms, shoulders, and head and neck.

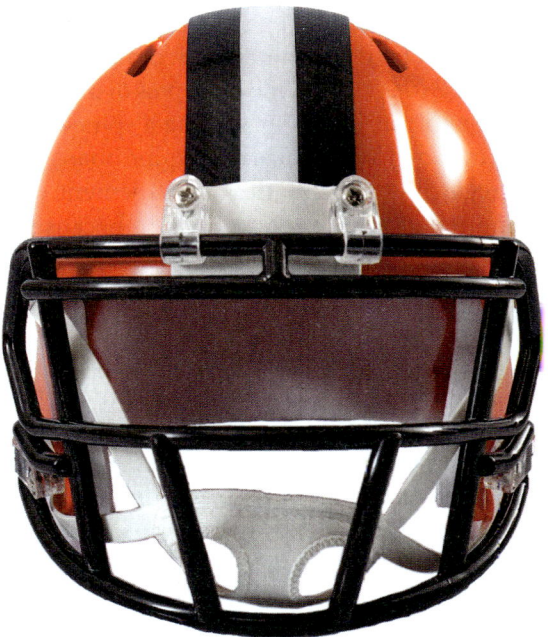

Figure 9.16 The loop, strap, and screw system is still a common football helmet type.
© Victor Moussa/Shutterstock.

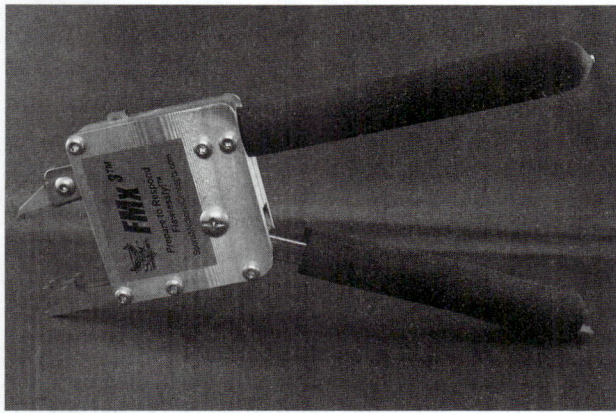
(a)

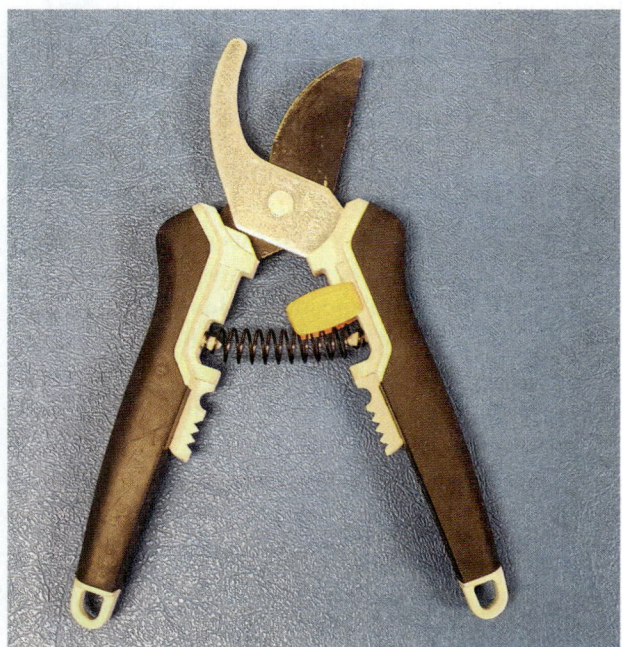
(b)

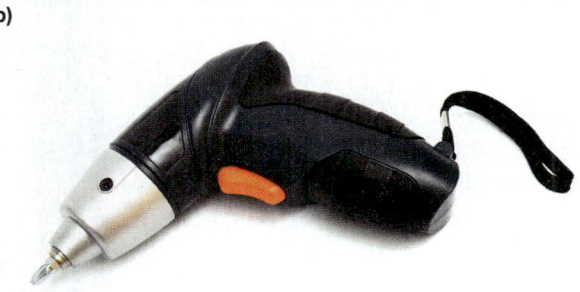
(c)

Figure 9.17 In the event of an injury, qualified personnel can use cutting tools, such as **(a)** the FM Extractor (FME) or **(b)** handheld pruners, to cut the straps on each side of the player's face mask or **(c)** a cordless screwdriver to unscrew the attachments for the face clips.
(a) © Sports Medicine Concepts, Inc.; (b) Courtesy of Cindy Trowbridge; (c) © terekhov igor/Shutterstock.

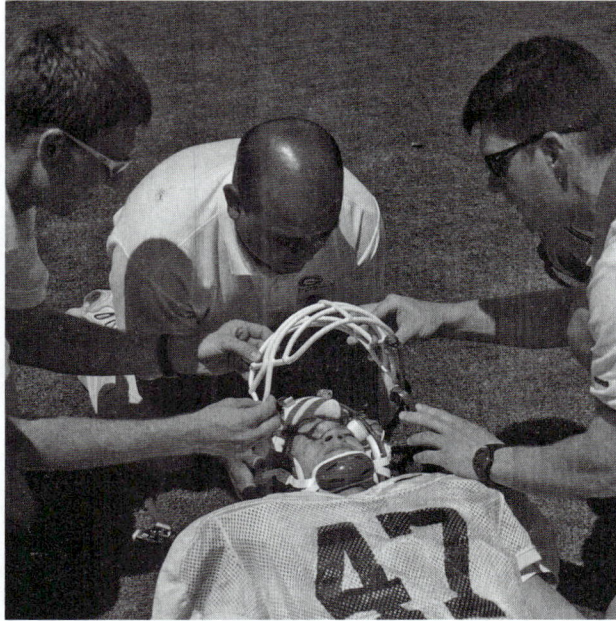

Figure 9.18 Once the face mask has been released, it can be lifted up and away from the player's face and then completely removed from the area.

face-mask clip system and whether it has been altered from the manufacturer's specifications. However, the recommended technique is to use a cordless screwdriver (assuming the face mask is attached to the helmet and is secured with screws). A further recommendation is that if this fails for some reason, the first responder should have an appropriate cutting tool on hand to cut the straps (Swartz et al., 2009; Swartz et al., 2010). A critical point to remember is that the head and neck must be stabilized at all times, including during removal of the face mask (Figure 9.18).

Remember, in most instances, there is no reason to move an injured player from the field before EMS personnel arrive. No game or practice is so important that it cannot be delayed to ensure proper first aid for an injured player.

Injuries to the Maxillofacial Region

A variety of injuries can occur to the maxillofacial region of the body, which includes the jaw and teeth, eyes, ears, nose, throat, facial bones, and facial skin, but estimates of facial injury rates are complicated because of a lack of or inconsistent reporting on specific types of injury (Black, Eliason, et al., 2017). Fortunately, with the advent of modern technology, protective equipment has been developed for use in high-risk sports; however, not all athletes playing high-risk sports adopt prevention methods (Black, Patton, et al., 2017). Athlete comfort and risk perception and utility and a lack of awareness or enforcement are often reasons athletes may not adopt preventive measures (Black, Patton, et al., 2017).

Dental Injuries

There are 32 teeth in the human adult upper and lower jaws, the majority of which are located just inside the front and sides of the mouth, where they are vulnerable to external blows common in collision and contact sports. Teeth are firmly secured into either the maxilla (upper jaw) or mandible (lower jaw) by way of the root, which is cemented into the sockets of the jaws with a specialized form of bone known as cementum. In addition, the sockets are lined with periosteum, which aids in securing the teeth to the jaw. The consequences of dental trauma for child and adolescent athletes include pain, psychological effects, and financial burdens (Spadinger, 2019).

Specific Injuries

In the United States, more than 5 million teeth are avulsed every year, costing hundreds of millions of dollars for proper care, with football, hockey, basketball, and martial arts experiencing the most risk of dental injuries (Young et al., 2015). The majority of dental injuries in sports are from direct blows resulting in orofacial lacerations and tooth trauma, such as tooth displacement; a fracture or avulsion; and in extreme cases, fracture or dislocation of the jaw or fractures of other facial bones (Anitha et al., 2020). Signs and symptoms of dental injury are listed in **Time Out 9.6**, along with the most likely injury.

Initial Check and Treatment: Guidelines

Whenever rendering first aid to someone suffering a dental injury, an important point to remember is that prognosis depends on the time between the injury and advanced dental care. For this reason, including immediate dental injury management in the EAP is highly recommended, specifically identifying an oral health care specialist for athletes to be referred. For high school and younger athletes, the referral can be to their pediatric dentist, and for collegiate athletes,

TIME OUT 9.6

Dental Injuries

Type of Injury	Signs and Symptoms
Tooth displacement	A single tooth or several displaced teeth pushed either forward or backward, with bleeding along the gum line.
Tooth fracture	Defects (missing fragments) are obvious along the crown of the tooth or a vertical fracture line is visible in the tooth. Less severe fractures are not painful when breathing through the mouth, whereas more severe fractures (at or below the gum line) are extremely painful, and the tooth is often loose.
Fractures of the jaw and other bones	Fractures of the jaw (mandible or maxilla) result in loosening of adjacent teeth, along with bleeding gums and numbness. In the case of fracture of the mandible, obvious deformity and an inability to open or close the mouth are apparent.
Tooth avulsion	Missing tooth with bleeding from the exposed socket.

the referral is usually to a team dentist as part of the sports medicine team. This oral healthcare specialist is then able to refer athletes to an endodontist, orthodontist, or oral and maxillofacial surgeon (Gould et al., 2016).

The recommendation is that a dental kit containing the following items be kept in a sealed, container separate from other supplies within the athletic training kit:

- Adhesive tape
- Biohazard bags
- Cotton rolls and applicators
- Dental floss
- Extra mouth guards
- Gauze, gloves, goggles, mask
- Tongue depressor
- Tooth kit
- Scissors
- Penlight

In the college setting, the team dentist may request and/or supply dental-specific items for this kit (Gould et al., 2016).

Because blood is common with oral injuries, protective gloves (latex) and eye protection, such as goggles, should be worn. Collecting the history of the accident is important by identifying where the injury is within the mouth and noting any symptoms, such as sharp or throbbing pain versus tooth sensitivity (Gould et al., 2016).

During the physical examination, the athlete should be checked to see whether they can open and close their mouth without pain or difficulty. The general symmetry of their teeth should be assessed by looking for irregularities visible in adjacent teeth, and the upper and lower teeth should be examined separately and carefully by noting any bleeding around the gum line or teeth as well as obvious chips or fractures.

Treatment for dental injuries includes direct finger pressure with sterile gauze over any area of bleeding. In the case of jaw fractures, misaligned teeth, or severe bleeding, athletes should be immediately referred to an oral healthcare specialist, and further damage should be prevented with stabilization and application of ice to reduce inflammation. In the case of tooth avulsions, every effort should be made to locate the tooth and protect it by placing it into either a commercially prepared dental kit, cool milk, or the athlete's saliva in a cup (Anitha et al., 2020; Young et al., 2015), after which the athlete should immediately be sent to a dentist or physician to have the tooth effectively put back into place. Time is of the essence in these situations, and the prognosis for the original tooth is poor if more than 30 minutes pass between the time of the injury and time of replantation in the socket (Anitha et al., 2020). Another important point to remember is that concussions can accompany dental injuries; thus, a neurological assessment should also be performed. Finally, RTP decisions are determined by the treating oral healthcare specialist (Gould et al., 2016).

Protection Against Injury

Obviously, in high-risk sports such as tackle football and ice hockey, a well-fitted mouth guard should be utilized to protect athletes from dental injuries. However, athletes often lack knowledge regarding the occurrence of dental injuries and the proper immediate treatment. The use of either stock or custom-made mouth guards is strongly recommended by the American Dental Association for protection in a variety of sports, including acrobatics, ice hockey, soccer, gymnastics, field hockey, rugby, wrestling, boxing, basketball, lacrosse, skiing, weightlifting, shot-putting, racquetball, softball, baseball, discus throwing, volleyball, and horseback riding (American Dental Association, 2019). In the United States, the use of mouth guards has been required in high school football since 1966, and in 1974 the NCAA mandated their use in tackle football. Since then, ice hockey, field hockey, men's and women's lacrosse, and wrestling have been added to the list of sports that require a mouth guard at the high school level (Lloyd et al., 2017; National Federation of State High School Associations, 2018), but the collegiate level requires mouth guards for only football, lacrosse, and field hockey. However, the NCAA does recommend all athletes in high-risk sports wear a mouth guard, as per the American Dental Association recommendations.

Mouth guards help to prevent lacerations and lessen applied forces to the jaw and teeth area. They separate the upper and lower teeth and absorb or redistribute the shock during a facial or head impact and can stabilize the mandible during a traumatic jaw closure (Green, 2017). However, whether mouth guards prevent mild brain injury (e.g., concussions) has not been thoroughly documented; therefore, mouth guards are not fully recommended for concussion prevention (Green, 2017). Mouth guards have been found to have no adverse effects on strength, performance, or ventilation (Gould et al., 2016), with the only drawback seeming to be speech impairment (Green, 2017). Properly fitted, a mouth guard can significantly reduce or even prevent many dental injuries and dislocations of the temporomandibular joint as well as jaw fractures. (Green, 2017; Gould et al., 2016; Young et al., 2015). All mouth guards fall into one of three groups: stock, mouth formed (boil and bite), and custom (Green, 2017). Stock versions are the least expensive; however, they are generally thought to be the least effective. The most commonly used are the mouth-formed type, and they are probably the most cost-effective for junior and senior high school athletes. The custom-fitted mouth guard provides the best possible fit and protection; however, the cost can be prohibitive for many athletes because specialized equipment and a trained oral health specialist are necessary. Ultimately, a mouth guard should be fitted, bilateral, balanced, and laminated and should cover to the maxillary's first permanent molar with a minimum thickness of 3 millimeters over the gum line and 2 millimeters over the palate (Lloyd et al., 2017). Athletes should not alter the mouth guard for comfort purposes (Gould et al., 2016); they should clean it regularly with an appropriate cleaning agent and store it in a clean environment such as a container. Athletes should also inspect the mouth guard on a daily basis and report any issues to medical personnel (Gould et al., 2016).

Eye Injuries

The human eye is an incredibly complex structure in the orbit of the skull (Figure 9.19). The front of the eye consists of clear tissue known as the cornea, behind which are the iris (pupil) and lens. In the eyeball is the vitreous body, consisting of transparent, semigelatinous material that essentially fills the globe of the eye. The posterior surface of the inside of the eye is covered by the retina, which contains the specialized neural cells of vision known as rods

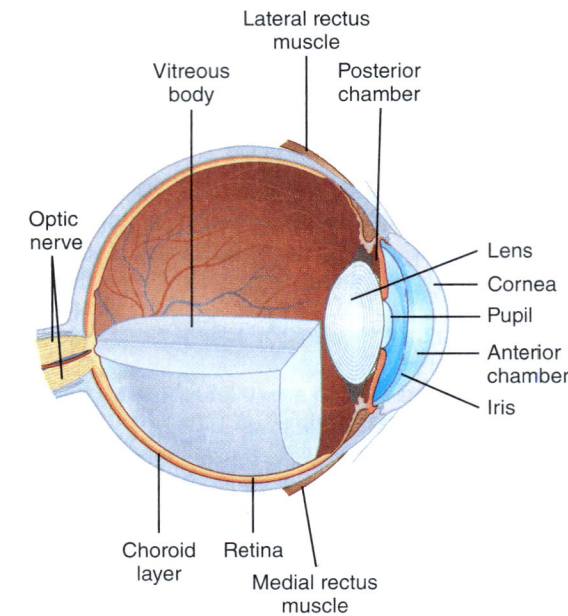

Figure 9.19 Anatomy of the eye.

and cones. With the exception of the clear tissue on the anterior surface of the eye, the majority of the eyeball is encased in a tough tissue known as the sclera.

Approximately 40,000 sports-related eye injuries occur annually in the United States, and it is believed that 90% of these injuries are preventable (Dashtevska & Ivanova, 2020). One-third of the victims are under the age of 16 years, and many of these injuries lead to vision loss and permanent blindness (Boden et al., 2017; Prevent Blindness, 2020). In high school sports, close to 90% of eye injuries were caused by contact, and in college sports close to 86% of eye injuries were contact related. The most common contact mechanism was player contact, followed by contact with a sports ball (Boden et al., 2017). The average cost of an eye injury to a child can be around $3,000–$7,000 (Brophy, Sinclair, Hostetler, Xiang, 2006). The sports with the highest associated risks are basketball, baseball, hockey, racket sports, lacrosse, fencing, paintball, boxing, water polo, soccer, football, and downhill skiing. Perhaps most distressing is the conclusion by medical experts that the majority of these eye injuries (90%) would have been preventable with properly fitting eye protection (Black, Patton, et al., 2017; Dashtevska & Ivanova, 2020; Rodriguez et al., 2003).

With their increasing popularity, sports such as racquetball, squash, and badminton have produced an increase in eye trauma as well. Problems related to these sports include the small size of the striking objects (balls and shuttlecocks), their velocity (Table 9.7), and the sometimes confined areas (squash) in which the games are played. Together, these factors greatly increase the probability of injury.

Specific Injuries

Eye injuries fall into two categories: contusional and penetrating (Dashtevska, 2018). A contusional injury is the result of a blow from a blunt object such as a squash or tennis ball. Contusional injuries vary greatly in severity, ranging from simple corneal abrasions to major distortions of the eyeball that result in rupture of the eye, fracture of the inner orbit, or a combination of the two. Additionally, the retina may be torn away from the inside of the eye, resulting in an injury commonly known as a detached retina. Penetrating injuries of the eye are less common but can occur in shooting sports or even as the result of defective protective eye equipment. Signs and symptoms of eye injury are listed in **Time Out 9.7**.

Table 9.7
Potential Speed of Sports Objects

Sports Object	Potential Speed
Shuttlecock (badminton birdie)	332–493 km/h
Golf ball	235–339 km/h
Jai alai (3/4 size of baseball)	302 km/h
Squash or racquetball	281 km/h
Tennis ball	249–263 km/h
Soccer ball	211 km/h
Hockey puck	184 km/h
Baseball	174 km/h
Cricket ball	161 km/h
Table tennis ball	113 km/h

Data from Nadolny, M. (2014, September 11). *Shuttlecock and balls: The fastest moving objects in sport.* Retrieved from https://olympic.ca/2014/09/11/shuttlecock-and-balls-the-fastest-moving-objects-in-sport/

TIME OUT 9.7

Eye Injuries

Type of Injury	Signs and Symptoms
Corneal abrasion/small foreign object	Pain, irritation, reddening, abrasion, and excessive tearing. In some cases, an object can be visible if the eyelid is pulled upward.
Orbital hematoma (contusion or black eye)	Discoloration around eyelid and surrounding tissue. Vision may be distorted or blurred.
Fractured orbit	Signs and symptoms for orbital hematoma but often includes double vision (diplopia) and rapid swelling above the eyes. Difficulty moving eye with potential that eye is trapped in downward position (unable to move eye up).
Hyphema	Severe contusion to eye. Blood will pool in the anterior portion of the eye and appear as if the pupil is filling with blood. Blurred or blocked vision is common.
Retinal detachment	Often an insidious onset after a contusion or a "whipping of the head." Abrupt changes in the amount of light or visual field occur: flashing lights, blurred vision, floating particles in the field of vision, and a "curtain over the eye" are commonly reported.

Initial Check and Treatment: Guidelines

Before administering treatment for any eye injury, consider whether an ophthalmological (eye physician) referral is needed (Pujalte, 2010). Referral is needed if there is visual field obstruction or physical damage to the anatomy of the eye. A simple penlight can be used to investigate and compare the injured eye with the uninjured eye. The majority of sports-related eye problems involve either simple corneal abrasions or a small foreign object in the eye, which will likely not need referral if there are no visual changes. The symptoms for each are often nearly identical: pain, irritation, and excessive tearing. The eye can be quickly examined by gently holding the upper eyelid up and away from the eye while checking the anterior of the eyeball for any problems (Figure 9.20). Small foreign bodies are usually washed away from the center of the eye by tears. Therefore, the particle may be below the lower eyelid or on the side of the eyeball at a site known as the medial canthus. If the foreign object can be seen, it can usually be carefully removed with a moist cotton swab or piece of gauze. If no object can be seen in the eye, the injury is most likely a *corneal abrasion*. Do not allow athletes to continue participation until the symptoms abate. If they persist or vision is severely disturbed, athletes should be referred to the appropriate medical specialist for further evaluation. If the small object appears to be imbedded in the eye tissue, both eyes should be carefully covered with clean gauze and transport of the athlete to a medical facility should be immediately arranged. Covering the uninjured eye is important to avoid movement of the damaged eye because the eyes normally move together to produce a visual image, which is known as "sympathetic eye movement."

When the eye receives a significant blow, or contusion (e.g., from being hit by an elbow in a game of basketball or by a squash ball or racquetball), vision is

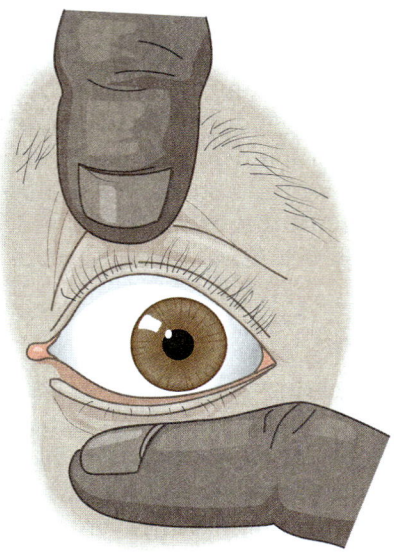

Figure 9.20 Proper positioning of fingers when initially examining the eye.

usually at least temporarily disturbed. In most cases, such an injury causes a black eye (**orbital hematoma**), which results from hemorrhaging of the tissue surrounding the eye. The immediate care of this injury is periodically applying cold until the acute signs of inflammation resolve. In the case of severe contusions, bleeding into the anterior portion of the eye (**hyphema**) may occur quickly and typically results in the visual field being completely or partially blocked. This is a potentially serious sign because it may indicate vascular damage in the eyeball. Athletes with a hyphema should have both eyes patched and be referred immediately for appropriate medical evaluation. Ice should not be applied to a suspected hyphema because the pooled blood may clot, which can cause further damage.

Additionally, contusions to the eye area can cause the eyeball itself to rupture (globe rupture), the orbit to fracture (orbital blowout), or the retina to detach. Athletes with any of these injuries should be immediately referred for further medical evaluation. With a ruptured globe, the eyes should be patched. Its symptoms include pain (especially when attempting to move the eye), double vision (**diplopia**), poor visual acuity, and possibly irregular pupils (Pujalte, 2010). An *orbital blowout* happens when pressure inside the eye increases, then causes the floor of the orbit to fracture. Diplopia, pain, swelling, and discoloration around the eye structure are evident, along

Orbital hematoma Bruising and bleeding associated with a blow to the eye and eye orbit; commonly referred to as a black eye.

Hyphema Accumulated blood in the anterior chamber of the eye from torn blood vessels within anterior eye structures.

Diplopia Double vision.

with restricted movement of the eye (Pujalte, 2010). Because the floor of the orbit is often what fractures, the inferior tissue structure may also become trapped, and athletes will be unable to move the eye upward. Injuries resulting in a **detached retina** can be caused by the mechanisms previously described; however, the symptoms may not be immediately apparent. An **insidious** aspect of this injury is that the retina may slowly fall away from the posterior section of the eye over a period of days, weeks, or even months in some cases. Early symptoms include seeing particles floating inside the eye, distorted vision, and abrupt changes in the amount of light or visual field seen. Athletes with a history of blunt trauma to the eye who later complain of any of these symptoms may have a retinal detachment and should be referred to a medical specialist. Table 9.7 has a list of signs and symptoms.

Contact Lens Problems

Many athletes are fitted with either hard or soft contact lenses, and few difficulties occur with these visual aids. However, if problems do arise, they are more often with hard lenses, mostly resulting from the lens slipping out of place or dust getting trapped between the lens and the eye. On the contrary, soft lenses cover the entire anterior portion of the eye and are less able to migrate around on the eye surface. The materials necessary to deal with problems involving contact lenses should be handy in the first aid kit, including a commercially prepared wetting (saline) solution, a small mirror, and perhaps a contact-lens case.

Protection Against Injury

Although presently not required for all high-risk sports by either the NCAA or high school sports regulatory bodies, protective eyewear is strongly recommended and is growing in popularity (NEI, 2019). Mandatory eye protection has been instituted at the high school and college levels for female lacrosse players, but only high school sports have mandated protective eyewear in field hockey and a batting helmet with an attached face mask for softball (Boden et al., 2017). The primary forms of protective eyewear are goggles, used in sports such as basketball and racket sports, and face shields attached to helmets, used in sports such as football, ice hockey, and baseball/softball (Dashtevska & Ivanova, 2020; NEI, 2019). Although many of these products are made of plastic, the best material is polycarbonate, which is extremely strong and protects well against impacts. The recommendation is that protective eye devices be approved by the American Society for Testing and Materials (ASTM International; http://www.astm.org/) or the Canadian Standards Association (CSA Group; http://www.csagroup.org/).

Nose Injuries

The human nose is, by nature of its location, often subjected to trauma in sports. The classic nosebleed (**epistaxis**) may well be one of the most common facial injuries in sports. Anatomically, the nose consists of a framework of bone and cartilage, over which the skin is attached. The nose consists mostly of soft tissue (cartilage and skin) and can absorb significant amounts of force. The bones of the nose include the right and left nasal bones and the frontal processes of the maxilla (Moini, 2020). The superior portions of the nasal bones meet with the frontal bone between the orbits. The nose has two openings, commonly called nostrils (nares), which are separated in the middle by the cartilaginous septum. The areas immediately inside the nares contain hairs that trap large particles during respiration. Farther up, the nares tissue is covered with mucous membrane.

Initial Check and Treatment: Guidelines

When athletes receive a blow to the nose that results in bleeding, the nose should immediately be examined for the possibility of fracture and airway compromise. Other injuries to the eye socket, cervical spine, or concussion must also be ruled out (Patel et al., 2017). The signs of such a fracture include an obvious deformity of the bridge of the nose, which usually swells quickly. Fractures of the nasal bones constitute the most frequent fractures of the facial region (Patel et al., 2017). If one is suspected, the first thing is to control

---

Detached retina The retina in the back of the eye pulls away from the blood vessels and is deprived of oxygen and nutrients; this is a medical emergency.

Insidious Slow onset or signs and symptoms occur with no obvious mechanism.

Epistaxis Nosebleed.

the nosebleed, then immediately refer the athlete for medical evaluation by a QMP. A physician can easily correct uncomplicated nasal fractures, whereas any complicated fractures will need to be addressed by a specialist (otolaryngologist) after the swelling goes down. Initially, after an injury, the recommendation is for athletes to use ice and take only acetaminophen if they have pain because aspirin and nonsteroidal anti-inflammatories are blood thinners and may promote further bleeding. An isolated nasal fracture does not usually influence an athlete's ability to perform and return to play that day; however, it comes with a risk of further insult to the nose and worsening of the condition. Patel and colleagues (2017) recommended that to return a player to play on the same day of injury, hemostasis (stopping of nosebleed) must be satisfactory, with no presence of airway blockage, facial fractures, visual field disturbances, concussion symptoms, or signs of cervical spine damage. After a more significant nasal fracture, athletes should be cautious and wear a protective face shield for up to 4 to 6 weeks (Patel et al., 2017).

Care of a simple nosebleed should include application of finger pressure directly against the nostril that is bleeding. The person rendering first aid should wear a latex glove for protection against exposure to blood. If the bleeding persists, application of a cold compress against the nasal region is usually effective in causing immediate vasoconstriction of the affected vessels. In addition, athletes should be instructed to lean forward or lie on the same side as the bleeding nostril to prevent blood from moving to the mouth and throat. If they need to continue participation, their nose can be packed with gauze, which should be allowed to protrude slightly from the nose to aid with extraction later.

Septal injuries present unique problems and the possibility of later complications. As a result of external blows, the septum can be bruised, and bleeding can occur between the septum and the mucous membrane covering it. This injury is referred to as a septal hematoma and can lead to serious septal erosion if not corrected. The signs of a septal hematoma are swelling that is usually visible both inside and outside the nose. In addition, the nose may appear red and infected externally, and athletes will complain of pain, especially when their nose is gently palpated. This injury should be referred to the appropriate medical specialist for diagnosis and correction. The septal hematoma should not be drained because the likelihood of infection and permanent damage is high (Patel et al., 2017).

Ear Injuries

Anatomically, the human ear shares a common characteristic with the nose. Externally, it appears as a cartilaginous framework covered with a layer of skin, but it also has an extensive internal structure. The ear can be divided into several anatomic components. The external ear consists of the large, expanded portion, called the pinna (auricle), and the opening into the ear canal, known as the external acoustic meatus. The middle ear, which is a small space within the temporal bone, contains a small group of bones that transmit vibrations to the tympanic membrane (eardrum). The inner ear comprises the complex structure known as the labyrinth, or specialized bones (vestibule, semicircular canals, and cochlea), and it is innervated by the vestibulocochlear nerve (Moini, 2020). The fluid within the structures of the inner ear also plays a major role in the maintenance of equilibrium (Moini, 2020). Thus, injuries to this area often affect not only hearing but also balance.

With the exception of aquatic sports, the majority of sports-related medical problems of the ear affect its external parts (Osetinsky et al., 2017). Sports such as wrestling, which involves a great deal of body contact between opponents and the playing surface, result in a large number of abrasions and contusions to the pinna. Although the use of protective equipment has reduced the overall numbers of such injuries, they do still occur. Because the tissues of the pinna have a fairly high degree of vascularity, trauma can lead to the development of a hematoma between the skin and underlying cartilage, known technically as an auricular hematoma (Osetinsky et al., 2017). If this condition is not treated properly or is repeatedly irritated before treatment, a serious cosmetic problem known as **cauliflower ear** can occur. In extreme cases, the cartilage of the pinna may even begin to break down, thereby complicating the problem. Signs and symptoms of auricular hematoma include skin redness, local

---

Cauliflower ear Blood and fluid accumulates in the pinna (auricle) of the ear due to friction or pressure and disrupts normal blood flow, resulting in excessive scarring and deformity; common in wrestlers.

increase in tissue temperature, pain, and/or a burning sensation. This condition should be treated immediately with a cold pack. If swelling in the auricula occurs, athletes should be referred to a physician so that the fluid can be removed via aspiration. The ear will then be packed with a special material to prevent swelling from returning. Athletes with a history of this injury or those involved in high-risk sports such as wrestling should be required to wear properly fitted protection.

Athletes who receive a blow to the ear region that is immediately followed by a sudden reduction in hearing and/or occurrence of dizziness require immediate referral to a physician. Blows to the outer ear can produce dramatic increases in pressure in the ear, resulting in ruptures of either the eardrum or a specialized structure known as the oval window (Osetinsky et al., 2017). When such an injury occurs, the immediate effects are significant reduction in hearing and transient loss of equilibrium. Other signs and symptoms may include bleeding from the ear and persistent and intense ringing in the ear. Damage to the oval window may require surgical intervention to correct the problem (Osetinsky et al., 2017).

Athletes can also acquire ear infections caused by unhealed skin lacerations or swimming (e.g., external ear infections) or the common cold (e.g., middle ear infection). Athletes with external or middle ear infections should see a physician so the proper medication can be prescribed or over-the-counter medications recommended. Those with ear infections are advised not to participate in aquatic sports until the problem has resolved itself. This is particularly true in diving because the infection and subsequent inflammation in the ear may make it impossible for athletes to clear the pressure that develops in ears while underwater, which often results in injury to the eardrum.

Fractures of the Face (Non-Nasal)

Though fractures can occur almost anywhere on the face, certain sites are more often involved in sports-related injuries. A relatively common form of facial fracture involves the mandible and occurs in boxing and other collision sports (Black, Eliason, et al., 2017). The signs and symptoms of such an injury include obvious pain and swelling at the site of the fracture, observable deformity, and malocclusion (misalignment of the maxillary and mandibular teeth). Treatment entails gentle application of a cold pack and immediate referral to a physician. If a fracture has occurred, the jaw will be treated by wiring the mouth closed; in severe cases, surgical fixation may be required until the fracture is healed (Black, Eliason, et al., 2017).

A related injury is dislocation of the jaw, which can result from the same type of mechanism. Here, the joint involved is the **temporomandibular joint (TMJ)**, which is classified as ellipsoid and is formed by the union of the mandibular condyle and the mandibular fossa of the temporal bone (Figure 9.21). The TMJ is held together by numerous ligaments and joint capsules. Because of its bony configuration, this joint tends to dislocate relatively easily. The signs and symptoms of this injury include extreme pain and deformity in the region of the TMJ and the inability to move the lower jaw; in some cases, the mouth may be locked in an open position. Treatment for jaw dislocation is essentially the same as for any other fracture—stabilization and referral. On-site reductions (putting the joint back in place) must not be attempted for a jaw dislocation.

Other bones of the face may be fractured, including the zygomatic (cheek) bone. Generally, the signs and symptoms include pain and swelling at the site of injury. In the case of the zygomatic bone, swelling and discoloration may also spread to the orbit of the eye, and athletes may experience diplopia and numbness (Black, Eliason, et al., 2017). Athletes with a history of a blow to the face who have some or all of the previous signs and symptoms should be referred immediately to a physician for diagnosis and treatment.

Wounds of the Facial Region

Wounds to the face may take many forms; in general, their treatment should be based on basic first aid guidelines. The wound should be carefully cleaned with mild soap and warm water and a sterile, commercially prepared dressing (not loose cotton), such as an adhesive bandage, applied. For minor injuries, referral to a physician is required only if there are signs of an infection.

Facial wounds take on greater significance than injuries to other parts of the body primarily because

> **Temporomandibular joint (TMJ)** The joint created by the temporal and mandibular bones; it allows our jaw to open and close.

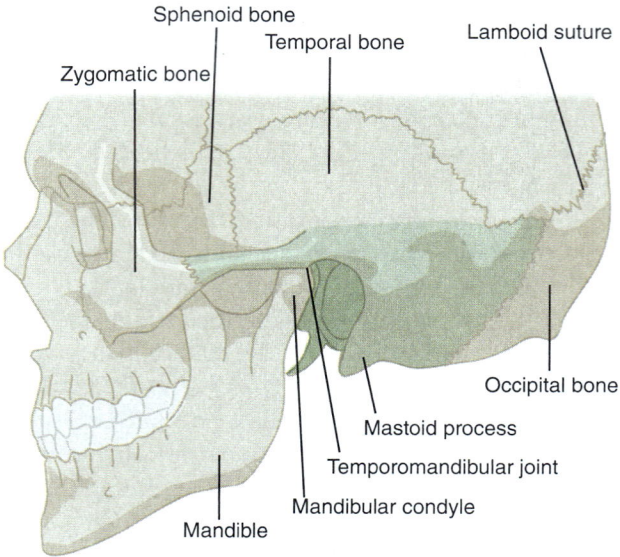

Figure 9.21 The temporomandibular joint.

of cosmetic reasons. Thus, any wound to the face, whether it be a simple **abrasion** (scraped skin), a more serious incision (smooth edged, bleeds freely), or a laceration (skin cut with jagged, irregular edges), should be evaluated relative to the potential long-term cosmetic effects. Generally, any incision or laceration resulting in an observable space between the margins of the skin should be seen by a physician for suturing. Facial wounds typically have a lower risk of infection and may be closed up to 24 hours following the injury; however, many patients are concerned about scarring and request more immediate treatment, including suturing by a plastic surgeon (DeLemos, 2021; Hyden & Tennison, 2020). Usually, athletes can return to participation after the wound has been treated and when necessary sutured. Sutures in the face are usually removed within 3 to 5 days owing to the rich blood supply and fast healing compared to the rest of the body. The decision to release such athletes to return to activity is best determined by the attending physician.

WHAT IF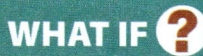

You are asked to provide first aid care to a high school basketball player who just received a blow to his mouth from an opponent's elbow. She notes that two teeth have been completely knocked out of their sockets. The teeth were recovered by the athlete and are in her hand. What would you do for this athlete? What would change if the teeth were avulsed but still in the sockets?

Abrasions Rubbing or scraping off of skin.

Review Questions

1. List the names of the cranial bones and give a description of their anatomic relationship.
2. What are the correct names of specialized tissues known collectively as the cerebral meninges?
3. What is located in the subarachnoid space?
4. What is the approximate weight in pounds of a human adult's brain?
5. What are the three basic components of the human brain?
6. What are some of the differences between a child's and an adult's brain?
7. List the correct number of cervical, thoracic, lumbar, sacral, and coccygeal nerves.
8. According to the chapter, what is a concussion?
9. What are the four categories of signs and symptoms for a concussion? Name one in each category.
10. What percentage of concussions result in LOC?
11. What percentage of concussions result in PTA?
12. How many days does it take for the typical concussion to resolve?
13. How long can athletes experience signs and symptoms if they are diagnosed with postconcussive syndrome?
14. True or false? An athlete can return to play the same day after receiving a concussion.

15. True or false? More than three-quarters of the states in the United States have laws that dictate the care and treatment of concussed athletes.

16. Describe the condition known as anisocoria.

17. What is anterograde amnesia as it relates to a head injury?

18. Define *subdural*, *epidural*, and *intracerebral hematomas*; also define *cerebral contusion*.

19. When rendering first aid to an athlete with a suspected head injury, what are the top three objectives?

20. True or false: The single most important indicator of the severity of head injury is the level of consciousness.

21. True or false? Baseline computerized neuropsychological testing is recommended for all high school athletes.

22. True or false? Athletes with a concussion history are more likely to experience a lower extremity injury.

23. What are the general areas of neurocognitive function that are assessed by the SCAT5?

24. What is the most likely mechanism of a sports-related injury to the cervical spine?

25. What conditions must be assumed present whenever treating an unconscious athlete?

26. What types of information should be obtained when treating a conscious athlete with a suspected head and/or neck injury?

27. True or false? Having two tools that can remove a football face mask are recommended in case one fails.

28. True or false? Experts agree that 90% of eye injuries could be prevented if athletes wore adequate eye protection.

29. What is the cause of the majority of dental injuries?

30. What is a simple, practical form of dental protection in sports?

31. True or false? The majority of sports-related eye injuries occur in basketball.

32. What is the recommended method of removing a small, nonembedded object from an athlete's eye?

33. What is an orbital blowout?

34. What materials should the coach have available in a first aid kit for treating problems related to athletes wearing contact lenses?

35. Define the term *epistaxis*.

36. Describe the appropriate method for controlling a nosebleed.

37. True or false? A facial laceration needs to be sutured within 2 hours to prevent infection and scarring.

38. True or false? With the exception of aquatic sports, the majority of sports-related medical problems with the ear involve the auricula.

39. Briefly describe the process leading to the condition known as cauliflower ear.

40. Why are facial wounds of greater significance than wounds on other areas of the body?

References

Agur, A. M., & Dalley, A. F. (2018). *Moore's essential clinical anatomy*. Philadelphia, PA: Lippincott Williams & Wilkins.

American Dental Association. (2019). *Oral health topics: Mouth guards*. Retrieved from https://www.ada.org/en/member-center/oral-health-topics/mouthguards

Anitha, N., Malathi, L., Babu, N. A., & Anjuga, E. S. (2020). Common dental injuries in athletes: A review. *European Journal of Molecular & Clinical Medicine, 7*(5), 1436–1440.

Bagley, A. F., Daneshvar, D. H., Schanker, B. D., Zurakowski, D., d'Hemecourt, C. A., Nowinski, C. J., Cantu, R. C., & Goulet, K. (2012). Effectiveness of the SLICE program for youth concussion education. *Clinical Journal of Sport Medicine, 22*(5), 385–389.

Black, A. M., Eliason, P. H., Patton, D. A., & Emery, C. A. (2017). Epidemiology of facial injuries in sport. *Clinical Sports Medicine, 36*(2), 237–255.

Black, A. M., Patton, D. A., Eliason, P. H., & Emery, C. A. (2017). Prevention of sport-related facial injuries. *Clinical Sports Medicine, 36*(2), 257–278.

Boden, B. P., Pierpoint, L. A., Boden, R. G., Comstock, R. D., & Kerr, Z. Y. (2017). Eye injuries in high school and collegiate athletes. *Sports Health, 9*(5), 444–449.

Boden, B. P., Tacchetti, R. L., Cantu, R. C., Knowles, S. B., & Mueller, F. O. (2006). Catastrophic cervical spine injuries in high school and college football players. *American Journal of Sports Medicine, 34*(8), 1223–1232.

Brigham, C. D., & Capo, J. (2013). Cervical spinal cord contusion in professional athletes: A case series with implications for return to play. *Spine, 38*(4), 315–323.

Broglio, S., Macciocchi, S., & Ferrara, M. (2007). Sensitivity of the concussion assessment battery. *Neurosurgery, 60*(6), 1050–1058.

Broglio, S. P., Cantu, R. C., Gioia, G. A., Guskiewicz, K. M., Kutcher, J., Palm, M., & Valovich McLeod, T. C. (2014). National Athletic Trainers' Association position statement: Management of sport concussion. *Journal of Athletic Training, 49*(2), 245–265. Retrieved from https://www.nata.org/sites/default/files/concussion_management_position_statement.pdf

Broglio, S. P., Collins, M. W., Williams, R. W., Mucha, A., & Kontos, A. (2015). Current and emerging rehabilitation for concussion: A review of the evidence. *Clinical Sports Medicine, 34*(2), 213–231.

Brophy, M., Sinclair, S. A., Hostetler, S. G., & Xiang, H. (2006). Pediatric eye injury–related hospitalizations in the United States. *Pediatrics, 117*(6), e1263–e1271.

Broshek, D. K., Kaushik, T., Freeman, J. R., Erlanger, D., Webbe, F., & Barth, J. T. (2005). Sex differences in outcome following sports-related concussion. *Journal of Neurosurgery, 102*(5), 856–863.

Carson, A. (2017). Concussion, dementia and CTE: Are we getting it very wrong? *Journal of Neurology, Neurosurgery and Psychiatry, 88*(6), 462.

Centers for Disease Control and Prevention (CDC). (2019). *National Concussion Surveillance System.* Retrieved from https://www.cdc.gov/traumaticbraininjury/ncss/

Centers for Disease Control and Prevention (CDC). (2021, May 12). *Get the facts about TBI.* Retrieved from https://www.cdc.gov/traumaticbraininjury/get_the_facts.html.

Chatelin, S., Vappou, J., Roth, S., Raul, J., & Willinger, R. (2012). Towards child versus adult brain mechanical properties. *Journal of the Mechanical Behavior of Biomedical Materials, 6*, 166–173.

Cleveland Clinic. (2022). *Concussion test.* Retrieved from https://my.clevelandclinic.org/health/diagnostics/22267-concussion-test

Collins, M. W., Kontos, A. P., Okonkwo, D. O., Almquist, J., Bailes, J., Barisa, M., Bazarian, J., . . . Zafonte, R. (2016). Statements of agreement from the targeted evaluation and active management (TEAM) approaches to treating concussion meeting held in Pittsburgh, October 15–16, 2015. *Neurosurgery, 79*(6), 912–929.

Committee on Sports-Related Concussions in Youth; Board on Children, Youth, and Families; Institute of Medicine; & National Research Council. (2014). *Sports-related concussions in youth: Improving the science, changing the culture.* Washington, D.C.: National Academies Press.

Comstock, R. D., & Pierpoint, L. A. (2020). *National High School Sports-Related Injury Surveillance Survey (2018–2019).* Retrieved from https://coloradosph.cuanschutz.edu/research-and-practice/centers-programs/piper/research-practice/research-projects

Courson, R., Ellis, J., Herring, S. A., Boden, B. P., Henry, G., Conway, D., . . . Walpert, K. P. (2020). Best practices and current care concepts in prehospital care of the spine-injured athlete in American tackle football March 2–3, 2019, Atlanta, GA. *Journal of Athletic Training, 55*(6), 545–562.

Dashtevska, E. G. (2018). Eye injuries in sports. *Research in Physical Education, Sport and Health, 7*(1), 45–48.

Dashtevska, E. G., & Ivanova, M. (2020). Prevention of eye injuries in sports. *Research in Physical Education, Sport and Health, 9*(2), 107–110.

Davis, G. A., Purcell, L., Schneider, K. J., Yeates, K. O., Gioia, G. A., Anderson, V., . . . Kutcher, J. S. (2017). The Child Sport Concussion Assessment Tool 5th Edition (Child SCAT5): Background and rationale. *British Journal of Sports Medicine, 51*(11), 859–861.

DeLemos, D. M. (2021, January 4). *Skin laceration repair with sutures.* Retrieved from https://www.uptodate.com/contents/skin-laceration-repair-with-sutures

Eagle, S. R., Kontos, A. P., Pepping, G. J., Johnson, C. D., Sinnott, A., LaGoy, A., & Connaboy, C. (2020). Increased risk of musculoskeletal injury following sport-related concussion: A perception–action coupling approach. *Sports Medicine, 50*(1), 15–23.

Echemendia, R. J., Meeuwisse, W., McCrory, P., Davis, G. A., Putukian, M., Leddy, J., . . . Herring, S. (2017). The Sport Concussion Assessment Tool 5th Edition (SCAT5): Background and rationale. *British Journal of Sports Medicine, 51*(11), 848–850.

Eckersley, C. P., Nightingale, R. W., Luck, J. F., & Bass, C. R. (2019). The role of cervical muscles in mitigating concussion. *Journal of Science and Medicine in Sport, 22*(6), 667–671.

Ellis, M. J., Leddy, J., & Willer, B. (2016). Multi-disciplinary management of athletes with post-concussion syndrome: An evolving pathophysiological approach. *Frontiers in Neurology, 7*, 136.

Fallows, R. R., Mullane, A., Smith Watts, A. K., Aukerman, D., & Bao, Y. (2020). Normal variability within a collegiate athlete sample: A rationale for comprehensive baseline testing. *The Clinical Neuropsychologist*, 1–17.

Field, M., Collins, M., Lovell, M., & Maroon, J. (2003). Does age play a role in recovery from sports-related concussion? A comparison of high school and collegiate athletes. *Journal of Pediatrics, 142*, 546–553.

Gilchrist, I., Storr, M., Chapman, E., & Pelland, L. (2015). Neck muscle strength training in the risk management of concussion in contact sports: Critical appraisal of application to practice. *Journal of Athletic Enhancement, 4*(2), 1–19.

Giza, C. C., & Hovda, D. A. (2014). The new neurometabolic cascade of concussion. *Neurosurgery, 75*(Suppl. 4), S24–S33.

Glang, A., Koester, M., Beaver, S., Clan, J., & McLaughlin, K. (2010). Online training in sports concussion for youth sports coaches. *International Journal of Sports Science & Coaching, 5*(1), 1–11.

Glasgow, B. (2017, September 20). *Concussion law: Where does your state stand?* Retrieved from https://blogs.usafootball.com/blog/4450/concussion-law-where-does-your-state-stand

Gould, T. E., Piland, S. G., Caswell, S. V., Ranalli, D., Mills, S., Ferrara, M. S., & Courson, R. (2016). National Athletic Trainers' Association position statement: Preventing and managing sport-related dental and oral injuries. *Journal of Athletic Training, 51*(10), 821–839.

Green, J. I. J. (2017). The role of mouthguards in preventing and reducing sports-related trauma. *Primary Dental Journal, 6*(2), 27–34.

Guskiewicz, K., Marshall, S. W., Bailes, J., McCrea, M., Cantu, R. C., Randolph, C., & Jordan, B. D. (2005). Association between recurrent concussion and late-life cognitive impairment in retired professional football players. *Neurosurgery, 57*(4), 719–726.

Guskiewicz, K. M., Weaver, N. L., Padua, D. A., & Garrett, W. E., Jr. (2000). Epidemiology of concussion in collegiate and high school football players. *American Journal of Sports Medicine, 28*(5), 643–650.

Halstead, M. E., McAvoy, K., Devore, C. D., Carl, R., Lee, M., & Logan, K. (2013). Returning to learning following a concussion. *Pediatrics, 132*(5), 948–957.

Harmon, K. G., Clugston, J. R., Dec, K., Hainline, B., Herring, S., Kane, S. F., Kontos, A. P., Leddy, J. J., McCrea, M., Poddar, S. K., Putukian, M., Wilson, J. C., & Roberts, W. O. (2019). American Medical Society for Sports Medicine position statement on concussion in sport. *British Journal of Sports Medicine, 53*(4), 213–225.

Hart, J., Kraut, M. A., Womack, K. B., Strain, J., Didehbani, N., Bartz, E., . . . Cullum, C. M. (2013). Neuroimaging of cognitive dysfunction and depression in aging retired national football league players. *JAMA Neurology, 70*(3), 326–335.

Harvey, H. (2013). Reducing traumatic brain injuries in youth sports: Youth sports traumatic brain injury state laws, January 2009–December 2012. *American Journal of Public Health, 103*(7), 1249–1254.

Heck, J. F. (1996). The incidence of spearing during a high school's 1975 and 1990 football seasons. *Journal of Athletic Training, 31*, 31–37.

Herman, D. C., Jones, D., Harrison, A., Moser, M., Tillman, S., Farmer, K., . . . Chmielewski, T. L. (2017). Concussion may increase the risk of subsequent lower extremity musculoskeletal injury in collegiate athletes. *Sports Medicine, 47*(5), 1003–1010.

Herman, D. C., Zaremski, J. L., Vincent, H. K., & Vincent, K. R. (2015). Effect of neurocognition and concussion on musculoskeletal injury risk. *Current Sports Medicine Reports, 14*(3), 194.

Hyden, A., & Tennison, M. (2020). Evaluation and management of sports-related lacerations of the head and neck. *Current Sports Medicine Reports, 19*(1), 24–28.

Jordan, B.D. (1989). Head injury in sports. In B. D. Jordan, P. Tsairis, & R. R. Warren (Eds.), *Sports neurology* (pp. 75–83). New York, NY: Aspen Publishers.

Kerr, Z. Y., Roos, K. G., Djoko, A., Dalton, S. L., Broglio, S. P., Marshall, S. W., & Dompier, T. P. (2017). Epidemiologic measures for quantifying the incidence of concussion in National Collegiate Athletic Association sports. *Journal of Athletic Training, 52*(3), 167–174.

Kirkwood, M. W., Randolph, C., & Yeates, K. O. (2009). Returning pediatric athletes to play after concussion: The evidence (or lack thereof) behind baseline neuropsychological testing. *Acta Paediatrica, 98*(9), 1409–1411.

Kontos, A. P., Collins, M. W., Holland, C. L., Reeves, V. L., Edelman, K., Benso, S., . . . Okonkwo, D. (2018). Preliminary evidence for improvement in symptoms, cognitive, vestibular, and oculomotor outcomes following targeted intervention with chronic mTBI patients. *Military Medicine, 183*(Suppl. 1), 333–338.

Kontos, A. P., Sufrinko, A., Sandel, N., Emami, K., & Collins, M. W. (2019). Sport-related concussion clinical profiles: Clinical characteristics, targeted treatments, and preliminary evidence. *Current Sports Medicine Reports, 18*(3), 82–92.

Kucera, K. L., & Cantu, R. C. (2020). *Catastrophic sports injury research: Thirty-seventh annual report, Fall 1982-Spring 2019.* Retrieved from https://nccsir.unc.edu/wp-content/uploads/sites/5614/2021/05/2019-Catastrophic-Report-AS-37th-AY2018-2019-FINAL2.pdf

Kucera, K. L., Klossner, D., & Cantu, R. C. (2020). *Annual survey of catastrophic football injuries, 1977–2019.* Retrieved from https://nccsir.unc.edu/wp-content/uploads/sites/5614/2020/09/Annual-Football-Catastrophic-2019-FINAL.pdf

Leddy, J. J., Baker, J. G., & Willer, B. (2016). Active rehabilitation of concussion and post-concussion syndrome. *Physical Medicine and Rehabilitation Clinics of North America, 27*(2), 437–454.

Leddy, J. J., Haider, M. N., Ellis, M. J., Mannix, R., Darling, S. R., Freitas, M. S., . . . Willer, B. (2019). Early subthreshold aerobic exercise for sport-related concussion: A randomized clinical trial. *JAMA Pediatrics, 173*(4), 319–325.

Lloyd, J. D. Nakamura, W. S., Maeda, Y., Takeda, T., Leesungbok, R., Lazarchik D., . . . Rock, J. B. (2017). Mouthguards and their use in sports: Report of the 1st International Sports Dentistry Workshop, 2016. *Dental Traumatology, 33*(6), 421–426.

Lovell, M. R. (2002). The relevance of neuropsychological testing. *Current Sports Medicine Reports, 1*(1), 7–11.

Lumba-Brown, A., Yeates, K. O., Sarmiento, K., Breiding, M. J., Haegerich, T. M., Gioia, G. A., . . . Timmons, S. D. (2018). Centers for Disease Control and Prevention guideline on the diagnosis and management of mild traumatic brain injury among children. *JAMA Pediatrics, 172*(11), e182853–e182853.

MacFarlane, M. P., & Glenn, T. C. (2015). Neurochemical cascade of concussion. *Brain Injury, 29*(2), 139–153.

Maroon, J. C., Winkelman, R., Bost, J., Amos, A., Mathyssek, C., & Miele, V. (2015). Chronic traumatic encephalopathy in contact sports: A systematic review of all reported pathological cases. *PloS One, 10*(2), e0117338.

McCrea, M., Guskiewicz, K., Randolph, C., Barr, W. B., Hammeke, T. A., Marshall, S. W., . . . Kelly, J. P. (2013). Incidence, clinical course, and predictors of prolonged recovery time following sport-related concussion in high school and college athletes. *Journal of the International Neuropsychological Society, 19*(1), 22–33.

McCrory, P., Meeuwisse, W., Dvorak, J., Aubry, M., Bailes, J., Broglio, S., . . . Vos, P. E. (2017). Consensus statement on concussion in sport: The 5th International Conference on Concussion in Sport held in Berlin, October 2016. *British Journal of Sports Medicine, 51*(11), 838–847.

McLendon, L. A., Kralik, S. F., Grayson, P. A., & Golomb, M. R. (2016). The controversial second impact syndrome: A review of the literature. *Pediatric Neurology, 62*, 9–17.

Mills, B. M., Conrick, K. M., Anderson, S., Bailes, J., Boden, B. P., Conway, D., . . . Courson, R. (2020). Consensus recommendations on the prehospital care of the injured athlete with a suspected catastrophic cervical spine injury. *Journal of Athletic Training, 55*(6), 563–572.

Moini, J. (2020). *Anatomy and physiology for health professionals* (3rd ed.). Burlington, MA: Jones & Bartlett Learning.

Morrissey, J. (2013). Research suggests time for change in prehospital spinal immobilization. *Journal of Emergency Medical Services, 38*(3).

Mucha, A., Collins, M. W., Elbin, R. J., Furman, J. M., Troutman-Enseki, C., DeWol, R. M., . . . Kontos, A. P. (2014). A brief vestibular/ocular motor screening (VOMS) assessment to evaluate concussions: Preliminary findings. *American Journal of Sports Medicine, 42*(10), 2479–2486.

Mueller, F., & Cantu, R. (2011). *Catastrophic sports injury research: 29th Annual report Fall 1982–Spring 2011*. Retrieved from https://nccsir.unc.edu/wp-content/uploads/sites/5614/2014/05/2011Allsport.pdf

Mueller, F., & Cantu, R. (2012). *Annual survey of catastrophic football injuries, 1977–2012*. Retrieved https://nccsir.unc.edu/wp-content/uploads/sites/5614/2014/05/FBAnnual2012.pdf

Murray, D. A., Meldrum, D., & Lennon, O. (2017). Can vestibular rehabilitation exercises help patients with concussion? A systematic review of efficacy, prescription and progression patterns. *British Journal of Sports Medicine, 51*(5), 442–451.

National Athletic Trainers' Association (NATA). (2014, June). *Official statement: EMS changes to pre-hospital care of the athlete with acute cervical spine injury*. Retrieved from https://www.nata.org/sites/default/files/c-spine-management.pdf

National Athletic Trainers' Association (NATA). (2015, August 5). *Appropriate prehospital management of the spine-injured athlete updated from 1998 document*. Retrieved from https://www.nata.org/sites/default/files/Executive-Summary-Spine-Injury-updated.pdf

National Collegiate Athletic Association (NCAA). (n.d.). *Concussion educational resources*. Retrieved http://www.ncaa.org/sport-science-institute/concussion-educational-resources

National Eye Institute (NEI). *Protective eyeware*. Retrieved from https://www.nei.nih.gov/learn-about-eye-health/nei-for-kids/protective-eyewear

National Federation of State High School Associations (NFHS). (2018). *Position statement and recommendations for mouthguard use in sports*. Retrieved from https://www.nfhs.org/media/1014750/position-statement-and-recommendations-for-mouthguard-use-in-sports-october-2018-final.pdf

National Spinal Cord Injury Statistical Center (NSCISC). (2021). *Spinal cord injury: Facts and figures at a glance*. Retrieved from https://www.nscisc.uab.edu/Public/Facts%20and%20Figures%20-%202021.pdf

Newman, J. A. (2020). Biomechanics of brain injury in athletes. In M. R. Lovell, R. J. Echemendia, J. T. Barth, & M. W. Collins (Eds.), *Traumatic brain injury in sports* (pp. 35–44). Oxfordshire, United Kingdom: Taylor & Francis.

O'Neill, J. A., Cox, M. K., Clay, O. J., Johnston, J. M., Jr., Novack, T. A., Schwebel, D. C., & Dreer, L. E. (2017). A review of the literature on pediatric concussions and return-to-learn (RTL): Implications for RTL policy, research, and practice. *Rehabilitation Psychology, 62*(3), 300–323. https://doi.org/10.1037/rep0000155

Osetinsky, L. M., Hamilton, G. S., & Carlson, M. L. (2017). Sport injuries of the ear and temporal bone. *Clinical Sports Medicine, 36*(2), 315–335.

Patel, Y., Goljan, P., Pierce, T. P., Scillia, A., Issa, K., McInerney, V. K., & Festa, A. (2017). Management of nasal fractures in sports. *Sports Medicine, 47*(10), 1919–1923.

Peterson, A. B., Likang, X., Daugherty, J., & Breiding, M. J. (2014). *Surveillance report of traumatic brain injury-related emergency department visits, hospitalizations, and deaths*. Retrieved from https://www.cdc.gov/traumaticbraininjury/pdf/TBI-Surveillance-Report-FINAL_508.pdf

Pop Warner Little Scholars. (2019, February 28). *Pop Warner becomes first national football organization to eliminate 3-point stance*. Retrieved from https://www.popwarner.com/Default.aspx?tabid=1403205&mid=1475016&newskeyid=HN1&newsid=279263&ctl=newsdetail

Potteiger, K. L., Potteiger, A. J., Pitney, W., & Wright, P. M. (2018). An examination of concussion legislation in the United States. *Internet Journal of Allied Health Sciences and Practice, 16*(2), 6.

Prevent Blindness. (2020). *Sports-related eye injuries by age–2019*. Retrieved from https://preventblindness.org/wp-content/uploads/2020/06/FS09_SportsInjuriesbyAge-detailed2020.pdf

Pujalte, G. (2010). Eye injuries in sports. *Athletic Therapy Today, 15*(5), 14–18.

Resch, J. E., Brown, C. N., Schmidt, J., Macciocchi, S. N., Blueitt, D., Cullum, C. M., & Ferrara, M. S. (2016). The sensitivity and specificity of clinical measures of sport concussion: Three tests are better than one. *BMJ Open Sport & Exercise Medicine, 2*(1).

Resch, J., Driscoll, A., McCaffrey, N., Brown, C., Ferrara, M. S., Macciocchi, S., . . . Walpert, K. (2013). ImPact test-retest reliability: Reliably unreliable? *Journal of Athletic Training, 48*(4), 506–511.

Reynolds, E., Collins, M. W., Mucha, A., & Troutman-Ensecki, C. (2014). Establishing a clinical service for the management of sports-related concussions. *Neurosurgery, 75*(Suppl. 4), S71–S81.

Rodriguez, J. O., Lavina, A. M., & Agarwal, A. (2003). Prevention and treatment of common eye injuries in sports. *American Family Physician, 67*(7), 1481–1488.

Roebuck-Spencer, T., Vincent, A. S., Schlegel, R. E., & Gilliland, K. (2013). Evidence for added value of baseline testing in computer-based cognitive assessment. *Journal of Athletic Training, 48*(4), 499–505.

Rowson, S., Duma, S. M., Greenwald, R. M., Beckwith, J. G., Chu, J. J., Guskiewicz, K. M., . . . Brolinson, P. G. (2014). Can helmet design reduce the risk of concussion in football? *Journal of Neurosurgery, 120*(4), 919–922.

Russo, M. J., Salvat, F., Sevlever, G., & Allegri, R. F. (2022). Acute and subacute clinical markers after sport-related concussion. *Neurology, 98*(1 Suppl. 1), S16.

Saladin, K. (2007). *Anatomy and physiology: The unity of form and function*. Columbus, OH: McGraw-Hill.

Sarmiento, K., Mitchko, J., Klein, C., & Wong, S. (2010). Evaluation of the Centers for Disease Control and Prevention's concussion intuitive for high school coaches: "Heads Up: Concussion in High School Sports." *Journal of School Health, 80*(3), 112–118.

Schneider, K. J. (2019). Concussion part II: Rehabilitation: The need for a multifaceted approach. *Musculoskeletal Science and Practice, 42*, 151–161.

Schroeder, G. D., & Vaccaro, A. R. (2016). Cervical spine injuries in the athlete. *Journal of the American Academy of Orthopaedic Surgeons, 24*(9), e122–e133.

Scorza, K., Raleigh, M., & O'Connor, F. (2012). Current concepts in concussion: Evaluation and management. *American Family Physician, 85*(2), 123–132.

Spadinger, A. (2019). Sports dentistry and mouth protection. In A. J. Nowak, J. R. Christensen, T. R. Mabry, J. A. Townsend, & M. H. Wells (Eds.), *Pediatric dentistry: Infancy through adolescence* (6th ed., pp. 610–616). Philadelphia, PA: Elsevier.

Stamm, J. M., Post, E. G., Baugh, C. M., & Bell, D. R. (2020). Awareness of concussion-education requirements, and management plans and concussion knowledge in high school and club sport coaches. *Journal of Athletic Training, 55*(10), 1054–1061.

Stein, T. D., Alvarez, V. E., & McKee, A. C. (2015). Concussion in chronic traumatic encephalopathy. *Current Pain and Headache Reports, 19*(10), 47.

Strelzik, J., & Langdon, R. (2017). The role of active recovery and "rest" after concussion. *Pediatric Annals, 46*(4), e139–e144.

Swartz, E. E., Belmore, K., Decoster, L., & Armstrong, C. (2010). Emergency face-mask removal effectiveness: A comparison of traditional and nontraditional football helmet face-mask attachment systems. *Journal of Athletic Training, 45*(6), 560–569.

Swartz, E. E., Boden, B. P., Courson, R. W., Decoster, L. C., Horodyski, M., Norkus, S. A., . . . Waninger, K. N. (2009). National Athletic Trainers' Association position statement: Acute management of the cervical spine-injured athlete. *Journal of Athletic Training, 44*(3), 306–331.

Swartz, E. E., Myers, J. L., Cook, S. B., Guskiewicz, K. M., Ferrara, M. S., Cantu, R. C., . . . Broglio, S. P. (2019). A helmetless-tackling intervention in American football for decreasing head impact exposure: A randomized controlled trial. *Journal of Science and Medicine in Sport, 22*(10), 1102–1107.

Tomei, K., Doe, C., Prestigiacomo, C., & Gandhi C. (2012). Comparative analysis of state-level concussion legislation and review of current practices in concussion. *Neurosurgical Focus, 33*(6), 1–9.

Van De Graaff, K. M. (1998). *Human anatomy* (5th ed.). Dubuque, IA: William. C. Brown.

Van Ierssel, J., Osmond, M., Hamid, J., Sampson, M., & Zemek, R. (2021). What is the risk of recurrent concussion in children and adolescents aged 5–18 years? A systematic review and meta-analysis. *British Journal of Sports Medicine, 55*(12), 663–669.

Van Kampen, D. A., Lovell, M. R., Pardini, J. E., Collins, M. W., & Fu, F. H. (2006). The "value added" of neurocognitive testing after sports-related concussion. *American Journal of Sports Medicine, 34*(10), 1630–1635.

Wetjen, N. M., Pichelmann, M. A., & Atkinson, J. L. (2010). Second impact syndrome: Concussion and second injury brain complications. *Journal of the American College of Surgeons, 211*(4), 553–557.

Wilkerson, G. B., Grooms, D. R., & Acocello, S. N. (2017). Neuromechanical considerations for postconcussion musculoskeletal injury risk management. *Current Sports Medicine Reports, 16*(6), 419–427.

Wilkerson, G. B., Nabhan, D. C., & Crane, R. T. (2020). Concussion history and neuromechanical responsiveness asymmetry. *Journal of Athletic Training, 55*(6), 594–600.

Young, E. J., Macias, C. R., & Stephens, L. (2015). Common dental injury management in athletes. *Sports Health, 7*(3), 250–255.

Zuckerman, S. L., Kerr, Z. Y., Yengo-Kahn, A., Wasserman, E., Covassin, T., & Solomon, G. S. (2015). Epidemiology of sports-related concussion in NCAA athletes from 2009–2010 to 2013–2014: Incidence, recurrence, and mechanisms. *American Journal of Sports Medicine, 43*(11), 2654–2662.

CHAPTER 10

Injuries to the Thoracic Through Coccygeal Spine

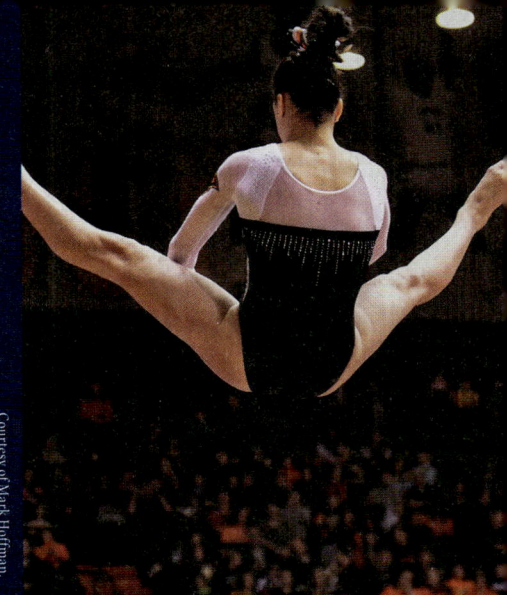

MAJOR CONCEPTS

This chapter presents a brief review of the gross anatomy of the thoracic spine, thoracic cage, lumbar spine, and sacral and coccygeal spine along with a discussion of possible injuries to these regions. Although relatively uncommon in sports, injuries to the thoracic spine and cage do occasionally occur. These injuries are usually strains and sprains but often involve fractures. The chapter covers typical mechanisms of injury as well as common signs and symptoms and recommended initial treatment for strains, sprains, fractures, and nerve injuries. Injuries to the lumbar spine in sports are quite common due to the impact loads and rotational forces placed on the spine during sports. Low back pain (including the lumbar, sacral, and coccygeal spines) is the most common global disability and both acute, and chronic cases are common in athletes due to the mechanics and duration of loading (Zemková et al., 2020). This chapter provides descriptions of the common problems associated with these parts of the spinal column, along with information regarding the signs and symptoms of related lumbar, sacral, and coccygeal spinal disorders. It also discusses sprains, strains, fractures, and intervertebral disk injuries, with a focus on recognition and initial management.

Anatomy Review of the Thoracic Spine

The portion of the human vertebral column known as the thoracic spine consists of 12 vertebrae that articulate at the top with the cervical spine and at the bottom with the lumbar, sacral, and coccygeal spine. Viewed from the side, the human vertebral column includes several curvatures that correspond with specific regions of the spine. Both the cervical and lumbar portions of the spine represent concave curves, whereas the thoracic, sacral, and coccygeal portions of the vertebral column are convex, curving in the opposite direction to both the cervical and lumbar components. The curves of the spine, along with the ligaments, muscles, and intervertebral disks, are important to the overall strength of the spinal column (Figure 10.1). The thoracic vertebrae are commonly numbered 1 through 12, beginning with the uppermost vertebra and ending with the 12th at the junction with the lumbar

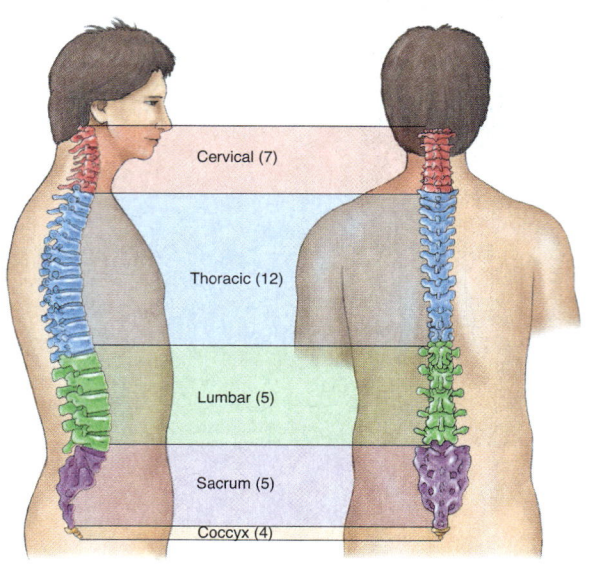

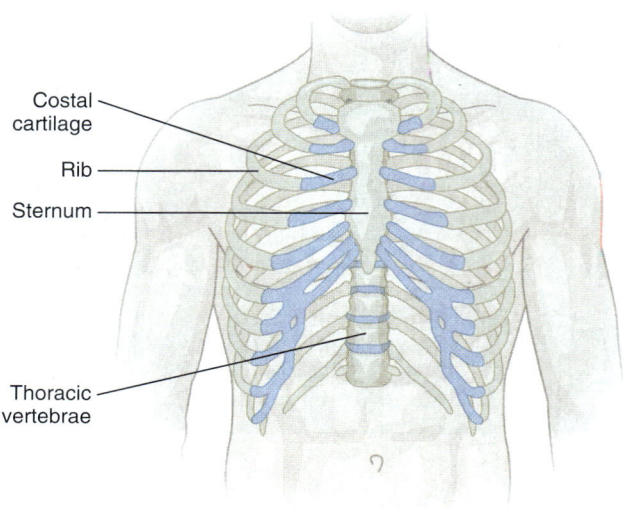

Figure 10.1 Lateral and posterior view of human vertebral column.

Figure 10.2 The thoracic cage (anterior view).

spine. An intervertebral disk is located between each thoracic vertebra. A unique aspect of the thoracic vertebrae is their relationship with the 12 pairs of ribs in the human skeleton. The thoracic vertebrae, their corresponding ribs, and the sternum form a strong **thoracic cage** (Figure 10.2), which serves as an attachment for several muscles and to protect the internal organs of the region, including the heart and lungs (Moini, 2020).

Because of the bony union of the ribs and adjacent vertebrae, the thoracic spine is much less mobile than either the cervical or lumbar sections of the spine. The majority of movements in the thoracic region of the spine result from the process of respiration (Moini, 2020), but achieving end range motion of the shoulder girdle and glenohumeral joint is dependent on extension of the thoracic spine (Johnston & Drake, 2021). Although injuries to the thoracic spine and thoracic cage are uncommon, they can be very severe and result in life-threatening situations. However, the lack of thoracic extension motion or a slouched posture is the biggest problem for athletes participating in upper extremity–dominant sports, such as pitching, throwing, swimming, or rowing.

Thoracic cage Thoracic vertebrae, their corresponding ribs, and the sternum.

Common Sports Injuries for the Thoracic Spine and Thoracic Cage

Sports injuries to the spine are rare, accounting for less than 15% of sports-related injuries. Thoracic spine injuries are less common than both cervical and lumbar injuries (Maslak & Savage, 2020). Those sports-related injuries that do occur can be divided into two groups: skeletal (i.e., bone) and soft tissue (i.e., ligaments, muscles, and tendons). Available data demonstrate that bone-related injuries (i.e., fractures) in this region are more serious than those involving soft tissues (i.e., contusions and muscular strains). Stress fractures in spinous processes and transverse processes often result from overuse mechanisms, whereas compression-type fractures are the result of high-energy mechanisms, including axial loading and flexion of the thoracic spine (Menzer et al., 2015). Epidemiological reports from high school seasons between 2005–2006 and 2013–2014 demonstrate that the injury rate was higher in competition than practice and boys' sports had a higher rate than girls' sports. Football (47.7%) accounted for the highest proportion of injuries, followed by wrestling (18.5%) and then boys' and girls' soccer. Because most of the injuries were to the soft-tissue structures, around 60% of injured athletes were able to return to play within 1 week (Johnson & Comstock, 2017).

Skeletal Injuries

The most common injury to the thoracic spine involves a compression fracture to the vertebral body (O'Toole et al., 2019). This injury is usually related to violent, ballistic movements that are unique to sports involving high velocities. An athlete with a history of recent trauma to the thoracic spine who complains of severe pain in the region or perhaps even neurological signs (e.g., pain, numbness, or lack of muscle function) should be referred to a medical doctor immediately for evaluation (Table 10.1).

Another problem related to the vertebrae of the thoracic spine is Scheuermann's disease, which is sometimes seen in adolescents and is characterized by **kyphosis** (an abnormal amount of convexity of the spine). Children involved in activities that subject the spine to severe bending, such as gymnastics, may develop this condition. A child who complains of recurrent pain in the region of the thoracic spine that is associated with activity should be evaluated. A quick visual examination may confirm an abnormal amount of spinal curvature, which is made worse when the child bends forward as if to touch the toes. In some cases, related spinal problems, such as **scoliosis** (lateral curvature), may also be present. Children with either of these disorders need to be referred to a doctor for extensive evaluation. If a diagnosis of Scheuermann's disease is made, treatment will involve both prescribed exercises and spinal bracing.

Table 10.1
Thoracic Nerve Distribution

Thoracic Nerve Section	Area of Body Affected and Area of Neurological Dysfunction*
T1	Inside of arm and elbow
T2–T5	Upper chest skin and muscles
T6–T8	Lower chest and abdominal skin and muscles
T9–T12	Abdominal skin and muscles

*Neurological dysfunction includes lack of sensation, hypersensitivity, pain, or muscle weakness.
Data from Rajasekaran, S., Kanna, R. M., & Shetty, A. P. (2015). Management of thoracolumbar spine trauma: An overview. *Indian Journal of Orthopedics*, 49(1), 72–82.

Vertebral Fractures

Fractures involving the thoracic spine are extremely rare; however, they can result from either a direct blow to the posterior thorax or extreme flexion of the thoracic spine, resulting in a compression of the vertebral body. In spite of the fact that neurological complications related to vertebral fractures in this region are rare, significant soft-tissue damage can occur to the skin and underlying muscles. The mechanism of injury described earlier can occur in a tackle in football, a collision in soccer, or while landing on the opponent's knee during a takedown move in wrestling.

Signs and symptoms of vertebral fractures include the following:

- Pain in the area of the injury.
- Although the athlete may be able to stand and even move about, any motion specific to the trunk, such as extension, flexion, or rotation, will be extremely painful.
- Swelling and discoloration in the area of injury may be apparent.
- Muscle spasm over the injured area.
- Palpable deformity of vertebral body.

First aid care of vertebral fractures involves the following:

1. Immediately apply rest, ice, compression, and elevation (RICE) (generally best accomplished with a 6-inch-wide elastic wrap and a bag of crushed ice).
2. Remove the athlete from participation, and schedule a follow-up evaluation with an athletic trainer or a physician.
3. If symptoms persist despite treatment, including rest, referral to a physician is warranted.
4. If neurological symptoms (Table 10.1) are present during the initial evaluation, stabilize the athlete and activate the emergency action plan.

Rib Fractures

Another type of fracture that may occur in the thoracic spine involves the ribs. These fractures can be "simple nondisplaced fractures or displaced fractures

---

Kyphosis Exaggeration of the normal curve of the thoracic spine.

Scoliosis Lateral and/or rotary curvature of the spine.

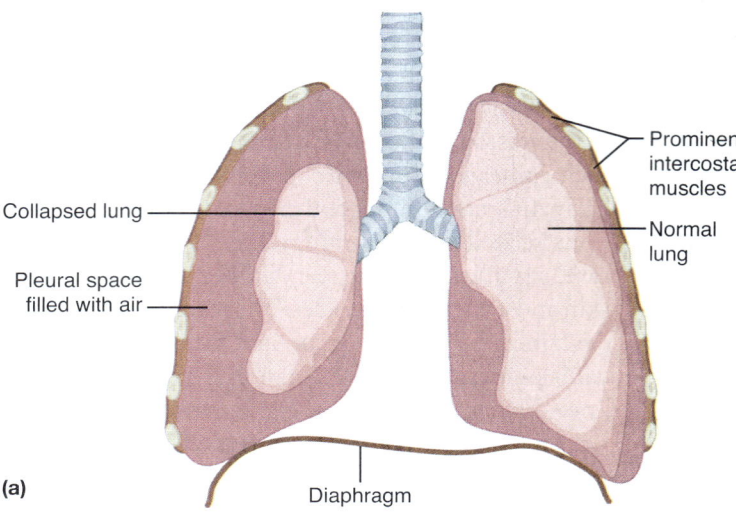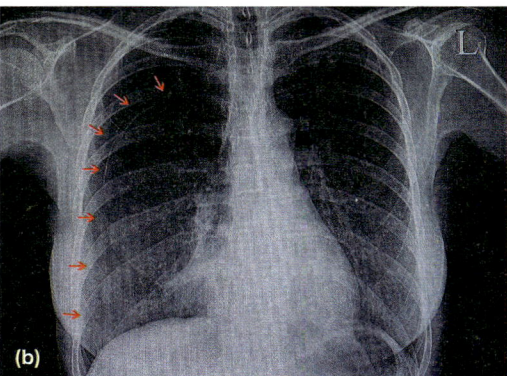

Figure 10.3 (a) Pneumothorax. (b) Pneumothorax X-ray; red arrows indicate separation of the visceral pleura from the parietal pleura.
(b) © Tomatheart/Shutterstock.

and may involve one rib or multiple ribs" (Gundersen et al., 2021). The mechanism for this injury is typically a direct blow to the lateral or posterior thorax from a kick or block; however, an indirect fracture can occur from general compression or stress on the rib cage (Dixit & Chang, 2018). Fractures may occur anywhere along the rib; however, the angle of the rib is the anatomically weakest point. A direct fracture causes the most damage because pieces of the rib can penetrate the chest cavity, causing severe damage. Displaced rib fractures may damage internal thoracic structures, particularly the lungs, resulting in either a traumatic **pneumothorax** (Figure 10.3a & b) or **hemothorax**. Both involve air within the chest cavity which causes lung collapse, but a hemothorax includes blood and other fluid in the chest cavity. Such injuries will result in significant changes in breathing and may also induce shock. For more detailed information on the care and management of these injuries, refer to Chapter 13, *Injuries to the Thorax and Abdomen*.

Pneumothorax Air collects in the pleural cavity (space between the lungs and chest wall) causing the lung to collapse.

Hemothorax Blood collects in the pleural cavity (space between the lungs and chest wall).

Flail chest A portion of the rib cage is separated from the rest of the chest wall, usually due to trauma, making breathing very difficult.

Signs and symptoms of a simple rib fracture include the following:

- Painful respiration.
- Deformity in the region of the injury, including a protruding rib or a depression where the normal contour of the rib should be.
- Swelling and discoloration.
- Pain when the rib cage is compressed gently by the examiner.
- In severe cases, lung damage may result in symptoms associated with pneumothorax.

First aid care of a simple rib fracture involves the following:

1. Immediately apply RICE (generally best accomplished with a 6-inch-wide elastic wrap and a bag of crushed ice).
2. Treat for any signs and symptoms of shock.
3. Refer for medical evaluation by a physician. Oftentimes, an injured athlete is more comfortable with light compression over the rib cage (best accomplished with a 6-inch-wide elastic wrap or rib belt).

Complications of these injuries are rare; however, when they do occur, they can be quite dangerous, so always monitor an athlete for changes in vitals, difficulty breathing, or signs and symptoms of shock. If athletes experience multiple rib fractures, they can experience a **flail chest**—separation of a portion of the rib cage from the rest of the chest wall, which causes difficulty breathing and requires immediate medical attention.

Sprains

Sprains occur whenever a joint is forced through an abnormal range of motion (ROM) that results in damage to supporting structures, such as ligaments and joint capsules. Because the thoracic spine is well supported, limited movement is allowed, thereby reducing the incidence of sprains. However, joint sprains can occur on the anterior surface at the costochondral joint (i.e., rib and cartilage), sternocostal joints (i.e., cartilage and sternum), or the vertebrocostal joint (i.e., rib and thoracic vertebrae). Evaluation of a sprain to the thoracic spine is difficult and must be based on a detailed history of the injury. An athlete with such an injury will usually report having sustained an unusual movement or overuse of the thoracic spine that is associated with localized pain, a feeling of popping or snapping, and in some cases swelling. A consistent symptom of injury to the thoracic area is painful respiration, which is associated with many different injuries to the region, including rib fractures and contusions. First aid for sprains to the thoracic spine includes the application of RICE and light compression to the rib cage. If significant symptoms, such as **dyspnea** (i.e., difficulty breathing), persist for more than 24 hours, the athlete should be referred to a medical doctor.

Strains

Strains involve primarily contractile tissues and their support structures—muscles, fascia, and tendons. The muscles of the thoracic spine region include the erector spinae, latissimus dorsi, pectoral, serratus, and intercostal muscles. Strains may occur related to maximum exertion in sports requiring large amounts of force, such as tackle football, wrestling, and ice hockey. Muscular strains can also occur in sports that require end ROM activities, such as baseball (Gerrie, Harris, Lintner, & McCulloch, 2016), golf, gymnastics, and rowing (Thornton et al., 2017). Signs and symptoms of strains may be difficult to differentiate from sprains. Often, the injury mechanism will be identical to that of a sprain. Muscle spasms of the affected muscle may be noticeable, and these muscles may also be sensitive to touch (i.e., palpation) and should be inspected for swelling. First aid for suspected strains of this region is the same as that for sprains: application of RICE and light compression to the rib cage.

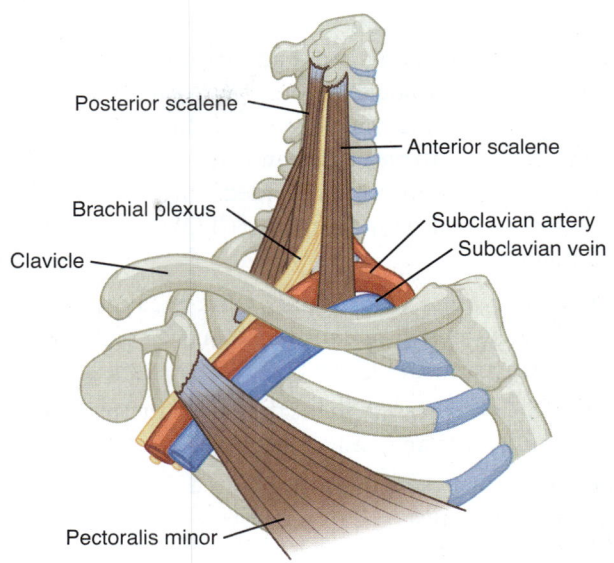

Figure 10.4 The brachial plexus and vascular network associated with the thoracic outlet.

Thoracic Outlet Syndrome

Thoracic outlet syndrome (TOS) (Figure 10.4) is a diverse group of disorders in which blood vessels and/or nerves (i.e., brachial plexus) are compressed in the space between the collarbone (i.e., clavicle) and the first rib (also called the thoracic outlet) or between the scalene muscles of the neck, thereby causing pain, tingling, or numbness in the upper extremities (Jones et al., 2019). TOS injuries are classified based on their symptoms; however, over 80% of cases are typically nerve related (Illig et al., 2021). A forceful trauma to the thoracic outlet can cause a TOS, but bony pathologies around the cervical and thoracic vertebrae or an extra rib (i.e., cervical rib) are usually associated with TOS. However, postural stressors associated with repetitive overuse in certain sports create soft-tissue adaptations, such as hypertrophy in some muscles and atrophy in others, creating a muscle imbalance around the thoracic outlet and brachial plexus (Jones et al., 2019). These muscle imbalances basically change the size and shape of the thoracic outlet and promote compression

Dyspnea Difficult or painful breathing.

Thoracic outlet syndrome (TOS) A group of disorders that occur when nerves or blood vessels in the space between the collarbone (clavicle) and the first rib are compressed, causing pain in the shoulders and neck and possibly numbness in the fingers.

of blood vessels and nerves (Jones et al., 2019). TOS can be difficult to diagnose and treat because its origins can be neurologic, venous, or arterial, and its signs and symptoms can vary between patients. Therefore, consultation with physicians and other sports medicine providers is highly recommended.

Signs and symptoms of TOS include the following:

- Complaints of a "dead" arm; weakness; cold hands/fingers; or numbness and tingling in the arm, hand, and fingers.
- Pain with pressure in the thoracic outlet area under the clavicle and above the first rib.
- Muscle spasms over the injured area and in the neck muscles.
- Vascular changes, including diminished pulse at the radial artery in the wrist with arms overhead.
- Neurological changes, including changes in sensation in the arm, hand, and fingers, as well as weakness with grip strength and other hand and wrist movements.

First aid care of TOS involves the following:

1. Rest from aggravating activity, and limit overhead activity.
2. Ice (generally best accomplished with a 6-inch-wide elastic wrap and a bag of crushed ice) over the thoracic outlet.
3. Schedule a follow-up evaluation with an athletic trainer or a physician.

Athletic Trainers SPEAK OUT

What is it like to be an athletic trainer for professional tennis?

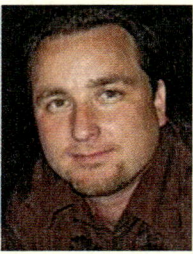

Courtesy of Robert Walls.

Being an athletic trainer in professional tennis is quite different than other traditional sports. I work in a field of athletes who are independent entities. We don't own or manage our players in the same way as most team sports. We are looked upon as advisors, and while most of our athletes listen and follow our advice, they are not bound to follow any guidelines that we set up. Also, in professional tennis, we are not typically called athletic trainers, but the broader term of "physio" is used. It's more recognizable in other countries and more accepted.

For me, I work out of a facility on the West Coast. I am the lone athletic trainer onsite completely dedicated to tennis. My typical day is 7:30 am through the last practice of the day.

I work not only on the rehabilitation side, but I work with the strength and conditioning staff to make sure all athletes are in proper form and are on preventative programs for natural dysfunctions due to the sport that they play. Tennis season is nearly year-round and we need to keep athletes playing at their peak levels. We recommend that players incorporate rest and recovery into their programs so that they can maintain their fitness levels without injury. We also assess our athletes prior to the start of each year and multiple times throughout the year to see if their potential for injury has increased or decreased based on the training and prevention programs that we assign to each player.

Tournament days are much longer than training days because of the tournament structure. When I am at a tournament, I am onsite prior to any American player and there until they finish competition. Each tournament is different and brings its own challenges. Unfortunately, I don't always have a dedicated space for me to work and I have to balance patient privacy with functionality in order to give the best care for any immediate issues. Tennis has really pushed me to be the best I can at manual therapy and at all the different taping techniques players prefer. We also have to be really innovative and think outside the box when coming up with programs when the players travel both domestically and internationally as they will still need to maintain their different regimens.

—**Robert Walls, MA, AC, CES, PES, FRCms**

Robert "Bobby" Walls is an athletic trainer for the United States Tennis Association in Los Angeles, California.

Intervertebral Disk Injuries in Thoracic Vertebrae

Although extremely rare in the thoracic region of the spine, injuries can occur to the intervertebral disks located between each of the vertebrae. Disk problems may be secondary to a compression fracture of thoracic vertebrae or can result from extreme flexion of the spine with a tackle or falls at high speeds (e.g., skiing, luge, and skeleton). Any athlete who complains of persistent neurological symptoms (Table 10.1), such as numbness or pain radiating around the thoracic region or into one or more of the extremities, should be stabilized and the emergency action plan should be activated so the injured athlete can be referred immediately to a physician for a more detailed evaluation.

Anatomy Review of the Lumbar, Sacral, and Coccygeal Regions of the Spine

The lumbar spine consists of five vertebrae that articulate superiorly with the thoracic vertebral column and inferiorly with the sacrum and coccyx. The lumbar vertebrae have the largest vertebral bodies because they bear a significant portion of body weight (Moini, 2020). The lumbar vertebrae are numbered L1 to L5, from proximal to distal, and have a concave curve when viewed from the side. Excessive lumbar curvature is called **lordosis** and can cause painful ailments. As is the case with the thoracic and cervical sections of the spine, intervertebral disks are located between each of the lumbar vertebrae as well as between T12 and L1 and L5 and S1 (the first sacral vertebra). Additionally, large, strong ligaments assist in stabilization of the lumbar vertebrae (Figure 10.5) along with the thoracic spine and the sacrum. The anterior and posterior longitudinal ligaments are located on the anterior and posterior surfaces of the vertebral bodies (Figure 10.6), respectively. Both of these important ligaments span the vertebral column from the level of C2 (i.e., axis) distal to the sacrum.

The sacrum, consisting of five fused vertebrae in a triangular shape, is located between the two pelvic bones posteriorly. In essence, the sacrum serves to

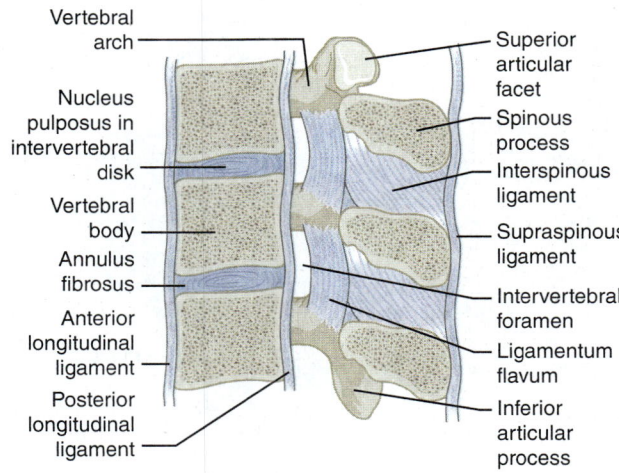

Figure 10.5 The lumbar vertebrae (sagittal view).

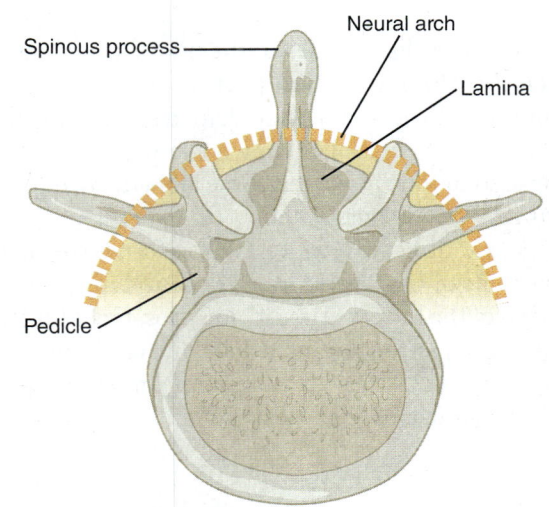

Figure 10.6 Overhead view of the neural arch of a typical lumbar vertebra.

connect the spinal column to the pelvis (Figure 10.7). Two articulations, the right and left sacroiliac joints, are formed by the union of the sacrum and the pelvis. There are no intervertebral disks between the sacral vertebrae, but strong ligaments serve to stabilize the area along with the pelvis. Blood vessels and nerves pass through tiny holes (called sacral foramina) and

Lordosis Abnormal curvature of the lumbar vertebrae.

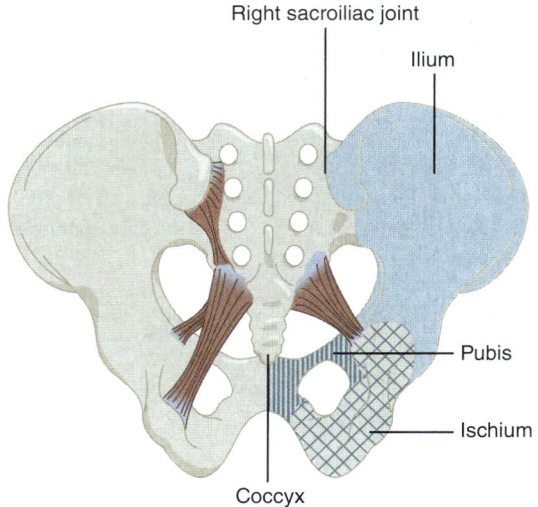

Figure 10.7 The pelvic girdle (posterior view).

serve many of the muscles in the buttocks and lower extremity. The most distal portion of the vertebral column is a small, arrowhead-shaped structure called the coccyx, which is also known as the tailbone. It is composed of four fused vertebrae and attached to the sacrum by strong ligaments.

The sciatic nerve (Figure 10.8) is formed from the nerve roots of L4–S3 and supplies neural innervation to many of the lower extremity muscles, including the hamstrings, gastrocnemius, soleus, and ankle muscles. Table 10.2 identifies areas of body innervation by lumbar, sacral, and coccygeal nerves.

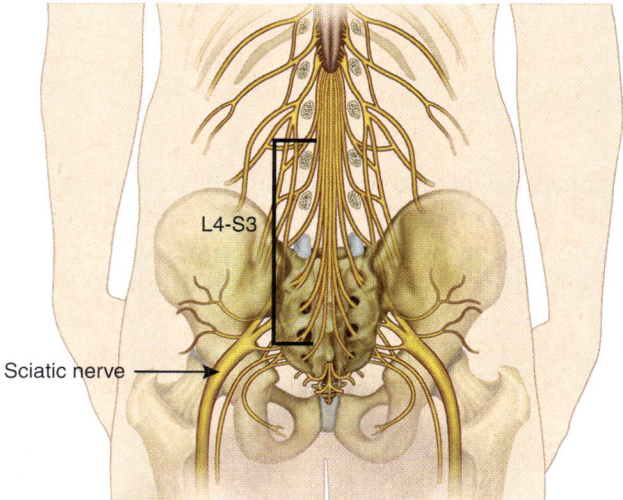

Figure 10.8 The sciatic nerve composed of nerve roots from L4–S3.
© ilusmedical/Shutterstock.

Table 10.2
Lumbar, Sacral, and Coccygeal Nerve Innervations

Lumbar/Sacral/Coccyx Nerve Section	Area of Body Affected and Area of Neurological Dysfunction*
L1	Anterior superior hip near inguinal line
L2	Anterior mid thigh
L3	Anterior distal thigh and medial thigh (groin)
L4	Medial lower leg
L5	Lateral lower leg and great toe
S1	Lateral foot/ankle, heel, Achilles tendon
S2	Posterior thigh and lower leg
S3, S4, S5, C1	Buttocks moving inward to anal region

*Neurological dysfunction includes lack of sensation, hypersensitivity, pain, or muscle weakness.

Common Sports Injuries

Injuries are more common to the lumbar than to the thoracic spine. In a recent survey of injuries in collegiate athletes from 2009 to 2015, collegiate men's football and women's gymnastics were the top two sports with the highest rate of lumbar spine injury, but men's and women's track and men's wrestling also had higher rates than other sports. The preseason was the most common time of injury across all sports, and most injuries were noncontact and did not result in significant time loss to participation. Overall, general pain was the most common reported injury, with strains, disk injuries, and stress fractures being frequently reported (Hassebrock et al., 2019). Stress fractures to the lumbar spine and pelvis were the third most common stress fracture injury reported from high school athletes from 2005 to 2013 (Changstrom, Brou, Khodaee, Braund, & Comstock, 2015). Collegiate athletes also experience lumbar stress fractures, and data from 2004–2014 shows that they were most common in men's wrestling and second most common in football (Rizzone et al., 2017).

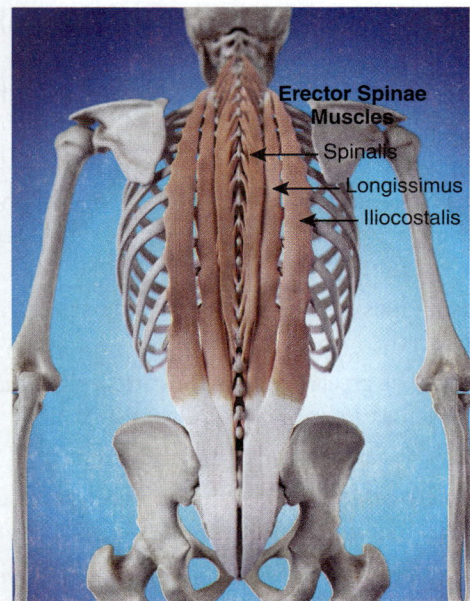

Figure 10.9 The erector spinae muscles of the upper and lower back.
© SciePro/Shutterstock.

Sprains and Strains

Very common soft-tissue injuries to the lumbar region are strains and sprains (Dowdell, Mikhail, Robinson, & Allen, 2018). Strains typically involve the global erector spinae muscles (Figure 10.9); however, there are many muscle groups that are local and run between two or three vertebrae (e.g., multifidus, rotatores, and interspinales), and these can also be strained. Muscle strains occur frequently, particularly in sports that place significant stress on the lumbar spine. Activities such as gymnastics, tackle football, and weight lifting can place the athlete in situations in which abnormal loads are exerted on the lumbar region of the spine.

Sprains involve the many ligaments and joint capsules of the region. As previously mentioned, there are large ligaments (i.e., the anterior and posterior longitudinal ligaments) that bind the vertebral bodies together. In addition, there are ligaments and capsules binding the joints between adjacent neural arches (i.e., facet joints). Major joints in the region include the lumbosacral, sacroiliac, and the sacrococcygeal. Generally, injuries to the joints are rare in this region.

Signs and symptoms of sprains and strains include the following:

- Localized muscle spasm.
- Pain that is increased with trunk movements.
- Postural abnormality of the trunk, which often involves a lateral tilting of the trunk away from the affected side.
- The athlete can link a specific incident with the onset of symptoms.
- In simple strains or sprains, pain will *not* radiate into the buttock or lower extremities.

First aid care of sprains and strains involves the following:

1. Remove the athlete from participation with assistance because any voluntary attempts to move will usually increase the pain.
2. Place the athlete in a position of lying supine, with the legs parallel and both knees drawn up so the knees and hips are flexed (Figure 10.10).
3. Place a rolled towel or some other soft material under the lumbar region for support.
4. Place a bag of crushed ice under the lumbar region.
5. The athlete should be instructed to sleep in a comfortable position and use ice to reduce pain.
6. If symptoms are not significantly reduced during the first 24 hours after the injury, medical referral is warranted.

It is important to remember that an injury mechanism of sufficient magnitude to cause a strain may also have caused more severe injury. It is always better to refer such athletes for further evaluation by a physician (Dowdell et al., 2018). This is especially important in cases in which the athlete complains of pain radiating into one or both legs (Table 10.2). Such

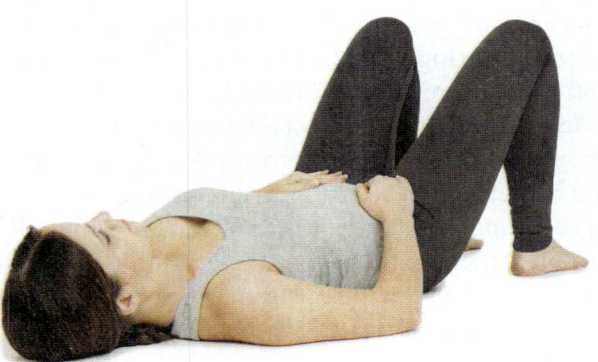

Figure 10.10 Hook lying position for relief of acute lower back pain in athletes. Knees and hips are bent to a position that relieves pain (this may be different for each person).
© fotandy/Shutterstock.

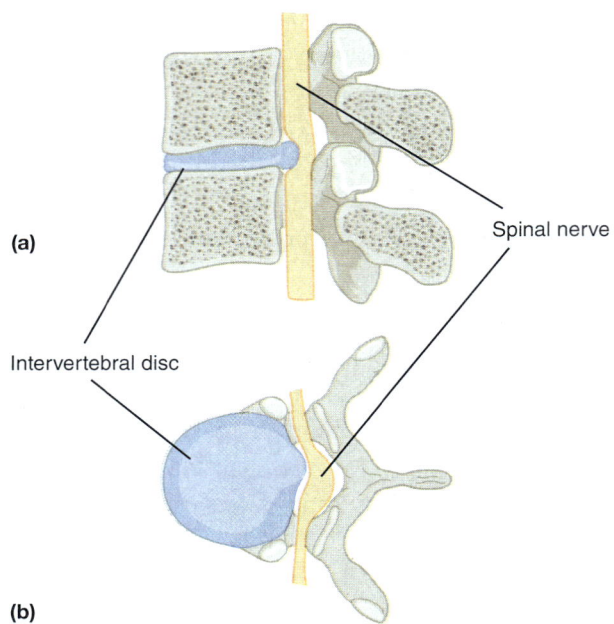

Figure 10.11 Disk protrusion/herniation at lumbar vertebrae. **(a)** Lateral view. **(b)** Cross-sectional view.

symptoms can indicate a significant injury involving a nerve, such as a herniated disk (Dowdell et al., 2018).

Lumbar Disk Injuries

A more serious form of soft-tissue injury to the lumbar region involves damage within an intervertebral disk, commonly known as a **herniated disk**. Though such injuries can occur to any of the disks of the spine, those most commonly injured in the lumbar region are L4 and L5 (Jenkins & Sasso, 2020). Most often, these injuries occur when an athlete is subjected to a great deal of force while in an awkward position. The anatomy of a typical intervertebral disk consists of an outer ring, called the annulus fibrosus, and a softer, inner portion, known as the nucleus pulposus (Moini, 2020). In the case of a herniation, a weakness develops in the annulus fibrosus, which then allows the nucleus pulposus to protrude through the wall of the annulus as if jelly was squeezed out of the jelly donut. Depending on the exact location of the herniation, pressure may be placed directly on the large spinal nerves (e.g., sciatic) passing through the region (Figure 10.11).

Herniated disk Rupture or protrusion of the nucleus pulposus through the annulus fibrosus of an intervertebral disk.

Signs and symptoms of lumbar disk injuries include the following:

- Intense local pain that is aggravated with any attempts to sit up, walk, or stand.
- Pain radiating into the buttock and lower extremity—radiating pain follows the distribution of the sciatic nerve down the back of the leg and into the foot (Table 10.2).
- Sensory loss or tingling/burning sensation radiating into the lower extremity.
- Pain will be greatly increased by attempting maneuvers such as a straight-leg raise or a sit-up.
- Muscle spasm and postural abnormalities.
- In severe cases, disk herniation may interfere with normal bladder and/or bowel function.

First aid care of lumbar disk injuries involves the following:

1. Remove the athlete from participation with assistance because any voluntary attempts to move will usually increase the pain.
2. Place the athlete in a supine position, with the legs parallel and both knees drawn up so the knees and hips are flexed (Figure 10.10); if this position is uncomfortable, allow the athlete to assume a position that is the least painful.
3. Place a rolled towel or some other soft material under the lumbar region for support.
4. Place a bag of crushed ice under the lumbar region.
5. Arrange for transport to a medical facility for evaluation.
6. Although little can be done in the field for such injuries, much can be done to alleviate long-term symptoms with a combination of physical therapy and drug therapy. The major goal of such a strategy is to return the athlete to participation and avoid the need for surgery.

WHAT IF ?

You are coaching gymnastics. One of your athletes just overrotated on a "double-back" on the floor. As soon as she hit the mat, she collapsed to the floor, complaining of severe pain in her lumbar region. In addition, she complains of a burning sensation in the back of her thigh and lower leg. What type of injury might she have? What type of first aid care would you provide?

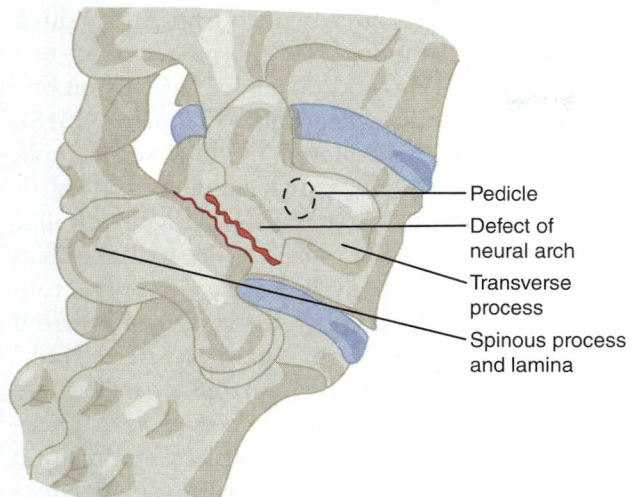

Figure 10.12 Defect of the neural arch that causes spondylolysis.

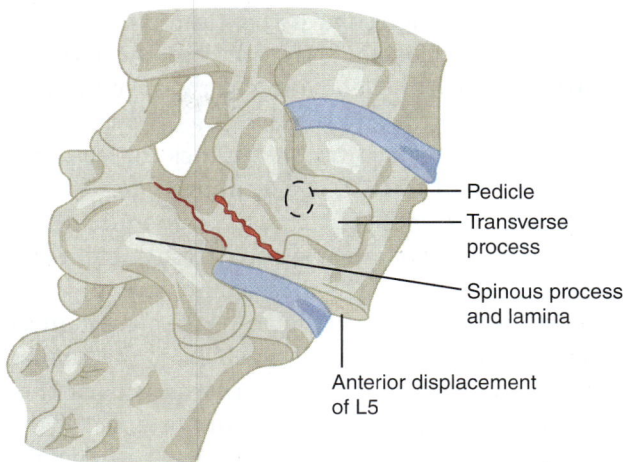

Figure 10.13 Anterior displacement of the L5 vertebra that induces spondylolisthesis.

Spondylolysis and Spondylolisthesis

Spondylolysis (Figure 10.12) is a defect (stress fracture) in the part of a vertebra that forms the bony ring around the spinal cord, known as the neural arch (Figure 10.6). Spondylolysis involves the portion of the neural arch known as the pars interarticularis (there are two on each vertebra, one each on the right and left sides). The significance of bony defects in this region relates to superior articulations with adjacent vertebrae. Thus, any defect of the neural arch in this area can compromise the integrity of the articulation between any two vertebrae.

In cases in which both the right and left neural arches are affected, the involved vertebra has the potential to slide forward, thus producing a condition known as **spondylolisthesis**. As can be seen in Figure 10.13, the most common site for this condition is between L5 and the sacrum (Sairyo et al., 2020). Given the normal slope of the sacrum, bony instability of the last lumbar vertebra makes anterior displacement possible, especially when the lumbar region is subjected to abnormal amounts of stress, such as the stress that occurs in gymnastics, tackle football, or competitive weight lifting.

The exact **etiology** of spondylolysis is not clear; however, evidence suggests that the bony defects may be either congenital (i.e., present at birth) or related to excessive stress to the bones during childhood and puberty. The symptoms of spondylolysis include low back pain, which becomes particularly acute when the lumbar spine is placed into **hyperextension**. When the defect is unilateral (one side only), standing on one leg in conjunction with lumbar hyperextension will elicit pain only on the side of the defect (Jenkins & Sasso, 2020). If spondylolysis progresses to spondylolisthesis, symptoms may become more severe. Pain in the lumbar region may increase during activity, and in some cases radiating pain may occur in the buttocks and upper thighs (Jenkins & Sasso, 2020).

Any athlete complaining of symptoms of this type, particularly those involved in high-risk sports for lumbar injuries (e.g., gymnastics, tackle football, and weight lifting), should be referred to a medical doctor for further evaluation. Treatment for spondylolysis and spondylolisthesis may include rest, drug therapy, lumbar bracing, exclusion from certain sports, and in very severe cases surgical spinal fusion.

Traumatic Fractures

Traumatic fractures of the lumbar vertebrae are infrequent in sports. Such injuries will normally be associated with a history of a severe blow to the

---

Spondylolysis Defect in the neural arch (i.e., pars interarticularis) of the vertebrae.

Spondylolisthesis Forward slippage of vertebra, usually between the fifth lumbar and the sacrum.

Etiology Science dealing with causes of disease or injury.

Hyperextension Extreme stretching of a body part. Joint range of motion beyond normal extension of the vertebral joints where there is compression on posterior bony structures.

lumbar region that results in a contusion (i.e., bruise) or falling from a height and landing on the buttocks (Davis et al., 2020). Depending on the specific location and type of fracture, neurological symptoms, such as radiating pain into the buttocks or legs, may be present (Table 10.2). Such injuries need to be treated initially with great care via immobilizing the athlete on a spine board or scoop stretcher and transporting him or her to a medical facility, where a complete evaluation by a physician can take place. It must be remembered that an external blow to the lumbar region may also cause injury to internal organs, specifically the kidneys. Thus, it is important that the athlete be evaluated for such an injury. Special attention should be given to the signs and symptoms of internal injury, such as deep abdominal pain, blood in the urine (known as **hematuria**), or shock.

Sacral and Coccyx Injuries

Because of the sacroiliac joints (right and left), formed between the sacrum and the pelvis, most injuries to this region are sprains and strains. However, contusions to the sacrum or coccyx by direct blows or falling backward are common. Most injuries occur due to a twisting or rotating motion, landing heavily on one leg, or lifting with locked knees (Schnebel, 2018). Sports with repetitive rotating motions, such as golf, baseball, dancing, punting, high jumping, hurdling, or gymnastics, put athletes at the most risk of sacroiliac dysfunction. Contusions, sprains, and strains result in palpable tenderness to the sacroiliac joints or sacrum bone. Most pain occurs when changing position from sitting to standing, and, sometimes, the pain will radiate down the thigh (Schnebel, 2018). Such injuries are normally self-limited and require both muscle stretching or strengthening to improve athletic motions and protection from future trauma. Treatment guidelines for lumbar strains and sprains can be followed. One notable exception is a severe blow to the coccyx, which may result in a fracture or severe bruise. This injury can occur when an athlete falls backward, landing hard on the buttocks and impacting the coccygeal region. The signs and symptoms of this injury involve an observable bruise in the coccygeal region, severe point tenderness, and swelling. This injury needs to be evaluated by a medical doctor because a fracture may be present. Protection from future trauma is essential with appropriate padding.

Hematuria Blood, which can appear red or brown, in the urine.

Review Questions

1. True or false: Because of the bony relationship between the ribs and adjacent vertebrae, the thoracic spine is much less mobile than either the cervical or lumbar region of the spine.

2. True or false: Available data indicate that soft-tissue injuries of the thoracic spine are more frequent than bone-related injuries.

3. Describe briefly the condition known as Scheuermann's disease, along with its signs and symptoms.

4. Define scoliosis, kyphosis, and lordosis.

5. What is a posterior rib fracture, and what are its common signs and symptoms?

6. What is a consistent symptom related to sprains in the thoracic spine?

7. True or false: Intervertebral disk injuries are extremely common to the thoracic spine.

8. Anatomically, the sacrum consists of how many fused vertebrae?

9. What nerve roots form the sciatic nerve?

10. Describe the condition known as spondylolysis.

11. Describe briefly the condition known as spondylolisthesis, including both the signs and symptoms and recommended treatment.

12. What is the recommended immediate treatment for a suspected strain or sprain of the lumbar spine?

13. Describe briefly the normal anatomy of a typical lumbar intervertebral disk as well as the process of disk herniation.

14. What are the signs and symptoms of lumbar disk herniation?

15. What are common mechanisms of a sacroiliac joint injury?

References

Changstrom, B. G., Brou, L., Khodaee, M., Braund, C., & Comstock, R. D. (2015). Epidemiology of stress fracture injuries among US high school athletes, 2005-2006 through 2012-2013. *American Journal of Sports Medicine, 43*(1), 26-33.

Davis, E. P., Showery, J. E., Prasarn, M. L., & Dodwad, S. N. M. (2020). Traumatic lumbar injuries in athletes. In W. K. Hsu & T. J. Jenkins (Eds.), *Spinal conditions in the athlete* (pp. 249-262). New York, NY: Springer, Cham.

Dixit, S., & Chang, C. J. (2018). Thorax and abdominal injuries. In C. C. Madden, M. Putukian, E. C. McCarty, & C. C. Young (Eds.), *Netter's sports medicine* (2nd ed., pp. 402-414). Philadelphia, PA: Elsevier.

Dowdell, J., Mikhail, C., Robinson, J., & Allen, A. (2018). Anatomy of the pediatric spine and spine injuries in young athletes. *Annals of Joint, 3*(4), 1-10.

Gerrie, B. J., Harris, J. D., Lintner, D. M., & McCulloch, P. C. (2016). Lower thoracic rib stress fractures in baseball pitchers. *The Physician and Sportsmedicine, 44*(1), 93-96.

Gundersen, A., Borgstrom, H., & McInnis, K. C. (2021). Trunk injuries in athletes. *Current Sports Medicine Reports, 20*(3), 150-156.

Hassebrock, J. D., Patel, K. A., Makovicka, J. L., Chung, A. S., Tummala, S. V., Peña, A. J., . . . Chhabra, A. (2019). Lumbar spine injuries in National Collegiate Athletic Association athletes: A 6-season epidemiological study. *Orthopaedic Journal of Sports Medicine, 7*(1), 1-10.

Illig, K. A., Rodriguez-Zoppi, E., Bland, T., Muftah, M., & Jospitre, E. (2021). The incidence of thoracic outlet syndrome. *Annals of Vascular Surgery, 70*, 263-272.

Jenkins, T. J., & Sasso, R. C. (2020). Lumbar disk herniation and degenerative disk disease in the athlete. In W. K. Hsu & T. J. Jenkins (Eds.), *Spinal conditions in the athlete* (pp. 201-213). New York, NY: Springer, Cham.

Johnson, B. K., & Comstock, R. D. (2017). Epidemiology of chest, rib, thoracic spine, and abdomen injuries among United States high school athletes, 2005/06 to 2013/14. *Clinical Journal of Sport Medicine, 27*(4), 388-393.

Johnston, H. A., & Drake, J. D. (2021). Multivariate shoulder and spine relationship using planar range of motion assessment. *Musculoskeletal Science and Practice, 54*, 102398.

Jones, M. R., Prabhakar, A., Viswanath, O., Urits, I., Green, J. B., Kendrick, J. B., Brunk, A. J., Eng, M. R., Orhurhu, V., Cornett, E. M., & Kaye, A. D. (2019). Thoracic outlet syndrome: A comprehensive review of pathophysiology, diagnosis, and treatment. *Pain and Therapy, 8*(1), 5-18.

Maslak, J. P., & Savage, J. W. (2020). Thoracic pathology in athletes. In W. K. Hsu & T. J. Jenkins (Eds.), *Spinal conditions in the athlete* (pp. 263-277). New York, NY: Springer, Cham.

Menzer, H., Gill, G. K., & Paterson, A. (2015). Thoracic spine sports-related injuries. *Current Sports Medicine Reports, 14*(1), 34-40.

Moini, J. (2020). *Anatomy and physiology for health professionals* (3rd ed.). Burlington, MA: Jones & Bartlett Learning.

O'Toole, J. E., Kaiser, M. G., Anderson, P. A., Arnold, P. M., Chi, J. H., Dailey, A. T., Dhall, S. S., Eichholz, K. M., Harrop, J. S., Hoh, D. J., Qureshi, S., Rabb, C. H., & Raksin, P. B. (2019). Congress of Neurological Surgeons systematic review and evidence-based guidelines on the evaluation and treatment of patients with thoracolumbar spine trauma: Executive summary. *Neurosurgery, 84*(1), 2-6.

Rajasekaran, S., Kanna, R. M., & Shetty, A. P. (2015). Management of thoracolumbar spine trauma: An overview. *Indian Journal of Orthopaedics, 49*(1), 72-82.

Rizzone, K. H., Ackerman, K. E., Roos, K. G., Dompier, T. P., & Kerr, Z. Y. (2017). The epidemiology of stress fractures in collegiate student-athletes, 2004-2005 through 2013-2014 academic years. *Journal of Athletic Training, 52*(10), 966-975.

Sairyo, K., Sakai, T., Takata, Y., Yamashita, K., Tezuka, F., & Manabe, H. (2020). Spondylolysis and spondylolisthesis in athletes. In W. K. Hsu & T. J. Jenkins (Eds.), *Spinal conditions in the athlete* (pp. 235-247). New York, NY: Springer, Cham.

Schnebel, B. E. (2018). Thoracic and lumbrosacral spine injuries. In C. C. Madden, M. Putukian, E. C. McCarty, & C. C. Young (Eds.), *Netter's sports medicine* (2nd ed., pp. 415-424). Philadelphia, PA: Elsevier.

Thornton, J. S., Vinther, A., Wilson, F., Lebrun, C. M., Wilkinson, M., Di Ciacca, S. R., . . . Smoljanovic, T. (2017). Rowing injuries: An updated review. *Sports Medicine, 47*(4), 641-661.

Zemková, E., Kováčiková, Z., & Zapletalová, L. (2020). Is there a relationship between workload and occurrence of back pain and back injuries in athletes? *Frontiers in Physiology, 11*, 894.

CHAPTER 11

Injuries to the Shoulder Region

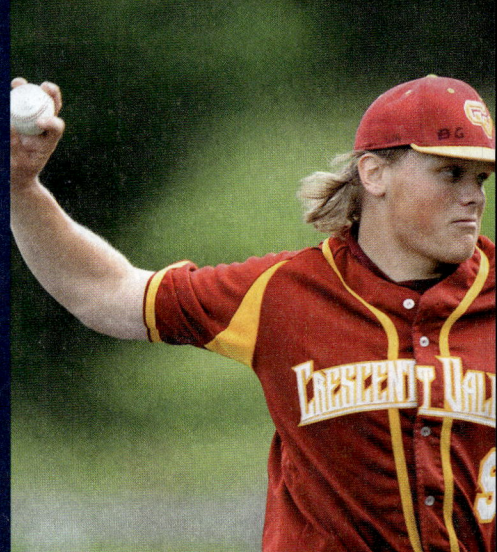

MAJOR CONCEPTS

The initial sections of the chapter review the gross anatomy and arthrology of the articulations of the shoulder, followed by a brief discussion of acute and chronic injuries common to the shoulder region. The chapter describes clavicular and proximal humeral fractures regarding the common mechanisms of injury, signs and symptoms, and recommended first aid care. It also covers injuries to the acromioclavicular (AC), sternoclavicular (SC), and glenohumeral (GH) joints, outlining the common mechanisms of injury, signs and symptoms, and recommended first aid care. Contusions to the shoulder area are also discussed regarding practical information about the signs and symptoms of this injury along with the suggested first aid.

Next, the chapter reviews musculotendinous injuries of the shoulder region regarding common mechanisms of injury, such as overhead throwing and swinging; it summarizes the basic kinesiology of the throwing or swinging motion with identification of the various types of muscle contractions during each phase of movement, followed by specific information regarding strains/tears to the rotator cuff and injuries to the biceps brachii tendon. Both of these injuries can be very debilitating and require surgical intervention. Shoulder impingement syndrome regarding its anatomy, signs and symptoms, and recommended treatments, including the role of altered functional movement of the glenohumeral joint commonly called scapular dyskinesis, is also discussed.

The chapter concludes with a short discussion of overuse shoulder injuries in the youth athlete and practical solutions demonstrated to reduce the risk of these injuries.

Anatomy Review

The shoulder allows for a great deal of movement while at the same time providing a point of attachment for the arm to the thorax. The skeleton of the shoulder (Figure 11.1) consists of the bones of the shoulder girdle and the humerus (upper arm bone). The clavicle and the scapula make up the shoulder girdle, so named because these two bones surround (girdle) the upper thorax. The head of the humerus combines with the shallow glenoid fossa of the scapula to form the highly mobile

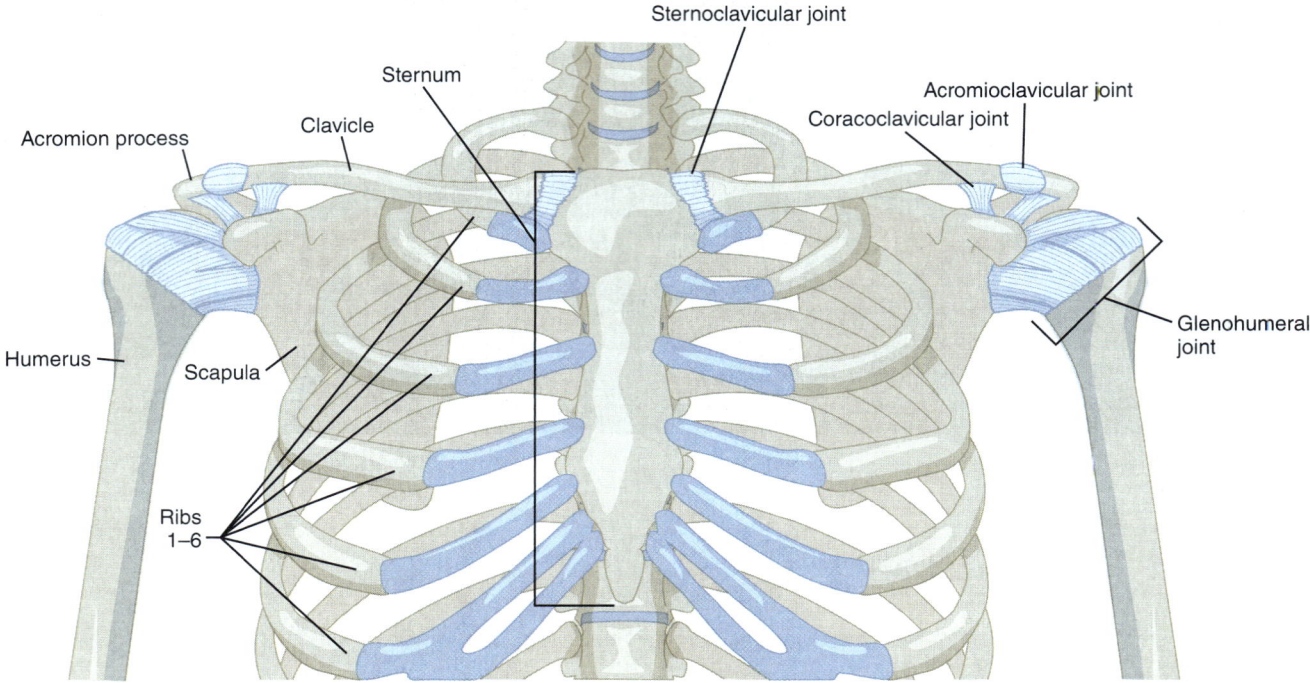

Figure 11.1 Skeleton of the shoulder region.

glenohumeral (GH) joint, commonly known as the shoulder joint (Figure 11.2). The GH joint is provided with additional stability by a fibrocartilaginous cuplike structure known as the glenoid labrum, which is directly attached to the glenoid fossa (Moini, 2020). The labrum makes the glenoid fossa a deeper receptacle for the head of the humerus. In addition, the long-head tendon of the biceps brachii muscle attaches to the superior labrum and to the supraglenoid tubercle at the top of the GH joint providing anterior stability to the GH joint. The shoulder region also includes the **acromioclavicular (AC) joint**, located between the distal end of the clavicle and the acromion of the scapula (Figure 11.2), and the **sternoclavicular (SC) joint**, located between the proximal end of the clavicle and the manubrium of the sternum (Figure 11.3). Each of these joints is held together with ligaments and joint capsules that provide stability while also allowing for necessary movement, which is quite limited.

Glenohumeral (GH) joint Articulation (spheroid) formed by the head of the humerus and the glenoid fossa of the scapula.

Acromioclavicular (AC) joint Articulation (arthrodial) formed by the distal end of the clavicle and the acromion process.

Sternoclavicular (SC) joint Articulation (arthrodial) formed by the union of the proximal clavicle and the manubrium of the sternum.

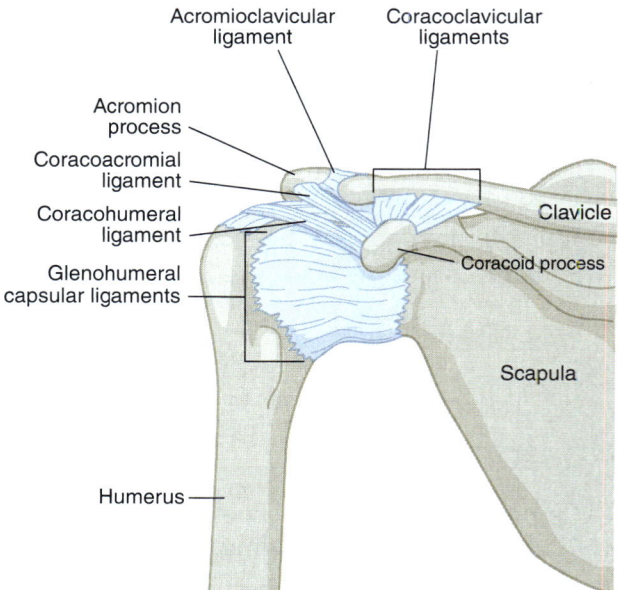

Figure 11.2 Ligaments of the coracoclavicular, acromioclavicular, and glenohumeral joints.

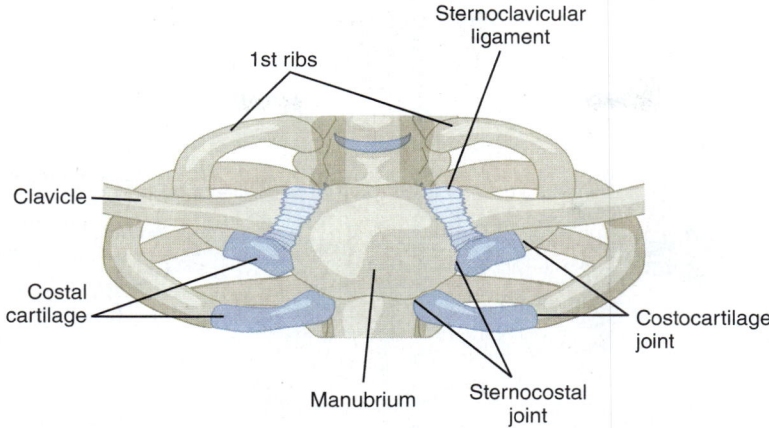

Figure 11.3 Ligaments of the sternoclavicular joint.

Many muscles move both the shoulder girdle and the GH joint in a multitude of directions. In nearly all motions the shoulder girdle and the GH joint work together to move the arm. Consequently, any limitation from injury to the shoulder girdle will indirectly affect the GH joint. The muscles in the region of the shoulder can be divided into two groups—those that act on the shoulder girdle and those that act on the GH joint (Figures 11.4a and b, 11.5a and b, and 11.6a and b). The muscles of the shoulder girdle are the levator scapulae; upper, middle, and lower trapezius; rhomboid minor and major; subclavius; pectoralis minor; and serratus anterior. These muscles collectively contribute to the movements of the shoulder girdle, which include scapular retraction and protraction, upward and downward scapular rotation, elevation, and depression. The muscles are listed with their specific actions and innervations in Table 11.1.

The muscles that act on the GH joint include the pectoralis major; latissimus dorsi; anterior, middle, and posterior deltoid; teres major; rotator cuff muscles (i.e., supraspinatus, infraspinatus, teres minor, and subscapularis); and coracobrachialis. The GH joint enjoys an astounding amount of movement, virtually in any direction; however, following are the movements normally attributed to the GH joint: flexion, extension, horizontal flexion and extension, internal and external rotation, abduction, and adduction. The muscles are listed with their specific actions and innervations in Table 11.2.

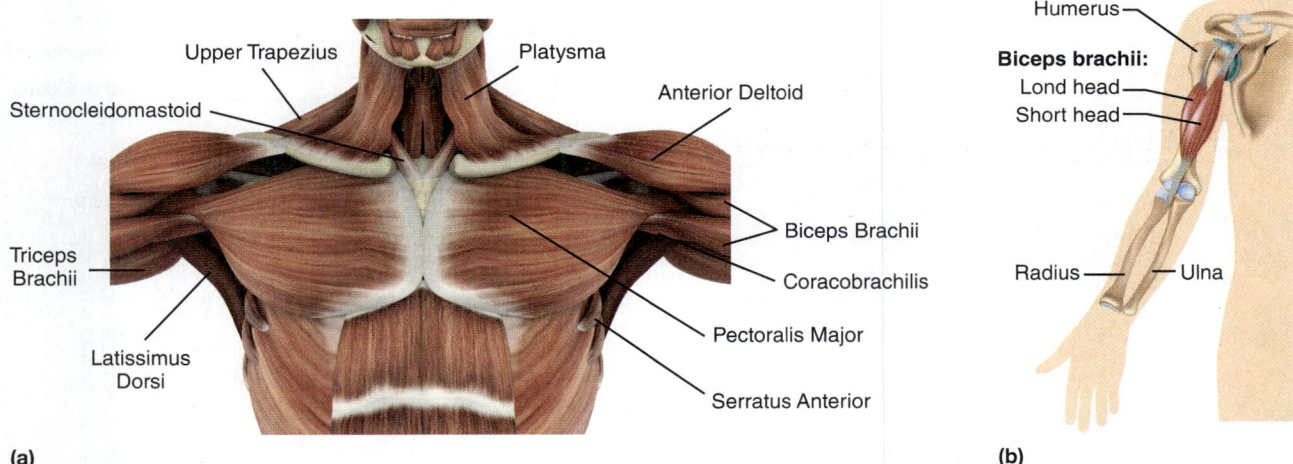

Figure 11.4 (a) Muscles of the anterior shoulder and trunk region. **(b)** Biceps brachii muscles (long and short heads).
(a) © Nerthuz/Shutterstock; (b) © Alila Medical Media/Shutterstock.

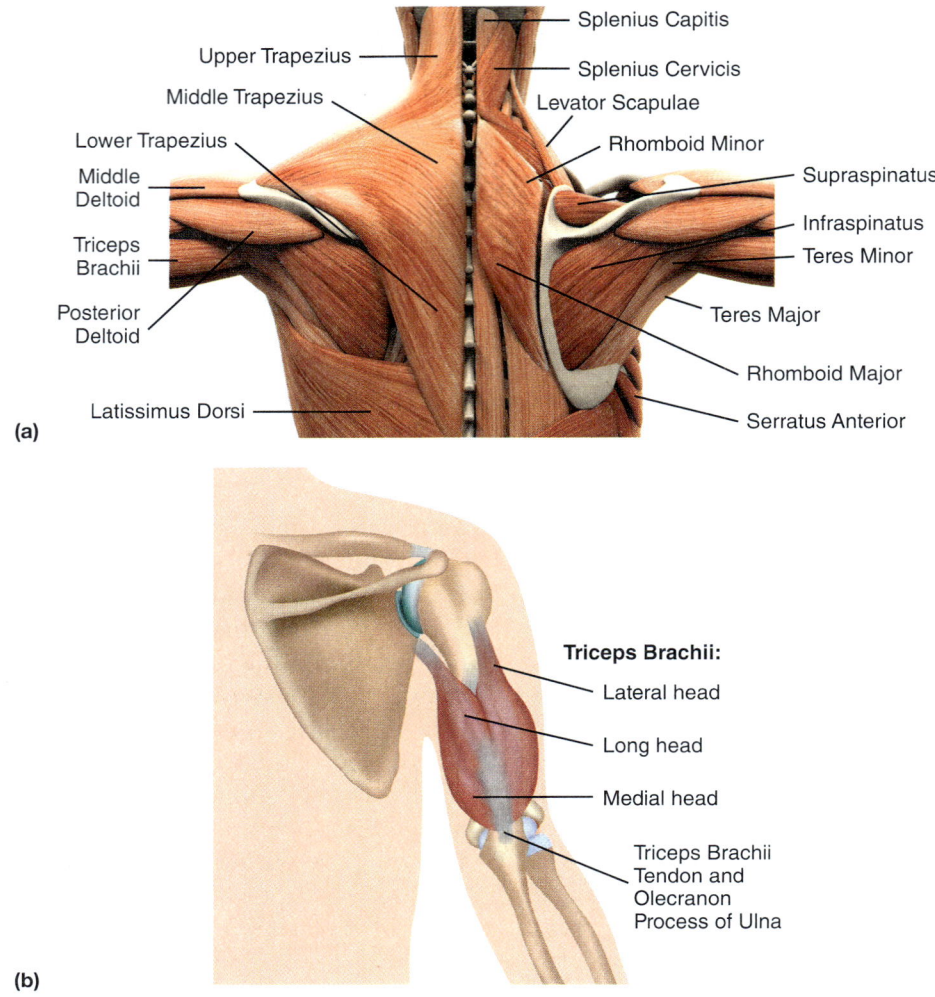

Figure 11.5 (a) Muscles of the posterior shoulder and trunk region. **(b)** Triceps brachii muscles (lateral, long, and medial heads).
(a) © Nerthuz/Shutterstock; (b) © Alila Medical Media/Shutterstock.

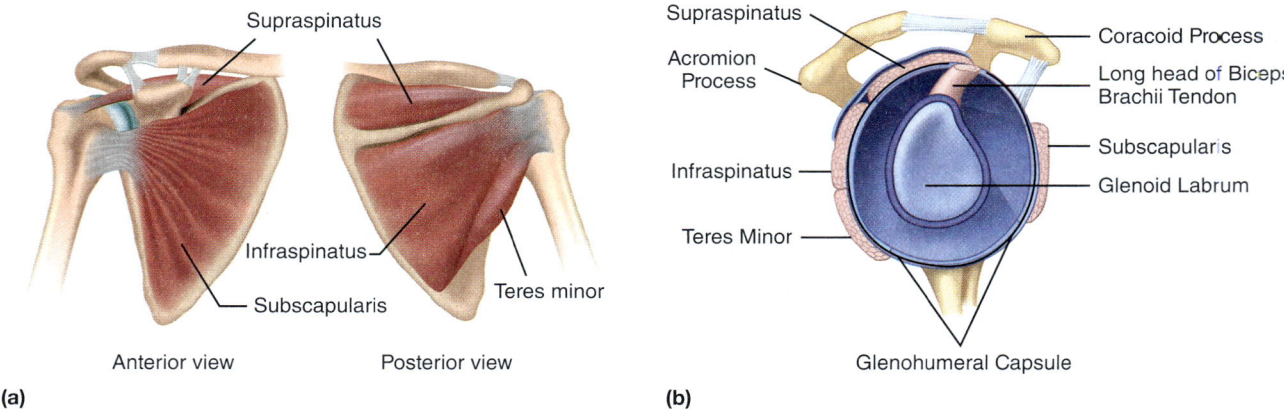

Figure 11.6 (a) Muscles of the rotator cuff. **(b)** Sagittal view of glenohumeral joint with humerus bone removed.
(a) © Alila Medical Media/Shutterstock; (b) © derter/Shutterstock.

Table 11.1
Muscles, Actions, and Innervations of the Shoulder Girdle

Muscle	Action	Innervation
Levator scapulae	Scapular elevation	Dorsal scapular
Rhomboid minor and major	Scapular retraction Downward rotation	Dorsal scapular
Upper, middle, and lower trapezius	Elevation Retraction Depression Upward rotation of scapula	Spinal accessory
Pectoralis minor	Depression	Medial pectoral
Serratus anterior	Protraction Upward rotation of scapula	Long thoracic
Subclavius	Depression Stabilization of the SC joint	Subclavian

Table 11.2
Muscles, Actions, and Innervations of the Glenohumeral Joint

Muscle	Action	Innervation
Pectoralis major	Adduction Internal rotation Flexion Extension	Medial and lateral pectoral
Latissimus dorsi	Extension Adduction Internal rotation	Thoracodorsal
Anterior, middle, and posterior deltoid	Adduction Internal rotation Extension and lateral rotation Flexion and internal rotation	Axillary

(*continues*)

Table 11.2 (continued)
Muscles, Actions, and Innervations of the Glenohumeral Joint

Muscle	Action	Innervation
Teres major	Adduction Internal rotation	Lower subscapular
Coracobrachialis	Flexion Adduction	Musculocutaneous
Rotator Cuff		
Supraspinatus	Adduction	Suprascapular
Infraspinatus	External rotation	Suprascapular
Teres minor	External rotation	Axillary
Subscapularis	Internal rotation Adduction	Upper and lower subscapular

In athletes, a large amount of soft tissue covers both the shoulder girdle and the GH joint; as a result, they are somewhat protected from external blows. However, even in extremely muscular athletes, both the AC and SC joints lie just under the skin and are therefore more exposed to external blows and subsequent injury. The blood supply to the entire upper extremity, including the shoulder, originates from branches of the subclavian artery. As this artery passes into the axillary region, it becomes the axillary artery; it continues into the upper arm, becoming the brachial artery, which splits just distal to the elbow to extend into the forearm and hand (Figure 11.7). Injuries to the arteries can cause external or internal hemorrhage, and they can also experience **thrombosis**. The veins are used to return blood to central circulation from the upper extremity. The cephalic, basilic, and brachial veins drain into the axillary vein, which drains into the subclavian vein. Injuries to the veins are uncommon but can include thrombosis.

Thrombosis Local coagulation or clotting of the blood.

The major nerves of the shoulder and upper extremity originate from the group known collectively as the brachial plexus (Figure 11.8). The brachial plexus originates from the ventral primary divisions of the fifth through the eighth cervical nerves and

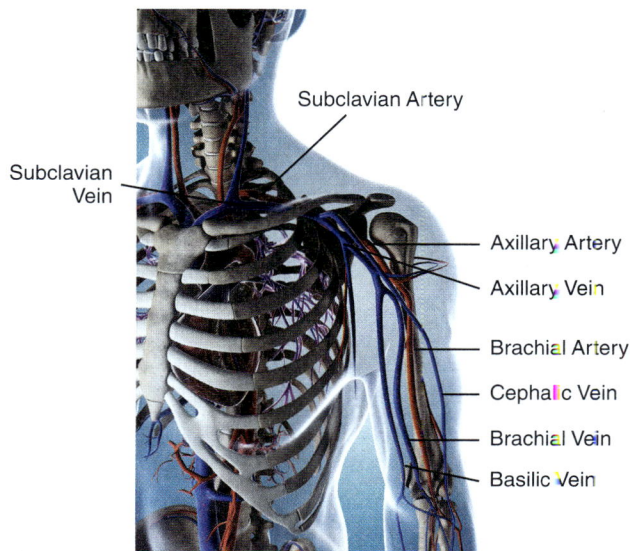

Figure 11.7 Major arteries and veins of the arm.
© SciePro/Shutterstock.

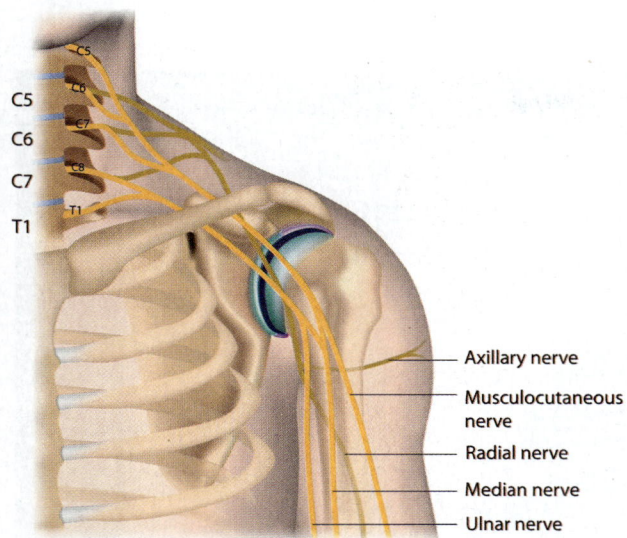

Figure 11.8 The nerves of the brachial plexus.
© Alila Medical Media/Shutterstock.

the first thoracic nerve. Through a complex series of divisions, the brachial plexus provides all the major nerves to the entire upper extremity, including nerve innervations to muscles of the shoulder girdle and GH joint (Moini, 2020).

Common Sports Injuries

Injuries to the shoulder region are common in many sports and in some cases are highly sport specific. For example, injuries to the GH and AC joints are quite common in wrestling. A recent epidemiology report cataloging wrestling injuries over the decade from 2005 to 2014 demonstrated that shoulder and clavicle injuries are the second most common injury in both practice and competition for high school athletes, behind head and face injuries, and they were the third most common injury for collegiate wrestling athletes, behind head and face and knee injuries (Kroshus et al., 2018). Sports that emphasize a throwing or swinging action often produce injuries caused by overuse or deconditioning of the muscles of the rotator cuff (i.e., infraspinatus, supraspinatus, teres minor, and subscapularis), which act on the GH joint (Lin et al., 2018). The rotator cuff muscles are extremely important to the stability of the GH joint because this large ball-and-socket structure lacks inherent strength owing to the combination of the geometry of the glenoid fossa and the extensive joint capsule. Epidemiological comparisons of high school softball and baseball demonstrated that in softball 16.7% of shoulder injuries were sustained by pitchers, whereas in baseball 39.6% of shoulder injuries were sustained by pitchers (Oliver et al., 2019; Saper et al., 2018). Interestingly, 21% of the baseball pitcher injuries required more than three weeks to return to sport, but only 2.3% of the softball pitcher injuries required as long (Oliver et al., 2019). Sports such as cycling, football, ice hockey, soccer, skateboarding, and snowboarding produce a large number of fractures of the clavicle brought about by falls (DeFroda et al., 2019; Frima et al., 2020). Injuries of the shoulder region can be classified as either acute (of sudden onset) or chronic (resulting from overuse). Sports involving heavy contact or collisions yield more acute injuries; those necessitating repeated movements tend to produce more chronic injuries (Lin et al., 2018). Shoulder injuries can have a significant effect on time lost from sport. Football, wrestling, men's ice hockey, and men's basketball had the highest incidence of season-ending shoulder injuries in collegiate athletes within a study covering 2009–2010 to 2013–2014 seasons (Goodman et al., 2018). In particular, out of all shoulder injuries, dislocations and subluxations resulting in instability (49.1% of 116 injuries) ended the most seasons, but when compared across all injuries, clavicular fractures (45.5% of 2,711) ended the most seasons (Goodman et al., 2018).

Skeletal Injuries

Fractured Clavicle

The most common fracture of the shoulder region is a fracture of the clavicle. Such fractures can result from direct blows to the bone; however, the majority occur as a result of falls that transmit the force to the clavicle either through the arm or shoulder. The majority of clavicular fractures occur about midshaft (Figure 11.9); the remainder involve either the proximal or distal end of the bone (Frima et al., 2020). Several classification systems for clavicle fractures have been developed based on the location and severity of the fracture (Moverley et al., 2020; Stenson & Baker, 2021). The classification systems are the Robinson, Edinburgh, Neer, and AO/IOTA (Axelrod et al., 2020; DeFroda et al., 2019; Ellis et al., 2020; Frima et al., 2020). In the adolescent

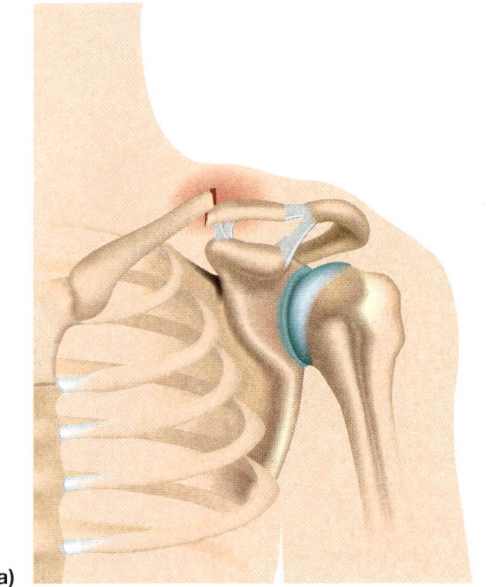
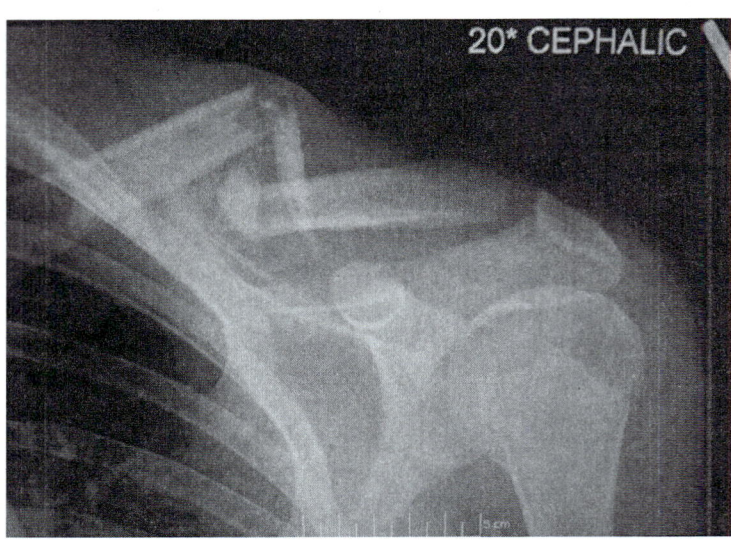

Figure 11.9 (a) Midshaft fracture of the left clavicle. (b) X-ray of fracture to the left clavicle.
(a) © Alila Medical Media/Shutterstock; (b) Courtesy of Kevin G. Shea, MD, Intermountain Orthopaedics, Boise, Idaho.

athlete, another type of clavicular fracture, commonly known as a greenstick fracture, can occur. This fracture occurs in immature bone and involves a cracking, splintering type of injury. Although a fractured clavicle is potentially dangerous given the close proximity of the bone to major blood vessels and nerves, the vast majority of these injuries cause few complications. Appropriate first aid must be applied to prevent unnecessary movement of the fracture, which can result in additional soft-tissue damage.

Signs and symptoms of a fractured clavicle include the following:

- Swelling and/or deformity of the clavicle
- Discoloration at the site of the fracture
- Possible broken bone end projecting through the skin
- Athlete reporting that a snap or pop was felt or heard
- Athlete holding the arm on the affected side under the elbow and bracing it to trunk to relieve pressure on the shoulder girdle

First aid care for a fractured clavicle involves the following:

1. Treat for possible shock. Determine whether any neurovascular compromise is present, such as arm or hand numbness, pale skin, ashen (gray) skin, or decreased capillary refill (Pollak, 2021).
2. Apply sterile dressings to any related wounds.
3. Carefully apply a sling-and-swathe bandage, as shown in Figure 11.10a and b.
4. Arrange for transport to a medical facility.

Fractured Scapula

A much less common type of fracture in the shoulder region involves the scapula. The location of the scapula behind the thorax and its musculature likely explains why fractures of the scapula are uncommon, representing only 1% of all fractures and 3–5% of upper extremity fractures (Burnier et al., 2019). Scapular fractures typically result from direct blows to the shoulder region. The symptoms of this type of fracture are less clear than those related to fractures of the clavicle. An athlete with a history of a severe blow to the shoulder region followed immediately by considerable pain and loss of function should be referred to a physician for further evaluation. This injury can be identified only by X-ray analysis. Treatment is determined by the specific location and extent of the fracture(s). Typically, the athlete's arm will be placed in a sling, and the player will be removed from sports participation for a period of 6 weeks.

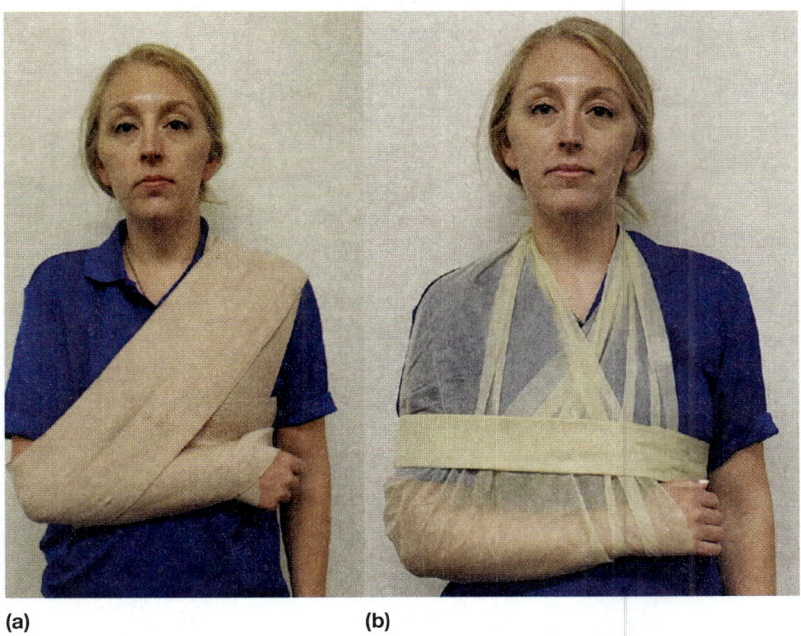

Figure 11.10 A sling-and-swathe bandage is effective for a variety of injuries to the upper extremity. **(a)** Using double-length elastic wrap. **(b)** Using cloth cravats.
Courtesy of Cindy Trowbridge.

Soft-Tissue Injuries

A variety of sprains and strains involving any number of specific ligaments and tendons occurs in this region of the body. Although any joint can sustain a sprain, the GH and AC joints are the most commonly injured in the shoulder region in sports.

Acromioclavicular Joint Injuries

Just under the skin on the lateral superior surface of the shoulder is the AC joint. This gliding synovial articulation is supported by the superior and inferior AC ligaments and contains an intra-articular cartilaginous disk (Wong & Kiel, 2018).). Additional support to the AC joint is provided by the coracoclavicular (CC) ligament (see Figure 11.2), which comprises the trapezoid and conoid ligaments. The CC ligament is attached between the superior coracoid process and the inferior lateral surface of the clavicle.

Shoulder injury data collected from NCAA quarterbacks from 2004–2014 demonstrated that acromoclavicular joint sprains were the most common injury reported (Tummala et al., 2018). The typical mechanism of injury for the AC joint is a downward blow, caused by falling or some external blow, other than a fall, to the distal end of the clavicle, which results in the acromion process being driven inferiorly while the distal clavicle remains in place. Another mechanism, resulting in what has been described as an "indirect" injury, is a fall forward on an outstretched arm, which then transmits the force up the extremity and results in the humeral head being driven up into the acromion, again, resulting in disruption of the supporting ligaments (Nordin et al., 2020).

Either of these two mechanisms can result in varying degrees of ligament damage. AC injuries can be classified according to the Rockwood classification system and the ISAKOS Upper Extremity Committee Consensus Statement (2014) into one of six types, with the least severe being type I with no AC ligament damage (sprain); type II involves a tear of the AC ligament with the CC ligaments intact; type III involves tearing of the AC and CC ligaments along with a dislocation of the AC joint (Figure 11.11); type IV is characterized by ligament disruption along with a gross displacement of the clavicle posteriorly, piercing the trapezius muscle; type V is characterized by a significant dislocation of the distal clavicle 100–300% from normal, along with additional damage to the deltotrapezial

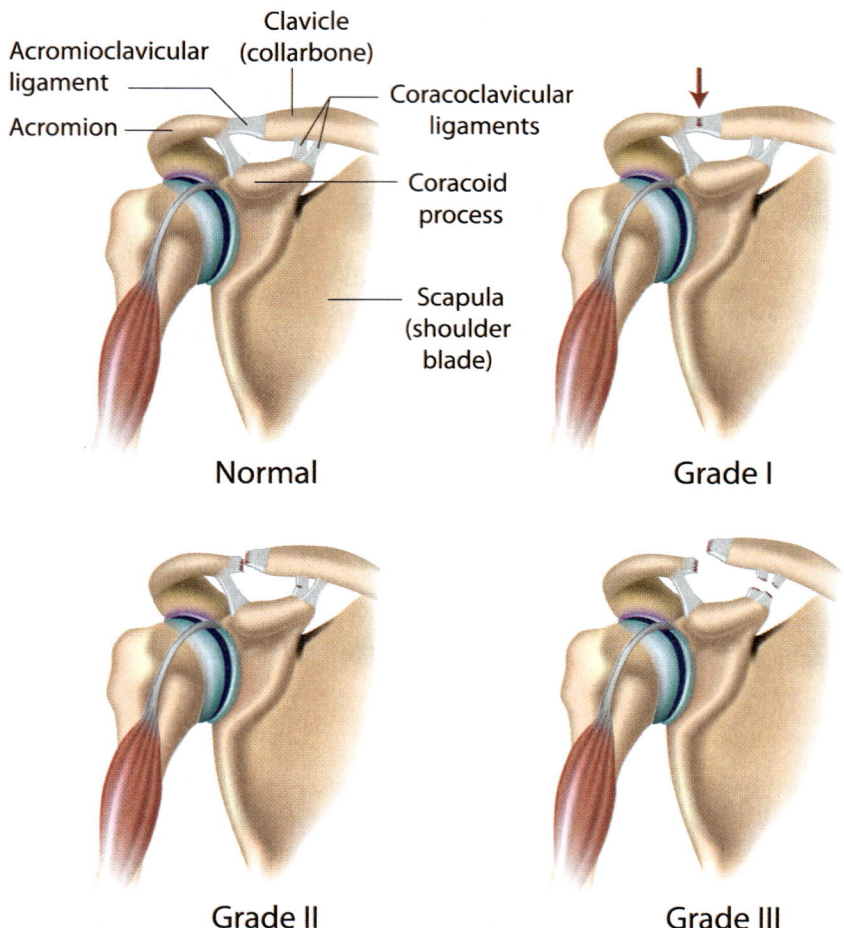

Figure 11.11 Separated shoulder injuries—types I, II, and III.
© Alila Medical Media/Shutterstock.

fascia; and type VI involves a complete dislocation of the distal clavicle to an inferior position (subacromial or subcoracoid; Beitzel et al., 2014; Gorbaty et al., 2017; Kiel & Kaiser, 2021; Wong & Kiel, 2018). The severity of the injury is graded based on the amount of damage to specific ligaments.

Signs and symptoms of AC joint sprains include the following:

- Types I and II sprains are characterized by mild swelling with point tenderness and discoloration around the AC joint. Type II sprains are normally characterized by more swelling and pain and likely a small deformity. Most movements, especially horizontal adduction of the shoulder will elicit pain.

- Type III and higher sprains are characterized by significant deformity in the region of the AC joint because these injuries involve complete ruptures of the AC and CC ligaments. Superior displacement of the clavicle results from the weight of the arm pulling down on the shoulder while the clavicle tends to move superiorly, creating the displacement that can easily be seen upon visual examination. The athlete may report having felt a snap or heard a pop.

First aid care for AC joint sprains involves the following:

1. Immediately apply ice and compression. This is best accomplished by placing a bag of crushed ice over the AC joint and securing it with an elastic wrap tied in a figure-eight configuration.

2. Once the ice and compression are in place, apply a standard sling-and-swathe bandage (Figure 11.10a and b). This is a critical step because the sling helps to remove the stress to the injured AC joint by supporting the weight of the arm in the sling.
3. Immediately refer the athlete to a medical facility for further evaluation. In the event of severe injury (types IV, V, and VI), arrange for transport and treat for shock. Monitor the sensory and vascular status of the upper extremity to rule out neurovascular compromise.

Long-term treatment for AC separations is dependent on the level of severity of the injury. Treatment for types I and II is typically nonsurgical and includes rest and nonsteroidal anti-inflammatory drugs, and in some cases, the athlete will be asked to wear a special sling that uses straps to support the AC joint while healing (Wong & Kiel, 2018). Once healed, depending on the sport, the athlete may be fitted with a sling-and-strap device that secures a protective pad over the AC joint.

Debate is ongoing within the medical community regarding the best treatment approach for type III AC joint injuries. However, recent research supports a nonsurgical approach, even for athletes, if the injury is uncomplicated (Frank et al., 2019). Given the extensive soft-tissue damage and clavicular displacement in more severe AC joint injuries (types IV–VI), surgery usually is indicated. Complications from acromioclavicular joint injuries can include continuing pain (30–50% of individuals) and the development of osteoarthritis (Kiel & Kaiser, 2021; Wong & Kiel, 2018).

Glenohumeral Joint Injuries

This articulation consists of the relatively large humeral head opposing the rather shallow glenoid fossa of the scapula. This bony arrangement is effective in giving the joint a great deal of mobility. As stated in the "Anatomy Review" section of the chapter, the stability of the joint is increased by the glenoid labrum. The GH joint is classified as a spheroidal articulation that moves within all three planes of motion: frontal, sagittal, and transverse. However, this mobility makes the GH joint very unstable (Bakhsh & Nicandri, 2018). The major soft-tissue structures of the GH joint include the capsular ligaments (Figure 11.6 b) and the coracohumeral ligament (Figure 11.2) (Moini, 2020).

The typical mechanism for a traumatic injury for the GH joint involves having the arm abducted and externally rotated. In this position, the anterior portion of the joint capsule, specifically the GH ligament, can be stressed beyond its capacity. If the ligament fails, the head of the humerus can move forward and out of place, resulting in the most common type of GH joint dislocation, an anterior dislocation (Figures 11.12 and 11.13). Depending on the severity, this injury may be either a subluxation (joint congruity is automatically restored) or a complete dislocation.

The joint capsule, ligaments, and supporting musculature are often stretched; therefore, as the athlete continues to participate in stressful activity, the joint becomes progressively less stable. The athlete typically will report that, during certain movements, often those placing the GH joint in abduction and external rotation, the joint will pop out and then return to its normal position. The risk of recurrence of anterior shoulder dislocations has received much discussion within the sports medicine literature (Provencher et al., 2021; Shanmugaraj et al., 2021). Young athletes are at risk for recurrent instability after first-time dislocation and have difficulties returning to sport (Shanmugaraj et al., 2021).

The humeral head can also move posteriorly, resulting in a posterior dislocation of the GH joint. This injury is not as common as anterior dislocations but does occur via acute traumatic loading and repetitive microtrauma causes. Sports that involve a load borne in front of the body are the most frequent

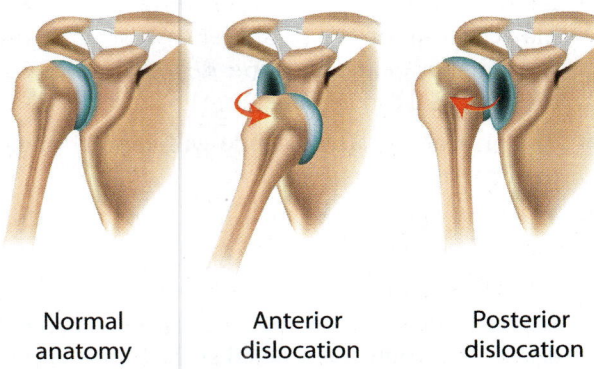

Figure 11.12 Anterior and posterior dislocation of glenohumeral joint compared to normal anatomy.
© Alila Medical Media/Shutterstock.

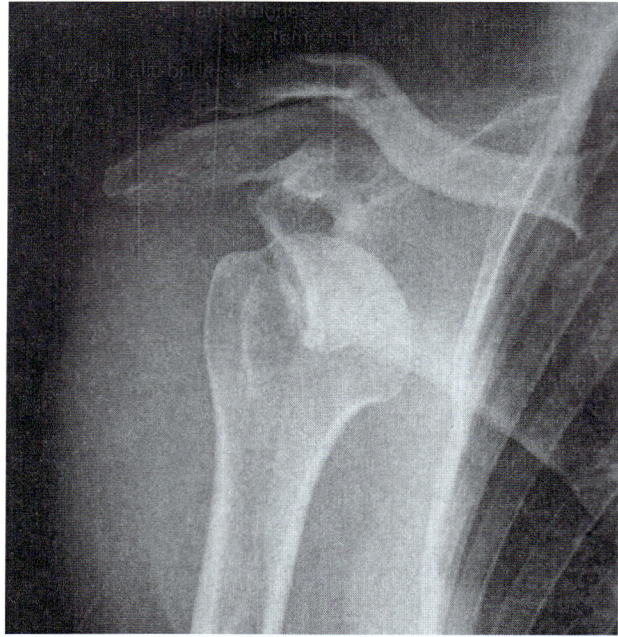

Figure 11.13 Anterior dislocation of the glenohumeral joint (right shoulder). Note the position of the humeral head relative to the glenoid fossa.
Courtesy of Kevin G. Shea, MD, Intermountain Orthopaedics, Boise, Idaho.

causes of posterior instability, and acute traumatic posterior dislocation typically involves a direct load on a flexed and internally rotated shoulder. Repetitive overhead weightlifting, bench pressing, playing as a blocking lineman in football, rowing, and swimming can result in repeated microtrauma to posterior structures of the shoulder and predispose athletes to posterior humeral dislocation (Merolla et al., 2016).

Signs and symptoms of an anterior GH joint dislocation include the following:

- Deformity of the shoulder joint: The normal contour of the shoulder is lost, and the shoulder appears to slope down abnormally (Figure 11.14a) (Pollak, 2021).
- The arm of the affected side will appear longer than normal.
- The head of the humerus will be palpable within the axilla.
- The athlete will be supporting the arm on the affected side with the opposite arm; the affected arm will be slightly abducted at the shoulder and flexed at the elbow (Figure 11.14b).
- The athlete will resist all efforts passively or actively to move the GH joint.

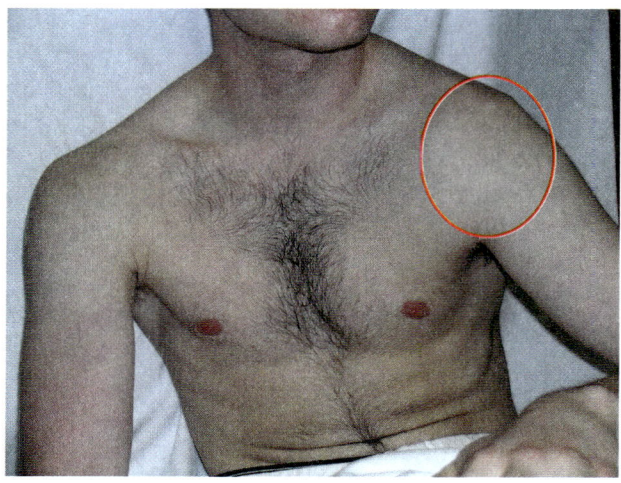

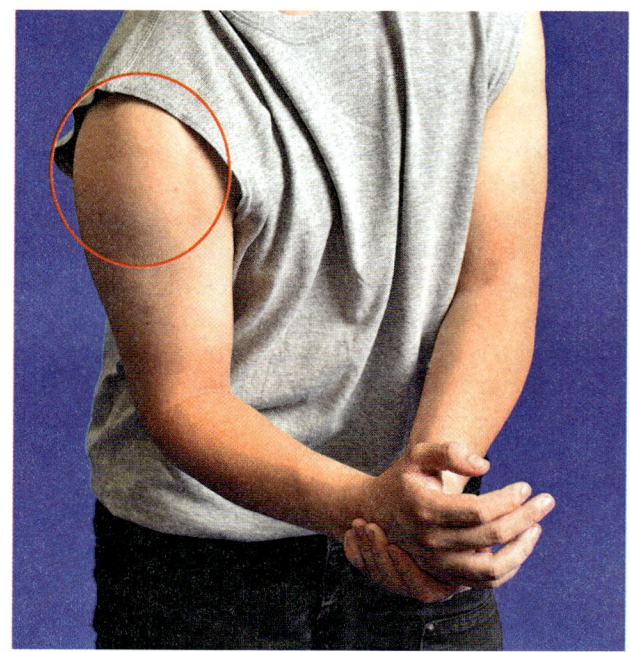

Figure 11.14 (a) Most shoulder dislocations are anterior. Notice the absence of the normal shoulder contour (circled area). **(b)** A patient with a dislocated shoulder will guard the dislocated shoulder (circled area) and protect it by holding the arm in a fixed position away from the chest wall.
(a) © E.M. Singletary. Used with permission.

- Special note: In cases of subluxations of the GH joint, the shoulder may appear normal. However, any movement, especially abduction and external rotation, will be extremely painful for the athlete. In addition, the joint may be point tender.

First aid care for an anterior GH joint dislocation involves the following:

1. Immediately apply ice and compression. Put a rolled towel in the axilla. Place a bag of crushed ice on the front and back of the shoulder joint and secure with an elastic wrap tied in a figure-eight configuration.
2. Once the ice and compression are in place, apply a standard sling-and-swathe bandage to support the arm in its most comfortable position (Figure 11.10a and b). This may require placing towels or a blanket under the arm to support it.
3. As a coach or physical educator, do not attempt to relocate the joint. Immediately refer the athlete to a medical facility for further evaluation.
4. Because soft-tissue injury may be extensive, rule out neurovascular compromise and treat for shock.

First-time anterior dislocations can be treated conservatively with rest and exercises that specifically focus on the muscles surrounding the joint, including those of the rotator cuff. Immobilization can include a variety of durations from 1 to 6 weeks. The consensus on management after the first anterior dislocation is that surgery lowers the reoccurence rate and has a higher return-to-play rate than nonoperative conservative management (Hurley et al., 2020; Kraentler et al., 2020; Shanmugaraj et al., 2020; Tokish et al., 2020). Surgical reconstructive procedures may be prescribed, but the timing depends on many factors, including extent of injury, age of athlete, mechanism of injury, athlete's symptoms, time in season, and future plans.

As described earlier in the chapter, the glenoid labrum serves to help make the GH joint more stable. In addition, the long head of the biceps brachii provides stability to the GH joint by passing across the top of the humeral head en route to its attachment on the superior labrum and supraglenoid tubercle. An injury that is unique to this specific area of the GH joint is known as a superior labrum, anterior and posterior (SLAP) lesion (Michener et al., 2018). The injury involves some level of damage to the superior labrum and in more severe cases also involves damage to the attachment of the long head of the biceps brachii. The mechanisms of injury most recognized are either traction, such as in overhead throwing, or compression of the head of the humerus into the glenoid, which could occur when falling forward and reaching out to break the fall (Michener et al., 2018). Even though SLAP lesions have multiple classifications, four types are most common in sports, and each is distinguished from the others based either on the level of damage or the specific structures involved. Type I lesions are the least severe and are essentially limited to degenerative changes to the superior labrum without any associated disruption of either the labrum or the biceps tendon. Type II lesions involve the same degenerative types of changes to the otherwise intact labrum; however, in this injury the biceps tendon is torn away from the supraglenoid tubercle. Type III lesions involve a tear of the superior labrum with an intact biceps tendon, and type IV lesions have labral damage like type III lesions but also have damage into the biceps tendon (Michener et al., 2018).

Signs and symptoms of a SLAP include the following:

- While this injury can result from a single incident, the symptoms are highly variable and may persist, demonstrating a pattern of periodic remissions followed by recurrence of symptoms.
- Vague pain in and around the GH joint that is sometimes associated with certain movements, including those overhead, such as throwing or reaching up.
- The athlete may complain of a snapping or popping sensation within the GH joint.
- The athlete may exhibit symptoms of a rotator cuff injury, deep pain, or "dead arm syndrome" (Michener et al., 2018).

First aid care for SLAP involves the following:

1. Immediately apply ice and compression. This is best accomplished by placing a bag of crushed ice over the GH joint and securing it with an elastic wrap tied in a figure-eight configuration.
2. Once the ice and compression are in place, apply a standard sling-and-swathe bandage (Figure 11.10a and b). This is a critical step because the sling helps to remove the stress to the injured GH joint and the long head of the biceps brachii tendon by supporting the weight of the arm in the sling.

3. Refer the athlete to a medical facility for further evaluation if the injury was from a single event or if the symptoms are more chronic in nature.

Both conservative and surgical treatment options are available for SLAP lesions. As noted in a position statement by the NATA (Michener et al., 2018), almost half of those with SLAP lesions did not require surgery and 67% of overhead athletes returned to preinjury activity level with nonoperative management. SLAP lesion surgical repair can involve various techniques and complex coexisting conditions in those with symptomatic shoulders. Most athletes were satisfied with the outcome after SLAP lesion repair, although there was less satisfaction in overhead athletes after repair (Michener et al., 2018).

WHAT IF ❓

You are at a high school wrestling tournament, and an athlete sustains a shoulder injury. You notice a large mass in the armpit area as well as a definite sloping of the shoulder's contour. The athlete is holding his arm in slight abduction and states that he felt his shoulder "pop out." What would you conclude based on all this information? How would you manage this injury?

Sternoclavicular Joint Injuries

The SC joint is formed by the union of the proximal end of the clavicle and the manubrium of the sternum. This synoviated articulation is strengthened by several ligaments (Figure 11.3). These include the joint capsule, the anterior and posterior SC ligaments, the interclavicular and costoclavicular ligaments, and an articular disk located within the joint (Moini, 2020).

Although fewer injuries occur to the SC joint than to either the AC or GH joints, the coach should be prepared to recognize and treat them correctly. The mechanism of injury for the SC joint involves an external blow to the shoulder region that results in a dislocation of the proximal clavicle, most commonly with the bone moving anteriorly and superiorly. A sprain to the SC joint can range in severity from minor stretching, with no actual tearing of tissues, to a complete rupture of ligaments and extensive soft-tissue damage. Fortunately, anterior and superior dislocations cause few additional problems and are easily treated. Occurring much less frequently, but potentially more dangerous, is a posterior SC dislocation. In this instance the proximal end of the clavicle is displaced posteriorly by a direct force over the anteromedial aspect of the clavicle or an indirect force to the posterolateral shoulder, which can cause direct pressure on soft-tissue structures in the region, including blood vessels or even the esophagus and trachea (Morell & Thyagarajan, 2016).

Signs and symptoms of SC joint injuries include the following:

- In most cases (second- and third-degree sprains), a gross deformity will be present at the SC joint.
- In all but the least severe cases, swelling will be immediate.
- Movement of the entire shoulder girdle will be limited owing to pain within the SC joint.
- The athlete will typically report having heard a snapping sound or may have experienced a tearing sensation at the SC joint.
- Note the body position of the athlete because in this injury the arm may be held close to the body and the head and neck may be tilted and flexed toward the injured shoulder (Morell & Thyagarajan, 2016).

First aid care for SC joint injuries involves the following:

1. Apply ice and compression, which is best accomplished using a plastic bag filled with crushed ice that is secured with an elastic wrap tied in a figure-eight configuration. Take care not to put pressure over the airway when wrapping the shoulder for compression of the SC joint.
2. Place the arm of the affected shoulder in a standard sling-and-swathe bandage (Figure 11.10a and b).
3. In cases of severe soft-tissue damage or a posteriorly displaced clavicle, immediately activate emergency care and treat the athlete for shock and the potential compromise of the neurovascular structures or trachea.

Medical treatment for the majority of SC joint sprains is conservative, that is, reduction of the dislocation if present followed by 2 to 3 weeks of support with a sling-and-swathe bandage. Rarely is any sort of surgical correction attempted, especially in the case of anterior dislocations. Obviously, a sound program of rehabilitation exercises prescribed by a competent sports medicine professional will be helpful in getting the athlete back into action.

Contusions of the Shoulder Region

External blows around the shoulder region are a common occurrence in a variety of sports, especially those that involve contact. Shoulder injury data collected from NCAA quarterbacks from 2004–2014 demonstrated that contusions were the second most common injury reported (Tummala et al., 2018). The GH joint is well protected by muscles crossing over the joint, such as the deltoid. The nearby AC joint, however, is exposed and quite vulnerable to external blows. If the athlete sustains a contusion to this joint, the result can be an extremely painful condition known as a **shoulder pointer**.

Signs and symptoms of shoulder contusions include the following:

- History of a recent blow to the shoulder, with resulting pain and decreased range of motion
- Spasm if muscle tissue is involved
- Discoloration and swelling, especially over bony regions such as the AC joint

First aid care of shoulder contusions involves the following:

1. Immediately apply ice and compression directly over the area(s) involved. This is best accomplished with a bag of crushed ice and an elastic wrap.
2. In cases of severe pain, apply an arm sling to relieve stress on the shoulder region.
3. If significant swelling persists for more than 72 hours in the region of the AC joint, refer the athlete to a physician. In some cases, the AC ligament may have sustained a sprain.

Strains of the Shoulder Region

A large number of muscles attach to the bones of the shoulder girdle, any one of which can suffer a strain. As mentioned earlier, certain sports produce very specific injuries to the shoulder. Perhaps the most common strain involves the muscles of the rotator cuff.

Rotator Cuff

The muscles of the **rotator cuff** (Figure 11.6a and b) serve a variety of purposes, including stabilization of the humeral head in the glenoid fossa as well as abduction and internal and external rotation of the GH joint. To better understand the mechanism of injuries involving the rotator cuff, a review of the kinesiology of the overhand throw and/or swing is necessary. Throwing has been described as a six-phase process involving windup, stride, arm cocking, acceleration, deceleration, and follow-through (Chalmers et al., 2017; Chu et al., 2016). Essentially, the windup and stride phases require putting the entire body into the best position to generate throwing forces. The arm-cocking stage involves pulling the throwing arm into an abducted and externally rotated position at the GH joint; this incorporates a **concentric contraction** of several of the rotator cuff muscles as well as other muscles of the shoulder region. The acceleration phase involves a sudden reversal of cocking: The arm is moved rapidly into internal rotation, horizontal flexion, and adduction of the GH joint via concentric contractions of muscles such as the pectoralis major, anterior deltoid, teres major, latissimus dorsi, and triceps. Depending on the skill and strength of the athlete, the forces generated during the acceleration phase can be substantial and must be dealt with effectively during deceleration and follow-through. The deceleration (release) phase is the shortest in the throwing cycle and involves timing the release at the point of maximum velocity. The follow-through phase requires that the entire upper extremity be decelerated immediately after the release. A critical point

---

Shoulder pointer Contusion and subsequent hematoma in the region of the acromioclavicular joint.

Rotator cuff Group of four muscles crossing the glenohumeral joint: subscapularis, supraspinatus, infraspinatus, and teres minor.

Concentric contraction Occurs when a muscle shortens and contracts resulting in joint movement.

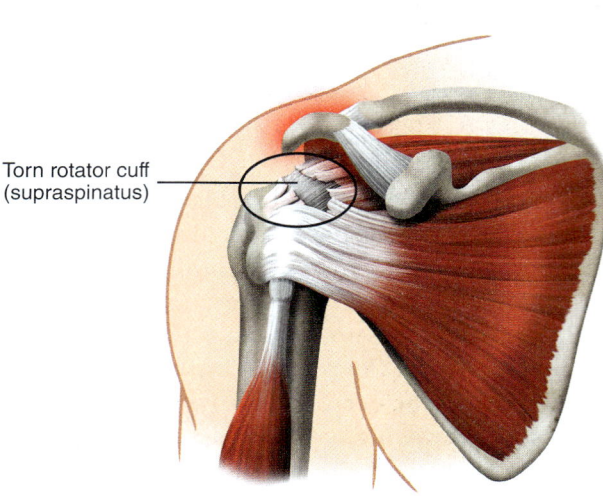

Figure 11.15 Torn rotator cuff.
© derter/Shutterstock.

to note is that several muscles of the rotator cuff are actively contracting eccentrically in an effort to slow the arm down.

The vast majority of strains to the rotator cuff occur during the deceleration and follow-through phases (Chu et al., 2016), specifically during the eccentric phase of the contraction. This problem is made worse when the muscles of the rotator cuff are significantly weaker than those muscles involved in the acceleration phase. This problem can best be addressed with a properly designed conditioning program aimed at strengthening the muscles of the rotator cuff. Unfortunately, many rotator cuff injuries and SLAP lesions coexist, making management challenging (Michener et al., 2018).

Strains and tears to the rotator cuff are normally the result of overuse (Figure 11.15). They develop slowly over many weeks or months. Athletes who are involved in sports that require throwing and swinging are at risk for this type of injury, especially athletes with improper biomechanics of throwing, weak rotator cuffs, and weak scapular stabilizers or those who are older. Proper warm-up of the throwing and/or swinging arm can help reduce the stress on the musculature of the shoulder girdle. Very frequently, errors in execution of the throw or swing can contribute to overuse injury (Chu et al., 2016). Therefore, athletes must learn correct techniques to reduce the chances of developing an injury.

Signs and symptoms of rotator cuff injuries include the following:

- Pain within the shoulder, especially during the deceleration and follow-through phases of a throw or swing
- Difficulty in bringing the arm up and back during the cocking phase of a throw or swing
- Pain and stiffness within the shoulder region 12 to 24 hours after a practice or competition that involved throwing or swinging
- Point tenderness around the region of the humeral head that appears to be deep within the deltoid muscle. (Note that rotator cuff injuries can mimic many others common to the shoulder region, including **bursitis** and **tendinitis**.)

Following are considerations in the care of rotator cuff strains:

1. Overuse injuries are difficult to treat effectively without a thorough medical evaluation. When symptoms occur, the application of ice and compression may prove helpful in reducing the pain and loss of function associated with the injury.
2. In the majority of cases, the athlete will report repeated episodes of symptoms spanning many weeks or even months. Therefore, medical referral for a complete evaluation is essential.

Any treatment program for a strained rotator cuff should be individualized with specific strengthening and flexibility exercises designed to achieve dynamic stability of the shoulder necessary for overhead throwing. Surgical repair is typically reserved for those who have not responded to rehabilitation and cannot return to pain-free throwing. Surgery would provide anatomical stabilization designed to salvage an athlete's career. Whether a conservative or surgical approach is chosen, a three-phase rehabilitation program that addresses the kinetic chain, shoulder mobility, and shoulder strengthening should be prescribed. Sports medicine specialists should focus not only on the shoulder but on the core and lower extremity because they play a significant role in force translation (Chalmers et al., 2017; Chu et al., 2016; Wilk et al., 2016).

Bursitis Inflammation of a bursa.

Tendinitis Inflammation of a tendon.

Glenohumeral Joint–Related Impingement Syndrome

To *impinge* means to be forced "upon or against something" (Guralnik & Friend, 1966). A **syndrome** is defined as "a number of symptoms occurring together and characterizing a specific disease" (Guralnik & Friend, 1966). Hence, an impingement syndrome of the shoulder, specifically the subacromial space, occurs when a soft-tissue structure, such as a ligament, bursa, or tendon, is squeezed between moving joint structures, resulting in irritation and pain. In the case of the GH joint, the most common impingement occurs to the tendon of the supraspinatus muscle as it passes across the top of the joint en route to its insertion (Dhillon, 2019). The normal anatomy of the GH joint is a tight fit relative to the amount of available space for structures above the joint capsule. This region, directly beneath the acromion process, is known as the subacromial space. The floor of the subacromial space is the GH joint capsule. The ceiling comprises the acromion process and the CC ligament, which form an arch across the top of the GH joint known as the coracoacromial arch (Figure 11.6b).

Any condition, whether related to sports or congenital, that decreases the size of the subacromial space may result in the development of an impingement syndrome (Figure 11.16). The most common causes of impingement syndromes found in the subacromial space are damage to rotator cuff tendons, altered GH or scapular motion, hook-shaped acromions, and/or physical activities that could lead to the aforementioned (Dhillon, 2019). Athletes who participate in sports that place an emphasis on arm movements above the shoulder level demonstrate a higher rate of impingement problems when compared with athletes who take part in sports not emphasizing such movements. Athletes in sports requiring repetitive arm motions, including baseball, tennis, volleyball, football, badminton, basketball, gymnastics, squash, swimming, table tennis, and track and field events, can be at risk of impingement (Lin et al., 2018; Figure 11.17).

Altered scapular motion has been described as a **SICK scapula**, which is a combination of scapular

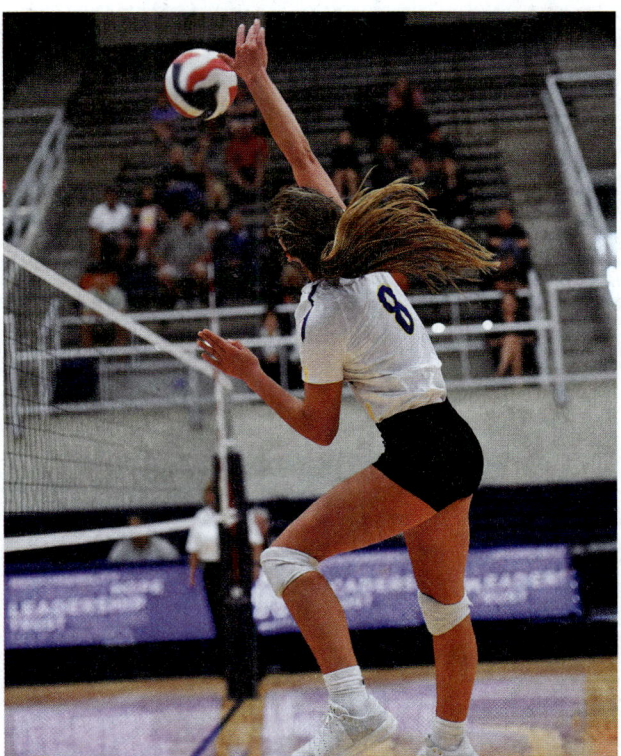

Figure 11.17 Overhead motions, such as spiking the ball in volleyball, place stress on the glenohumeral joint.
© Alila Medical Media/Shutterstock.

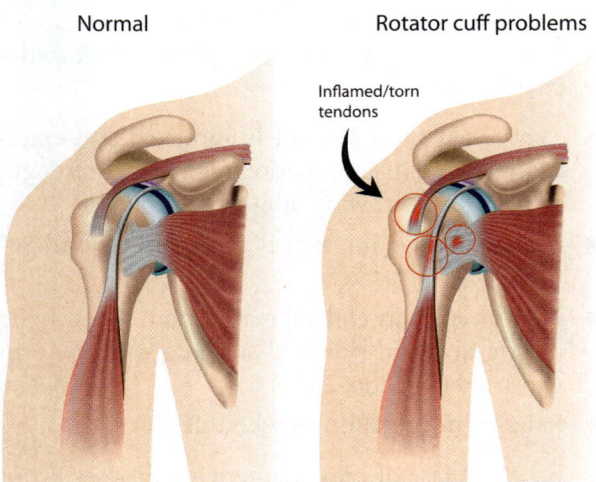

Figure 11.16 Glenohumeral joint–related impingement syndrome is common in overhead athletes.
© JoeSAPhotos/Shutterstock.

> **Syndrome** Group of typical symptoms or conditions that characterize a deficiency or disease.
>
> **SICK scapula** A combination of scapular malposition, inferior medial border prominence, coracoid process tenderness, and dyskinesis of scapular movement.

malposition, inferior medial border prominence, coracoid process pain and malposition, and dyskinesis of scapular movement. Altered scapular movement, or **scapular dyskinesis**, is implicated as a cause of GH joint–related impingement (Kibler & Sciascia, 2016). Dyskinesis represents an alteration of either the static or dynamic scapular position in coordination with arm motion, which reduces optimum shoulder function (Kibler & Sciascia, 2016). In essence, the scapula does not properly rotate upward with the progression of the overhead throwing motion (windup, arm cocking, and acceleration), nor does it properly rotate downward with the deceleration and follow-through phases. These dysfunctions are related to imbalances between muscle length and strength in the anterior and posterior muscles of the shoulder. One common muscle imbalance is caused by a weak serratus anterior muscle, which causes scapular winging, or medial border prominence (**Figure 11.18**). Also implicated as a cause of impingement are alterations in the balance of GH internal and external rotation motions in the throwing arm relative to the nonthrowing arm. Throwing athletes will often experience an ability to excessively externally rotate their throwing arm but be limited in the ability to internally rotate the arm, causing a deficit in internal rotation when compared to the nonthrowing arm. **Glenohumeral internal rotation deficit (GIRD)** is considered an adaptive process in which the throwing shoulder experiences a loss of internal rotation of >20° compared to the nonthrowing shoulder. GIRD is related to posterior capsular, rotator cuff tightness and anatomical changes in GH joint alignment and are often caused from the repetitive cocking within the overhead throwing

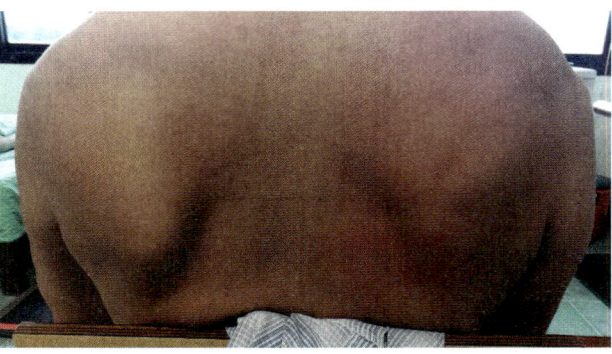

Figure 11.18 Left scapular winging caused by serratus anterior weakness, which is a common condition with shoulder dyskinesis.
© Piyada Jaiaree/Shutterstock.

motion (Rose & Noonan, 2018). GIRD has often been implicated as a cause of several overhead shoulder injuries, including impingement; however, more emphasis is now being placed on deficits in the sum of internal and external rotation within the shoulder, or **total glenohumeral rotation range of motion (TRM)**. Optimum shoulder joint function is dependent on a complex sequence of motions, loads, and forces, and research has demonstrated that a TRM deficit >8° between shoulders is associated with decreased shoulder strength and increased shoulder injury rates (Kibler & Sciascia, 2016; Rose & Noonan, 2018). Although a variety of other risk factors can contribute to overuse shoulder injuries, such as impingement, both GIRD and TRM can be predictive of a shoulder at risk for injury (Keller et al., 2018; Kibler & Sciascia, 2016).

Signs and symptoms of impingement syndromes include the following:

- Pain when the GH joint is abducted and externally rotated in conjunction with loss of strength in overhead throwing or athletic motions
- Pain whenever the arm is abducted beyond 80° to 90°
- Nocturnal pain and increased pain when lying on the involved side and sleeping with the arm overhead (Dhillon, 2019)
- Pain felt deep within the shoulder

First aid care of impingement syndromes is not required because they tend to develop over many days, weeks, or even months. Rather, any athlete

Scapular dyskinesis Abnormal mobility or function of the scapula both statically and dynamically.

Glenohumeral internal rotation deficit (GIRD) An adaptive process in which the throwing shoulder experiences a loss of internal rotation, usually caused by posterior capsular and rotator cuff tightness, owing to the repetitive cocking that occurs with the overhead throwing motion.

Total glenohumeral rotation range of motion (TRM) The entire measurement arc of passive range of motion of the shoulder, including external and internal rotation.

complaining of the signs and symptoms listed should be referred for a complete medical evaluation. Treatment will consist of rest, anti-inflammatory drugs, and directed physical therapy to correct the individual's kinetic chain imbalance through the application of kinetic chain exercises and shoulder mobility and shoulder strengthening interventions (Kibler & Sciascia, 2016). If these fail, surgery to correct the problem may be prescribed. In many cases, this can be done via arthroscopy; typically, it involves procedures such as removal of bone spurs from beneath the acromion process, release of the CC ligament, or a resectioning of a portion of the undersurface of the acromion process (Brabston et al., 2015; Dhillon, 2019).

Biceps Tendon Problems

The anatomy of the GH joint (Figure 11.19) includes the tendon of the long head of the biceps brachii muscle because it is a dynamic anterior stabilizer. The tendon passes into the joint capsule and is surrounded by a specialized portion of the synovium of the joint. As the tendon continues through the joint, it runs across the superior surface of the humeral head and down through the bicipital groove; in this position, the tendon helps to stabilize the humeral head when the joint is abducted. The tendon of the long head of the biceps brachii originates from the supraglenoid tubercle (Moini, 2020). The short head of the biceps brachii derives from the nearby coracoid process. This tendon, however, remains anatomically separate from the GH joint.

The tendon of the long head of the biceps brachii is located directly beneath the acromion process; therefore, it can suffer a type of impingement similar to that seen in the supraspinatus tendon. As the joint is abducted, the tendon may be compressed within the subacromial space. Consequently, symptoms similar to those of impingement of the supraspinatus will develop. Athletes at risk for this injury include those involved in sports that place an emphasis on repetitive overhead movements with the arms.

Another problem related to the long-head tendon of the biceps brachii is tendinitis, which may lead to a subluxation of the tendon from the bicipital groove. In most cases, tendinitis will develop slowly over a period of weeks or months as a result of kinetic dysfunctions during the overhead motion. Several of the dysfunctions already discussed, such as SICK scapula, GIRD, or TRM deficits, can cause undue stress on the long-head tendon of the biceps brachii. As the tendon enlarges from inflammation, it becomes less stable in the groove, where it is held by the transverse humeral ligament (Flanagin et al., 2015). In chronic cases, a sudden violent force such as is commonly generated in throwing may cause the tendon to subluxate out of the groove, thereby tearing the transverse humeral ligament. The athlete will notice significant symptoms if the tendon subluxates from the bicipital groove.

Signs and symptoms of biceps tendon problems include the following (Kibler et al., 2009):

- Painful abduction of the shoulder joint similar to that seen in impingement problems
- Pain while trying to hold the hand on top of the opposite shoulder while resistance is being applied to pull the hand off the shoulder
- Pain in the shoulder joint when the athlete performs a motion similar to a boxing upper cut

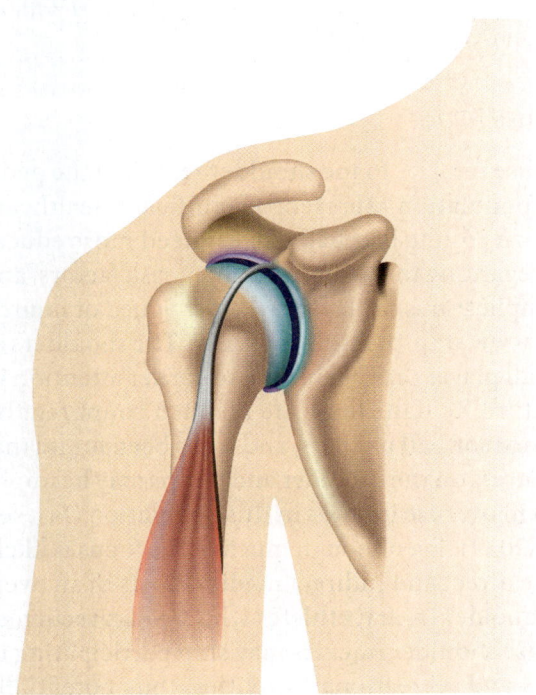

Figure 11.19 The bicipital tendon often suffers tears or avulsion from the glenohumeral labrum in overhead athletes.
© Alila Medical Media/Shutterstock.

punch where the elbow is flexed, forearm is supinated with a fist, and the motion is resisted

- The athlete may note a popping or snapping sensation as the tendon of the long head of the biceps brachii subluxates.

First aid care of biceps tendon problems is not a practical concern because they generally develop over time and fall into the category of a chronic injury. However, if the athlete should subluxate the biceps tendon from the bicipital groove, the initial episode of this injury can require first aid. In such cases, the immediate application of ice and compression is recommended. Long-term care for this injury includes rest, anti-inflammatory drugs, and gradually progressive exercise rehabilitation. If symptoms persist and the tendon continues to subluxate from the bicipital groove, then surgery may be required to stabilize the tendon. Any treatment should be directed specifically to the patient's goals and expectations and may involve controlling pitch counts or other overhead activities in addition to establishing dynamic and static shoulder stability (Flanagin et al., 2015).

Little League Shoulder

Little League shoulder was first described in the 1950s when a Little League pitcher reported a gradual onset of shoulder pain in the throwing shoulder (Carson & Gasser, 1998). It is commonly associated with a stress fracture or **osteochondrosis** of the proximal humeral **epiphyseal plate** or proximal humeral epiphysiolysis (Bednar et al., 2021; Carson & Gasser, 1998). Throwing athletes between the ages of 11 and 16 years are most commonly affected. The adolescent's growing humerus bone is more susceptible to both micro- and macrotrauma than an adult's humerus. A clinical evaluation and X-ray are the most common diagnostic tools. The cocking phase and the subsequent stresses of the rotation that occurs in the acceleration phase of throwing are most likely related to the development of Little League shoulder (Bednar et al., 2021). Athletes with a current or prior history of shoulder pain, altered throwing mechanics, GIRD, or TRM deficits are at most risk of developing this injury. The most common reported symptoms are pain with throwing, palpating over the proximal humerus lasting 2 weeks to 1 year, and actively or passively moving the shoulder. Specifically, a lack of glenohumeral internal rotation is notable. Imaging may show humeral physeal widening, Salter-Harris pathology, and/or periosteal edema (Bednar et al., 2021). Treatment is typically nonoperative with adequate rest from throwing, directed shoulder rehabilitation, and a progressive return to a throwing program. Little League shoulder is similar to Little League elbow (see Chapter 12, *Injuries to the Arm, Wrist, and Hand*) because they both affect growth plates of an adolescent's arm. Likewise, both can benefit from preventive techniques that include abiding by age-associated pitch counts and rest days (Bednar et al., 2021). More specific information on pitch counts is provided in Chapter 12, *Injuries to the Arm, Wrist, and Hand*.

Overuse Injuries

Overuse injuries to the shoulder region in the pediatric population represent a significant healthcare concern. Young baseball players need more education regarding throwing guidelines, risk factors, and the implications of playing with a fatigued or injured arm (www.stopsportsinjuries.org). The shoulders of softball players are beginning to garner attention in literature. To date, there are no pitch count regulations for softball pitchers, and it has been found that high stress on the shoulder and biceps may be implicated in overuse injuries in this population (Friesen et al., 2022). Even though much of the focus is likely on the direct and indirect medical costs of an overuse shoulder injury, athletes who sustain recurrent overuse shoulder injuries may stop participating in sports and recreational activities, thus potentially adding to the already increasing number of sedentary individuals and the obesity epidemic. The National Athletic Trainers' Association developed

Osteochondrosis Self-limiting derangement of normal bone growth in developing bone at the growth plate.

Epiphyseal plate A hyaline cartilage plate at the end of each long bone where the growth center of the bone resides.

a position statement, *Prevention of Pediatric Overuse Injuries*, to help coaches, parents, and physical educators understand the role that training errors, improper technique, excessive sports training, inadequate rest, muscle weakness and imbalances, and early specialization have on the occurrence of overuse injuries in a pediatric population (Valovich McLeod et al., 2011). Recommendations include high-quality injury surveillance (e.g., incidence and prevalence); identification of risk factors for injury, including preparticipation physical examinations, proper supervision, and education (both coaching and medical); effective sport alterations; appropriate training and conditioning programs based on age and experience level; delayed specialization; and appropriate rest between seasons (Valovich McLeod et al., 2011).

> **WHAT IF ❓**
>
> You have a youth baseball player on your team who is complaining of chronic pain in the front of his shoulder. He notices the pain especially after he throws a ball, and he is point tender in the region of the upper humerus. What structures could be involved in this case?

Athletic Trainers SPEAK OUT

What should coaches and parents know about sports specialization and the potential for shoulder injuries?

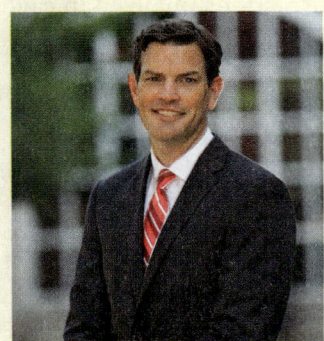

Courtesy of Kevin Laudner, PhD, ATC.

As participation in competitive youth sports rises, unfortunately, so does the number of athletes who choose to specialize in a sport. Sport specialization often consists of high-volume training among youth athletes, with little to no rest throughout the year, and has been associated with an increased risk of developing both psychological stress and physical injury. Athletes who participate in overhead sports that require repetitive and ballistic motions of the shoulder, such as swimming, baseball, softball, and tennis (just to name a few) may be even more susceptible to these overuse injuries owing to the general unstable nature of the GH joint.

Because of the strong relationship between sport specialization and shoulder injury, many youth sport organizations, in collaboration with clinicians and researchers, have implemented participation restrictions that include designated amounts of playing time during a year, a week, and an individual game. Such mandates indicate that overhead sport athletes should rest or participate in lower extremity intensive sports at least 2 to 4 months out of each year. The recommendation for these athletes is also not to participate in their sport for more hours per week than their age in years and no more than 16 total hours per week.

Youth athletes should be encouraged to help minimize stress placed on the shoulder during sport participation by developing proper sport biomechanics, strength, range of motion, and sensorimotor control. These physical traits should not be considered as means to allow for sport specialization. Rather, they should accompany adequate rest to minimize the stress placed on the shoulder during overhead sports.

Youth athletes should be strongly encouraged to rest appropriately and participate in a variety of sports that emphasize involvement of both the upper and lower extremities. This balance allows for a reduced risk of shoulder injury caused by the accumulation of stress from participating in a single sport year-round.

—**Kevin Laudner, PhD, ATC**

Kevin Laudner is the dean and a professor in the Beth-El College of Nursing and Health Sciences at the University of Colorado in Colorado Springs.

Review Questions

1. Which two bones make up the shoulder girdle?
2. To what structure is the glenoid labrum attached?
3. Which one of the following arteries provides the blood supply to the shoulder region and upper extremity?
    a. Common iliac
    b. Ulnar
    c. Internal carotid
    d. Subclavian
    e. Axillary
4. Which one of the following is the correct derivation of the brachial plexus?
    a. C-5/T-2
    b. C-3/T-1
    c. C-1/T-5
    d. C-1/T-1
    e. C-5/T-1
5. List the four muscles of the rotator cuff group and identify one action common to each muscle.
6. List four signs and/or symptoms of a fractured clavicle.
7. Describe and/or demonstrate the appropriate first aid procedures for a fractured clavicle.
8. Describe the major ligaments that form the AC joint.
9. Describe briefly the two mechanisms of injury for the AC joint as discussed in the chapter.
10. Describe the common signs and symptoms of AC joint injuries.
11. Explain and/or demonstrate the appropriate first aid care for AC joint injuries.
12. List the major ligaments of the GH joint.
13. True or false? The most common type of GH joint dislocation is posterior.
14. Describe the common signs and symptoms of a GH joint dislocation.
15. Explain and/or demonstrate the appropriate first aid treatment of an athlete with a suspected GH joint dislocation.
16. Define the condition known as chronic GH joint subluxation.
17. Describe the primary ligaments of the SC joint.
18. Describe the common signs and symptoms of injury to the sternoclavicular joint.
19. Explain and/or demonstrate the appropriate first aid treatment of an athlete with a suspected SC joint injury.
20. Explain the five phases of an overhand throw and/or swing and give a brief description of the types of muscle contractions involved in each.
21. True or false? The vast majority of strains of the rotator cuff occur during the windup and cocking phases of the throw and/or swing.
22. List several of the signs and symptoms of rotator cuff strain as described in the chapter.
23. What anatomic structure forms a ceiling for the subacromial space?
24. True or false? Athletes involved in sports placing a heavy emphasis on arm movements below the shoulder level demonstrate a higher incidence of impingement syndromes.
25. List four signs and/or symptoms of impingement syndrome of the GH joint.
26. Which one of the following structures (ligaments) holds the biceps (long-head) tendon in the bicipital groove?
    a. Annular ligament
    b. Medial collateral ligament
    c. Capsular ligament
    d. Transverse humeral ligament

References

Axelrod, D. E., Ekhtiari, S., Bozzo, A., Bhandari, M., & Johal, H. (2020). What is the best evidence for management of displaced midshaft clavicle fractures? A systematic review and network meta-analysis of 22 randomized controlled trials. *Clinical Orthopaedics and Related Research, 478*(2), 392.

Bakhsh, W., & Nicandri, G. (2018). Anatomy and physical examination of the shoulder. *Sports Medicine and Arthroscopy Review, 26*(3), e10–e22.

Bednar, E. D., Kay, J., Memon, M., Simunovic, N., Purcell, L., & Ayeni, O. R. (2021). Diagnosis and management of Little League shoulder: A systematic review. *Orthopaedic Journal of Sports Medicine, 9*(7), 23259671211017563.

Beitzel, K., Mazzocca, A. D., Bak, K., Itoi, E., Kibler, W. B., Mirzayan, R., ... & Upper Extremity Committee of ISAKOS. (2014). ISAKOS Upper Extremity Committee consensus statement on the need for diversification of the Rockwood classification for acromioclavicular joint injuries. *Arthroscopy: The Journal of Arthroscopic & Related Surgery, 30*(2), 271–278.

Brabston, E. W., Galdi, B., & Ahmad, C. S. (2015). Posterosuperior and anterosuperior impingement in overhead athletes. In J. Y. Park (Ed.), *Sports injuries to the shoulder and elbow* (pp. 167–183). Berlin, Germany: Springer-Verlag Berlin Heidelberg.

Burkhart, S. S., Morgan, C. D., & Kibler, W. B. (2003). The disabled throwing shoulder: Spectrum of pathology part III: The SICK scapula, scapular dyskinesis, the kinetic chain, and rehabilitation. *Arthroscopy, 19*(6), 641–661.

Burnier, M., Barlow, J. D., & Sanchez-Sotelo, J. (2019). Shoulder and elbow fractures in athletes. *Current Reviews of Musculoskeletal Medicine, 12*(1), 13–23.

Carson, W. G., & Gasser, S. I. (1998). Little Leaguer's shoulder. *American Journal of Sports Medicine, 26*(4), 575–580.

Chalmers, P. N., Wimmer, M. A., Verma, N. N., Cole, B. J., Romeo, A. A., Cvetanovich, G. L., & Pearl, M. L. (2017). The relationship between pitching mechanics and injury: A review of current concepts. *Sports Health, 9*(3), 216–221.

Chu, S. K., Jayabalan, P., Kibler, W. B., & Press, J. (2016). The kinetic chain revisited: New concepts on throwing mechanics and injury. *PM&R, 8*(3), S69–S77.

DeFroda, S. F., Lemme, N., Kleiner, J., Gil, J., & Owens, B. D. (2019). Incidence and mechanism of injury of clavicle fractures in the NEISS database: Athletic and non athletic injuries. *Journal of Clinical Orthopaedics and Trauma, 10*(5), 954–958.

Dhillon, K. S. (2019). Subacromial impingement syndrome of the shoulder: A musculoskeletal disorder or a medical myth? *Malaysian Orthopaedic Journal, 13*(3), 1–7.

Ellis, H. B., Li, Y., Bae, D. S., Kalish, L. A., Wilson, P. L., Pennock, A. T., ... Heyworth, B. E. (2020). Descriptive epidemiology of adolescent clavicle fractures: Results from the FACTS (function after adolescent clavicle trauma and surgery) prospective, multicenter cohort study. *Orthopaedic Journal of Sports Medicine, 8*(5), 2325967120921344.

Flanagin, B. A., Fitzpatrick, K., Garofalo, R., Moon, G. H., & Krishnan, S. G. (2015). Biceps instability: With versus without rotator cuff lesions. In J. Y. Park (Ed.), *Sports injuries to the shoulder and elbow* (pp. 281–292). Berlin, Germany: Springer-Verlag Berlin Heidelberg.

Frank, R. M., Cotter, E. J., Leroux, T. S., & Romeo, A. A. (2019). Acromioclavicular joint injuries: Evidence-based treatment. *The Journal of the American Academy of Orthopaedic Surgeons, 27*(17), e775–e788.

Friesen, K. B., Saper, M. G., & Oliver, G. D. (2022). Biomechanics related to increased softball pitcher shoulder stress: Implications for injury prevention. *American Journal of Sports Medicine, 50*(1), 216–223.

Frima, H., van Heijl, M., Michelitsch, C., van Der Meijden, O., Beeres, F. J., Houwert, R. M., & Sommer, C. (2020). Clavicle fractures in adults: Current concepts. *European Journal of Trauma and Emergency Surgery, 46*(3), 519–529.

Goodman, A. D., DeFroda, S. F., Gil, J. A., Kleiner, J. E., Li, N. Y., & Owens, B. D. (2018). Season-ending shoulder injuries in the National Collegiate Athletic Association: Data from the NCAA Injury Surveillance Program, 2009–2010 through 2013–2014. *American Journal of Sports Medicine, 46*(8), 1936–1942.

Gorbaty, J. D., Hsu, J. E., & Gee, A. O. (2017). Classifications in brief: Rockwood classification of acromioclavicular joint separations. *Clinical Orthopaedics and Related Research, 475*, 283–287.

Guralnik, D. B., & Friend, J. H. (Eds.). (1966). *Webster's new world dictionary of the American language.* Cleveland, OH: World Publishing Company.

Hurley, E. T., Manjunath, A. K., Bloom, D. A., Pauzenberger, L., Mullett, H., Alaia, M. J., & Strauss, E. J. (2020). Arthroscopic Bankart repair versus conservative management for first-time traumatic anterior shoulder instability: A systematic review and meta-analysis. *Arthroscopy, 36*(9), 2526–2532.

Keller, R. A., De Giacomo, A. F., Neumann, J. A., Limpisvasti, O., & Tibone, J. E. (2018). Glenohumeral internal rotation deficit and risk of upper extremity injury in overhead athletes: A meta-analysis and systematic review. *Sports Health, 10*(2), 125–132.

Kibler, W. B., & Sciascia, A. (2016). The shoulder at risk: Scapular dyskinesis and altered glenohumeral rotation. *Operative Techniques in Sports Medicine, 24*(3), 162–169.

Kibler, W. B., Sciascia, A. D., Hester, P., Dome, D., & Jacobs, C. (2009). Clinical utility of traditional and new tests in the diagnosis of biceps tendon injuries and superior labrum anterior and posterior lesions in the shoulder. *American Journal of Sports Medicine, 37*(9), 1840-1847.

Kiel, J., & Kaiser, K. (2022). Acromioclavicular joint injury. *StatPearls*. StatPearls Publishing. Retrieved January 2022 from https://www.ncbi.nlm.nih.gov/books/NBK493188/

Kroshus, E., Utter, A. C., Pierpoint, L. A., Currie, D. W., Knowles, S. B., Wasserman, E. B., . . . Kerr, Z. Y. (2018). The first decade of web-based sports injury surveillance: Descriptive epidemiology of injuries in US high school boys' wrestling (2005–2006 through 2013–2014) and National Collegiate Athletic Association men's wrestling (2004–2005 through 2013–2014). *Journal of Athletic Training, 53*(12), 1143–1155.

Lin, D. J., Wong, T. T., & Kazam, J. K. (2018). Shoulder injuries in the overhead-throwing athlete: Epidemiology, mechanisms of injury, and imaging findings. *Radiology, 286*(2), 370–387.

Lin, K. M., James, E. W., Spitzer, E., & Fabricant, P. D. (2018). Pediatric and adolescent anterior shoulder instability: Clinical management of first-time dislocators. *Current Opinion in Pediatrics, 30*(1), 49–56.

Merolla, G., Augusti, C. A., Paladini, P., De Santis, E., & Porcellini, G. (2016). Posterior shoulder instability. In P. Volpi (Ed.), *Arthroscopy and sport injuries* (pp. 153–161). Cham, Switzerland: Springer International Publishing.

Michener, L. A., Abrams, J. S., Bliven, K. C. H., Falsone, S., Laudner, K. G., McFarland, E. G., Tibone, J. E., Thigpen, C. A., & Uhl, T. L. (2018). National Athletic Trainers' Association position statement: Evaluation, management, and outcomes of and return-to-play criteria for overhead athletes with superior labral anterior-posterior injuries. *Journal of Athletic Training, 53*(3), 209–229.

Moini, J. (2020). *Anatomy and physiology for health professionals* (3rd ed.). Burlington, MA: Jones & Bartlett Learning.

Morell, D. J., & Thyagarajan, D. S. (2016). Sternoclavicular joint dislocation and its management: A review of the literature. *World Journal of Orthopedics, 7*(4), 244–250.

Moverley, R., Little, N., Gulihar, A., & Singh, B. (2020). Current concepts in the management of clavicle fractures. *Journal of Clinical Orthopaedics and Trauma, 11*, S25–S30.

Nordin, J. S., Olsson, O., & Lunsjö, K. (2020). Acromioclavicular joint dislocations: Incidence, injury profile, and patient characteristics from a prospective case series. *JSES International, 4*(2), 246–250.

Oliver, G. D., Saper, M. G., Drogosz, M., Plummer, H. A., Arakkal, A. T., Comstock, R. D., . . . Fleisig, G. S. (2019). Epidemiology of shoulder and elbow injuries among US high school softball players, 2005–2006 through 2016–2017. *Orthopaedic Journal of Sports Medicine, 7*(9), 1–7.

Pollak, A. N. (2021). *Emergency care and transport of the sick and injured* (12th ed.). Burlington, MA: Jones & Bartlett Learning.

Provencher, M. T., Midtgaard, K. S., Owens, B. D., & Tokish, J. M. (2021). Diagnosis and management of traumatic anterior shoulder instability. *Journal of the American Academy of Orthopaedic Surgeons, 29*(2), e51–e61.

Rose, M. B., & Noonan, T. (2018). Glenohumeral internal rotation deficit in throwing athletes: Current perspectives. *Open Access Journal of Sports Medicine, 9*, 69–78.

Saper, M. G., Pierpoint, L. A., Liu, W., Comstock, R. D., Polousky, J. D., & Andrews, J. R. (2018). Epidemiology of shoulder and elbow injuries among United States high school baseball players: School years 2005–2006 through 2014–2015. *American Journal of Sports Medicine, 46*(1), 37–43.

Shanmugaraj, A., Chai, D., Sarraj, M., Gohal, C., Horner, N. S., Simunovic, N., . . . Ayeni, O. (2021). Surgical stabilization of pediatric anterior shoulder instability yields high recurrence rates: A systematic review. *Knee Surgery, Sports Traumatology, Arthroscopy, 29*, 192–201.

Stenson, J., & Baker, W. (2021). Classifications in brief: The modified Neer classification for distal-third clavicle fractures. *Clinical Orthopaedics and Related Research, 479*(1), 205–209.

Tokish, J. M., Kuhn, J. E., Ayers, G. D., Arciero, R. A., Burks, R. T., Dines, D. M., . . . Cordasco, F. A. (2020). Decision making in treatment after a first-time anterior glenohumeral dislocation: A Delphi approach by the Neer Circle of the American Shoulder and Elbow Surgeons. *Journal of Shoulder and Elbow Surgery, 29*(12), 2429–2445.

Tummala, S. V., Hartigan, D. E., Patel, K. A., Makovicka, J. L., & Chhabra, A. (2018). Shoulder injuries in National Collegiate Athletic Association quarterbacks: 10-Year epidemiology of incidence, risk factors, and trends. *Orthopaedic Journal of Sports Medicine, 6*(2), 1–7.

Valovich McLeod, T. C., Decoster, L. C., Loud, K. J., Micheli, L. J., Parker, J. T., Sandrey, M. A., & White, C. (2011). National Athletic Trainers' Association position statement: Prevention of pediatric overuse injuries. *Journal of Athletic Training, 46*(2), 206–220.

Wilk, K. E., Arrigo, C. A., Hooks, T. R., & Andrews, J. R. (2016). Rehabilitation of the overhead throwing athlete: There is more to it than just external rotation/internal rotation strengthening. *PM&R, 8*, S78–S90.

Wong, M., & Kiel, J. (2018). Anatomy, shoulder and upper limb, acromioclavicular joint. Treasure Island, FL: StatPearls Publishing LLC.

CHAPTER 12
Injuries to the Wrist, Arm, and Hand

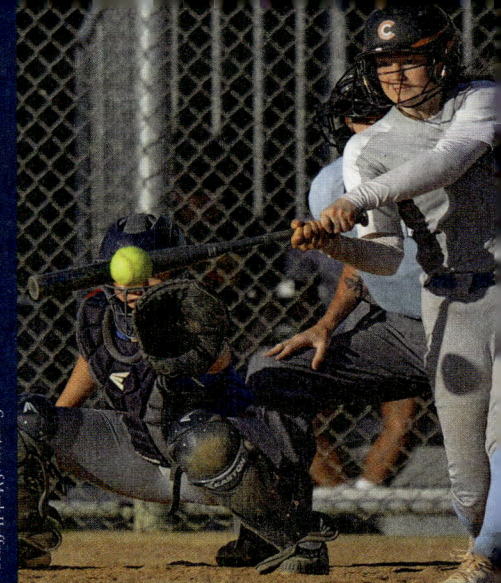

Courtesy of Mark Hoffman.

MAJOR CONCEPTS

The chapter begins with a brief review of the gross anatomy of the entire arm region with special emphasis on arthrology. It goes on to discuss upper arm (brachial region) injuries, focusing especially on contusions and fractures. Given the potentially serious consequences of fractures of the humerus, the chapter provides detailed instructions for proper first aid care of these injuries. Next, the chapter reviews elbow injuries, outlining current information regarding the typical mechanisms, signs and symptoms, and critical first aid procedures. Again, because there are potential catastrophic consequences of a mismanaged elbow injury, this section provides specific first aid instructions. It also discusses problems related to the muscle attachments surrounding the elbow, clinically known as epicondylitis, along with special attention paid to the possible causes, signs and symptoms, and care.

Although quite rare, forearm injuries do occasionally occur, and the chapter reviews the more frequent varieties, along with guidelines on signs and symptoms and first aid care. Next, it discusses injuries to the wrist, emphasizing relatively common injuries, such as fractures of the scaphoid bone and dislocations of the lunate bone. Nerve injuries of the wrist region are common, of which carpal tunnel syndrome is perhaps the most well-known. Therefore, the chapter outlines specific signs and symptoms for nerve problems involving the median and ulnar nerves.

Finally, the chapter discusses hand and finger injuries, which are both extremely common in sports and can result in debilitating injury if not managed correctly.

Anatomy Review

The bones of the arm are the humerus (upper arm), the radius, and the ulna (forearm). The proximal end of the humerus (head) articulates with the glenoid fossa of the scapula to form the shoulder (glenohumeral) joint. The distal end of the humerus articulates with both of the forearm bones to form the elbow joint, which actually comprises three specific articulations—the **humeroulnar**, **humeroradial**, and proximal **radioulnar** joints. The distal end of the forearm articulates with the wrist (carpal) bones,

> **Humeroulnar joint** Articulation (ginglymus) formed by the proximal end of the ulna, specifically the trochlear notch, with the distal end of the humerus, specifically the trochlea.

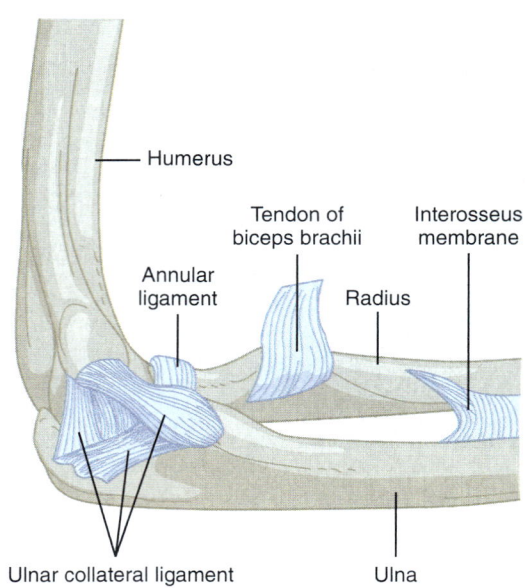

Figure 12.1 The elbow joint (medial view).

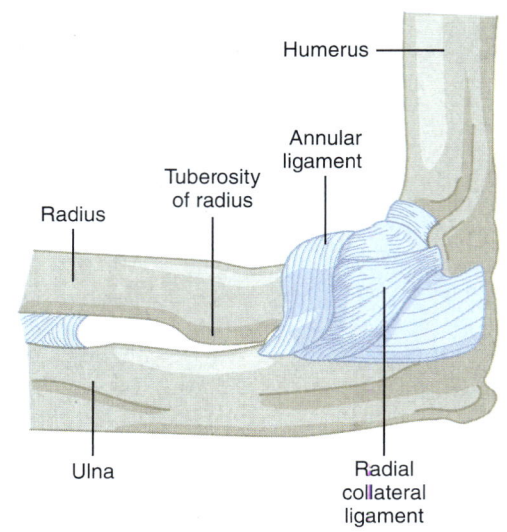

Figure 12.2 The elbow joint (lateral view).

forming the **radiocarpal** (wrist) and distal radioulnar joints. The joints of the arm allow for a great variety of motions, including flexion/extension and pronation/supination at the elbow as well as flexion/extension and radial and ulnar deviation at the wrist. The elbow (Figure 12.1) and wrist joints are held together with several ligaments, which may be subject to trauma related to sports participation. Certainly, one of the more distinctive ligament structures in the human body is the annular ligament of the elbow (Figure 12.2). This ligament holds the head of the radius in the proximal radioulnar joint; and in doing so, it allows that articulation to pronate and supinate while simultaneously allowing the radial head to articulate with the capitellum of the humerus.

Humeroradial joint Articulation (arthrodial) formed by the proximal end of the radius and the distal end of the humerus, specifically the capitellum.

Radioulnar joints Two articulations (pivot) formed by the proximal and distal radius and ulna, known commonly as the proximal and distal radioulnar joints.

Radiocarpal joint Articulation (ellipsoidal) formed by the distal end of the radius and three bones of the wrist: navicular, lunate, and triquetral.

As seen in Figure 12.3, the musculature of the upper arm is extensive. It is dominated by the elbow extensor and flexors, which include the biceps brachii, brachialis, triceps brachii, and anconeus. The muscles of the arm collectively contribute to several of the movements of the elbow: extension, flexion, and supination. The muscles are listed, along with their specific actions and innervations, in Table 12.1.

The forearm includes a large number of muscles for the movements of the forearm, wrist, hand, and fingers. The majority of the forearm muscles originate from the regions of the humeral epicondyles, either lateral or medial, which are located immediately proximal to the elbow joint. The muscles of the forearm can be divided into the extensor/supinator (Figure 12.4) and flexor/pronator groups (Figure 12.5). These muscles collectively contribute to the pronation and supination of the elbow, flexion and extension of the wrist and fingers, flexion and extension of the thumb, and radial and ulnar deviation of the wrist. The muscles are listed with their specific actions and innervations in Table 12.2.

Soft-Tissue Injuries to the Upper Arm

The majority of injuries to the upper arm are either contusions or fractures. Though strains do occur to this region, they are uncommon. Because

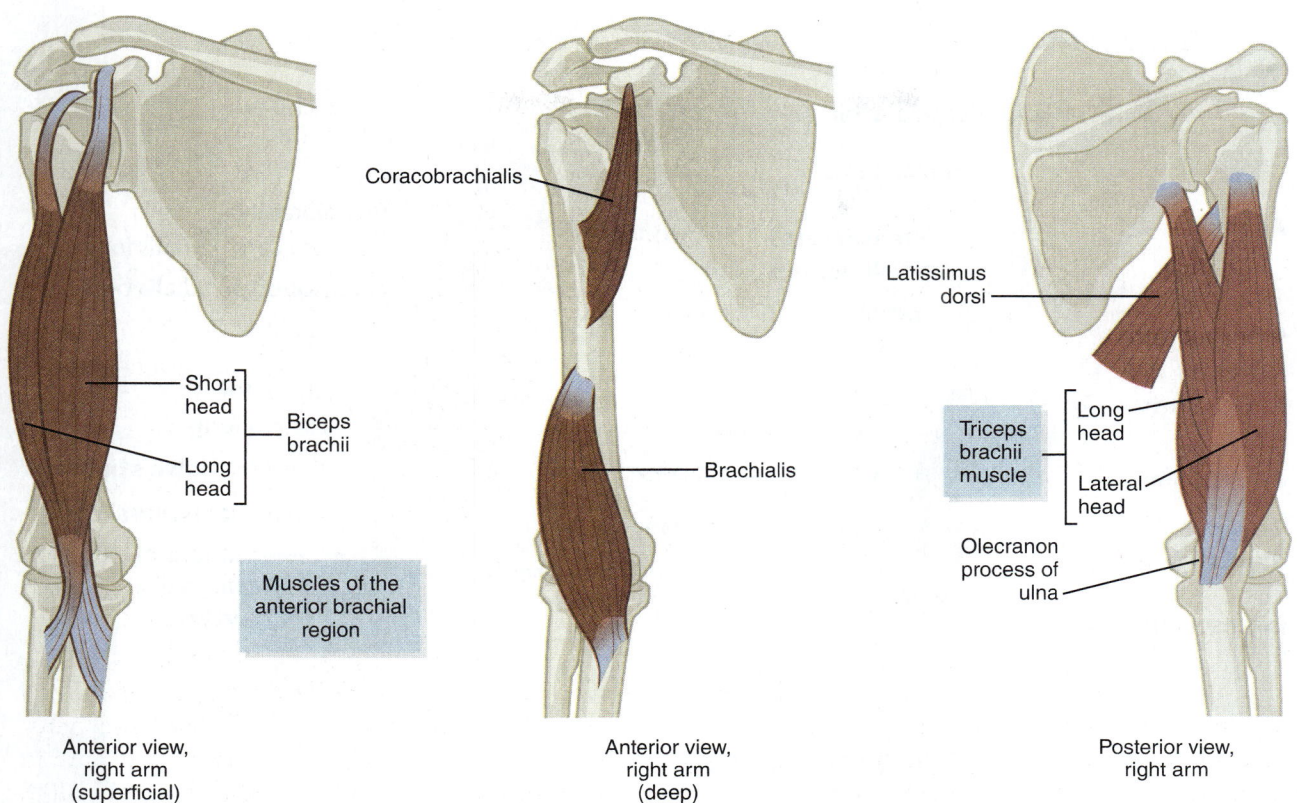

Figure 12.3 Muscles of the arm, anterior and posterior.

of the nature of contact sports, blows to the arm region are a common occurrence. A typical scenario involves a football lineman blocking with arms flexed at the elbows and receiving blows to the lateral surfaces of the upper arms. The underlying muscle tissue is compressed between the overlying skin and the bone of the humerus. Depending on the magnitude of the blow(s), damage to the muscle tissue may be significant. If such episodes are repeated, the athlete may develop a condition known as myositis ossificans traumatica.

Table 12.1
Muscles, Actions, and Nerves of the Arm

Muscle	Action	Innervation
Biceps brachii (long and short head)	Flexion of the forearm at the elbow Supination of the forearm	Musculocutaneous
Brachialis	Flexion of the forearm at the elbow	Musculocutaneous
Triceps brachii (long, lateral, and medial heads)	Extension of the forearm at the elbow	Radial
Anconeus	Extension of the forearm at the elbow	Radial

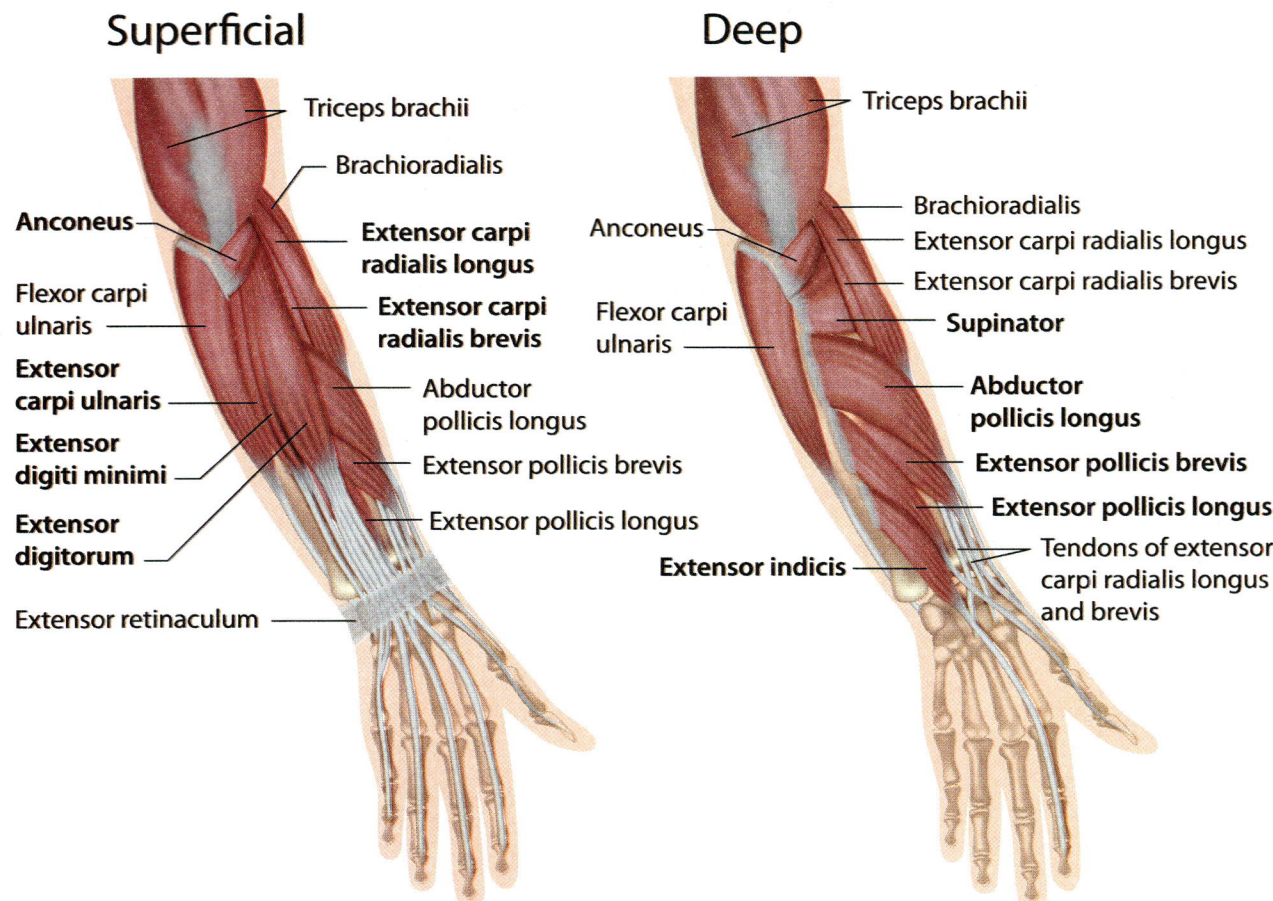

Figure 12.4 Extensor muscles of the forearm.
© Alila Medical Media/Shutterstock.

Myositis Ossificans Traumatica

Myositis ossificans traumatica involves chronic inflammation of a muscle after repeated blows and damage to the tissue. The chronic inflammation leads to the development of bonelike tissue in the muscle. It is quite common in football—so much so that the condition has become known as **tackler's exostosis** (McCarty et al., 2018). An **exostosis** is defined as "a benign growth projecting from a bone surface characteristically capped by cartilage". Myositis ossificans traumatica develops over a period of weeks or even months and therefore tends to be ignored in early stages of development, when it is typically dismissed as a simple bruise. It is important to recognize that such an injury can develop into a more serious one and evaluate it accordingly.

Signs and symptoms of upper arm contusions include the following:

- The athlete has a recent history of contusion to the region.

Myositis ossificans traumatica Inflammation of muscle as a result of repeated traumatic blows, which causes bleeding and then bony deposits to collect within muscle.

Tackler's exostosis Formation of a benign growth projecting from the humerus that is caused by repeated blows to the upper arm region; common in tackle football.

Exostosis Bony outgrowths that protrude from the surface of a bone where there is not typical bony formation.

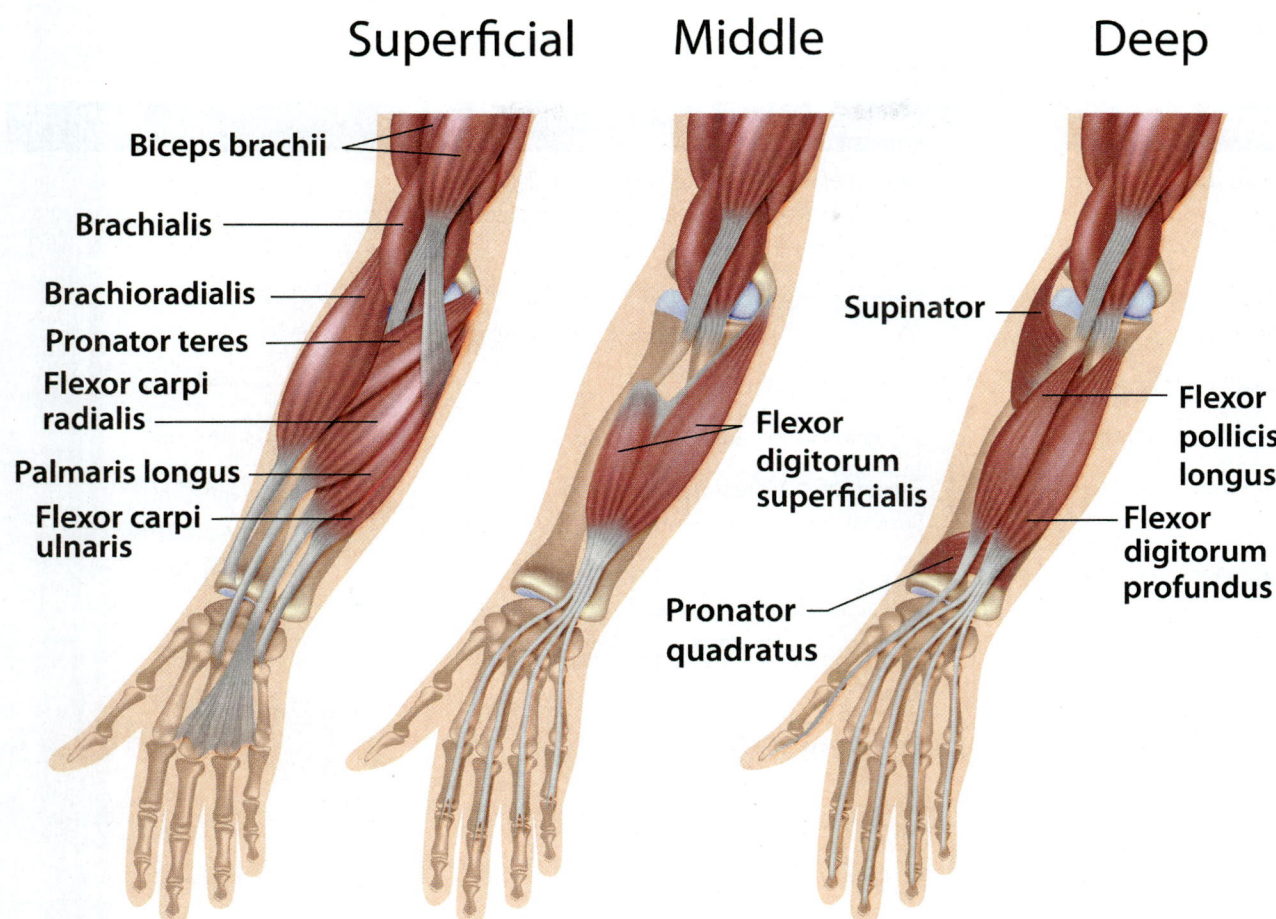

Figure 12.5 The three layers of the flexor muscles of the forearm.
© Alila Medical Media/Shutterstock.

- Pain, discoloration, and swelling in the region of the injury are present.
- Muscle spasm and subsequent loss of strength in the affected muscle are noted.
- Present are possible neurological symptoms, including loss of sensation or muscle function distal to the site of injury.

First aid care of upper arm contusions involves the following:

1. Immediately apply ice and compression. This is best accomplished by using a bag of crushed ice that is secured with a wide elastic wrap tied around the arm.
2. If it is extremely painful to move, place the arm in a sling to immobilize the limb for a period of 24 hours.

In cases of severe acute pain or symptoms that persist beyond 72 hours, refer the athlete for a complete medical evaluation.

Biceps Brachii Injuries

Injuries to the biceps brachii muscle at the elbow (Figure 12.3) can occur in a variety of sports and can be caused by direct blows or hyperextension of the elbow resulting in a strain. However, partial or complete ruptures of the muscle or tendon can occur when powerful concentric (shortening) or eccentric (lengthening) muscle actions are performed against large forces (40 kg or more; Chew & Giuffrè, 2005). A completely ruptured biceps brachii tendon at its attachment near the elbow will often result in a significant deformity where the muscle rolls up in the arm above the elbow. The muscle will appear as a

Table 12.2
Muscles, Actions, and Nerves of the Arm

Muscle	Action	Innervation
Flexor digitorum profundus	Flexion of the distal interphalangeal (DIP), proximal interphalangeal (PIP), and metacarpophalangeal (MCP) joints of the fingers	Median and ulnar
Flexor digitorum superficialis	Flexion of the proximal interphalangeal (PIP) and metacarpophalangeal (MCP) joints of the fingers	Median
Flexor pollicis longus	Flexion of the thumb	Median
Pronator quadratus	Pronation of forearm	Median
Brachioradialis	Flexion of the forearm at the elbow Supination of the forearm	Radial
Extensor carpi radialis longus	Extension of the hand at the wrist Radial deviation of the hand at the wrist	Radial
Extensor carpi radialis brevis	Extension of the hand at the wrist Radial deviation of the hand at the wrist	Radial
Extensor digitorum	Extension of the fingers Extension of the hand at the wrist	Radial
Extensor digiti minimi	Extension of little finger	Radial
Extensor indicis	Extension of index finger	Radial
Extensor carpi ulnaris	Extension of the hand at the wrist Ulnar deviation of the hand at the wrist	Radial
Supinator	Supination of forearm	Radial
Abductor pollicis longus	Abduction of thumb	Radial
Extensor pollicis longus	Extension of thumb	Radial
Extensor pollicis brevis	Extension of thumb	Radial

firm mass above the elbow crease and there will be a significant reduction in elbow flexion and forearm supination strength (Crellin et al., 2018).

Signs and symptoms of injuries to the biceps brachii muscle include the following:

- The athlete may report having experienced a sudden popping in the region of the anterior humerus or elbow.
- Significant pain is present in the elbow region or just proximal in the area of the biceps brachii tendon.
- Swelling and discoloration are likely present immediately but may be delayed for a period of hours after the injury.
- The muscle may roll up proximal to the elbow, producing a palpable mass and significant dysfunction.

First aid care of injuries to the biceps brachii muscle involves the following:

1. The treatment of choice for complete rupture of the distal biceps tendon is early surgical repair (Chew & Giuffrè, 2005).

2. For immediate management of pain and protection so the athlete can be referred to a physician, apply ice and an elastic wrap to the area and place the shoulder and elbow in sling.

Triceps Brachii Injuries

A less common group of injuries to the upper arm involves the triceps muscle. The mechanism of injury may be either a direct blow to the posterior elbow or a fall on an outstretched hand. Either mechanism can result in a partial or complete rupture in the muscle or its tendon. An avulsion fracture of the triceps insertion on the olecranon process of the ulna is a relatively rare injury, but it can be extremely disabling and may be associated with either a fracture of the radial head or the olecranon process (Limpisvasti et al., 2015). Triceps brachii avulsions can occur among a wide range of athletes, including competitive weightlifters, body builders, and football players, but is most common in males 30–50 years old and those who have used anabolic steroids or have a systemic inflammatory disease (Limpisvasti et al., 2015). By definition, all these injuries fall into the general category of muscle strains and/or avulsion fractures; depending on their relative severity and precise location, they may require immediate medical attention. In cases that involve partial or complete ruptures or avulsion fractures of the olecranon process, surgical intervention is necessary (Limpisvasti et al., 2015).

Signs and symptoms of injuries to the triceps brachii muscle include the following:

- The athlete may report having experienced a sudden popping in the region of the posterior humerus or elbow.
- Significant pain is present in the elbow region or just proximal in the area of the triceps tendon.
- A defect is visible in the triceps muscle or in the tendon near the olecranon process.
- Discoloration and possible swelling are present, although both may be delayed for a period of hours after the injury.

First aid care of injuries to the triceps muscle involves the following:

1. If pain is severe or there is a visible bony deformity or defect in the triceps muscle or its tendon, immediate medical referral is necessary. Apply an appropriate splint to minimize movement and check distal pulses (e.g., radial pulse and capillary refill by squeezing the nail and letting go to monitor how quickly the nail goes from white to normal color).
2. Apply ice with an elastic wrap for pain control. Be careful of application of ice over medial elbow as the ulnar nerve is very superficial. If it causes numbness or decreased circulation, remove the ice and wrap.

Fractures of the Upper Arm/Humerus

Little information is available about the frequency of proximal and midshaft humeral fractures related to sports. It would seem that activities involving collisions between participants, such as tackle football and ice hockey, or sports with a potential for high-speed falls, such as cycling or inline skating, would carry a higher risk for such injuries (Figure 12.6).

Signs and symptoms of humeral fractures include the following:

- Severe pain is present in the region of the upper arm with a recent history of trauma to the area.
- Deformity may be present and visible, especially when compared with the opposite extremity.
- The athlete may experience loss of function or be unwilling to use the extremity.
- Muscle spasm is present in the musculature surrounding the extremity.
- The athlete may report having felt a snap or heard a pop at the time of injury.
- If the radial nerve is involved there may be loss of sensation into the dorsum of the forearm and wrist. This may also result in loss of strength in the wrist extensors (AAOS, 1991).
- In cases of stress fracture, pain may not be associated with a specific traumatic incident. Instead, the athlete may report a change in a training program (e.g., a sudden increase in the intensity or volume of a strength training program).

First aid care of humeral fractures involves the following:

1. Immediately apply a properly constructed splint. Many commercial splints are available and will

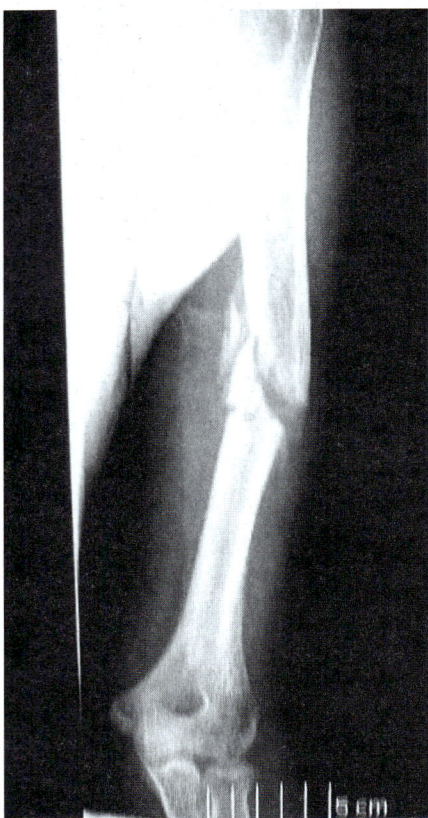

Figure 12.6 Midshaft fracture of the humerus (left arm).
Courtesy of Kevin G. Shea, MD, Intermountain Orthopaedics, Boise, Idaho.

work well when used according to the manufacturer's specifications. The application of ice and compression is best accomplished with a bag of crushed ice that is secured with a wide elastic wrap tied around the arm. Discontinue ice application if radial nerve involvement (weak wrist extensors or numbness) or a circulatory deficiency is observed.

2. Apply moldable splints that encircle both the humerus and forearm along with a standard sling-and-swathe bandage (Perrin and McLeod, 2018; Pollak, 2021) for the shoulder (Figure 12.7a and b) or a vacuum immobilization splint (Figure 12.7c).

3. As with any injury requiring the application of a splint, periodic evaluation of circulation distal to the site of the splint is essential to guarantee that blood flow has not been impaired. This can be accomplished simply by squeezing the nail bed of a finger and observing the return of blood to the fingertip.

4. Humeral fractures are serious injuries often associated with significant soft-tissue damage. In such instances, the athlete should be treated for shock and immediately transported to a healthcare facility.

Athletic Trainers SPEAK OUT

How can an athletic trainer's skills be translated into a public health position designed to prevent injuries?

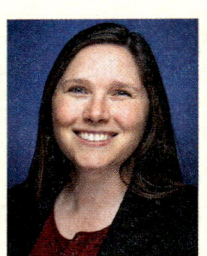

Courtesy of Beth Wolfe, DHS, ATC.

The first domain of the Board of Certification's *Practice Analysis* (7th ed.) is Injury and Illness Prevention and Wellness Promotion, which is defined as "promoting healthy lifestyle behaviors with effective education and communication to enhance wellness and minimize the risk of injury and illness." This domain does not state the population(s) with which, or field(s) in which, injury prevention must be performed, and this provides unlimited opportunities for athletic trainers to use their skills in a wide variety of public health and safety arenas.

Although a job title or position may not explicitly ask for a "certified athletic trainer," the duties, skills, and requirements that are often associated with public health and safety positions are directly transferrable to an athletic training skillset. For example, knowledge and experience on short- and long-term patient outcomes for orthopedic, brain, and musculoskeletal injuries are beneficial skills for the Injury Prevention Coordinator (IPC) position at American College of Surgeon's verified trauma centers. There are hundreds of IPCs across the United States, and to my knowledge, I was the first athletic trainer to work as an IPC for a Level 1 trauma center. As such, I worked collaboratively with physicians, surgeons, nurses, mental health and public health professionals to prevent injuries in our communities.

Working at the trauma center exposed me to many types of injuries that athletic trainers typically do not treat or see in an athletic setting (e.g., car crashes, falls, penetrating trauma), but my athletic training education gave me a foundation of knowledge so that I could be an active member of the trauma service team. Exposure to various types of traumatic injuries opened avenues for me to learn more about the roles, responsibilities, and evaluations that other professionals have in preventing injuries. For example, law enforcement officers use Standardized Field Sobriety Tests (SFST) to evaluate suspected impaired drivers, and the SFSTs are an abbreviated neurological assessment which overlaps with many elements of a concussion evaluation. This and many other overlaps in knowledge opened a new opportunity for me to work in the field of highway safety. Now each day I go to work to save lives by preventing traffic crashes related to impaired driving.

Athletic trainers have the knowledge and skills to work in almost any public health and safety field. We are not, and should not, be limited to only applying for jobs that have "athletic trainer" in the title or in the job description. Looking forward to the future, it would be great to have other athletic trainers by my side working to keep the U.S. safe in the federal government and beyond. Will you join me?

—**Beth Wolfe, DHS, ATC**

Beth Wolfe is a Highway Safety Specialist for the Impaired Driving Division of the National Highway Traffic Safety Administration in the US Dept. of Transportation in Washington, D.C.

WHAT IF ❓

You are asked to examine the elbow of a young softball pitcher. She has been suffering from elbow pain and reports that her elbow "locks" occasionally. When this happens she experiences sharp pain and swelling. What might be the cause of the problem, and what course of action would you recommend?

Elbow Injuries

Elbow injuries are common in sports and range from simple abrasions or contusions to sprains and complete dislocations or fractures. In sports involving repeated throwing or swinging actions, the elbow may develop an overuse injury related to muscular attachments on the humeral epicondyles, sometimes resulting in a condition known as

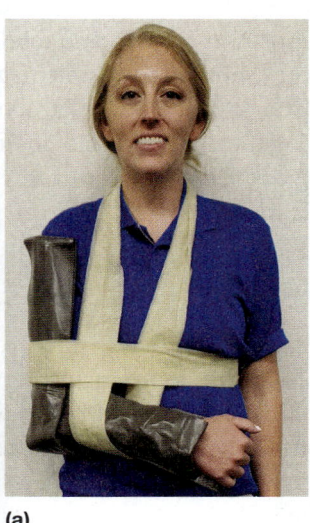
(a)

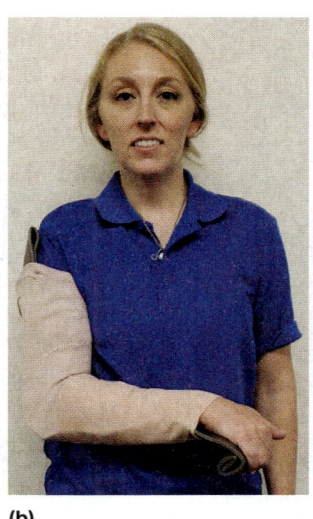
(b)

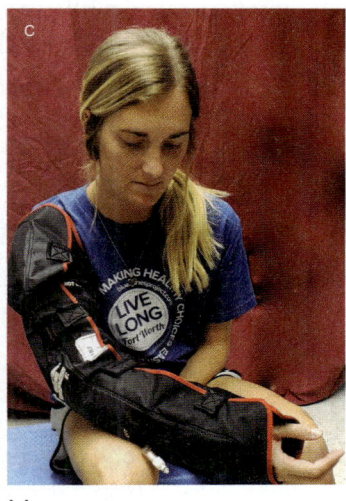
(c)

Figure 12.7 (a) Splinting of an elbow injury or humeral fracture with moldable splints and cravats. **(b)** Splinting of an elbow injury or humeral fracture with moldable splints and ace wrap. **(c)** Splinting of an elbow injury or humeral fracture with vacuum splint.
Courtesy of Cindy Trowbridge.

epicondylitis. The epicondyles in the pediatric aged athlete are anatomically immature and are therefore classified as growth plates because they are sites for muscle attachments. As such, when these structures are damaged resulting in inflammation, typically as in an overuse injury, the injury is technically called **apophysitis**. The joint can also sustain sprains, the most common involve hyperextensions in which the joint is forced beyond its normal locked position in extension. Dislocations and fractures are probably the most severe types of injuries to this complex joint; if not cared for properly, either can lead to permanent complications.

Elbow Sprains and Dislocations

The three articulations of the elbow are bound together by several ligaments that combine to give support to the joint throughout its wide range of motion. The joint capsule of the elbow is extensive and is reinforced both medially and laterally by the ulnar and radial collateral ligaments, respectively. These two ligaments serve to protect the elbow from **valgus** and **varus** forces acting across the joint. In addition, the radial head is held in position by the annular ligament described previously.

The elbow may be sprained through a variety of mechanisms, including falls, particularly when an athlete falls backward with the elbow locked in extension. This mechanism results in a stretching and/or tearing of the anterior joint capsule as well as other soft-tissue structures in the anterior portion of the joint. Two other mechanisms for elbow sprains are valgus and varus forces that can occur suddenly in situations in which the arm is trapped in a vulnerable position, such as can happen in tackle football or wrestling. A valgus force typically comes from the outside and strains the inside of the elbow and this may cause a sprain of the ulnar collateral ligament (UCL), whereas a varus force comes from the inside and strains the outside of the elbow and this may cause a sprain of the radial collateral ligament (RCL).

Dislocations of the elbow are sprains in the extreme sense as the joint capsule is completely disrupted, and they involve damage to significant soft-tissue structures around the joint. The mechanism of injury is typically a fall in which the elbow is in either an extended or flexed position. The force of the impact causes the forearm bones to be driven posteriorly out of their normal position, with the olecranon process of the ulna coming to rest well behind the distal end of the humerus. The deformity is obvious, which makes the initial evaluation relatively straightforward. This injury may be associated with a fracture of either the radius or the ulna, or both.

Signs and symptoms of elbow sprains and dislocations include the following:

- In cases of minor sprains, mild swelling and localized pain may be present, with difficulty in gripping objects or making a fist.
- In cases of dislocations, the elbow is grossly deformed, with abnormal positioning of the forearm bones behind the distal end of the humerus. (Figure 12.8a and b).
- The athlete reports severe pain and total dysfunction of the elbow joint and possible neurological symptoms distal to the elbow characterized by numbness along the distribution of major nerves. The ulnar nerve appears to be the most vulnerable to this specific injury (AAOS, 1991).

First aid care of elbow sprains and dislocations involves the following:

1. In cases of minor sprains, the immediate application of ice and compression, using a bag of crushed ice held in place with an elastic wrap, is effective. Once ice and compression are properly situated, the arm should be placed in a sling-and-swathe bandage.
2. In cases of obvious dislocations, the primary concern is to prevent complications, which can be extremely serious and include compression on the neurovascular structures in the elbow region.

Epicondylitis Inflammatory response of the soft tissue that attaches to the epicondyle.

Apophysitis Inflammation or stress injury where a tendon attaches near or around growth plates of bones resulting in pain and/or excessive pulling of the bone causing structural changes.

Valgus Outward force on a bone segment distal to a joint causing an opening on the medial (inside) of the joint.

Varus Inward force on a bone segment distal to a joint causing an opening on the lateral (outside) of the joint.

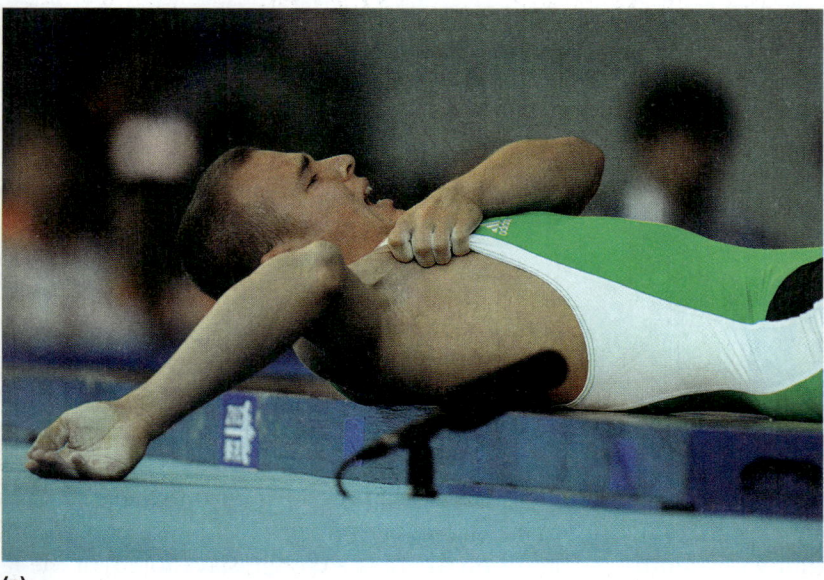 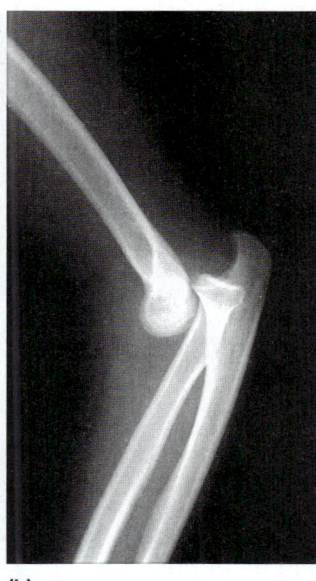

Figure 12.8 (a) Posterior dislocation of the elbow makes the olecranon process of ulna more prominent. (b) X-ray of posterior dislocation of the elbow.
(a) © JUNG YEON-JE/AFP/Getty Images; (b) © Medical Body Scans/Science Source.

Immediately apply a splint to immobilize area and if tolerated apply ice for pain control. Splinting of this injury requires special attention to avoid moving the displaced forearm bones and causing further injury. Moldable splints that encircle both the humerus and forearm along with a sling and swathe (Figure 12.7a and b) or a vacuum immobilization splint (Figure 12.7c) are the most appropriate.

3. Elbow dislocations are serious injuries. The athlete should be treated for shock, and arrangements must be made for transportation to a medical facility.

Elbow Fractures

Elbow fractures generally involve the distal humerus, just above the epicondyles, known as supracondylar fractures, or the proximal ulna or radius. Supracondylar fractures are reported to be common in young (pediatric and adolescent) athletes. Because of the complexity of the joint, any fracture represents potential problems for the athlete. As is the case with dislocations, neurovascular structures are in jeopardy when fractures result in displacement of bones. This is especially true if broken bones are moved inadvertently by the athlete or by someone else attempting to render first aid. A simple elbow fracture can easily be converted into an irreversible injury in such a situation. If the radial artery is compressed by broken bone ends, circulation to the forearm can be significantly reduced or stopped, resulting in a condition known as **Volkmann's contracture** (Figure 12.9). This condition involves the reaction of the forearm musculature to a lack of blood supply. If left uncorrected, it becomes a permanent deformity; therefore, it is imperative that elbow fractures be handled very carefully during the application of first aid procedures. Furthermore, it is important that the blood supply distal to the elbow be monitored until the athlete is transported to a medical facility.

The mechanisms of injury are similar to those of sprains and dislocations. Fractures of the olecranon process of the ulna are often associated with falls in which the elbow is in a flexed position and the impact occurs on the tip of the joint. When elbow fractures occur in adolescents, they require special attention to ensure that the injury will not adversely affect the growth centers of the bones involved.

> **Volkmann's contracture** Contracture of muscles of the forearm related to a loss of blood supply caused by a fracture and/or dislocation of either of the bones in the forearm or the humerus.

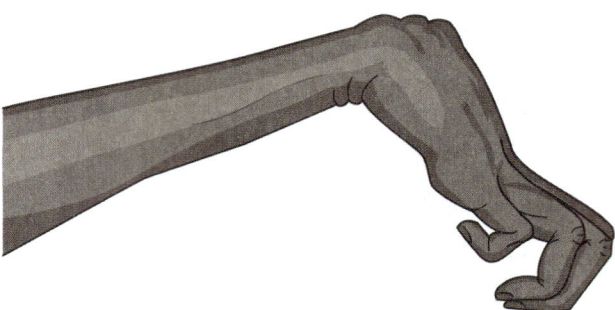

Figure 12.9 Volkmann's ischemic contracture.

Signs and symptoms of elbow fractures include the following:

- The athlete has a recent history of significant trauma to the elbow in association with significant pain and dysfunction.
- Immediate swelling in the region of the injury is present.
- In the case of displaced fractures, an obvious deformity will be noted.
- In cases of problems with the blood supply, a lack of proper blood flow will be noted in the forearm and hand, both of which will feel cold and clammy. In addition, the athlete will likely report pain or numbness in the hand.

First aid care of elbow fractures involves the following:

1. Apply an appropriate splint, taking great care to avoid moving the bones of the elbow, as shown in Figure 12.7 a–c. As mentioned previously, keep the fingers available to assess for circulation and sensation.
2. Treat the athlete for shock and arrange for transport to a medical facility.

Epicondylitis of the Elbow

The epicondyles of the humerus are located distally immediately proximal to the articular surfaces of the radius and ulna bone (Figure 12.10a). The more prominent medial epicondyle serves as the common site of attachment for flexor muscles of the forearm (Figure 12.5) as well as for the ulnar collateral ligament. The smaller lateral epicondyle serves as the common site of attachment for the extensor muscles (Figure 12.4) of the forearm as well as for the radial collateral ligament. As mentioned earlier in the chapter, in the pediatric-aged athlete, the epicondyles are anatomically immature and represent growth plates. Thus, when these become inflamed, the condition is known as apophysitis. Regardless of age, these bony prominences are easily located near the elbow joint with palpation and visual inspection.

Activities that require continuous gripping of an object along with simultaneous wrist actions, such as is common in racket and throwing sports, place considerable stress on the tissues of the epicondylar regions. With respect to baseball (overhead) pitching, the stresses exerted at the elbow are profound. Biomechanical analysis indicates that the elbow moves through extension in the acceleration phase achieving velocities of 3,000° per second. In addition, there is a compressive force on the lateral side of the elbow between the radial head and the humeral capitellum, whereas there is a distraction force on the medial side of the elbow between the ulna and the trochlea that can cause medial epicondylitis or inflammation/tears in the common flexor tendon (Figure 12.10b). While the phrase "Little League elbow" was first coined in 1960 (Brogden & Crow, 1960), the first major studies on the topic did not get published until more than a decade later. It was during the 1970s that two major papers on the topic were published, lending support to a national debate on the topic that included the medical community, sponsoring organizations, coaches, parents, and athletes (Gugenheim et al., 1976; Larson et al., 1976). During this time, considerable attention was given to identifying the contributors to these injuries, including type of pitch, appropriate technique, and total number of pitches thrown over the course of a game, a week, and an entire season. A major concern was that the throwing motion might cause degenerative changes and subsequent inflammation within the medial epicondyle (Amin et al., 2015). Elbows of young players experience apophysitis on the medial side of the elbow, whereas older player experience epicondylitis. Both conditions result in significant pain around the region of the medial epicondyle and can severely limit the athlete's ability to flex or pronate the wrist and hand. In the adolescent, extreme cases can lead to actual fracturing of the epicondyle away from the humerus, known as an avulsion fracture. As a result, rules that limited the maximum number of innings young pitchers could throw during a season

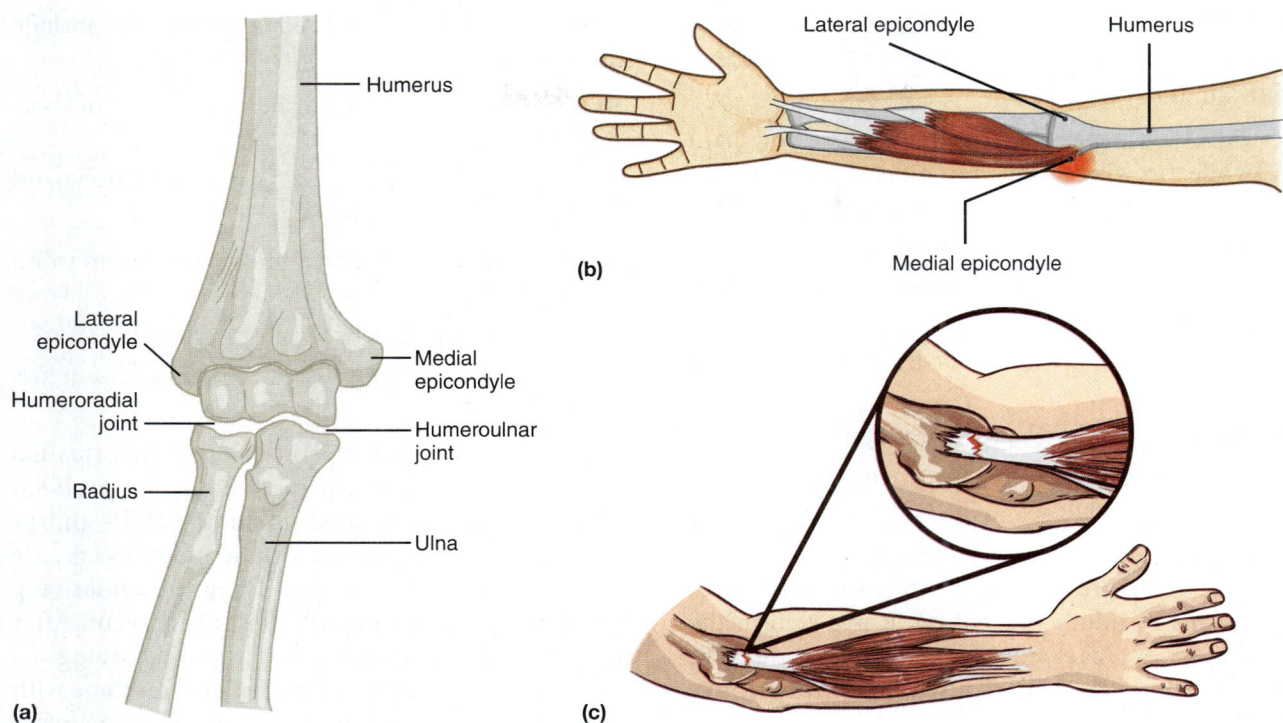

Figure 12.10 (a) Epicondyles of the elbow joint. (b) Little League or golfer's elbow—tear or inflammation in the common flexor tendon of the arm. (c) Tennis elbow—tear or inflammation in the common extensor tendon of the arm.
(b) © solar22/Shutterstock; (c) © Drp8/Shutterstock.

were instituted. In spite of the increased awareness of this problem within the youth baseball community, it is estimated that Little League elbow continues to affect youth pitchers. Recent epidemiological studies that examined high school baseball and softball players, demonstrated that high school baseball players have around a 2.1 times greater relative risk of getting an elbow injury when compared to high school softball players, and most of the elbow injuries in baseball were attributable to pitching (Pytiak et al., 2018).

Currently, there are pitch count recommendations as well as rest days after a certain number of pitches for different age groups. These guidelines were first developed in 1996 with subsequent revisions in 2006 and 2010 (Feeley et al., 2018). The pitch counts are based on age and range from 50 pitches/game for 7- to 8-year-olds to 105 pitches/game for 17- to 18-year-olds (Feeley et al., 2018). Rest days required are based on age and number of pitches. If fewer than 20 pitches are thrown then no rest is necessary before the next outing; however, up to age 16 if more than 60 pitches are thrown and after age 17 if more than 76 pitches are thrown, then 3 days of rest is recommended (Feeley et al., 2018). These guidelines are supported by orthopedic physicians, athletic trainers, and baseball coaching organizations, but must be implemented to be successful (Feeley et al., 2018). Regarding the type of pitch, there are recommendations as to when is the appropriate age to begin throwing different pitches such as the curve ball, but there has not been completely clear evidence as to a link between pitch type and elbow injury (Feeley et al., 2018). Additional prevention recommendations to avoid throwing-related injuries are to properly warm up, to not catch and pitch on the same days, to not pitch on multiple teams, to not play all year round, to not use a radar gun for pitch speed, and to emphasize control and good pitching mechanics.

Recent research has also emphasized the importance of educating parents, coaches, and baseball players on their potential risk for developing elbow injuries (Yukutake et al., 2015). After significant investigations and many iterations of questionnaires, the research team was able to develop a six-question preseason checklist that could accurately predict which players would be injured during a season (Yukutake et al., 2015). Players who answered yes to more than three questions on this checklist had a 33% chance of elbow injury.

- Have you experienced shoulder or elbow pain while throwing in the preceding 12 months?
- Have you ever experienced an elbow or shoulder injury requiring medical attention?
- Do you complete team training at least 4 days per week?
- Do you participate in self-training 7 days per week?
- Are you considered a regular player?
- Do you experience pitching arm fatigue while playing baseball?

Although it might be an exaggeration to suggest that use of only this checklist is the most effective means of injury prevention, it is a step in the right direction. Likely the most effective tactic is the combination of the checklist with other preventive measures listed above.

Another sport identified as a cause of medial epicondylitis in some athletes is golf. The condition, known as **golfer's elbow**, has been linked to players who faulty mechanics with their swing (Tucker, 2016; Figure 12.10b). However, repetitively gripping the club too tightly, performing repetitive and excessive muscular contractions, or after experiencing a single traumatic force such as inadvertently striking an immobile object with the club may also be the cause. The condition occurs more often in the trail arm and has been associated with the number of rounds played and practice balls hit per week, and other risk factors such as failure to warm up and poor conditioning (Tucker, 2016).

Tennis has also been identified as a cause of epicondylitis. Tennis elbow or lateral epicondylitis involves the lateral humeral epicondyle and the extensor carpi radialis brevis tendon (Tosti et al., 2013; Figure 12.10c). It is estimated that 50% of those who play tennis will experience some degree of lateral elbow pain in their lifetimes and the ncidence is higher in novice players and those who use a one-handed backhand stroke (Tosti et al., 2013). A variety of sports-related factors related to epicondylitis include the following:

- Overload related to the sheer frequency of shots played
- Incorrect technique, particularly on the backhand
- Too small a racket handle
- Recent change of racket, for instance, from wood to graphite
- Too tight a grip between shots
- Poor conditioning, muscle imbalance, and/or loss of flexibility

Regardless of the type of epicondylitis (medial or lateral), the first step in treating the problem is to identify the cause(s), including skill- and/or equipment-related problems. If the athlete treats only the symptoms without identifying the underlying problems, epicondylitis will most likely recur. After the causes are identified and adjusted accordingly, a program of aggressive treatment of symptoms with ice application or nonsteroidal anti-inflammatories for pain relief plus strengthening exercises and restoration of upper extremity muscle balance and flexibility is recommended. Strength exercises, including wrist curls and extensions with pronation and supination against mild resistance, may prove helpful. Recent evidence also suggests that exercises focusing on the eccentric phase are important in developing the tendon's resistance to injury (Tosti et al., 2013). During the early phase of treatment, exercises without weight may be advised, such as squeezing a tennis ball (finger flexors) and finger extension against the resistance of the opposite hand. Any rehabilitation program should be developed and supervised by a competent sports medicine practitioner such as an athletic trainer or a sports physical therapist.

Signs and symptoms of epicondylitis/apophysitis include the following:

- Pain is present in the region of either the medial or lateral epicondyle. Symptoms become worse during or immediately after participation.
- Pain radiates distally into either the flexor/pronator or extensor/supinator muscles, depending on which epicondyle is involved.
- Pain may be elicited in the region of the epicondyles during resisted wrist flexion or extension, depending on which epicondyle is involved.

Golfer's elbow Medial humeral epicondylitis related to incorrect golf technique.

- Swelling is present in the region of the painful epicondyle.
- In severe and chronic cases, crepitus (feeling hardened fragments through the skin) may be noted over the region of the affected epicondyle.

Care of epicondylitis/apophysitis involves the following:

1. Both medial and lateral epicondylitis tend to be chronic injuries resulting from overuse. When symptoms worsen, however, the application of ice and compression can be helpful; this is best accomplished with a bag of crushed ice that is secured with an elastic wrap. However, numbness and muscle function must be monitored as the radial and ulnar nerves are superficial and may experience damage with too long of a duration or too much compression of ice bag.
2. If symptoms persist, medical referral is necessary. Surgical intervention is rare but may be necessary.
3. Long-term treatment includes rest, reduced participation in the activity, and sometimes use of anti-inflammatory drugs.
4. The use of a counterforce brace along the proximal flexors and extensors of the wrist can theoretically inhibit full muscular expansion and can decrease the forces on the bony origin of the common extensor tendon (Tosti et al., 2013).
5. It is critical that the causes of the injury be identified, which likely include technique errors, overuse due to excessive participation in the absence of adequate rest, or equipment-related issues (tennis and golf; Amin et al., 2015).

Osteochondritis Dissecans of the Elbow

The mechanism of throwing can lead to a type of impingement syndrome in the elbow joint occurring between the radial head and the capitellum of the humerus. The anatomy of the radiocapitellar joint and the blood supply to the capitellum are thought to play a significant role in the development of these lesions. It is typical in youth between 11 and 17 years old especially those who participate in repetitive overhead activities such as baseball, gymnastics, football, javelin, or overhead weightlifting (Churchill et al., 2016). In young pitchers and throwers, the injury is associated with the late cocking and acceleration phases of the overhead throw, whereas axial loading is implicated in gymnastics, football, and weightlifting. With throwing, the action of high-velocity extension can cause the elbow to develop a valgus overload resulting in abnormal compression of the elbow on the lateral side of the joint (Churchill et al., 2016). Over time and with continued throwing or axial loading, the cartilage on the proximal end of the radius can become inflamed and even begin to fracture, resulting in a condition known as **osteochondritis dissecans (OCD)**. It has been reported that osteochondritis dissecans involving the capitellum, rather than the radial head, is a significant problem in adolescent athletes (Churchill et al., 2016).

Signs and symptoms of osteochondritis dissecans include the following:

- During the initial phases of development, the athlete will experience pain during participation, but it will not be self-limiting.
- Joint inflammation and stiffness may be noted, particularly 12 to 24 hours after participation.
- In well-established cases, cartilage fragments (loose bodies) may form in the joint; these are commonly known as joint mice.
- The athlete may experience a locking of the elbow, which occurs when a loose body is caught between the moving bone ends in the joint.
- In advanced cases, the elbow may develop osteoarthritis.

First aid care of osteochondritis dissecans involves the following:

1. An athlete with a history of trauma to the elbow joint associated with the symptoms just described should be referred to the appropriate physician for a thorough diagnostic evaluation.
2. Immediate symptoms are best treated with a bag of crushed ice held in place with an elastic wrap with caution for the radial and ulnar nerves.

Osteochondritis dissecans (OCD) Condition in which a fragment of cartilage and underlying bone are detached from the articular surface; also called "joint mice."

3. If fragments are identified in the joint, the physician may recommend arthroscopic surgery to remove the loose bodies.
4. The conservative (nonsurgical) treatment for this condition involves rest followed by an extensive period of rehabilitative exercise designed to concentrically and eccentrically strengthen the muscles surrounding the elbow and the ligaments of the joint.

Contusions of the Elbow

External blows to the elbow region are common in sports. Little protective equipment is available for the joint, and its large range of motion and irregular shape make taping and wrapping impractical. Fortunately, the vast majority of contusions result in only temporary discomfort, which normally improves in a few days. An exception, however, is the olecranon bursa, which is a large sac between the skin and the olecranon process of the ulna. Falling on a flexed elbow or sustaining repeated blows to the olecranon area can irritate this **bursa** and cause acute bursitis. Although bursitis does not directly affect the integrity of the elbow joint, persistent swelling, stiffness, and pain associated with this problem can reduce the quality of athletic performance. The risk of infection or sepsis also exists with olecranon bursitis, which can complicate the treatment and require antibiotics (Reilly & Kamineni, 2016).

Signs and symptoms of olecranon bursitis include the following:

- The most obvious sign of this injury is swelling around the olecranon process of the ulna. It typically looks like a golf ball is under the skin around the point of the elbow.
- Another sign is pain and stiffness, especially when the elbow is flexed.
- Skin over the olecranon process may appear taut, and the joint may show signs of internal hemorrhage. Skin temperature over the olecranon may be elevated, which would potentially indicate an infection. Tenderness, redness, fever, and a sign of external trauma are also linked with infections (Reilly & Kamineni, 2016).

First aid care of olecranon bursitis involves the following:

1. Immediate care of elbow contusions includes the application of a bag of crushed ice held in place with an elastic wrap.
2. If the signs and symptoms of olecranon bursitis do not subside and excessive warmth, redness, tenderness, and fever are present, refer the athlete to the appropriate physician.

Wrist and Forearm Injuries

The anatomy of the human wrist is highly complex. Within this compact joint exists a large number of tendons (for the wrist, fingers, and thumb) that are tightly bound together underneath bands of connective tissue known as retinaculum (transverse carpal ligaments). Also passing through this region are the major nerves and blood vessels of the hand and fingers (Figure 12.11).

Aside from simple contusions, injuries to the forearm in sports are relatively uncommon. Usually, contusions can be easily treated with ice, compression, and elevation, which can be followed later with the application of protective padding and taping. Probably the most serious forearm injuries involve fractures distal in the forearm, just proximal to the wrist joint. The most well-known of these is a **Colles' fracture**, which involves a transverse fracture of the distal radius (Figure 12.12). Variations of this fracture include simultaneous fractures of both the radius and ulna as well as compound fractures of either bone; such injuries are serious and must be properly cared for to avoid complications. The mechanism of injury is highly variable, but the injury is often caused by falling on an outstretched arm. When a high amount and rate of force is encounter in the wrist, many soft-tissue structures will also be damaged in conjunction with the fracture.

Signs and symptoms of distal forearm fractures include the following:

- The athlete will have a recent history of significant trauma to the wrist region associated with having heard a popping sound and/or felt a snapping of the bones.

Bursa Small, fluid-filled sac, typically located over bony prominences, that assists in cushioning and reducing friction.

Colles' fracture Transverse fracture of the distal radius.

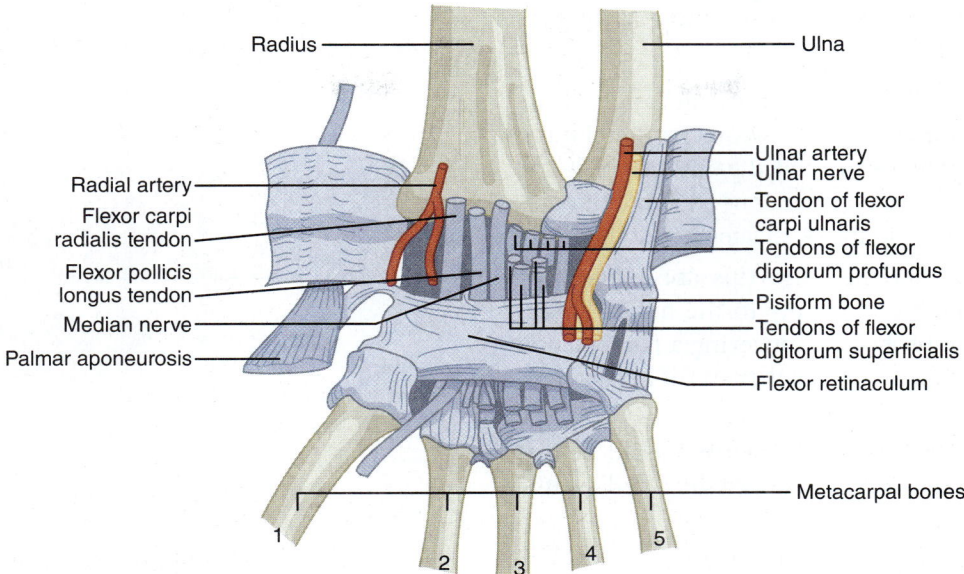

Figure 12.11 Right wrist (palmar view).

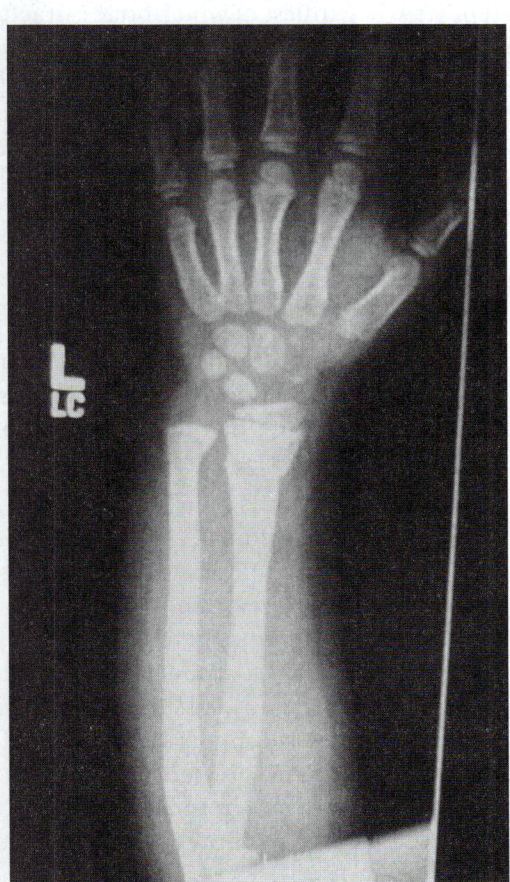

Figure 12.12 Distal forearm fracture (Colles' fracture).
Courtesy of Kevin G. Shea, MD, Intermountain Orthopaedics, Boise, Idaho.

- A deformity, known as the silver fork deformity, between the arm and wrist is typical; in the case of a Colles' fracture, the hand is driven backward and outward (radial deviation) (Figure 12.13).
- Swelling, often severe, develops quickly and may affect the hand and fingers.
- Pain is generally severe, and motion of the wrist, hand, or fingers will be significantly curtailed.
- In cases in which a broken bone puts pressure on nerves, loss of sensation may be noted in the hand and/or fingers. If there is pressure on arteries, the skin will appear pale or gray, and capillary refill will be impaired.

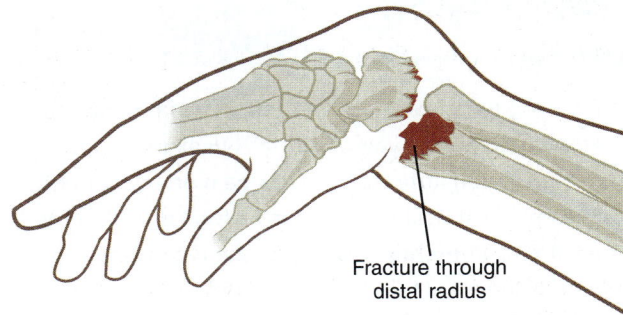

Figure 12.13 A Colles' fracture demonstrating the silver fork deformity.

First aid care of distal forearm fractures involves the following:

1. Immediately immobilize with an appropriate splint to protect the area from further injury. You can apply ice to reduce pain but not if you suspect either the vascular or nerve supply is compromised (see Figure 12.25 later in the chapter).
2. Make sure that the fingertips are exposed to monitor the blood supply to the hand. This is easily accomplished by squeezing a nail bed and noting the return (or lack thereof) of normal reddish color to the tissue.
3. Once immobilized, the forearm should be elevated carefully using a standard sling-and-swathe bandage.
4. Because of the pain and damage associated with this type of injury, the athlete must be treated for shock and transported to a medical facility immediately.

Wrist Fractures

Fractures of the carpal bones do occur in sports. According to multiple authors (Limpisvasti et al., 2015; Prentice, 2017), the most common fractures involve the scaphoid bone (Figure 12.14). This bone can receive considerable force when the wrist is placed into extension in sports, such as tackle football (blocking) and gymnastics (vaulting and floor exercise). Simple falls can also cause fractures to this critical bone of the wrist. The fracture generally occurs in a specific site on the scaphoid bone known as the waist, which is the narrowest section of the bone.

Other bones of the wrist can also be fractured; fractures of the lunate, pisiform, and hamate have been reported. Regardless of which bone is fractured, the signs and symptoms will be similar. Because the carpal bones are small, gross deformity is typically not present, and evaluation of these injuries is difficult. When doubt exists about the extent or nature of the injury, the best policy is to refer the athlete to a physician for a more complete diagnostic evaluation.

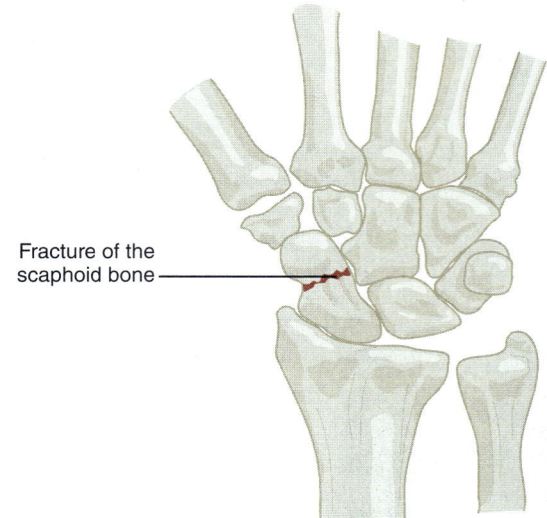

Figure 12.14 Fracture of the scaphoid bone is common in sports.

Signs and symptoms of wrist fractures include the following:

- The athlete has a recent history of trauma to the wrist, specifically forced extension associated with a snapping or popping sensation in the wrist.
- The athlete experiences pain in the wrist, which is aggravated by movement. A simple test for the integrity of the scaphoid bone involves pressing lightly into the region at the base of the thumb known as the anatomic snuffbox (Figure 12.15), which is bordered by several tendons that attach within the thumb. The radial surface of the scaphoid bone is located within the anatomic snuffbox. Consequently, external pressure in this region may elicit a painful response from the athlete, which is a positive sign of a fracture of that bone.
- The athlete may be unable or unwilling to move the wrist, and doing so may result in considerable pain.

WHAT IF ?

A young gymnast grabs her left wrist immediately after completing a vault. During your examination of her wrist, you note that she has pain on movement. She reports that she felt a snap as soon as her hands hit the vaulting horse and that she is tender in the region known as the anatomic snuffbox. What would you conclude happened, and what would you do for initial care?

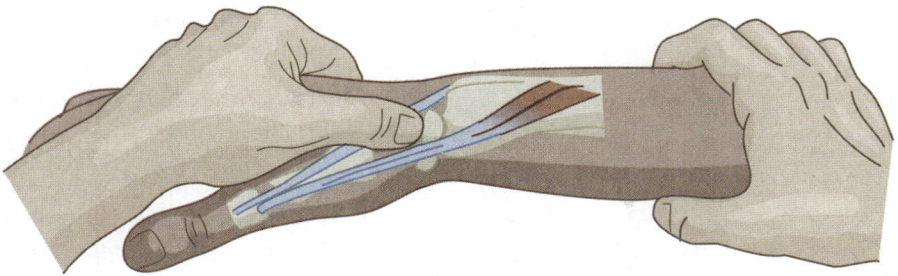

Figure 12.15 Palpation in the anatomic snuffbox.

- The athlete may state that the wrist feels locked in a certain position, which can be an indication of a displaced fracture.

First aid care of wrist fractures involves the following:

1. Immediately apply an appropriate splint to immobilize the wrist joint (see Figure 12.25 later in the chapter). Leave the fingertips exposed to facilitate monitoring blood flow to the hand beyond the level of the splint.
2. Once immobilized, the wrist should be elevated carefully by way of a standard sling-and-swathe bandage.
3. Ice can be applied to help with pain control, and an orthopedic evaluation should be obtained soon.

Wrist Sprains and Dislocations

The mechanism producing a fracture of the wrist may also produce a sprain or dislocation in that region when it is of lesser severity. Essentially, the wrist (radiocarpal) joint is bound together by a network of large, strong ligaments known as the palmar and dorsal radiocarpal ligaments (Figures 12.16a and b; Figure 12.17a and b). In addition, several smaller ligaments bind the remaining bones of the wrist to form a well-supported series of joints known collectively as the intercarpal joints.

The most common sprain of the wrist is caused by forced hyperextension, which results in a stretching and possible tearing of the palmar radiocarpal ligament. Such an injury can, if severe enough, result in a dislocation of one or more of the carpal bones. In the case of a simple sprain, the carpal bones will remain in their normal position.

The most common dislocation of the wrist involves the lunate bone, which is located between the distal end of the radius and the capitate bone (Limpisvasti et al., 2015; Prentice, 2017). The mechanism of injury is forceful hyperextension, which causes the bone to shift out of its normal position and slide toward the palmar side of the wrist. In severe cases, the lunate will put pressure on the tendons and nerves of a region of the wrist known as the carpal tunnel, resulting in significant symptoms in the hand and fingers.

Signs and symptoms of wrist sprains and dislocations include the following:

- The athlete will report having sustained a forced hyperextension of the wrist in conjunction with

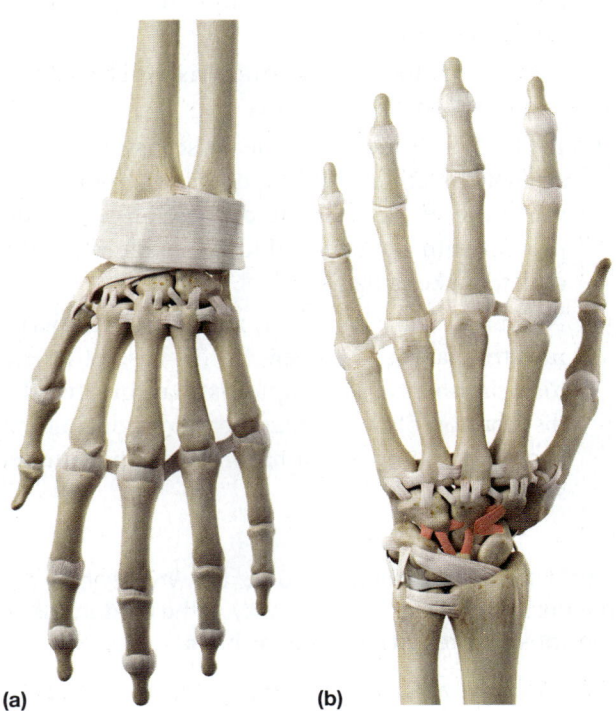

(a) (b)

Figure 12.16 (a) Superficial dorsal wrist ligaments and retinaculum. (b) Deep dorsal wrist ligaments.
© SciePro/Shutterstock.

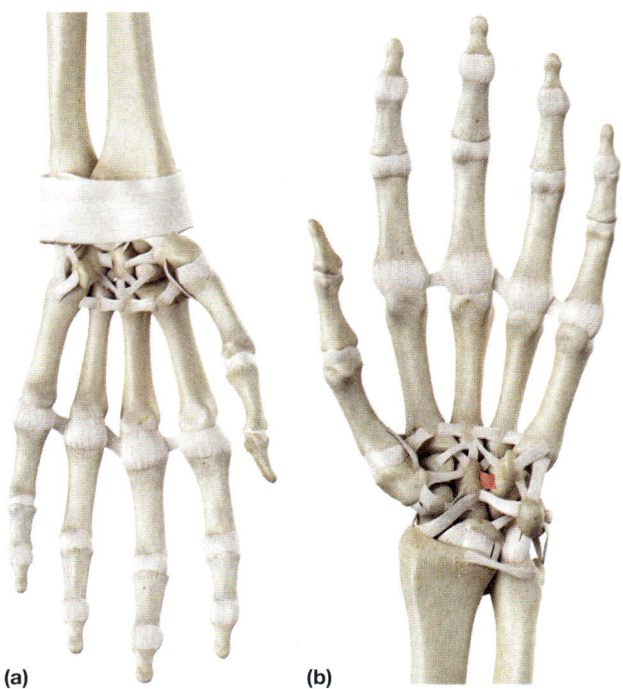

Figure 12.17 **(a)** Superficial palmar wrist ligaments and retinaculum. **(b)** Deep palmar wrist ligaments.
© SciePro/Shutterstock.

a snapping or popping sensation in the bones of the joint.

- Attempted movements of the wrist will be painful and meet with little success.
- In cases of dislocations, the wrist may be locked so that the athlete will be unable to voluntarily move the wrist. A lunate dislocation will often present with a sunken middle knuckle when the athlete makes a fist.
- Numbness and/or pain may radiate from the wrist into the hand and fingers. In the case of lunate dislocations, these symptoms may involve the distribution of the median nerve, producing the symptoms known commonly as carpal tunnel syndrome.

Carpal tunnel Anatomic region of the wrist where the median nerve and the majority of the tendons of the anterior forearm pass into the hand.

Carpal tunnel syndrome A complex set of symptoms resulting from pressure on the median nerve as it passes through the carpal tunnel of the wrist, causing soreness and numbness.

- Swelling of the wrist may be limited owing to the nature of the ligaments of the region.

First aid care of wrist sprains and dislocations involves the following:

1. Immediately apply an appropriate splint designed to immobilize the wrist joint (Figure 12.25 later in the chapter). To help control pain, a bag of crushed ice, held in place by an elastic wrap, should be applied. Do not apply ice if you suspect that either the vascular or nerve supply is compromised.
2. Elevation is best achieved using a standard sling-and-swathe bandage.
3. In cases of significant pain or a possible dislocation, the athlete must be referred to a healthcare facility for further evaluation and treatment.

Nerve Injuries to the Wrist

Three major nerves cross the wrist from the forearm into the hand to supply sensation and motor function to the hand and fingers. These nerves are the radial, the median, and the ulnar. Though any of these nerves may be damaged in a sports-related injury, the most commonly injured nerve is the median (Padua et al., 2016). This nerve passes through a region of the wrist known as the **carpal tunnel** (Figure 12.18), which also houses eight flexor tendons that pass into the hand. The tunnel is surrounded by dense, strong ligaments and bone.

The exact cause of **carpal tunnel syndrome** is unknown, but it probably involves swelling within the tunnel caused by tendinitis or sprains of the region. In any event, the pressure of the swelling has a negative effect on the median nerve. Although carpal tunnel syndrome can be caused by a single traumatic episode, such as a dislocated lunate bone, the majority of cases involving athletes tend to be the result of chronic overuse injuries. Sports with a high incidence include racket sports and those requiring the participant to grip an object tightly for extended periods. Unless treated properly, carpal tunnel syndrome can be extremely disabling and can often preclude an athlete from returning to the sport.

Another nerve-related injury in the wrist involves the ulnar nerve as it passes through the region on the ulnar side of the forearm. Specifically, the ulnar nerve is in the vicinity of the pisiform bone and the hook of

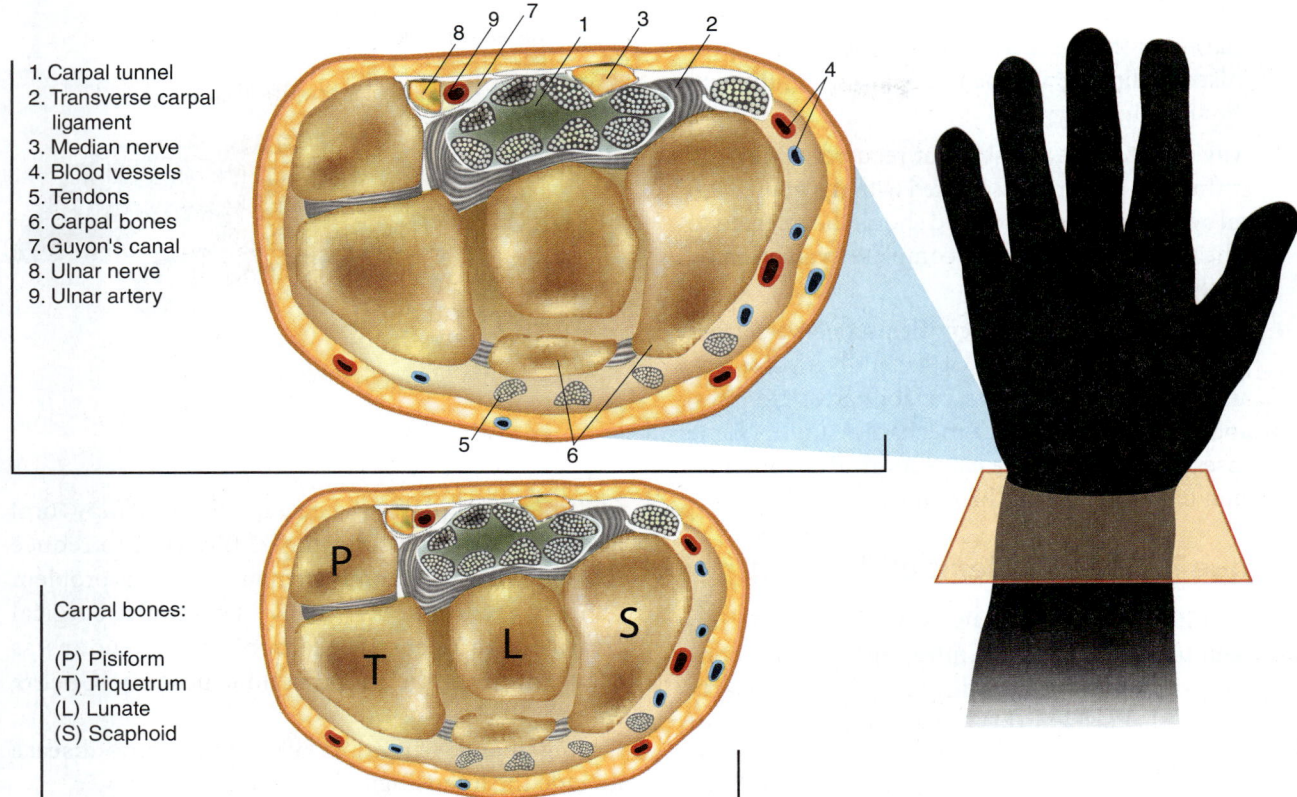

Figure 12.18 Cross-section view of the forearm at the wrist showing the carpal tunnel. Note the position of the median nerve.
© Sakurra/Shutterstock.

the hamate bone within the **tunnel of Guyon** (Maroukis et al., 2015). A blow to the wrist, nerve compression, or tendinitis in the tendon of the flexor carpi ulnaris can result in irritation to the ulnar nerve and a variety of symptoms, which include loss of sensation to a portion of the hand and fingers as well as loss of muscle strength in the fingers affected by the ulnar nerve. The region of the hand that receives sensory impulses from the ulnar nerve is the medial portion of the palm, including the region known as the hypothenar eminence, as well as the medial half of the ring finger and the entire little finger (Maroukis et al., 2015).

Signs and symptoms of nerve injuries to the wrist include the following:

- The athlete experiences loss of sensation to a portion of the hand and/or fingers that follows the distribution of a major nerve in the region. In some cases, pain may also radiate into the forearm.
- Pain and tenderness are noted around the region of the wrist on the palm side.
- The athlete has associated tendinitis of the wrist or a recent history of trauma to the area, such as a contusion or sprain.
- Symptoms may become worse when the wrist is fully flexed or extended and there is compression from equipment or from gripping an object too tightly with the hand.

Care of nerve injuries to the wrist involves the following:

1. This type of injury tends to develop slowly over time. The exception is when a nerve of the wrist is aggravated by an acute injury, such as a severe contusion (compression) or sprain.
2. When associated with an acute trauma, the best approach is the immediate application of ice for

Tunnel of Guyon Anatomic region formed by the hook of the hamate bone and the pisiform bone, whereby the ulnar nerve passes into the hand.

inflammation relief. Do not apply ice if you suspect that either the vascular or nerve supply is compromised. Splinting may be necessary depending on the specific injury.

3. Any athlete with a history of recurrent pain and stiffness in the wrist associated with the neurological symptoms just described should be referred to a healthcare facility for a complete evaluation by a medical doctor.

4. If the medical diagnosis confirms a nerve-related problem, the initial care will generally involve rest, anti-inflammatory drugs, rehabilitative exercises, and correction of faulty mechanics and in some cases a splint. In severe cases surgical decompression of the nerve may be required.

Unique Tendon Problems of the Wrist

By definition, **tenosynovitis** is an "inflammation between tendon and surrounding tissues with consequent loss of smooth gliding motion" (McCarty et al., 2018). Perhaps the most common form of tenosynovitis in the wrist involves the tendons of the thumb (Figure 12.19) and is known as **de Quervain's disease**. In reality this is not a disease in the classic sense but rather a type of overuse injury specific to the wrist. De Quervain's disease most commonly involves the tendons of the extensor pollicis brevis and the abductor pollicis longus muscles as they pass across the radial styloid process. A third tendon is in the region, the extensor pollicis longus; however, it is rarely involved in this condition.

The mechanism of injury for de Quervain's disease is vague, but it probably involves overuse of the wrist and/or thumb (Goel & Abzug, 2015). Initially, the tendons and the synovial sheath around the tendons become inflamed, resulting in pain, swelling, and stiffness. As the injury progresses the tendons begin catching within the anatomic tunnel, at times with such force that the athlete will feel them as they break free. Using the thumb, particularly in flexion and extension, will be extremely painful, and even wrist movements will be impeded. Conservative

Tenosynovitis Inflammation of the sheath of a tendon.

de Quervain's disease Inflammation of sheaths surrounding the extensor tendons of the thumb.

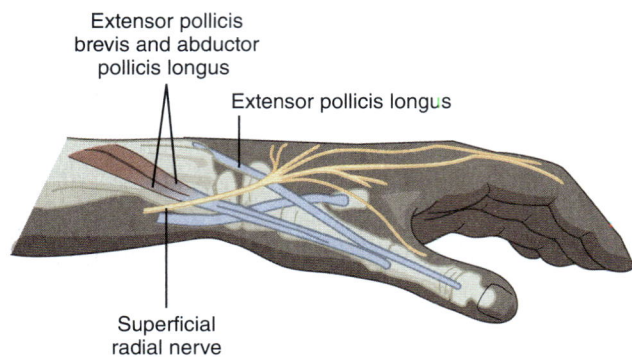

Figure 12.19 Tendons of the thumb.

treatment includes rest, heat, and drug therapy (oral and injection) and splinting of the wrist to reduce movements of the thumb. In many cases this problem tends to recur and eventually may require surgical treatment to release (decompress) the tendons as they pass near the radial styloid process (Goel & Abzug, 2015).

Signs and symptoms of de Quervain's disease include the following:

- Pain and tenderness are present within the region of the radial styloid process, specifically involving the tendons of the abductor pollicis longus and the extensor pollicis brevis.
- Swelling is present in the area of the radial styloid process, and, in advanced cases, a nodule develops on one or more of the tendons.
- The athlete may report that the tendons are catching within the wrist during activity.
- Thumb flexion in conjunction with ulnar deviation of the wrist will cause a significant increase in pain and related symptoms.

Care of de Quervain's disease involves the following:

1. If diagnosed early, the condition is treated with rest, immobilization with an appropriate splint, and drug therapy.

2. In advanced or recurring cases, surgical treatment for compartment release has been found to be highly effective with this condition. The basic surgical objective is to create more room within the tunnel for the tendons (Goel & Abzug, 2015).

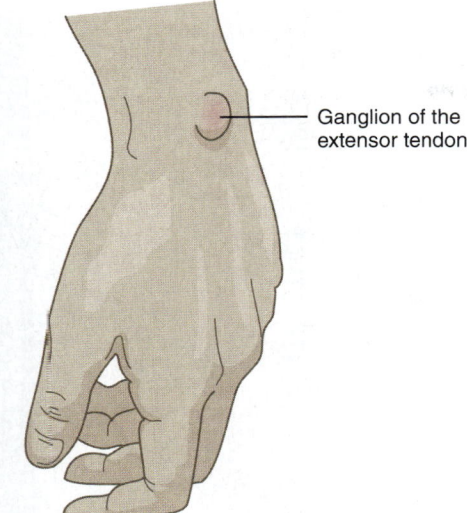

Figure 12.20 Ganglion of the wrist.

Another unique tendon-related wrist problem is known as a ganglion cyst. Technically, a **ganglion** is a herniation of the synovium surrounding the tendons, often at the wrist. When this occurs, the herniated tissue will gradually begin to fill with synovial fluid, producing a protrusion often visible as a bump on the surface of the wrist (Figure 12.20). The most common site for wrist ganglions is on the extensor tendon (dorsal) side of the wrist, although cases have been reported on the flexor tendon side of the wrist as well. They appear to be related to the chronic strain of wrist tendons but also can occur spontaneously with a traumatic force. Ganglions are highly variable in appearance. Some appear as soft, apparently fluid-filled masses just under the skin, and others materialize as hard, painful masses over a tendon. Depending on their specific location, ganglions may interfere with an athlete's performance, but in most cases the problem is seen as primarily cosmetic (Lee et al., 2018).

Signs and symptoms of a ganglion include the following:

- The most obvious symptom is a visible swelling through the skin of the wrist in the region of the extensor or flexor tendons.
- In more advanced cases a painful, hardened nodule may be present directly over a tendon (see Figure 12.20).

Care of a ganglion involves the following:

1. In some cases, ganglions regress on their own spontaneously.
2. In cases in which the ganglion does not interfere with performance, most physicians recommend leaving it alone.
3. In cases in which the ganglion does interfere with performance or is cosmetically unattractive, surgical aspiration is recommended as a primary approach with steroid or other drug injection to decrease inflammation and encourage recession. Repair of the synovial hernia is an option, but often, even after surgery, ganglions may recur.

Hand Injuries

The hand, fingers, and thumb are often injured in sports, with some of the highest frequencies occurring in sports such as baseball, softball, basketball, and football. The variety of injuries seen is nearly infinite; however, those described in this section represent the most common ones (Limpisvasti et al., 2015).

The hand contains 19 bones: the five metacarpals and the 14 **phalanges** of the fingers (Figure 12.21). The joints of the hand include the carpometacarpal joints at the base of the hand, the metacarpophalangeal joints (knuckles), and the interphalangeal joints of the fingers and thumb. All these joints are freely movable and supported by many ligaments and capsular tissues. Movements at each of these joints are affected by the many muscles originating from the forearm that pass tendons into the hand and fingers. Also within the hand are small, intrinsic (i.e., originating within the hand) muscles that precisely move the thumb and fingers (Figure 12.5). The nerves and vessels of the hand are continuations of the major structures that cross the wrist: the radial, median, and ulnar nerves and the radial and ulnar arteries.

> **Ganglion** Herniation of the synovium surrounding a tendon and subsequent filling of the area with synovial fluid, resulting in a visible bump seen through the skin.
>
> **Phalanges** Anatomic name for the bones of the fingers and toes.

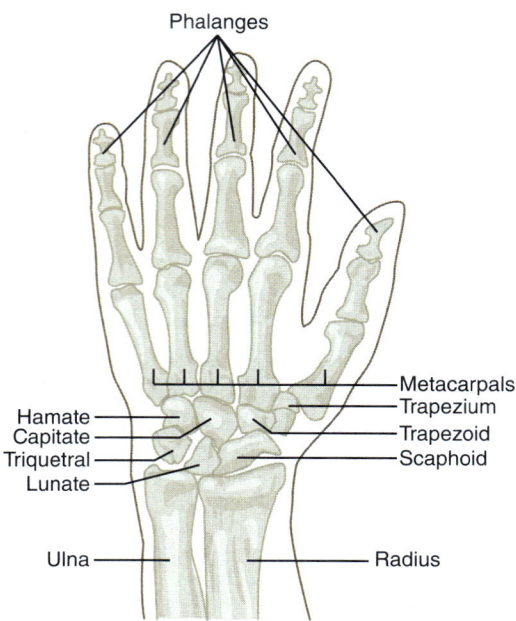

Figure 12.21 Bones of the hand and wrist.

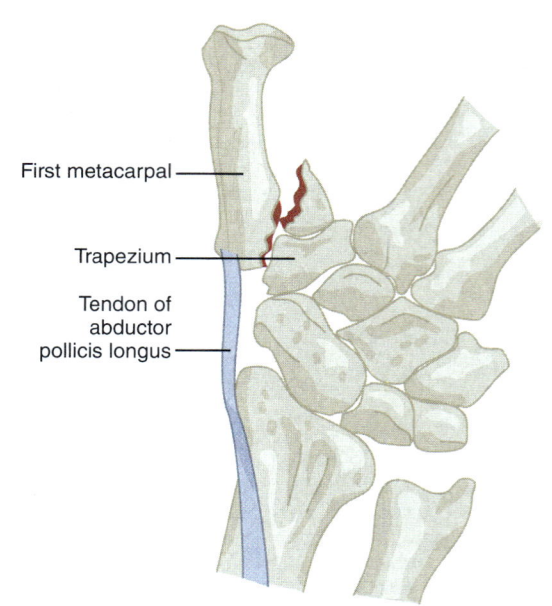

Figure 12.22 Bennett's fracture.

Hand Fractures

Fractures can occur to any of the 19 bones of the hand; however, certain types of fractures are seen more commonly in sports. An injury unique to the thumb is a **Bennett's fracture** (Figure 12.22). This injury often results from a blow to the hand while it is in a clenched-fist position; the force of the mechanism causes the proximal end of the first metacarpal bone to be driven into the wrist. The result is a **fracture-dislocation** of the first metacarpal bone away from the greater multangular (trapezium) bone of the wrist by the pull of the abductor pollicis longus (Jones et al., 2012). An obvious deformity appears with this injury, characterized by the thumb's being shorter in appearance when compared with that of the opposite hand. Significant swelling will also be present near the base of the thumb over the carpometacarpal joint.

Bennett's fracture Fracture and/or dislocation of the base of the first metacarpal bone (thumb) and trapezium (wrist).

Fracture-dislocation An injury resulting in both the fracture of a bone and dislocation at the joint.

Boxer's fracture Fracture of the proximal or neck section of the fourth and/or fifth metacarpal bones.

Fractures of the metacarpal bones of the fingers can also occur via a mechanism similar to that described for a Bennett's fracture, that is, a blow with a clenched fist. The most common injury involves the fourth and/or fifth metacarpal bone near the proximal end (base) and is known as a **boxer's fracture** (Meals & Meals, 2013). Because of the ligamentous structure of this area, displaced fractures are rare; consequently, deformity is usually not a common sign of injury. Another mechanism of injury for metacarpal fractures is a crushing force, such as having the hand stepped on by another athlete, which is common in sports such as tackle football. When acceptable alignment cannot be achieved with immobilization or immobilization cannot be tolerated for the athlete, operative fixation is occasionally considered (Avery et al., 2016).

Fractures of the phalanges also occur frequently in sports, particularly fractures of the proximal phalanges (Avery et al., 2016; Limpisvasti et al., 2015). Most of these fractures remain undisplaced (stable) and are relatively easily treated with splinting, requiring 2 to 8 weeks of recovery before returning to activity; few if any long-term complications ensue (Avery et al., 2016). In cases in which phalangeal fracture resists fixation and remains unstable with cast or splint immobilization, surgically implanted fixation is effective. This is critical because a serious complication of

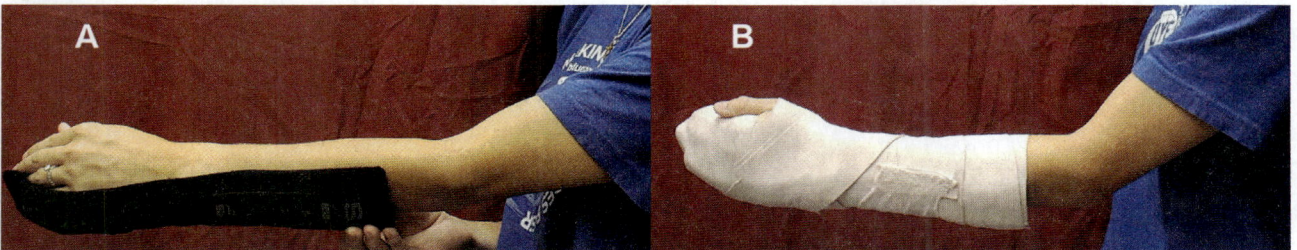

Figure 12.23 (a) Ulnar gutter splint provides immobilization for fractures of the forearm, wrist, and hand. **(b)** Ace wrap is used to secure splint for transport.
Courtesy of Cindy Trowbridge.

a finger fracture is rotational deformity, which results when the broken bone ends fail to unite in the correct position (Avery et al., 2016).

Signs and symptoms of hand fractures include the following:

- The athlete has a recent history of significant trauma to the hand, followed immediately by specific pain and dysfunction of the hand and/or finger(s).
- In cases of displaced fractures, deformity may be observable either as a bump or protrusion in the hand or as an oddly shaped finger.
- In cases of compound fractures, the skin will be broken over the region of the fracture.
- Significant inflammation will be associated with any fracture in the hand or finger.

First aid care of hand fractures involves the following:

1. Immediately apply an appropriate splint. Take care to leave the nonaffected fingernails exposed so circulation can be monitored. Fractures of the metacarpal bones are best treated by immobilization of the entire hand and wrist. A boxer's fracture is best stabilized with an ulnar gutter splint (Figure 12.23), and a Bennett's fracture is best stabilized with a radial splint (Figure 12.24); however, a palmar splint (Figure 12.25) can also effectively be used for a hand or some proximal finger fractures. Typically, fractured fingers should be splinted in a position of comfort with the finger relaxed in flexion and protected on the dorsal surface (see Figure 12.33a later in the chapter).
2. Ice can be applied for control of inflammation, and elevation can be easily achieved by placing the arm in a standard sling-and-swathe bandage.
3. If a rigid splint is not necessary, such as in the case of an isolated phalangeal fracture, a procedure known as buddy taping can be used, which simply involves taping the fractured finger to an adjacent one (see Figure 12.33b later in the chapter).
4. The athlete should be transported to the appropriate healthcare facility for further medical evaluation and treatment. Fractures of the hand must be treated as serious injuries.

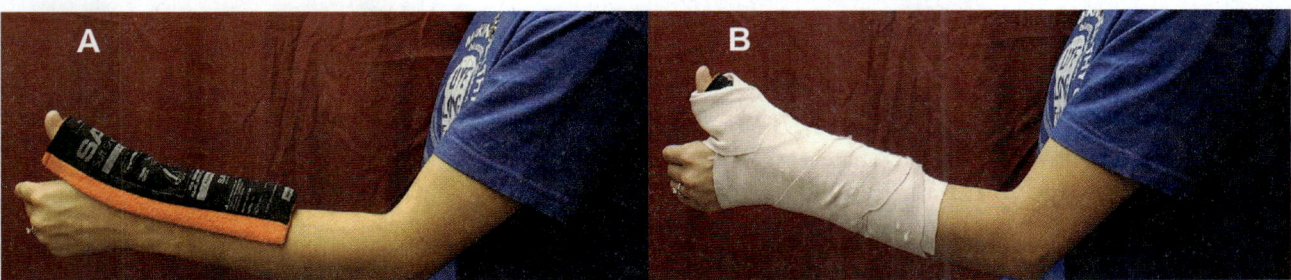

Figure 12.24 (a) Radial splint provides immobilization for fractures of the forearm, wrist, thumb, and hand. **(b)** Ace wrap is used to secure splint for transport.
Courtesy of Cindy Trowbridge.

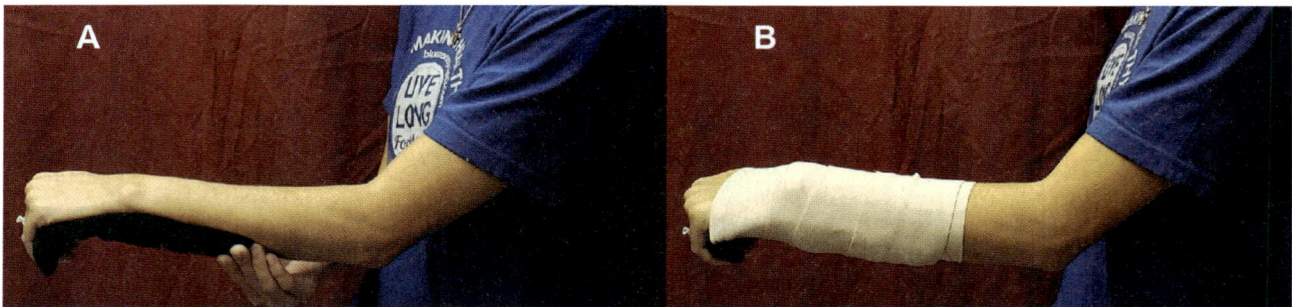

Figure 12.25 (a) Palmar splint provides immobilization for fractures of the forearm, wrist, and hand. (b) Ace wrap is used to secure splint for transport.
Courtesy of Cindy Trowbridge.

Sprains, Dislocations, and Muscle Avulsions of the Hand

Any of the many joints in the hand can be subject to sufficient trauma to cause a sprain of the supporting ligaments. If the force is severe enough, a dislocation of the joint may occur as well. Although virtually any of the joints of the hand may be injured, available information regarding sports-related injuries indicates that certain types are quite common. These injuries include gamekeeper's thumb, mallet (baseball) finger, jersey finger, boutonnière deformity, and swan neck deformity.

Gamekeeper's Thumb

The MCP joint of the thumb is a large, condyloid joint that allows a considerable range of motion in flexion and extension plus a slight amount of abduction and adduction. The joint is supported by both capsular and collateral ligaments. The latter are named according to their location relative to the radius and ulna; the collateral ligament on the lateral side of the joint is the radial collateral ligament, and the one on the medial side is the ulnar collateral ligament (Figure 12.26).

The term **gamekeeper's thumb** originated in the 1950s to describe an injury unique to gamekeepers, whose profession required them to break the necks of rabbits. Apparently, this procedure resulted in considerable damage to the ulnar collateral ligament of the thumb, causing chronic instability of the MCP joint (Madan et al., 2014). Although there are few gamekeepers today, the injury occurs with surprising frequency in sports such as alpine skiing and football (Avery et al., 2016). The mechanism of injury involves a valgus (i.e., force applied to the medial side of the joint) stress across the MCP joint of the thumb, which results in stretching, partial tearing, or even complete rupture of the ulnar collateral ligament.

Injury to the ulnar collateral ligament can produce a grossly unstable thumb, particularly when an athlete attempts to grasp or hold an object. In skiing,

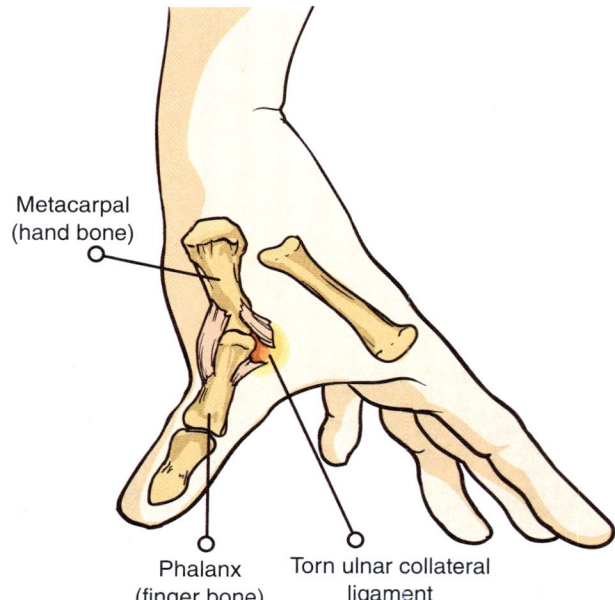

Figure 12.26 Damage to the ulnar collateral ligament of the metacarpophalangeal joint can result in gamekeeper's thumb.
© Drp8/Shutterstock.

Gamekeeper's thumb Sprain of the ulnar collateral ligament of the metacarpophalangeal joint of the thumb.

certain types of pole grips place considerable stress on the MCP joint of the thumb when planting a pole to execute a turn. Evidence suggests that 30% of the cases of ligament injuries occur in conjunction with an avulsion fracture of a bone fragment from the base of the proximal phalanx (Madan et al., 2014). Regardless of the specific type of injury, any significant sprain of the ulnar collateral ligament within the MCP joint of the thumb must be carefully evaluated by a physician to determine the extent of joint laxity and bony integrity. If left uncorrected, this injury can lead to a chronically unstable joint that can negatively affect use of the hand.

Signs and symptoms of gamekeeper's thumb include the following:

- The athlete reports significant point tenderness over the region of the ulnar collateral ligament.
- The athlete may report having felt a snap during the initial injury.
- Significant swelling is present over the MCP joint of the thumb.
- The athlete is not able and/or is unwilling to move the thumb.

First aid care of gamekeeper's thumb involves the following:

1. Use a radial splint to provide support to the thumb if the athlete is uncomfortable (Figure 12.24).
2. Apply ice to reduce inflammation. This is best accomplished by placing a small bag of crushed ice around the injured joint and securing it with an elastic wrap.
3. Provide elevation by placing the arm in a simple sling.
4. Refer the athlete to a healthcare facility for further evaluation and treatment of the injury.

Mallet (Baseball) Finger

Mallet finger involves the distal phalanx of a finger, often the index or middle finger. The injury is so named because the resulting deformity gives the distal segment of the finger the appearance of a mallet. The term *baseball finger* arose because the injury is so common in that sport—getting hit on the fingertip by a ball is a frequent occurrence (Avery et al., 2016; Meals & Meals, 2013).

> **WHAT IF ?**
>
> You are coaching a junior high basketball game. During the second half, your starting point guard injures her finger when receiving a passed ball. On examination, you note obvious deformity with the distal phalanx pushed up so that the distal interphalangeal joint is dislocated. What is this injury, and how would you care for it initially?

The anatomy of the distal finger includes the **distal interphalangeal (DIP) joint**, which functions as a hinge. The muscles acting at this joint are the flexor digitorum profundus and the extensor digitorum.

These two muscles are located in the forearm; however, their tendons pass through the hand, inserting into the bases of the distal phalanges of each of the four fingers (Figure 12.27). The mechanism of injury for mallet finger is quite precise: The tip of the finger

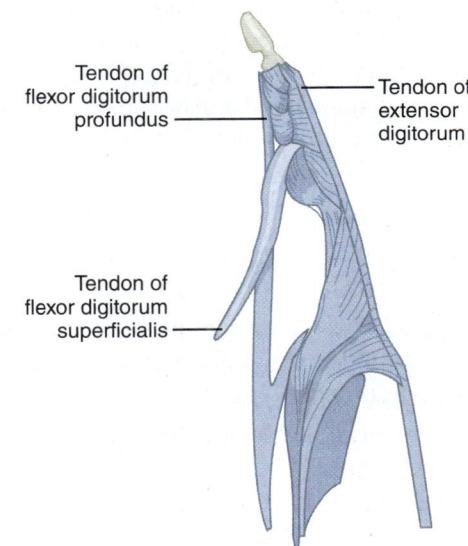

Figure 12.27 Tendons of the finger.

Mallet finger Deformity of the distal interphalangeal joint of the finger caused by an avulsion of the tendon of the extensor digitorum muscle from the distal phalanx.

Distal interphalangeal (DIP) joint The joint formed by the articulation between the middle and distal phalanges of the digits (hinge type of joint).

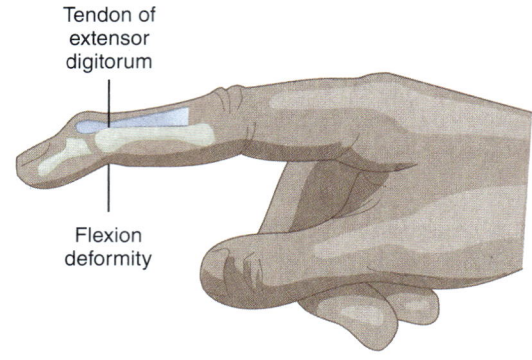

Figure 12.28 Mallet finger.

must receive a blow at the time the finger is extending from a flexed position. The result is that the distal phalanx is suddenly forced into flexion against the action of the extensor digitorum muscle. This can lead to an avulsion of the extensor tendon, with or without a small fragment of bone, from the insertion at the base of the distal phalanx (Avery et al., 2016; Meals & Meals, 2013). After this injury occurs, the athlete is unable to extend the affected finger; it remains in a flexed position at the DIP joint (Figure 12.28). Conservative care using a splint will last six to eight weeks.

Signs and symptoms of mallet finger include the following:

- The single most important sign is the deformity itself (flexed DIP), which is associated with a recent history of trauma to the fingertip.
- Point tenderness is present on the dorsal surface of the base of the distal phalanx, directly over the site of insertion of the extensor digitorum tendon.
- The athlete is not able to extend the DIP joint in isolation.

First aid care of mallet finger involves the following:

1. Immediately splint the finger, with the DIP joint extended. Do not let the distal phalanx fall back into the flexed position (see Figure 12.33c later in the chapter).
2. The easiest method of achieving elevation is to place the arm in a simple sling.
3. Immediately apply ice to reduce inflammation. This is best accomplished by placing a small bag of crushed ice around the involved finger and holding it in place with a small elastic wrap.
4. Refer the athlete to a healthcare facility for further evaluation and treatment of the injury.

Jersey Finger

Jersey finger, much like mallet finger, involves a tearing away of a finger tendon from its attachment (Avery et al., 2016; Meals & Meals, 2013). In this case, however, the mechanism of injury involves catching a finger in an opponent's clothing, for example, a football jersey. In the attempt to grip the clothing, as the opponent pulls away, the tendon of the flexor digitorum profundus (FDP) is torn away from its attachment on the distal phalanx (Figure 12.29). The most common finger to be injured is the fourth finger (ring finger), but any of the fingers can be affected. Because the FDP is the only muscle that flexes the distal phalanx at the distal interphalangeal joint, this injury results in an inability to flex the DIP joint, and surgery is essential to restore the pulley system to the flexor tendons. The timing of the surgery is dependent on the type of avulsion, including the amount of tendon retraction and whether any of the bony attachment was avulsed. For jersey finger cases in which the FDP retracts all the way into the palm, surgery should be performed within 10 days, whereas, in cases that do not involve significant tendon retraction, surgery can be delayed.

Signs and symptoms of jersey finger include the following:

- The athlete is not able to flex the DIP joint of the affected finger.

Jersey finger Torn flexor tendon of finger typically due to the finger being caught in a jersey and pulled forcefully into extension.

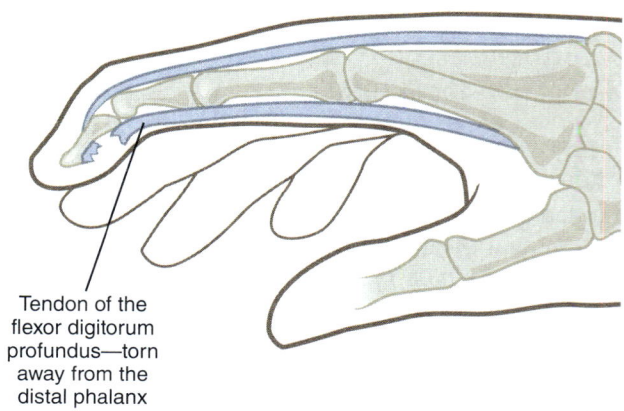

Figure 12.29 Jersey finger.

- The athlete reports having felt something snap or tear away at the area of the fingertip.
- Point tenderness is present on the volar surface of the distal phalanx of the finger.

First aid care of jersey finger involves the following:

1. Splint the finger in a position of flexion at the DIP and PIP (see Figure 12.33d later in the chapter).
2. Provide a sling, apply ice with compression, and refer as mentioned in treatment for mallet finger.

Boutonnière Deformity

Boutonnière deformity (French for "buttonhole") involves the **proximal interphalangeal (PIP) joint** of the fingers (Avery et al., 2016; Meals & Meals, 2013). The structure of the extensor digitorum tendon is unique because it crosses the dorsal surface of the PIP joint. The tendon is divided into three distinct bands: one central and two lateral bands (Figure 12.30). This arrangement allows for full flexion of the PIP joint without interference from the extensor digitorum muscle.

The mechanism for this injury is characterized by severe forced finger flexion, such as having the hand contact a playing surface during a fall with the fingers in a flexed position while simultaneously extending the fingers. This results in tearing the central portion of the extensor tendon. Initial symptoms are limited; the athlete will be able to extend the injured PIP joint but with limited strength (Avery et al., 2016; Meals & Meals, 2013). If left uncorrected, the PIP joint will eventually pop through the opening in the central portion of the tendon like a button popping up through

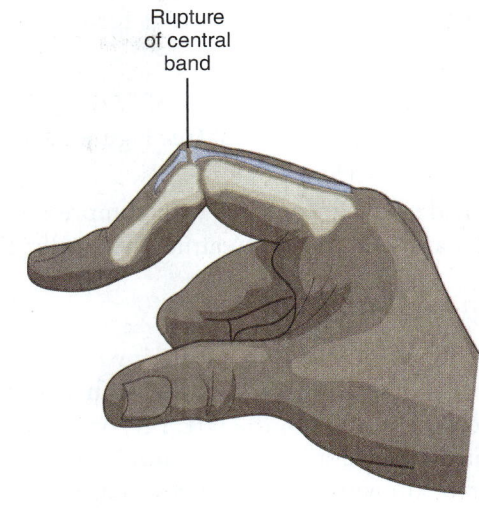

Figure 12.31 Boutonnière deformity.

a buttonhole. This results in a deformity that places the finger in a position of flexion at the PIP joint in conjunction with hyperextension at both the MCP and DIP joints (Figure 12.31). Treatment for the injury consists of splinting the finger for up to 8 weeks to allow the central portion of the extensor tendon to heal. Surgical correction is not recommended (Avery et al., 2016; Meals & Meals, 2013).

Signs and symptoms of boutonnière deformity include the following:

- The athlete will report a violent flexion to the finger, perhaps associated with the sensation of tearing or popping over the PIP joint.
- The injury will be followed immediately by significant weakness in extending the injured finger at the PIP joint.
- The PIP joint will become painful and swollen, then stiff.
- If left unattended, the injury may progress to the classic deformity, which is characterized by hyperextension of the MCP and DIP joints, with flexion of the PIP joint.

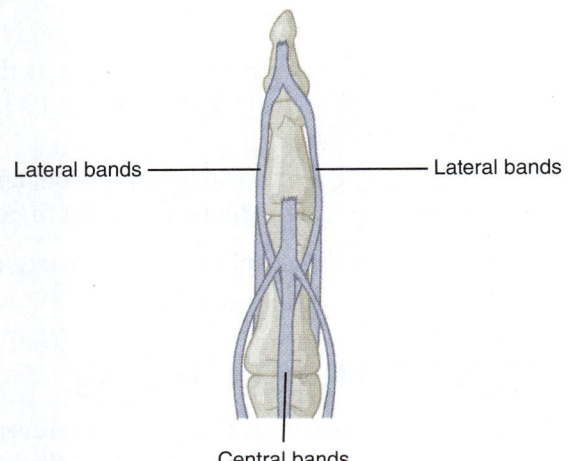

Figure 12.30 Bands of the extensor tendons.

Boutonnière deformity Buttonhole deformity whereby the proximal interphalangeal joint of the finger is forced through the central band of the tendon of the extensor digitorum muscle.

Proximal interphalangeal (PIP) joint The joint formed by the articulation between the proximal and middle phalanges of the digits (hinge type of joint).

First aid care of boutonnière deformity involves the following:

1. Splint the finger in a position of flexion at the DIP and extension at PIP joint (see Figure 12.33e later in the chapter).
2. Provide a sling, apply ice with compression, and refer as mentioned in treatment for mallet finger.

Phalangeal Dislocations

Violent forces of sporting events involving contact with other players or equipment can result in a complete dislocation of the DIP, PIP, or MCP joints. The joint capsule and the collateral ligaments are disrupted, allowing the phalanges to move either in a palmar or dorsal direction relative to the closest proximal phalanx. The phalanx can also rotate and appear radially or ulnarly deviated. Dorsal dislocations of the middle phalanx are common injuries (Figure 12.32). Because a dislocation can be associated with a fracture, coaches and physical educators are encouraged to splint the finger as it presents and immediately refer the athlete to a physician. Athletic trainers experienced in joint reduction may reduce the injury using guidelines learned in their formal education.

Swan Neck Deformity

Another common injury to the fingers is a volar plate separation as a result of hyperextension at the PIP joint. The volar plate is a thick ligament that helps to reinforce the joint capsules at the PIP and MCP joints, enhance joint stability, and limit hyperextension. Often, the initial trauma to the PIP is usually dismissed as trivial because it is a mild hyperextension and can be well tolerated, but over time, as the fingers are continually exposed to violent forces, the volar plate becomes increasingly unstable, which causes dorsal subluxation (Melone et al., 2010). The imbalance of ligament support at the PIP joint causes hyperextension and tension on the FDP, which pulls on the DIP and moves it into a position of flexion. This deformity is called a **swan neck deformity** because the bent DIP looks like a swan's head and the hyperextended

Swan neck deformity A rupture to the volar plate of the PIP joint causing a deformity that resembles a swan's neck with the head (bent DIP) and long neck (hyperextended PIP).

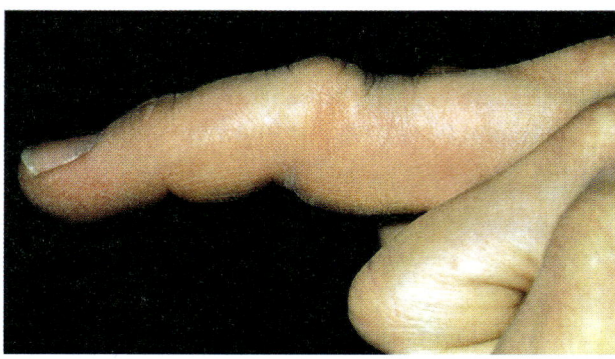

Figure 12.32 Dorsal dislocation of PIP joint.
© Dr. P. Marazzi/Science Source.

PIP looks like the swan's long neck (Melone et al., 2010). Treatment of an initial injury involves splinting for 2 to 3 months, but a repeated injury will most likely need surgery to correct the volar plate (Melone et al., 2010).

Signs and symptoms of swan neck deformity include the following:

- The athlete will report a violent hyperextension to the finger and sometimes indicate there was a tear or pop under the PIP joint.
- The volar side of the PIP joint will become painful and swollen, and the DIP joint will flex owing to the tension on the FDP tendon (swan neck deformity).
- The injury may present with a *V* sign, where the distal end of the middle phalanx and the head of the proximal phalanx hyperextend and form the tip of the *V*. The joint may also be locked or click in and out of position.

First aid care of swan neck deformity involves the following:

1. Splint the finger in a position of flexion at the PIP and extension at the DIP joint (Figure 12.33f later in the chapter).
2. Provide a sling, apply ice with compression, and refer as mentioned in treatment for mallet finger.

Figure 12.33 summarizes splinting of a variety of finger injuries.

Wrist and Thumb Taping

One of the taping procedures that can help prevent injuries in athletes involved in contact and collision sports is wrist and thumb taping. Taping the wrist and thumb before activity can help reduce excessive movement from contact, thus reducing the number of sprains to the area. Taping is both a science and an art that requires learning and practice. Once coaches or athletic trainers learn the basic concepts of a taping procedure, they need to practice its application. Books are available that demonstrate different taping procedures for different joints. These books depict how the tape should be applied, but to really understand the reasons behind the procedures and to become a proficient applicator of the tape, an educational background is most helpful. The thumb-taping pictures presented in Figures 12.34 through 12.41 provide an overview of a preventive thumb procedure that can be applied. Wrist taping can be designed to limit hyperflexion (Figure 12.42) or hyperextension (Figure 12.43) or be combined with thumb taping to provide maximum support (Figure 12.44).

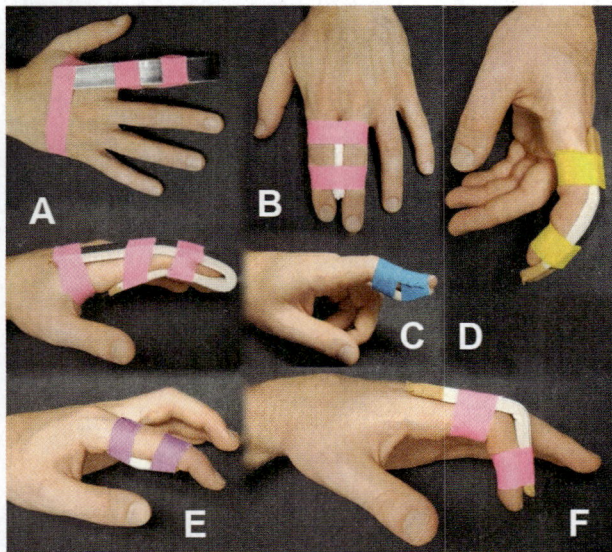

Figure 12.33 Splinting of a variety of finger injuries. **(a)** Full finger splint. **(b)** Buddy taping. **(c)** Mallet finger. **(d)** Jersey finger. **(e)** Boutonnière deformity. **(f)** Swan neck deformity.
Courtesy of Cindy Trowbridge.

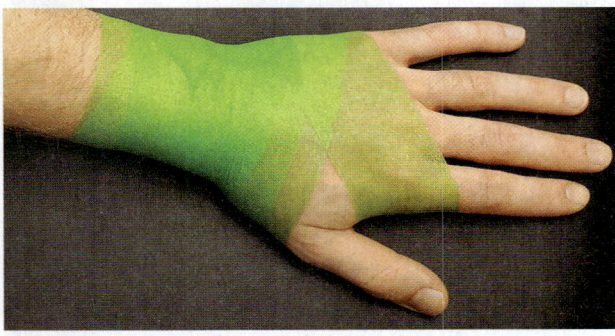

Figure 12.34 Start by applying prewrap to protect skin.
Courtesy of Cindy Trowbridge.

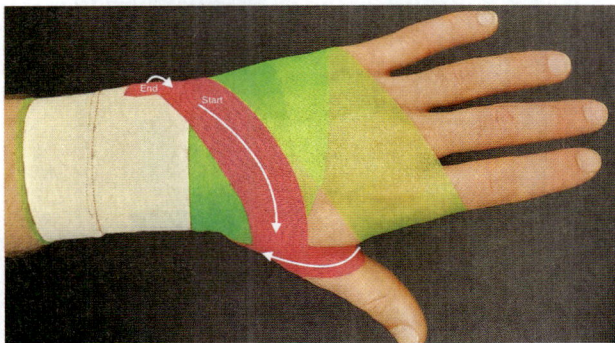

Figure 12.36 Apply thumb spica strips in an alternating pattern, moving from the base of the thumb to the nail. Start on the ulnar side of the wrist so that the tape is pulling the thumb into slight flexion and adduction.
Courtesy of Cindy Trowbridge.

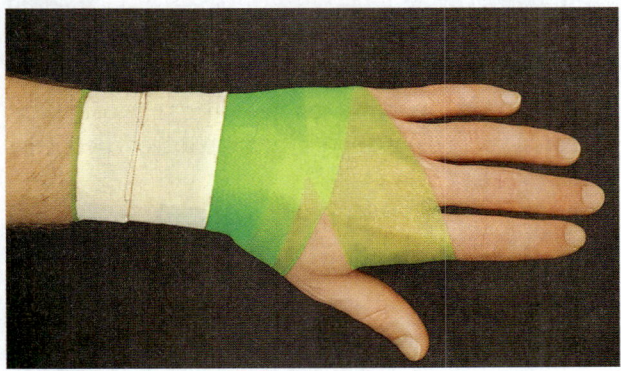

Figure 12.35 Apply anchor strips to the distal wrist.
Courtesy of Cindy Trowbridge.

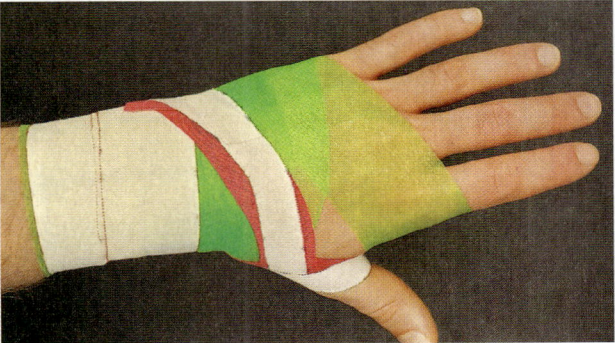

Figure 12.37 Alternate spica strips, overlapping each one as you move distally. Do not pull tightly as you bring the tape around the thumb so that blood flow is not compromised.
Courtesy of Cindy Trowbridge.

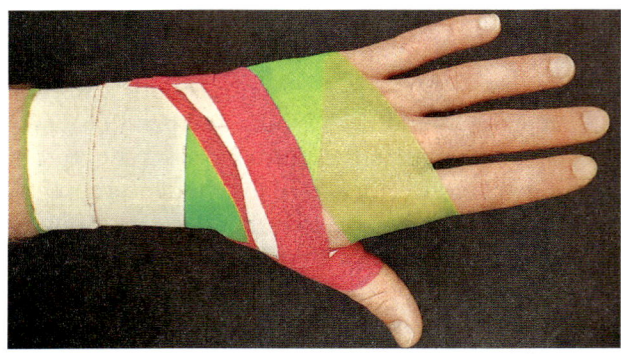

Figure 12.38 Thumb spica strips should be applied so that thumb extension and abduction are limited.
Courtesy of Cindy Trowbridge.

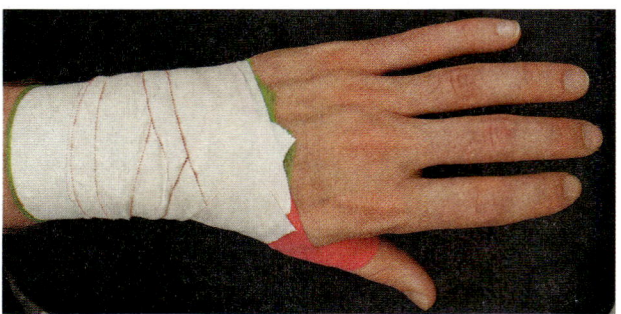

Figure 12.41 Apply anchor strips to close the tape job and remove excess prewrap.
Courtesy of Cindy Trowbridge.

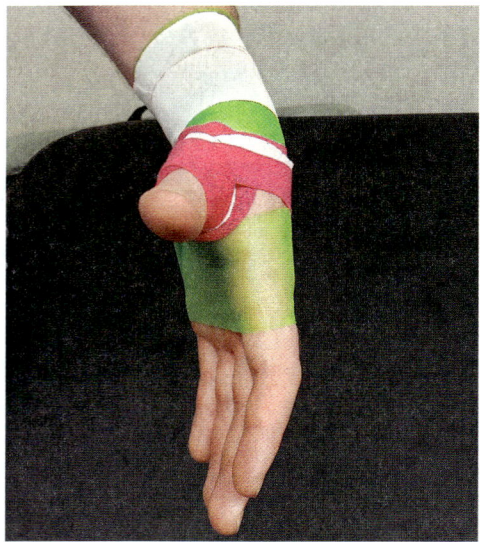

Figure 12.39 Spica strips applied correctly will prevent thumb hyperabduction.
Courtesy of Cindy Trowbridge.

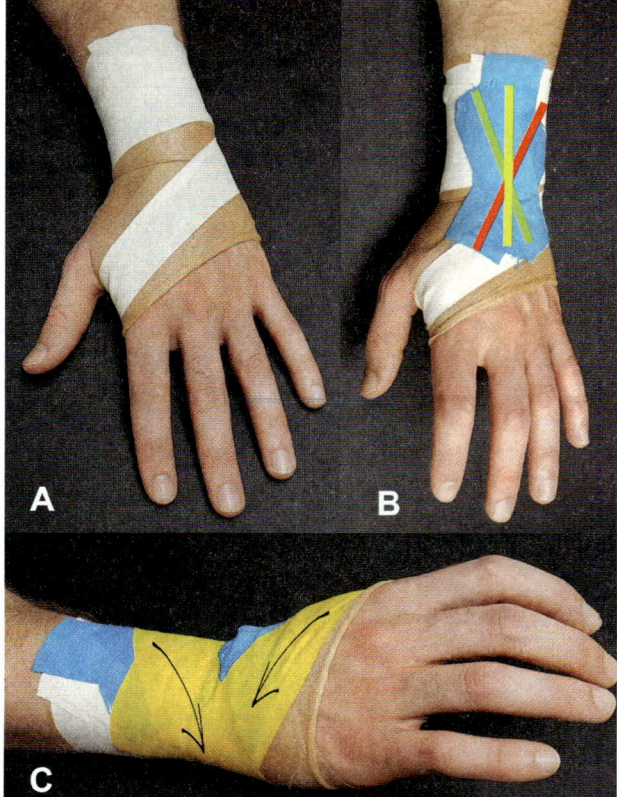

Figure 12.42 (a) Anchors applied to the wrist and palm. **(b)** Dorsal check reins provide resistance to hyperflexion. **(c)** Dorsal figure eight applied over the top of check reins to close the tape job.
Courtesy of Cindy Trowbridge.

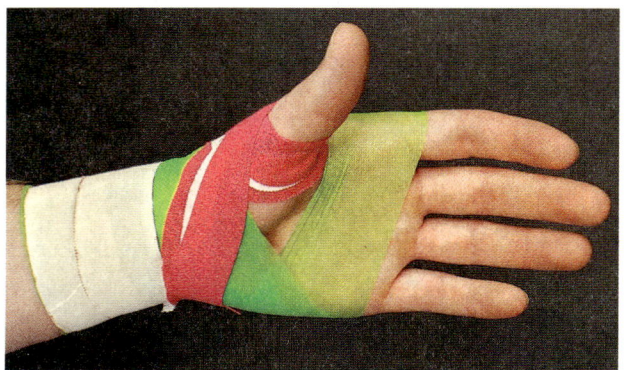

Figure 12.40 Spica strips applied correctly will prevent thumb hyperextension.
Courtesy of Cindy Trowbridge.

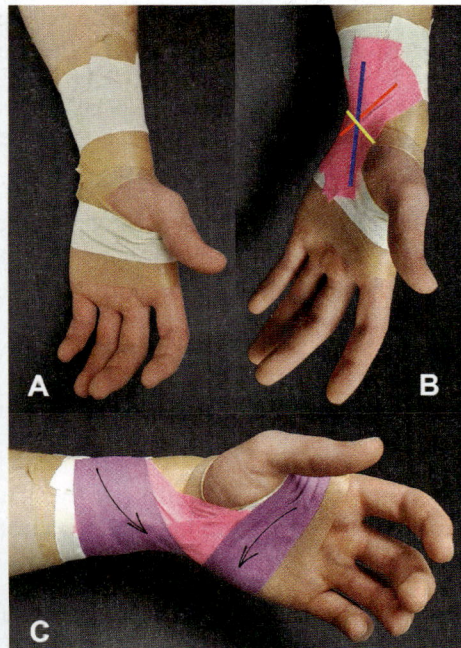

Figure 12.43 (a) Anchors applied to the wrist and palm. **(b)** Palmar check reins provide resistance to hyperextension. **(c)** Palmar figure eight applied over the top of the check reins to close the tape job.
Courtesy of Cindy Trowbridge.

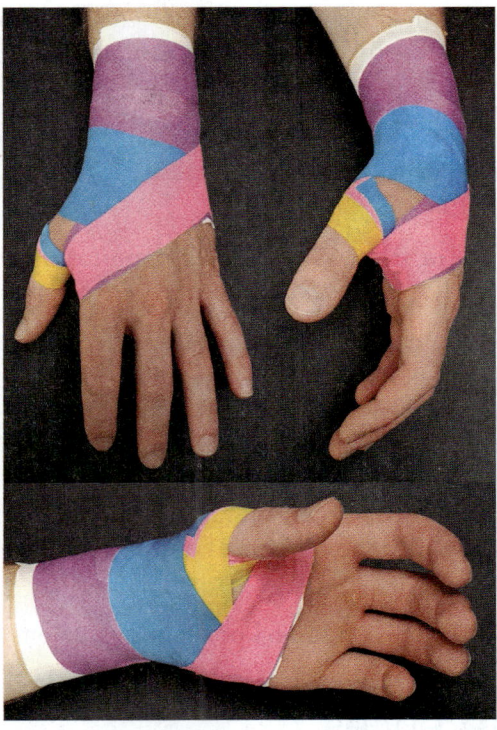

Figure 12.44 Complete thumb and wrist tape job designed to prevent injury.
Courtesy of Cindy Trowbridge.

Review Questions

1. List the three articulations of the elbow.
2. Explain the term *myositis ossificans traumatica* as it relates to a condition of the upper arm known as tackler's exostosis.
3. List the signs and symptoms of a humeral fracture.
4. Explain and/or demonstrate the first aid procedures for an athlete with a suspected fracture of the humerus.
5. Briefly describe the mechanism of injury for a posterior dislocation of the elbow.
6. List the signs and symptoms of a dislocation of the elbow.
7. True or false? The ulnar nerve is the most commonly damaged nerve in a dislocation of the elbow.
8. Explain and/or demonstrate the appropriate first aid care for an athlete with a suspected dislocation of the elbow.
9. Define the term *Volkmann's contracture*.
10. Review the signs and symptoms of either medial or lateral epicondylitis of the elbow.
11. Define *osteochondritis dissecans*.
12. What are the signs and symptoms of osteochondritis dissecans of the elbow?
13. What is the location of the olecranon bursa of the elbow?
14. True or false? A Colles' fracture involves the carpal bones of the wrist.
15. Describe the signs and symptoms of a Colles' fracture.

16. Explain and/or demonstrate the appropriate first aid procedures for an athlete with a suspected Colles' fracture.

17. What carpal bone can be located within a region at the base of the thumb known as the anatomic snuffbox?

18. True or false? The most common form of wrist sprain is the result of forced hyperextension.

19. What anatomic structures in the wrist form the tunnel of Guyon?

20. Which major nerve passes through the tunnel of Guyon?

21. What musculotendinous unit is most often involved in the condition known as de Quervain's disease?

22. Define the condition known as a ganglion.

23. Explain and demonstrate the appropriate first aid care for a suspected phalangeal fracture of the hand.

24. Which specific ligamentous structure is damaged in the condition known as gamekeeper's thumb?

25. Describe the signs and symptoms of gamekeeper's thumb; explain and demonstrate the appropriate first aid for an athlete suspected of having sustained such an injury.

26. Explain the mechanism of injury and the structures involved in the condition known as mallet finger.

27. Explain the mechanism of injury and the structures involved in the condition known as boutonnière deformity.

28. Explain the mechanism of injury and the structures involved in the condition known as jersey finger.

References

Amin, N. H., Kumar, N. S., & Schickendantz, M. S. (2015). Medial epicondylitis: Evaluation and management. *Journal of American Academy of Orthopaedic Surgeons, 23*(6), 348–355.

Avery, D. M., Rodner, C. M., & Edgar, C. M. (2016). Sports-related wrist and hand injuries: A review. *Journal of Orthopaedic Surgery and Research, 11*(1), 99.

Brogden, B. S., & Crow, M. D. (1960). Little Leaguer's elbow. *American Journal of Roentgenology, 83*, 671–675.

Chew, M. L., & Giuffrè, B. M. (2005). Disorders of the distal biceps brachii tendon. *Radiographics, 25*(5), 1227–1237.

Churchill, R. W., Munoz, J., & Ahmad, C. S. (2016). Osteochondritis dissecans of the elbow. *Current Reviews in Musculoskeletal Medicine, 9*(2), 232–239.

Crellin, C. T., Honig, K. M., McCarty, E. C., & Bravman, J. T. (2018). Shoulder injuries. In C. C. Madden, M. Putukian, E. C. McCarty, & C. C. Young (Eds.), *Netter's sports medicine* (2nd ed., pp. 367–381). Philadelphia, PA: Elsevier.

Feeley, B. T., Schisel, J., & Agel, J. (2018). Pitch counts in youth baseball and softball: A historical review. *Clinical Journal of Sport Medicine, 28*(4), 401–405.

Goel, R., & Abzug, J. M. (2015). De Quervain's tenosynovitis: A review of the rehabilitative options. *Hand, 10*(1), 1–5.

Gugenheim, J. J., Stanley, R. F., Woods, G. W., & Tullos, H. S. (1976). Little League survey: The Houston study. *American Journal of Sports Medicine, 4*(5), 189–200.

Jones, N. F., Jupiter, J. B., & Lalonde, D. H. (2012). Common fractures and dislocations of the hand. *Plastic and Reconstructive Surgery, 130*(5), 722e–736e.

Larson, R. L., Singer, K. M., Bergstrom, R., & Thomas, S. (1976). Little League survey: The Eugene study. *American Journal of Sports Medicine, 4*(5), 201–209.

Lee, A. H., Ellenbecker, T. S., & Safran, M. R. (2018). Tennis. In C. C. Madden, M. Putukian, E. C. McCarty, & C. C. Young (Eds.), *Netter's sports medicine* (2nd ed., pp. 590–597). Philadelphia, PA: Elsevier.

Limpisvasti, O., Karvak, B. J., Albohm, M. J., Wadsworth, L. T., Herring, S. A., & Provencher, M. T. (Eds.). (2015). *The sports medicine field manual.* https://www5.aaos.org/store/product/?productId=7952897&ssopc=1

Madan, S. S., Pai, D. R., Kaur, A., & Dixit, R. (2014). Injury to ulnar collateral ligament of thumb. *Orthopaedic Surgery, 6*(1), 1–7.

Maroukis, B. L., Ogawa, T., Rehim, S. A., & Chung, K. C. (2015). Guyon canal: The evolution of clinical anatomy. *Journal of Hand Surgery, 40*(3), 560–565.

McCarty, E. C., Walsh, W. M, Hald, R. D., Peter, L. E., & Mellion, M. B. (2018). Musculoskeletal sports injuries. In C. C. Madden, M. Putukian, E. C. McCarty, & C. C. Young (Eds.), *Netter's sports medicine* (2nd ed., pp. 317–321). Philadelphia, PA: Elsevier.

Meals, C., & Meals, R. (2013). Hand fractures: A review of current treatment strategies. *Journal of Hand Surgery, 38*(5), 1021–1031.

Melone, C. P., Jr., Polatsch, D. B., Beldner, S., & Khorsandi, M. (2010). Volar plate repair for posttraumatic hyperextension deformity of the proximal interphalangeal joint. *American Journal of Orthopedics, 39*(4), 190–194.

Moini, J. (2016). *Anatomy and physiology for health professionals* (2nd ed.). Burlington, MA: Jones & Bartlett Learning.

Padua, L., Coraci, D., Erra, C., Pazzaglia, C., Paolasso, I., Loreti, C., . . . Hobson-Webb, L. D. (2016). Carpal tunnel syndrome: Clinical features, diagnosis, and management. *The Lancet Neurology, 15*(12), 1273–1284.

Perrin, D. H., & McLeod, I. A. (2018). *Athletic taping, bracing, and casting* (4th ed.). Champaign, IL: Human Kinetics.

Pollak, A. N. (2021). *Emergency care and transport of the sick and injured* (12th ed.). Burlington, MA: Jones & Bartlett Learning.

Prentice, W. E. (2017). *Principles of athletic training: A guide to evidence-based practice* (16th ed.). New York, NY: McGraw-Hill.

Pytiak, A. V., Kraeutler, M. J., Currie, D. W., McCarty, E. C., & Comstock, R. D. (2018). An epidemiological comparison of elbow injuries among United States high school baseball and softball players, 2005–2006 through 2014–2015. *Sports Health, 10*(2), 119–124.

Reilly, D., & Kamineni, S. (2016). Olecranon bursitis. *Journal of Shoulder and Elbow Surgery, 25*(1), 158–167.

Tosti, R., Jennings, J., & Sewards, J. M. (2013). Lateral epicondylitis of the elbow. *American Journal of Medicine, 126*(4), 357e1–357e6.

Tucker, C. J. (2016). *Golf injuries*. Retrieved from https://www.sportsmed.org/AOSSMIMIS/members/downloads/SMU/2016MayJun.pdf

Yukutake, T., Kuwata, M., Yamada, M., & Aoyama, T. (2015). A preseason checklist for predicting elbow injury in Little League baseball players. *Orthopaedic Journal of Sports Medicine, 3*(1), 1–7.

CHAPTER 13
Injuries to the Thorax and Abdomen

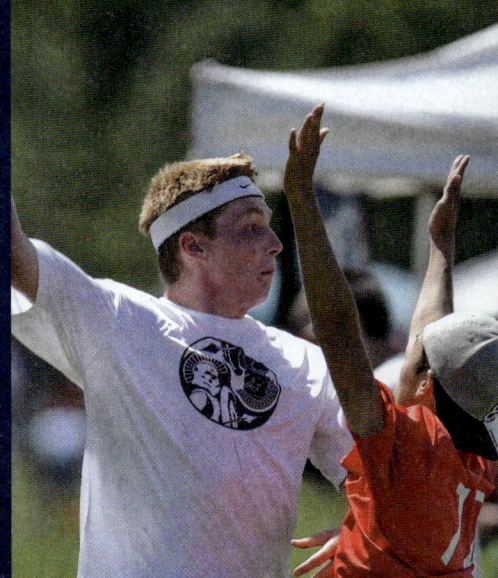

MAJOR CONCEPTS

The chapter begins with an overview of the gross anatomy of the thorax and abdomen. It also discusses the internal organs and structures associated with the thorax and abdomen that can be injured through sports participation, including the heart and lungs, liver, kidneys, spleen, stomach, and diaphragm.

External injuries are also discussed, such as fractures to the ribs, various joint-related problems, and breast injuries and contusions. The chapter gives signs and symptoms of internal injuries to the heart, lungs, liver, kidneys, spleen, and bladder. At times, coaches overlook serious injuries to the internal organs; however, many injuries can have debilitating and even life-threatening effects if proper care is not applied.

Anatomy Review

The thorax and abdominal cavities contain the majority of the vital organs of the body. This area is enclosed by the spinal column, the rib cage, and the clavicle, all of which provide bony protection for the area. The vertebrae in this area include the 12 thoracic vertebrae and the 5 lumbar vertebrae located posterior to the abdomen. There are 12 pairs of ribs in males and females. Anteriorly, the first through seventh ribs articulate with the sternum directly from their costal cartilage and are connected to the spinal column posteriorly; therefore, they are known as true ribs. The anterior connection of the true ribs is made via a costal cartilage for each rib (Moini, 2020). The remaining ribs, specifically ribs 8 through 10, connect via a common costal cartilage. Ribs 11 and 12 do not connect to the sternum anteriorly; thus, they are called floating ribs. The 8th to 12th pairs are sometimes referred to as false ribs (Figure 13.1). All the joints between the ribs and the spinal column are reinforced with strong ligamentous support. This area is further strengthened by the anterior longitudinal ligament, which runs on the anterior surface of the spinal column from the occipital bone of the skull to the pelvic surface of the sacrum.

The main joints of the thorax include the intervertebral joints, the vertebral and rib joints, the sternocostal and costochondral joints, and the sternoclavicular joints. The intervertebral joints are those between each of the vertebral bodies. These joints are stabilized by ligaments and the intervertebral disks located between each vertebral body. The intervertebral disks are mostly fibrocartilaginous and play an important role in the weight-bearing ability of the spine. The ribs articulate with the vertebrae in

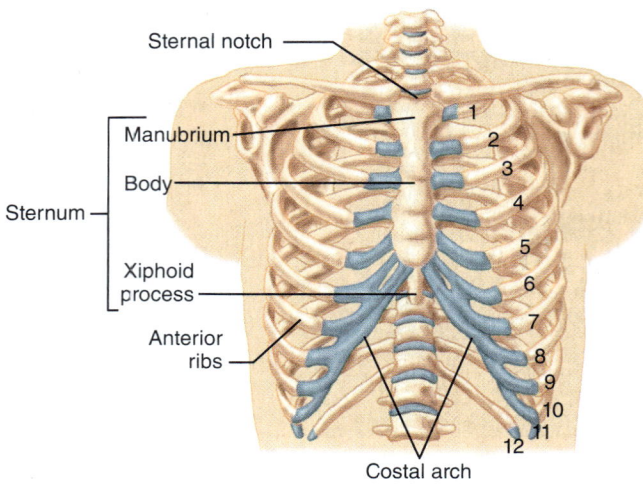

Figure 13.1 The thoracic cage (anterior view).

an interesting manner. Each rib articulates with two adjacent vertebrae and the intervertebral disk. These vertebrocostal joints are strengthened by ligaments that allow the gliding movements of the ribs at the vertebral column. The anterior joints are known as the sternocostal joints, which is where the ribs articulate with the sternum via costal cartilage. The point at which the rib attaches to the costal cartilage is known as the costochondral joint. Typically, no movement occurs at these costochondral joints (Moini, 2020).

One of the main joints of the thorax is the sternoclavicular joint, which is an articulation between the clavicle and the sternum. This joint is the only bony articulation between the thorax and the arm, and it is supported by strong ligaments. Movement occurs at this joint even though it is not viewed as a major site of movement, as are other joints within the region. Several muscles surround the thorax and abdomen. The main thoracic muscles include the external and internal intercostal muscles, which function primarily to lift and lower the rib cage and assist with inhalation and exhalation. More superficially, the pectoralis major and minor are located in the upper chest area and mainly control arm movement. In the posterior thorax, several muscles running the length of the spinal column are responsible for a variety of movements and stabilization of the spine. Most of the deep muscles running the length of the back, including the spinalis, longissimus, and iliocostalis as well as others, are responsible for keeping the spine erect. More superficially, muscles of the trunk, such as the latissimus dorsi, rhomboids, and trapezius, are mainly responsible for movements of the upper extremity. See Table 13.1 for specifics of muscle activity and innervation.

Several important muscles are also in the abdominal region. The main muscles of the anterior abdominal region are the external and internal obliques and the rectus abdominis. The transversus abdominis is a deep muscle that is essential for core stability. The oblique muscles help to flex and rotate the trunk as well as assist with support of the abdominal viscera. The rectus abdominis is the main muscle of the anterior abdominal wall; it acts to support the abdominal viscera and to flex the trunk. All the abdominal muscles are important, but the transversus abdominis is a key muscle because it assists the lower extremity by helping to fixate the pelvis during movement, which allows the muscles of the lower extremity to function more effectively.

Internal Organs

The two main organs in the thorax (Figure 13.2) are the lungs and the heart (Moini, 2020). Each lung is encased in a separate and closed space called the pleural sac, which assists the lungs by helping to transmit the forces of the chest wall muscles to the lungs, making respiration an efficient process. The lungs oxygenate blood as it circulates; they are normally light, soft, spongy, and pinkish in a healthy person. The left lung has two lobes, and the right has three, which makes it a little larger and heavier than the left. Located directly between the two lungs is the heart. The heart is situated in an area called the mediastinum, which also houses major blood vessels and parts of the respiratory and digestive systems (i.e., trachea and esophagus) along with nerve and lymphatic tissues. Inferior to the pleural cavities and the mediastinum is a muscle called the diaphragm, which essentially separates the thoracic and abdominal cavities and is considered the main muscle of respiration. The diaphragm is basically a circular muscle with a tendon in the middle that allows the muscle to contract and assist with breathing. Several openings allow the blood vessels, nerves, and digestive structures to pass through the diaphragm.

For descriptive purposes, the abdominal region (Figure 13.3a and b) is typically divided into four quadrants: the right upper and lower quadrants and the left upper and lower quadrants, with the umbilicus serving as the center point. The main organs in the

Table 13.1
Main Muscles, Actions, and Innervations of the Thorax and Abdomen

Muscle	Action	Innervation
Latissimus dorsi	Adducts, extends, and medially rotates the arm	Thoracodorsal
Rhomboids	Scapular adduction	Dorsal scapular
Trapezius (upper, middle, lower)	Elevates, rotates, and retracts scapula	Accessory and C3–4
Pectoralis major	Adduction and medial rotation of arm	Lateral and medial pectoral
Pectoralis minor	Draws shoulder anteriorly and inferiorly	Medial pectoral
External oblique	Tenses abdominal wall and lateral flexes trunk to same side and rotates trunk to opposite side	T6–12
Internal oblique	Tenses abdominal wall and rotates trunk to same side	T6–12 and T1
Rectus abdominis	Tenses abdominal wall and flexes trunk	T7–12
Diaphragm	Inspiration	Phrenic
Transverse abdominis	Tenses abdominal wall	T6–12 and L1
External intercostals	Raise the rib cage upward and outward and contribute to the expansion of the thoracic cavity, which allows air into the lungs	Intercostal nerves
Internal intercostals	Depression of the ribs and bending them inward causing a decrease in the transverse dimensions of the thoracic cavity and assisting in exhalation	Intercostal nerves

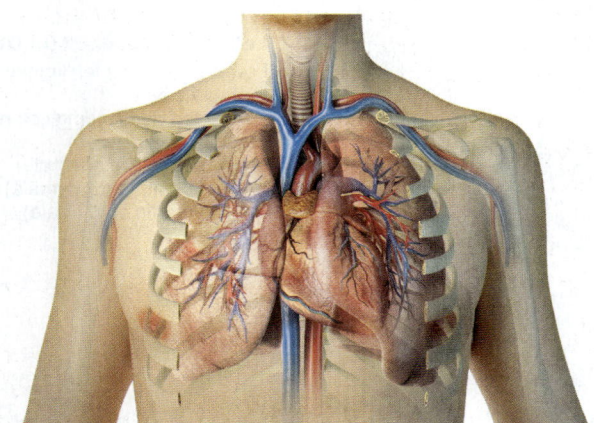

Figure 13.2 The internal organs of the thorax.
© Matis75/Shutterstock.

right upper quadrant are the liver, gallbladder, and right kidney; in the right lower quadrant, the ascending colon and the appendix; and in the left upper quadrant, the stomach, spleen, pancreas, and left kidney. In the left lower quadrant, the only organ is the descending colon (Moini, 2020).

Common Sports Injuries

Sports injuries to the thorax and abdomen are relatively uncommon in children and adolescents. However, some injuries to the region require immediate attention to prevent long-term disability and possibly even death. The discussion focuses first on external injuries involving the skeletal, muscular,

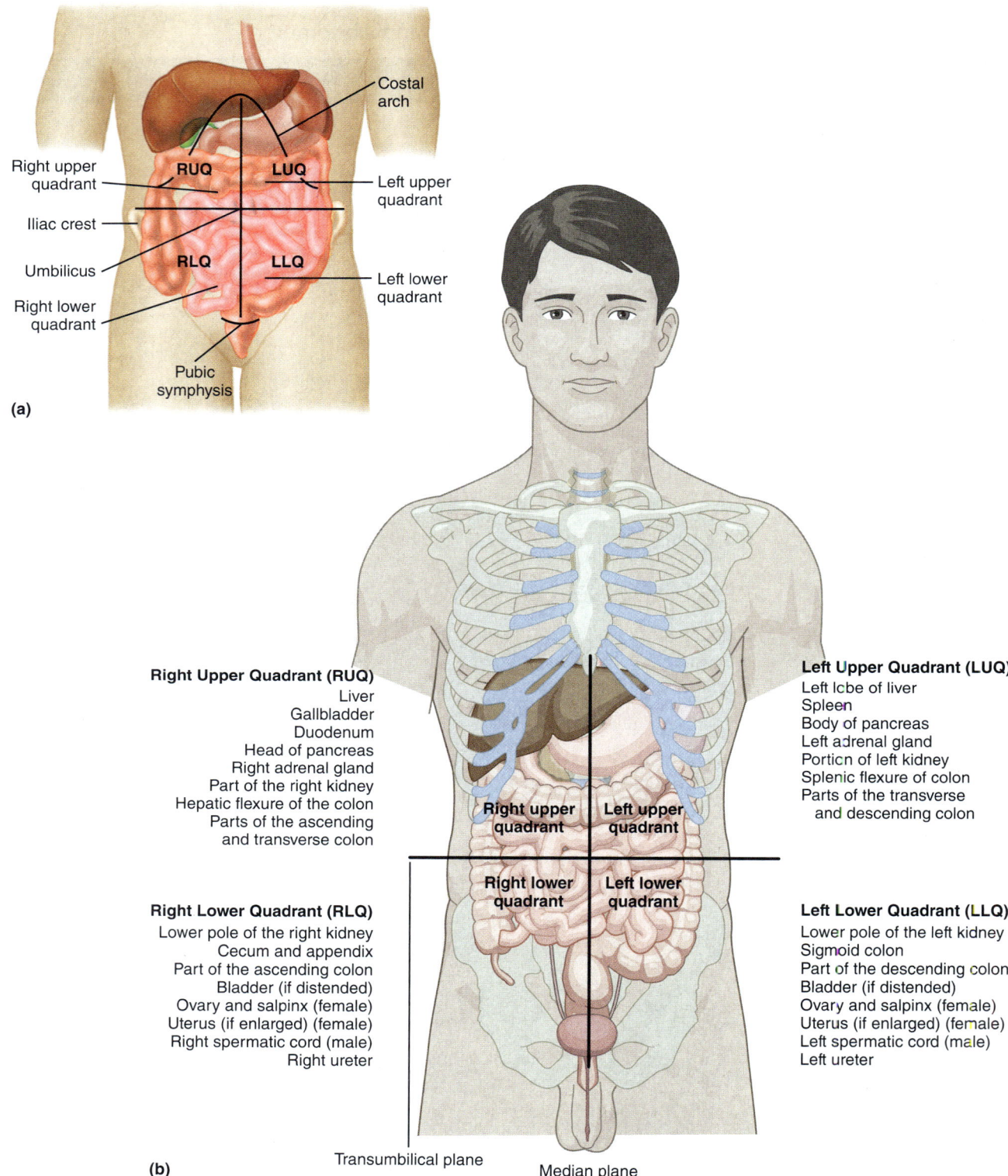

Figure 13.3 (a) The four quadrants of the abdomen (RUQ: right upper quadrant; LUQ: left upper quadrant; RLQ: right lower quadrant; LLQ: left lower quadrant). (b) The four quadrants of the abdomen and the organs they house.

and other external components of the region, then reviews injuries to the internal organs of the thorax and abdomen.

External Injuries

Fractures

Fractures to the bones of the skeleton can occur as a result of direct trauma. An athlete may fracture a rib, the sternum, the clavicle, or part of a vertebra. Fractures to any of these structures should be cared for immediately. Without proper care, complications can occur; the athlete may develop a pneumothorax or hemothorax, both of which are life-threatening conditions. A **pneumothorax** is the presence of air in the pleural cavity, and a **hemothorax** is the presence of blood in the pleural cavity. The lung injuries section that follows provides more detail on both of these pathologies.

In the case of a sternal fracture, which is infrequent in sports, two complications may arise. First, if the manubrium is dislocated and moves posteriorly, the possibility of an airway obstruction exists. Second, if the sternum and ribs are separated completely, the likelihood of a **flail chest** (i.e., loss of stability to the thoracic cage) exists; the possible complications of this condition include a pneumothorax or hemothorax.

The other type of fracture to this region, which is more common in sports, is a rib fracture (see Chapter 10). Most often, ribs are fractured in contact sports when two players collide and the rib cage is violently compressed. The fifth through ninth pairs of ribs are generally more susceptible to fracture as they are often exposed to contact in a variety of sports. However, any of the ribs can be fractured under forceful circumstances, such as tackling or falling. As with other bones in the body, the ribs can be broken in varying degrees of severity, from greenstick to displaced fractures. If a rib fracture is suspected, the athlete must be referred to the appropriate physician as soon as possible.

Signs and symptoms of a sternum or rib fracture include the following:

- At the site of injury, extreme localized pain is present, which is typically aggravated by sneezing, coughing, forced inhalation, or sometimes movement.
- The athlete may grasp the chest wall at the point of injury.
- Mild swelling may occur at the site, and a bony deformity may be present.
- The athlete may complain of breathing difficulties and take rapid, shallow breaths.

First aid care of a sternum or rib fracture involves the following:

1. Monitor the athlete's vital signs and watch for respiratory distress.
2. Keep the athlete immobile and treat for shock if necessary.
3. Arrange for transport to a healthcare facility.

The athlete may also experience subluxations and dislocations at various joints in the skeleton of the thorax. The discussion here focuses on **costochondral separation**, which involves some type of disunion of the sternum and ribs. In a costochondral separation, the cartilage portion of the costosternal union is separated from either the sternum medially or the rib laterally. Because such a separation requires a great deal of force, this type of injury is usually associated with contact or collision sports. Typically, the athlete with a costochondral separation experiences a great deal of pain at the time of the injury and in many cases will complain of pain for weeks after the injury.

Signs and symptoms of a costochondral separation include the following:

- The athlete will report that a pop or snap occurred.
- A palpable defect may be felt because deformity may or may not be present as well as swelling in the immediate area.

Pneumothorax Air collects in the pleural cavity (space between the lungs and chest wall) causing the lung to collapse.

Hemothorax Blood collects in the pleural cavity (space between the lungs and chest wall).

Flail chest A portion of the rib cage is separated from the rest of the chest wall, usually due to trauma, making breathing very difficult.

Costochondral separation Injury to the ribs at the attachment of the cartilage.

Athletic Trainers SPEAK OUT

How have athletic trainers (ATs) advanced the health care of our military service members?

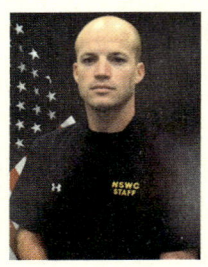

Courtesy of Steven Koch.

ATs are known as sports medicine rehabilitation specialists. The U.S. Air Force has adapted a sports medicine model of keeping its service members in the fight instead of being grounded, which is like being on the sidelines in the sporting world.

Musculoskeletal injuries are the leading cause of delayed graduation in the military. By bringing on ATs, we are able to use our advanced knowledge in orthopedic and musculoskeletal care to help reduce the risk of and prevent injuries. We can keep injuries less severe through the use of a variety of injury prevention techniques (e.g., flexibility, proper shoes, nutrition and hydration, and strength training) and by rehabilitating service members while keeping them in military training or service. Just like with athletes on a team, the AT in the military setting can provide a functional waiver so service members can remain in training through modifying their daily activities of running, rucking, or strength and conditioning. The military, just like sports, uses ATs to provide a functional waiver to modify service members' daily workload to keep them in the "fight" (game) so they are able to stay with their unit (team).

—Steven Koch, MS, ATC, LAT, CIDN, GT, CKTP, SMTC

Steven Koch is a staff AT for the U.S. Air Force.

- Maximum or near maximum inhalation may be very difficult.
- The athlete experiences localized pain and tenderness over the area of the costochondral junction.

First aid care of a costochondral separation involves the following:

1. Immediately apply ice and light compression.
2. Treat for shock if necessary.
3. Arrange for transport to a medical facility.

Muscle Strains

The muscles in the area of the thorax and abdomen can be strained, which may result in significant pain and movement limitations. Strains of the pectoral muscles can occur when athletes are training with heavy weights in a strength and conditioning center. They can also result from the athletes' putting their shoulders into an extended position carrying excessive weight or being in this position when an opponent applies a high-velocity stretch through some type of mechanism. When the intercostal muscles are strained, generally by a high-velocity stretching mechanism, the athlete may experience localized pain and breathing difficulty during exercise.

Abdominal muscle strains can be a significant problem for athletes because the athletes' movements during practice or competition can irritate the strained abdominal muscle, thus creating a chronic cycle of reinjury to the involved muscles. The incidence of abdominal muscle strains has increased over the years, especially in baseball players, and often results in significant time loss during the season (Gundersen et al., 2021). For example, on average, baseball players can take 4–5 weeks to return from the disabled list but pitchers often take longer (Gundersen et al., 2021). Even though the muscles in this area are not prime movers of any extremity, they do support the core and thus affect the athlete's overall movement capability.

Breast Injuries

Depending on the type of sport and the gender of the athlete, the breast is also subject to injury. Women do incur breast contusions as a result of contact in some sports. Sports bras typically do not provide protection from direct contact, but they do help to support the breast during activity. Women will have various preferences regarding the type and size of sports bra that will provide the required support

(Yu & Zhou, 2016). Conversely, some women will elect not to wear a bra during sports participation. This decision should be left up to the athlete, based on comfort and performance, but sports bras are effective in reducing excessive breast movement and can reduce discomfort during physical activities. However, if the athlete elects not to wear a sports bra, she should be aware of the possible long-term effects of not supplying proper breast support during activity. Most often the major long-term effect is that the breast tissue stretches, resulting in loss of stability and natural breast contour.

At times, both men and women will experience nipple irritation. This problem is easily remedied by either changing tops or (if that is not possible) placing a bandage over the nipple during competition so that irritation is reduced or eliminated.

Internal Injuries

Many organs and structures can be injured from direct trauma from collision during contact sports, but determining whether an internal injury has occurred is not always easy to do; therefore, the coach or AT must be educated and knowledgeable about the signs and symptoms of possible injury to an internal organ. Anatomically, the heart and lungs are separated from the abdominal viscera by the diaphragm, which is an important distinction to understand. The heart and lungs are encapsulated by their own separate membranes within the thorax. The membranes that surround these organs are important in maintaining the proper function of the heart and lungs (discussed in more detail later in the chapter). This discussion begins with the heart and lungs and continues with the internal viscera.

Heart Injuries

Although considered a rare occurrence, sudden death among athletes has become a more publicized event in recent years. Many times, sudden death in an athlete is the result of a cardiac problem (Harmon, Asif, et al., 2015; Maron et al., 2016). In a report by the U.S. National Registry of Sudden Death in Young Athletes (instituted at Minneapolis Heart Institute Foundation), from 1980 to 2011, 2,406 sudden deaths in athletes were reported (Maron et al., 2016). During that 31-year reporting cycle, 36% of the reported sudden death events were due to hypertrophic cardiomyopathy (Maron et al., 2016). Sudden cardiac death in male athletes was also almost fourfold greater than in females athletes. In the National Collegiate Athletic Association (NCAA) athlete population, based on an analysis of 79 reported sudden cardiac deaths (SCDs) during a 10-year period, from 2003–2013, the death rate per year was estimated to be 1 in 43,703 for all athletes (Harmon, Asif, et al., 2015). These data indicated that male athletes had a 3.22 times higher risk of cardiac death compared to females, and Black athletes had a 3.18 times higher risk of cardiac death when compared to Caucasian athletes (Harmon, Asif, et al., 2015). Both men's basketball and football had the highest number of SCDs over the 10-year period studied, but basketball had the highest incidence in a 4-year career of 1 in 2,245 versus football, with an incidence of 1 in 8,988 (Harmon, Asif, et al., 2015). A variety of cardiac events can and do result in the death of an athlete, including hypertrophic cardiac myopathy, anomalous coronary arteries, cardiac contusions, myocarditis, and inherited genetic diseases. However, many of these cardiac events can be helped through the quick and appropriate actions of a first responder, including the use of an **automated external defibrillator (AED)** and the performance of **cardiopulmonary resuscitation (CPR)**.

One of the cardiac events that may be most responsive to early and appropriate response is **ventricular fibrillation**, in which the heart beats with rapid, erratic electrical impulses and is unable to effectively pump blood. Any time the heart is compressed between the sternum and the spinal column

> **Automated external defibrillator (AED)** A lightweight, portable device that delivers an electric shock through the chest to the heart. The shock can potentially reset an irregular heartbeat and allow a normal rhythm to resume following sudden cardiac arrest.
>
> **Cardiopulmonary resuscitation (CPR)** A technique involving repeated compression of a patient's chest and rescue breathing to restore the blood circulation of a person who has suffered cardiac arrest.
>
> **Ventricular fibrillation** The heart beats with rapid, erratic electrical impulses. The ventricles quiver, diminishing the effectiveness of expelling blood from the heart.

by a violent external force, such as might be caused by being hit by the helmet of an opposing player or a fast-moving baseball, lacrosse ball, or hockey puck, a cardiac contusion or other thoracic injury can result (Singh & Link, 2021). When athletes are hit in the chest and the impact is timed exactly with the repolarization phase of the contracting heart, they can experience ventricular fibrillation that leads to SCD. This injury is known as **commotio cordis** and can occur in both competitive and recreational sports (Singh & Link, 2021). Unfortunately, commotio cordis is usually fatal. Deaths have often been associated with bystanders' failure to initiate appropriately aggressive and timely resuscitation measures because they do not understand the life-threatening nature of the collapse (Singh & Link, 2021). Young male youths playing baseball, lacrosse, hockey, football, and basketball are most susceptible, and those children under 10 years of age are most likely not to survive an event (Singh & Link, 2021).

Trained professionals' early intervention using AED (Figure 13.4a and b) appears to be the most practical approach to saving lives threatened by commotio cordis (Casa, Guskiewicz, et al., 2012; Narayanan et al., 2017; Singh & Link, 2021). Many medical organizations continue to emphasize that sudden cardiac arrest is a situation for which a well-written and well-practiced plan of action must be available to avoid serious complications or even death in the athlete. Specifically, the National Athletic Trainers' Association (NATA) published a statement regarding the best practices for the overall prevention of sudden death in athletics programs (Casa, Guskiewicz, et al., 2012), secondary school athletics programs (Casa et al., 2013), and collegiate conditioning sessions (Casa, Anderson, et al., 2012). The NATA statements primarily outline a need for a well-defined emergency action plan at all venues and training in CPR and AED use for all likely early responders. According to the statements, an AED should be on-site and available for use within 3 minutes (1 minute is ideal) of an athlete's collapsing and prompt contact to emergency services for immediate transport. Any athlete who has collapsed and is unresponsive should be assumed to be in sudden cardiac arrest until proven otherwise. Each statement also points out the need for continual training for all members of the medical and coaching staff in the prevention and care for athletes in the area of sudden death (Casa, Anderson, et al., 2012; Casa, Guskiewicz, et al., 2012; Casa et al., 2013). A well-executed emergency action plan in a time of need can save an athlete's life. An important point to remember is that the early use of an AED has been shown to increase the success rates of life-saving

Commotio cordis A rare, lethal disruption of heart rhythm as a result of abrupt, blunt, nonpenetrating trauma to the chest/heart area.

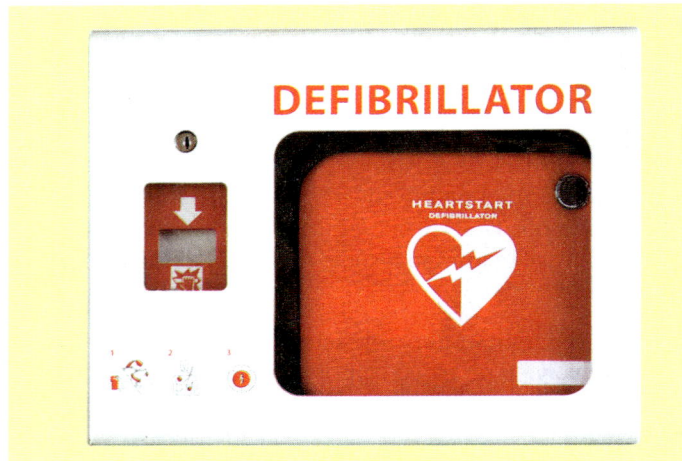
(a)

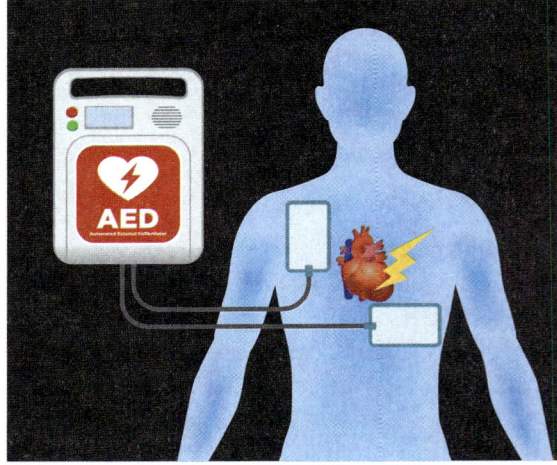
(b)

Figure 13.4 (a) Example of a commercially available AED for use by a trained individual. **(b)** Application of AED pads to the chest for defibrillation of the heart.
(a) © Flowersandtraveling/Shutterstock; (b) © metamorwork/Shutterstock.

measures in athletes and others experiencing specific cardiac problems.

Young and old athletes may also experience numerous other cardiac pathologies. The purpose of a preparticipation physical examination is to identify these conditions so the appropriate activity level and monitoring can be recommended. Athletes who have diagnosed cardiac pathology will often have specific directives from their personal cardiologist regarding participation in activity. However, **hypertrophic cardiomyopathy (HCM)** and anomalous coronary arteries are genetic disorders and are most often discovered after an athlete's death. Unfortunately, sudden death is often the first sign and symptom of these conditions. HCM is generally described as an excessive thickening of the left ventricular wall, resulting in a ventricle that is less efficient in pumping the necessary volume of blood (Figure 13.5).

Many parent groups now advocate that medical professionals be more diligent in determining methods to circumvent problems associated with injury or preexisting conditions of the heart. Although some athletes may have preexisting cardiac abnormalities, the use of echocardiogram or echocardiography during the preparticipation screening and the optimal preparticipation screening for cardiovascular disease is still debated, but the use of 12-lead electrocardiograms (ECGs) is gaining popularity (Harmon, Zigman, et al., 2015; Maron et al., 2014). Two recent papers took opposing views or the inclusion of ECGs in preparticipation exams. Sharma and Millar (2015) argued for the inclusion of ECGs because they are a valid and cost-effective way to prevent SCD; however, Wexler and Estes (2015) argued that ECGs are imprecise and result in too many false positives with only a few effective interventions. ECG in the preparticipation examination has been proposed in recent reports, arguing that the added cost is minimal, and the exam can lead to a greater ability to identify athletes at risk. However, a concern exists about the training of the physician providing the exam and reading the ECG. If the physician is not well trained in reading the ECG, errors can be made that result in either unnecessary costs or missed opportunities to refer an athlete for further testing (Emery & Kovacs, 2018). Unfortunately, a discussion of the outcome of many systematic reviews and the various opinions of physician groups as well as data from longitudinal studies that support both sides of the debate is beyond the scope of the chapter. However, a study that compared two very similar populations of athletes

Hypertrophic cardiomyopathy (HCM) The heart muscle becomes abnormally thick (i.e., hypertrophied), which makes it hard for the heart to pump blood.

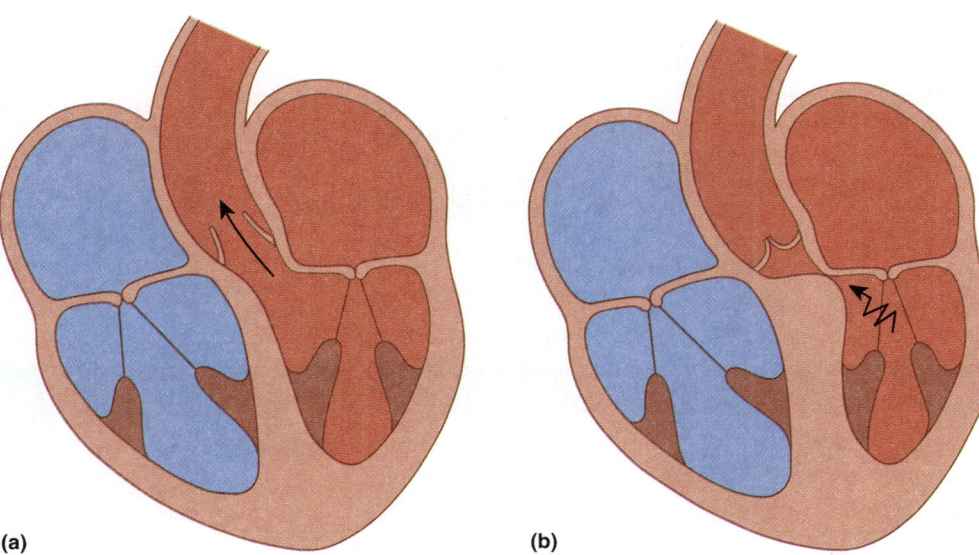

(a) (b)

Figure 13.5 A comparison of normal cardiac function with malfunction characteristic of hypertrophic cardiomyopathy.
(a) Normal heart, illustrating unobstructed flow of blood from left ventricle into aorta during ventricular systole.
(b) Hypertrophic cardiomyopathy, illustrating obstruction to outflow of blood from left ventricle by hypertrophied septum, which impinges on anterior leaflet of mitral valve.

with different preparticipation screening policies was unable to support a lower mortality rate when ECGs were included and administered by specially trained personnel (Maron et al., 2009).

Minimally, the 14-Element AHA Cardiovascular Screening Checklist for Congenital and Genetic Heart Disease (Hainline et al., 2016; Maron et al., 2014) should be used to assess risk and determine referral for follow-up with a cardiologist (see Table 13.2). The use of this 14-element assessment, which includes 10 personal and familial history questions plus four specific physical exam results, will assist healthcare providers in determining whether athletes may be at risk for SCD and need further testing by a cardiologist or other professional. The advice and direction of the team or personal physician are critical for the final decision regarding what testing should be implemented to ensure athletes' health. An important point is to review each athlete's history very closely to determine whether a cardiac or respiratory problem may be exacerbated by an increased level of athletic participation. If an athlete has a family or personal history of cardiac or respiratory problems, the physician providing the preparticipation examination must make an informed decision as to the appropriateness of additional specific medical testing and of participation in a specific sport or activity for that athlete.

The prevention of injuries to the heart, lungs, and chest is primarily a function of protective equipment as part of the sport or activity. In baseball and softball, the catcher is equipped with a chest protector (Figure 13.6). These days, chest protectors are made of materials that are much better at attenuating the shock from a ball traveling at high speeds.

In football, hockey, lacrosse, and some other contact sports, part of the uniform is protective equipment designed to reduce possible impact to the heart and

Table 13.2
The 14-Element AHA Cardiovascular Screening Checklist for Congenital and Genetic Heart Disease

Ten Questions Related to Personal and Family History Regarding Cardiac Medical Conditions
1. Do you experience chest pressure, discomfort, pain, or tightness related to exercising or exertion?
2. Do you experience unexplained fainting or almost fainting?
3. Do you experience unexplained fatigue, heart palpitations, or painful/excessive breathing related to exercising or exertion?
4. Have you had a heart murmur diagnosed by a physician?
5. Do you have high blood pressure?
6. Have you ever been restricted from participating in physical activity?
7. Have you ever had testing for the heart prescribed by a physician?
8. Has anyone in your family died prematurely (unexpected, sudden, or other) before age 50 and was the death attributable to a heart condition?
9. Has anyone in your family younger than age 50 experienced disability due to a heart condition?
10. Has anyone in your family experienced significant arrhythmias, long-QT syndrome, hypertrophic/dilated cardiomyopathy, Marfan syndrome, or genetic/acquired defects within the ion channels of the heart?

Diagnoses from Physical Examination by Qualified Medical Professional
1. Are there physical signs of Marfan syndrome (i.e., tall and slender build; disproportionately long arms, legs, and fingers; protruding or concave breastbone)?
2. Are there weak pulses in the femoral arteries?
3. Is there a nonorganic heart murmur or left ventricular outflow obstruction?
4. Is there abnormal brachial artery blood pressure in both arms while sitting?

Data from Maron, B. J., Friedman, R. A., Kligfield, P., Levine, B. D., Viskin, S. . . . Thompson, P. D. (2014). Assessment of the 12-lead electrocardiogram as a screening test for detection of cardiovascular disease in healthy general populations of young people (12–25 years of age). *Journal of the American College of Cardiology, 64*(14),1479–1514.

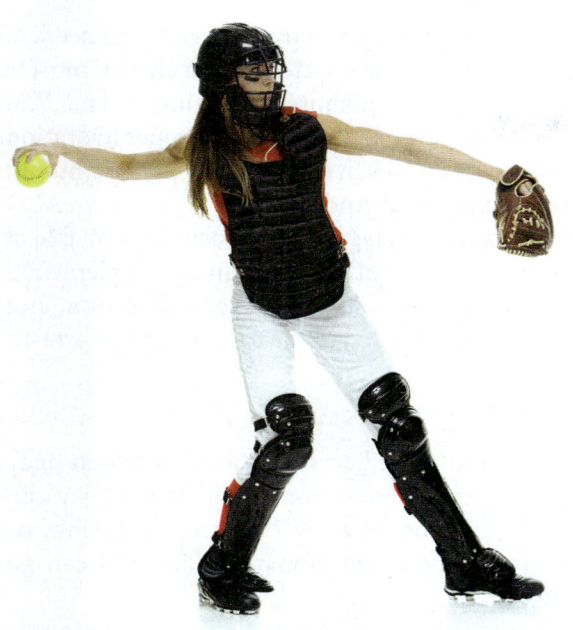

Figure 13.6 Softball chest protector.
© 4x6/iStock/Getty Images Plus/Getty Images.

chest area. Some sports, such as soccer and basketball, do not provide any preventive equipment protection from a blow to the chest area. In these sports, the athlete must be trained to protect the chest when specific situations arise. Certified ATs and other likely early care providers must be current in their CPR training and prepared with either an AED or an emergency action plan that would provide immediate care for a player experiencing signs and symptoms of sudden cardiac arrest.

Other Cardiac Defects

As discussed earlier, athletes should be screened properly by the team physician or their personal physician because a number of congenital defects need to be screened for and ruled out before athletes begin participation in sports (Table 13.2). Nassar, Saber, Farhan, Moussa, and Elsherif (2011) suggested that athletes' hearts go through changes as they grow, develop, and continue their performance training. This research group followed young World Cup soccer players for a year and documented that changes did occur in the cardiac structure and function in these young elite athletes. In addition to HCM, as noted earlier, some athletes are at a higher risk of SCD for problems associated with anomalous coronary arteries;

Marfan syndrome; use of anabolic androgenic steroids (AAS); sickle cell trait (SCT); and other less common disorders, such as long QT syndrome (Casa, Guskiewicz, et al., 2012; Far et al., 2012; Harris et al., 2012; Hoffman et al., 2012). **Marfan syndrome** is a connective tissue disorder, typically associated with the very tall athlete (male and female), that imposes a greater risk for SCD in athletes caused by a number of cardiac implications, including aortic rupture (Hoffman et al., 2012). Physicians doing the preparticipation physical exam should be well aware of the various cardiac syndromes and their associated warning signs. If an athlete exhibits multiple warning signs and/or indicated a personal or familial history during the exam, the physician needs to refer the athlete to a cardiologist for further testing before participating in high-level athletic practices or competitions (Erat, 2019; Hainline et al., 2016). Hainline and colleagues (2016) also indicated four cardiovascular priorities for all student-athletes: (1) identifying risk of SCD, (2) identifying regional centers for cardiac referral, (3) rehearsing emergency action plans, and (4) training all stakeholders in CPR and AED use.

Athletes who abuse AAS must be made aware of the possibility of SCD from the alterations in the heart after the use of these drugs in an illegal and abusive manner (Torrisi et al., 2020). By completing cardiac magnetic resonance (CMR) imaging on a control group, followed by a group of admitted AAS users all exercising regularly, researchers demonstrated that the AAS users had structural abnormalities in the right ventricle, left ventricle, and left ventricular wall that were consistent with impaired ventricular flow (Luijkx et al., 2012). Even more conclusive were the findings after autopsy of 87 deceased males who tested positive for AAS use, which demonstrated abnormal cardiac hypertrophy after comparison to 173 age-adjusted controls (who were also deceased males; Far et al., 2012). Cardiac hypertrophy in this study was a leading factor in a direct cardiotropic effect.

Athletes with ancestors from Sub-Saharan Africa, the Mediterranean basin, India, the Arabian Peninsula,

> **Marfan syndrome** Inherited disorder affecting connective tissue in the heart, blood vessels, eyes, and bones. Vision problems and defects in the large blood vessels leaving the heart are two primary conditions associated with this genetic disorder.

the Caribbean, or South and Central America who have the SCT are also susceptible to SCD. Harris and colleagues (2012) reported that SCT occurs in approximately 8–10% of African Americans and is generally a benign problem; however, in athletes working at high levels of physical capacity, most commonly college football players, the probability of SCD is higher. The report specifically points out the occurrence of SCD during conditioning activities with this specific population (Harris et al., 2012).

SCT is characterized by the inheritance of one copy of the normal beta-globin gene and one copy of the sickle variant. The red blood cells can change shape, or sickle, in situations of oxygen depletion caused by physical exertion, heat exhaustion, or dehydration. As a result, exertional sickling can occur where these odd-shaped, or sickled, red blood cells then experience trouble traveling through blood vessels, thereby potentially causing blood clotting or organ death (Baker et al., 2018). In 2010, the NCAA issued a policy that required all Division I student-athletes to confirm their SCT status or sign a liability waiver to opt out of testing (Baker et al., 2018). The intent was to ensure the safety of the athletes by providing essential medical information to ATs and team physicians. Being prepared for a potential episode of exertional sickling has allowed for modified activity levels when needed. Athletes with SCT are watched closely for muscle cramping, fatigue, and labored breathing, and medical and coaching staff must ensure that proper hydration and cooling occur when exercising in hot and humid environments (Casa, Anderson, et al., 2012). An AED and supplemental oxygen should also be available at practices and competitions at all times. Supplemental oxygen helps organs survive oxygen depletion, and an AED may be needed in the case of cardiac arrest.

Lung Injuries

In addition to a cardiac contusion, an athlete may experience a **pulmonary contusion**. This injury can be a complication of a rib fracture, contusion, or some other type of pulmonary injury and can go undetected.

Pulmonary contusion can also occur in athletes experiencing blunt chest trauma. The possibility also exists for the occurrence of spontaneous pneumothorax among athletes. Spontaneous pneumothorax occurs without a preceding traumatic event. This injury is significant and must be attended to by a physician. Ribs can also fracture and puncture the pleural sac that surrounds the lungs. If air gets into the pleural cavity, the possibility exists for a lung to collapse (Figure 13.7a and b). When a lung collapses in this way, it is termed a pneumothorax. A more general description of a pneumothorax is the presence of air

Pulmonary contusion A direct blow to the thorax that results in lung trauma.

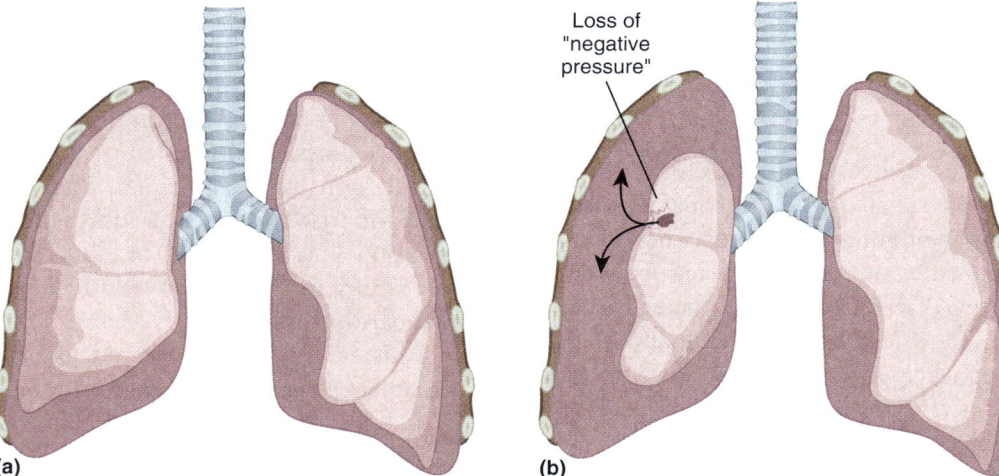

Figure 13.7 **(a)** Normal relation of lung to chest wall. Pleural space is exaggerated, and surfaces are normally in contact. "Negative pressure" is primarily a result of the tendency of the stretched lung to pull away from the chest wall.
(b) Pneumothorax caused by a perforating injury of lung, allowing the air under atmospheric pressure to escape into the pleural cavity.

or a gas in the pleural cavity (i.e., space between the lungs and chest wall), which may cause a partial or complete collapse of the lung. As we all know, air is inside the lungs; when outside air gets into the area of the chest cavity between the lungs and the ribs, it results in a loss of the appropriate pressure gradient between the inside and outside pressures, which affects the lung and inhibits the lung's ability to expand for normal breathing to occur (Figure 13.8). The surface of the lung pulls away and is no longer in contact with the chest wall.

Blood in the pleural cavity is commonly called a hemothorax; again, it can occur without a preceding traumatic event. Air and blood in the pleural cavity are called a **hemopneumothorax**. The coach or AT must be aware of the signs and symptoms of cardiac and pulmonary contusions and the potential occurrence of a pneumothorax, hemothorax, or a hemopneumothorax. The athlete's healthcare provider should monitor the progress of the athlete over a period of days because some injuries tend to exhibit complications later.

Signs and symptoms of a cardiac or pulmonary contusion and/or air and blood inside the pleural cavity include the following:

- The athlete will complain of severe pain in the chest area, sometimes radiating to the thoracic spine.
- The athlete will typically experience breathing problems, either shortness of breath or painful breathing exhibited by short, shallow breaths. Inspect for a loss of chest wall movement during breathing.
- The athlete may exhibit a nonproductive cough and may have a tachycardia (fast) heart rate.

First aid care of a cardiac or pulmonary contusion and/or a pneumothorax involves the following:

1. Treat the athlete for possible shock.
2. Monitor vital signs continuously.
3. Arrange for transport to a medical facility.

Respiratory problems can lead to or be a precursor for chest pain in the athlete. Whenever athletes report chest pain or have a heart condition, they should be seen immediately by the team physician or other medical doctor.

Liver

The liver aids in the production of plasma proteins and glucose for the bloodstream and the detoxification of alcohol and other substances; it also has various digestive functions (Reisner & Reisner, 2022). It is located in the upper right quadrant of the abdomen and can be susceptible to blunt trauma in collision sports, such as football (Dixit & Chang, 2018). The liver may be contused or lacerated if a rib fracture occurs in the upper right abdominal quadrant. Otherwise, the liver is fairly safe from injury associated with sports participation. The liver is, however, susceptible to various pathologies from the overuse of alcohol and drugs (especially massive amounts of steroids) as well as other insults from chemicals and diseases.

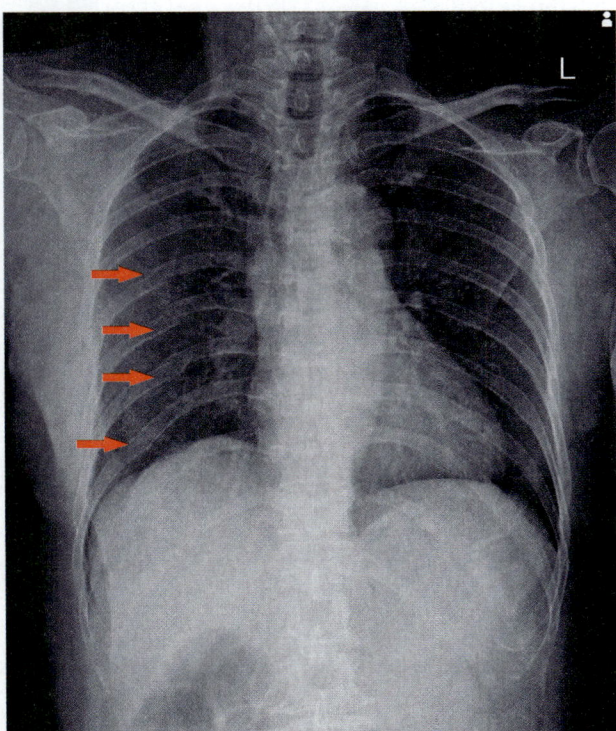

Figure 13.8 X-ray illustrating pneumothorax secondary to multiple rib fractures in which broken ends of fractured ribs have torn through the pleura and torn underlying lung. The arrows indicate the surface of the lung that is no longer in contact with the chest wall.
© April stock/Shutterstock.

Hemopneumothorax Blood and air collect in the pleural cavity (space between the lungs and chest wall).

Kidneys

The kidneys serve to maintain the proper levels of waste, gas, salt, water, and other chemicals in the bloodstream (Reisner & Reisner, 2022). The kidneys are located posteriorly and somewhat inferiorly on each side of the abdomen; they are susceptible to injury from blunt trauma or elevated core temperature (via extreme exercise in the heat of the day). The body can experience acute renal failure, and the kidneys will cease to function. An athlete who has **hematuria**, or blood in the urine, after being hit by an opponent in the lower back or after having exercised strenuously in the heat should be seen by a physician immediately. Both of these scenarios can indicate kidney problems or damage. The physician will determine how an athlete's exercise regimen will need to be modified until the urine is once again clear of any blood.

Spleen

The chief function of the spleen is to maintain a reserve of ready-to-use blood cells for the body (Reisner & Reisner, 2022). It is located in the upper left quadrant of the abdomen and is somewhat protected by the ribs on the lower left side. Like most of the other internal organs, the spleen is susceptible to injury from blunt trauma and internal disorders. A recent review of abdominal injuries in pediatric soccer players in Pennsylvania from 2001–2015 indicated that the spleen was the most frequently injured abdominal organ due to player-to-player contact (Khakimov et al., 2021). An athlete who gets hit quite hard in the abdomen over the spleen can suffer a lacerated spleen. Nevertheless, the spleen has the capacity to splint or patch itself at the site of the injury during the healing process because it is a reservoir of red blood cells. If the spleen does patch itself completely and the athlete is eventually allowed to participate, the possibility remains that the patch may be disrupted by even a small amount of trauma. This secondary trauma can allow internal bleeding to resume, and death can occur days after the original injury. **Kehr's sign** is when an athlete is hit hard in the upper left quadrant and later complains of pain in the abdomen and/or left shoulder and upper third of the left arm (sometimes the right shoulder). If Kehr's sign is present, the athlete should be referred to a physician as soon as possible.

Additionally, if an athlete is suffering from **mononucleosis**, an infectious illness, the spleen will probably be enlarged and susceptible to injury not only from blunt trauma but also from excessive movement during sports participation. The athlete with mononucleosis needs to be restricted in activity for at least 1 month until the physician can discern whether the spleen has returned to normal size. Current consensus supports that athletes be afebrile, well hydrated, and asymptomatic, with no palpable tenderness over liver or spleen, before a gradual and monitored return to competition (Sylvester et al., 2019).

Bladder

The bladder acts as a reservoir for the urine produced by the kidneys. It is located under the midline of the abdominal quadrants. Because this area is well protected, the bladder is rarely injured by participation in sports and athletics. If the athlete receives a direct blow to the area of the bladder and injury does occur, the signs are pain in the localized area and possibly blood in the urine (hematuria). Avoiding injury to the bladder is best accomplished by emptying it before practice or competition (Guttman & Kerr, 2013).

Abdominal Pain

Various types of abdominal pain occur in athletes before, during, and after competition. Some of the more common abdominal pain complaints can be linked to choices related to eating and drinking, bowel movement habits, and psychological stress. If an athlete is experiencing chronic pain in the same location, the athlete should see a physician as soon as possible. Another reason for abdominal pain is referred pain, as noted with the spleen or the diaphragm, either of which can be injured or irritated and result in shoulder tip pain. Esophageal problems are typically noted by the athlete as epigastric pain. Stomach problems, such as duodenal ulcers, are typically localized to the stomach area but have been known to produce low back pain complaints.

Hematuria Blood, which can appear red or brown, in the urine.

Kehr's sign Pain radiating into the left shoulder that is normally associated with an injury to the spleen.

Mononucleosis Viral illness that creates a variety of symptoms, including fever, muscle aches, and fatigue.

Exercise-related transient abdominal pain (ETAP) is a problem commonly called "side ache" or "stitch in the side" by athletes. This problem typically occurs during running early in an exercise regimen of an unconditioned athlete. The cause of this problem has not been definitively determined, but different hypotheses have been put forth to explain why this discomfort might occur in athletes (Wynne & Wilson, 2022). Some possible explanations are ischemia in the diaphragm, stress on the visceral connective tissues, or a cramping of the local musculature. Other theoretical explanations address the time of onset (early in the exercise program) and hypothesize that the acute increase in venous return from the lower extremities to the liver results in the extra blood flow stretching the vein near the liver. This acute stretching of the vein initiates a pain response to the brain, which then recognizes a pain in the right side. In response to the pain, athletes typically slow their running pace or even stop. Following this decrease in exercise, blood flow equalizes, which decreases the stretch to the vein, thus resulting in a decrease in the pain signal to the brain. When an athlete warms up appropriately, the incidence of this phenomenon reduces. Another theory for pain on the left side in the exercising athlete is that gas or fecal matter is being moved through the intestinal tract and that during exercise the timing is such that this movement is inhibited and could be stopped in one of the angles of the winding intestinal tract. Finally, recent research has revealed that anxiety and stress may be causes of ETAP in runners (Wynne & Wilson, 2022). Side aches do not appear to be a problem that eliminates athletes from participation in most sports, and most athletes learn how to deal with them on the rare occasions when they happen.

Right side pain, though, can occur for other reasons, such as being an early sign of **acute appendicitis**. Initially, the athlete has a loss of appetite, followed by generalized abdominal pain. When the problem progresses, the chief complaint of the athlete with acute appendicitis is severe pain in the lower right quadrant. At times, this pain can be excruciating, and the athlete rendered immobile. Additionally, the athlete experiences nausea and possibly vomiting and has a fever that increases over time. The athlete will be point tender to palpation in the lower right quadrant (McBurney's point) and should be taken to the hospital immediately. Without medical attention, the athlete can die from the complications associated with a ruptured appendix.

Preexisting conditions of the chest and abdomen that may disqualify an athlete from participation can include problems such as HCM; heart murmurs and arrhythmias; significantly decreased lung function from disease or a disorder, such as cystic fibrosis or chronic obstructive pulmonary disease; or mononucleosis. Disqualification from sports participation based on these conditions is dependent on the type of sport being considered, the amount of stress the activity will place on the dependent structures or systems, and the ability to control potential problems during the activity. Athletes with what might be considered a severe cardiac, abdominal, or respiratory disorder may be able to participate in specific activities depending on the control of their disorder, the type of activity, and the willingness of the physician to help the athlete make the necessary adjustments for participation at some level.

WHAT IF ❓

You are coaching a tackle football game at the high school level. On the last play, your quarterback was sacked and, in the process, received a severe blow to his abdomen. On further examination, he complains of extreme abdominal pain and pain radiating into his left shoulder and upper arm, and he has a rigid abdomen. Based on these signs and symptoms, could this athlete have a serious injury, and, if so, what?

Exercise-related transient abdominal pain (ETAP) Commonly called a "stitch in the side," pain that is benign and self-limiting but may be stabbing or sharp when severe or achier and cramping when less intense. It can be recurrent and tends to be resistant to treatment.

Acute appendicitis Severe inflammation of the appendix caused by trapped feces or an occurrence of a virus, bacteria, or parasite and accompanied by increasing symptoms (i.e., pain, fever, nausea) within 24 to 48 hours; is considered a medical emergency.

Review Questions

1. True or false? Men and women have the same number of ribs.
2. Explain the difference between true ribs and floating ribs.
3. List the five main joints of the thorax.
4. With what necessary function do the intercostal muscles assist in the thorax?
5. True or false? Both lungs are the same size and configuration.
6. What is the name of the enclosed space where each lung is located?
7. True or false? The diaphragm separates the heart and lungs from the abdominal viscera.
8. Explain the difference between a pneumothorax and a hemothorax.
9. List the signs and symptoms of a costochondral separation.
10. Which gender experiences more sudden cardiac deaths in athletics?
11. Which sport typically has seen the most sudden cardiac deaths in athletics?
12. What is the current opinion on including ECGs and cardiac-specific questions in preparticipation examinations?
13. How does sickle cell trait predispose an athlete to sudden cardiac death?
14. If an athlete experiences cardiac arrest, what is the time frame in which an automated external defibrillator should be applied?
15. What is the best indicator of kidney damage or disorder?
16. True or false? The spleen is able to splint itself if injured by blunt trauma.
17. Name the infection, prevalent among college-aged students, that causes the spleen to enlarge, requiring the athlete to reduce physical activity until the spleen is once again normal.
18. List four functions of the kidneys.
19. When pain occurs in the abdomen, what are some of the locations that the abdominal pain can be referred to?
20. Explain the best way to prevent bladder injury among athletes.

References

Baker, C., Powell, J., Le, D., Creary, M. S., Daley, L. A., McDonald, M. A., & Royal, C. D. (2018). Implementation of the NCAA sickle cell trait screening policy: A survey of athletic staff and student-athletes. *Journal of the National Medical Association, 110*(6), 564–573.

Buchanan, B. K., Siebert, D. M., Zigman Suchsland, M. L., Drezner, J. A., Asif, I. M., O'Connor, F. G., & Harmon, K. G. (2020). Sudden death associated with sickle cell trait before and after mandatory screening. *Sports Health, 12*(3), 241–245.

Casa, D. J., Almquist, J., Anderson, S. A., Baker, L., Bergeron, M. F., Biagioli, B., ... Valentine, V. (2013). The Inter-Association Task Force for Preventing Sudden Death in Secondary School Athletics Programs: Best-practices recommendations. *Journal of Athletic Training, 48*(4), 548–553.

Casa, D. J., Anderson, S. A., Baker, L., Bennett, S., Bergeron, M. F., Connolly, D., ... Thompson, C. (2012). The Inter-Association Task Force for Preventing Sudden Death in Collegiate Conditioning Sessions: Best practices recommendations. *Journal of Athletic Training, 47*(4), 477–480.

Casa, D. J., Guskiewicz, K. M., Anderson, S. A., Courson, R. W., Heck, J. F., Jimenez, C. C., ... Walsh, K. M. (2012). National Athletic Trainers' Association position statement: Preventing sudden death in sports. *Journal of Athletic Training, 47*(1), 96–118.

Dixit, S., & Chang, C. J. (2018). Thorax and abdominal injuries. In C. C. Madden, M. Putukian, E. C. McCarty, & C. C. Young (Eds.), *Netter's sports medicine* (2nd ed., pp. 402–414). Philadelphia, PA: Elsevier.

Emery, M. S., & Kovacs, R. J. (2018). Sudden cardiac death in athletes. *JACC: Heart Failure, 6*(1), 30–40.

Erat, A. (2019). Pre-participation evaluation for screening of health risks in leisure and young competitive athletes. *Sports & Exercise Medicine Switzerland, 67*(3), 6–11.

Far, G. R. M., Agren, G., & Thiblin, I. (2012). Cardiac hypertrophy in deceased users of anabolic androgenic steroids: An investigation of autopsy findings. *Cardiovascular Pathology, 21*, 312–316.

Gundersen, A., Borgstrom, H., & McInnis, K. C. (2021). Trunk injuries in athletes. *Current Sports Medicine Reports, 20*(3), 150–156.

Guttmann, I., & Kerr, H. A. (2013). Blunt bladder injury. *Clinics in Sports Medicine, 32*(2), 239–246.

Hainline, B., Drezner, J. A., Baggish, A., Harmon, K. G., Emery, M. S., Myerburg, R. J., ... Thompson, P. D. (2016). Interassociation consensus statement on cardiovascular care of college student-athletes. *Journal of American College of Cardiology, 67*(25), 2981-2995.

Harmon, K. G., Asif, I. M., Maleszewski, J. J., Owens, D. S., Prutkin, J. M., Salerno, J. C., . . . Drezner, J. A. (2015). Incidence, etiology, and comparative frequency of sudden cardiac death in NCAA athletes: A decade in review. *Circulation, 132*(1), 1-21.

Harmon, K. G., Zigman, M., & Drezner, J. A. (2015). The effectiveness of screening history, physical exam, and ECG to detect potentially lethal cardiac disorders in athletes: A systematic review/meta-analysis. *Journal of Electrocardiology, 48*(3), 329-338.

Harris, K. M., Haas, T. S., Eichner, E. R., & Maron, B. J. (2012). Sickle cell trait associated with sudden death in competitive athletes. *American Journal of Cardiology,* 110, 1185-1188.

Hoffman, B. A., Rybczynski, M., Rostock, T., Servatius, H., Drewitz, I., Steven, D., . . . Willems, S. (2012). Prospective risk stratification of sudden cardiac death in Marfan's syndrome. *International Journal of Cardiology, 167*(6), 2539-2545.

Khakimov, S., Zaki, P., Hess, J., & Hennrikus, W. (2021). Abdominal organ injuries in youth soccer: A case series and review of literature. *Current Sports Medicine Reports, 20*(2), 69-75.

Luijkx, T., Velthuis, B. K., Backx, F. J., Buckens, C. F., Prakken, N. H., Rienks, R., . . . Cramer, M. J. (2012). Anabolic androgenic steroid use is associated with ventricular dysfunction on cardiac MRI in strength trained athletes. *International Journal of Cardiology, 167*(3), 664-668.

Maron, B. J., Doerer, J. J., Haas, T. S., Tierney, D. M., & Mueller, F. O. (2009). Sudden deaths in young competitive athletes: Analysis of 1866 deaths in the United States, 1980-2006. *Circulation,* 119, 1085-1092.

Maron, B. J., Friedman, R. A., Kligfield, P., Levine, B. D., Viskin, S., Chaitman, B. R., ... & Council on Quality of Care and Outcomes Research, and American College of Cardiology. (2014). Assessment of the 12-lead electrocardiogram as a screening test for detection of cardiovascular disease in healthy general populations of young people (12-25 years of age): A scientific statement from the American Heart Association and the American College of Cardiology. *Journal of the American College of Cardiology, 64*(14), 1479-1514.

Maron, B. J., Haas, T. S., Ahluwalia, A., Murphy, C. J., & Garberich, R. F. (2016). Demographics and epidemiology of sudden deaths in young competitive athletes: From the United States National Registry. *American Journal of Medicine, 129*(11), 1170-1177.

Maron, B. J., Haas, T. S., Doerer, J. J., Thompson, P. D., & Hodges, J. S. (2009). Comparison of U.S. and Italian experiences with sudden cardiac deaths in young competitive athletes and implications for preparticipation screening strategies. *American Journal of Cardiology, 104,* 276-280.

Moini, J. (2020). *Anatomy and physiology for health professionals* (3rd ed.). Burlington, MA: Jones & Bartlett Learning.

Narayanan, K., Bougouin, W., Sharifzadehgan, A., Waldmann, V., Karam, N., Marijon, E., & Jouven, X. (2017). Sudden cardiac death during sports activities in the general population. *Cardiac Electrophysiology Clinics, 9*(4), 559-567.

Nassar, Y. S., Saber, M., Farhan, A., Moussa, A., & Elsherif, A. (2011). One year cardiac follow up of young World Cup football team compared to nonathletes. *Egyptian Heart Journal, 63,* 13-22.

Reisner, H., & Reisner, E. (2022). *Crowley's an introduction to human disease* (11th ed.). Burlington, MA: Jones & Bartlett Learning.

Sharma, S., & Millar, L. (2015). Should preparticipation cardiovascular screening of athletes include ECG? Yes: Screening ECG is cost-effective. *American Family Physician, 92*(5), 338-340.

Singh, M., & Link, M. S. (2021). Commotio cordis in athletes. In D. J. Engel & D. M. Phelan (Eds.), *Sports cardiology* (pp. 375-381). New York, NY: Springer, Cham.

Sylvester, J. E., Buchanan, B. K., Paradise, S. L., Yauger, J. J., & Beutler, A. I. (2019). Association of splenic rupture and infectious mononucleosis: A retrospective analysis and review of return-to-play recommendations. *Sports Health, 11*(6), 543-549.

Torrisi, M., Pennisi, G., Russo, I., Amico, F., Esposito, M., Liberto, A., Cocimano, G., Salerno, M., Rosi, G. L., Di Nunno, N., & Montana, A. (2020). Sudden cardiac death in anabolic-androgenic steroid users: A literature review. *Medicina, 56*(11), 587.

Wexler, R., & Estes, N. A. (2015). Should preparticipation cardiovascular screening of athletes include ECG? No: There is not enough evidence to support including ECG in the preparticipation sports evaluation. *American Family Physician, 92*(5), 343.

Wynne, J. L., & Wilson, P. B. (2022). Thorn in your side or thorn in your head? Anxiety and stress as correlates of exercise-related transient abdominal pain. *Clinical Journal of Sport Medicine,* 1-5.

Yu, W., & Zhou, J. (2016). Sports bras and breast kinetics. In W. Yu (Ed.), *Advances in women's intimate apparel technology* (pp. 135-146). Philadelphia, PA: Woodhead Publishing.

CHAPTER 14

Injuries to the Hip and Pelvis

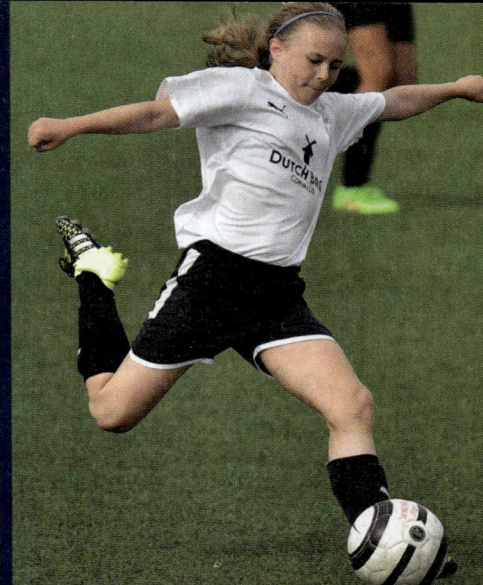

MAJOR CONCEPTS

This chapter includes a basic overview of the anatomy in the region of the hip and pelvis and a brief description of movements by the joints and actions of the musculature in the area. It discusses some of the more common hip and pelvis injuries incurred in sports and outlines emergency procedures. The chapter also includes a section about injuries to the areas that are less common in athletes. Coaches need to be aware of these types of injuries because of the possibility of negative long-term consequences that can result from improper care. The chapter reviews injuries to the male genitalia, including testicular contusion and torsion. It also covers hernia and nerve problems and discusses proper referral.

Anatomy Review

The hip and pelvis resemble a square in the way they are constructed. This area comprises the two large, irregularly shaped pelvic bones on the lateral sides, the sacrum and coccyx posteriorly, and the articulation of the pubic bones anteriorly. The pelvic bones are also known as the innominate bones and are made up of three distinct parts: the ilium, the ischium, and the pubis. In the adult, the three parts are fused and come together at a lateral point called the acetabulum, which is where the head of the femur articulates with the hip to form the hip joint (Figure 14.1).

The bony pelvis has several functions in the body: The lower extremities attach here, muscle attachments are prevalent, and it provides substantial protection of organs in the entire pelvic region. In the female, the pelvis becomes important in the birth process (Moini, 2020).

The major articulations of the bony pelvis include the hip joints, the sacroiliac joints, and the symphysis pubis. The hip joint is the articulation of the head of the femur and the acetabulum in the hip bone; it is a true ball-and-socket joint and is well supported by strong ligaments. The sacroiliac joints are formed by the sacral bones and the iliac portion of the hip bones. The symphysis pubis is formed by the two pubic bones meeting in the anterior portion of the bony pelvis. All of these joints have strong ligamentous support that assists in joint stability.

Several nerves and blood vessels course through the bony pelvis (Figures 14.2 and 14.3). Some of the more important nerves that course down the lower extremity are subdivisions that make up the cauda equina. The spinal cord ends at the L2 level, and the cauda equina exits the spinal cord beginning at L2 and proceeding inferiorly (Moini, 2020). Nerves exiting the spinal cord below the L1 level typically pass

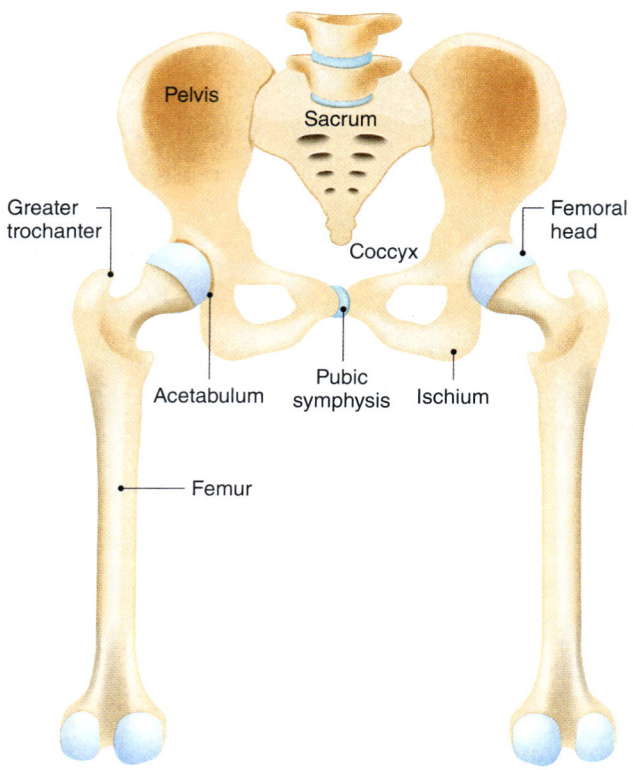

Figure 14.1 The ball-and-socket structure of the hip joint.
© Designua/Shutterstock.

through the bony pelvis. These nerves include the formation of the lumbar plexus, the sacral plexus, the coccygeal plexus, and other individual nerves. Probably the most well known of these nerves is the sciatic nerve, which is the largest in the body and is made up of nerve roots L4 through S3. The sciatic nerve passes through the posterior portion of the bony pelvis and down the posterior aspect of the leg. The blood vessels of the area include both arteries and veins that supply the pelvis and lower extremities. The more well known of these vessels include the iliac artery and vein and the femoral artery and vein.

Many of the muscles that attach to the bony pelvis are ones that move the lower extremities. The smaller muscles consist of the medial and lateral rotators of the femur. Some of the medial rotators include the tensor fasciae latae and gluteus minimus. These muscles are quite active in many movements of the lower extremity. The lateral rotators of the hip are small muscles located deep within the hip area, which are also quite active in many movements of the lower extremity. One of the muscles more commonly injured is the piriformis, which attaches to the anterior surface of the sacrum and to the greater trochanter of the femur. The piriformis is a lateral rotator of the thigh; the sciatic nerve runs directly

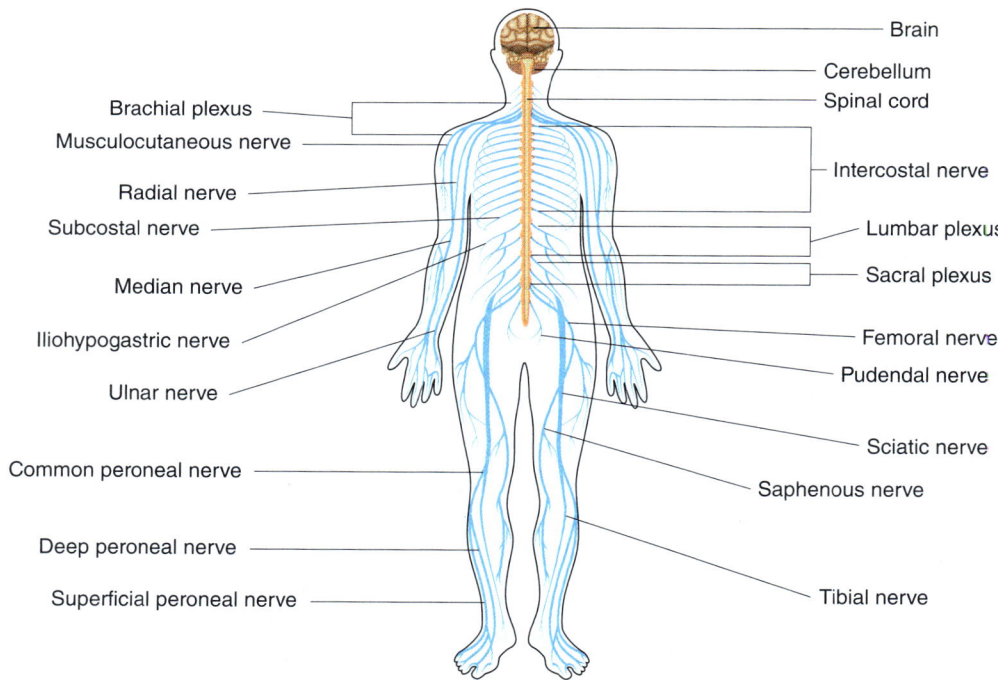

NERVOUS SYSTEM

Figure 14.2 The nerves of the lower extremities.
© stockshoppe/Shutterstock.

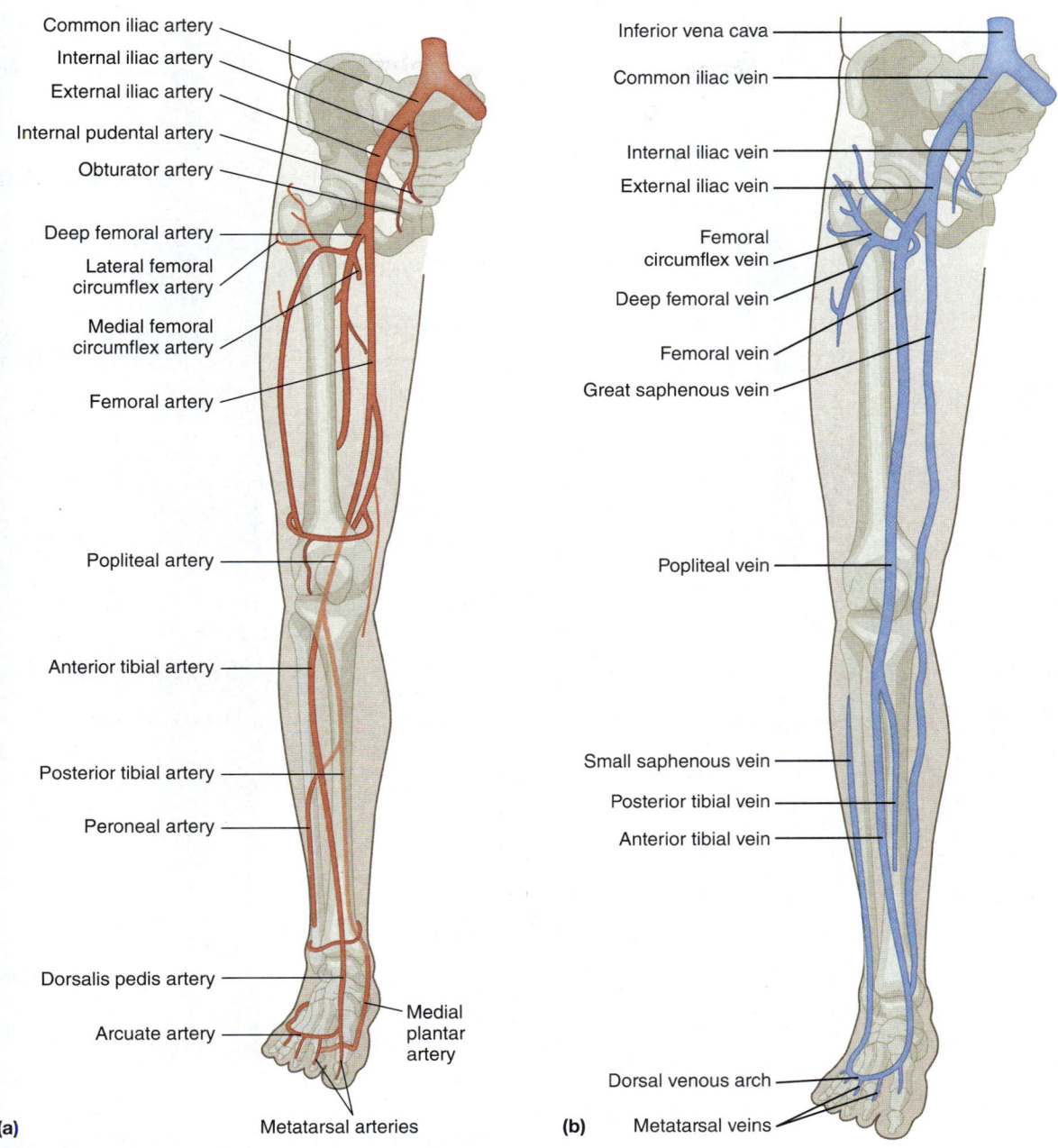

Figure 14.3 (a) Arteries of lower extremity. (b) Veins of lower extremity.

beneath the piriformis and can be irritated by the overuse of this muscle. Other external rotators of the thigh include the gemelli (superior and inferior), which attach on the ischium and run to the greater trochanter of the femur. All of these muscles are small in comparison to the surrounding muscles, but they play an important part in the proper functioning of the hip and leg.

Many muscles attach on the pelvis and provide musculature for the leg, back, and abdomen. The muscles responsible for many of the large movements at the hip joint include flexors, extensors, adductors, and abductors. The main hip flexors include the rectus femoris, the iliopsoas group, the tensor fasciae latae, and the sartorius (Figure 14.4). The rectus femoris attaches at the anterior inferior iliac spine and runs down the front of the leg to the common attachment of the quadriceps group at the patellar tendon. The iliopsoas group is a combination of the iliacus and the psoas muscles, which attach on the anterior lumbar spine and iliac crest and come together as they run down to the lesser trochanter of the femur. The tensor fasciae latae and sartorius attach on the anterior iliac spine. The tensor fasciae latae runs to the lateral condyle of the tibia, whereas the sartorius runs across

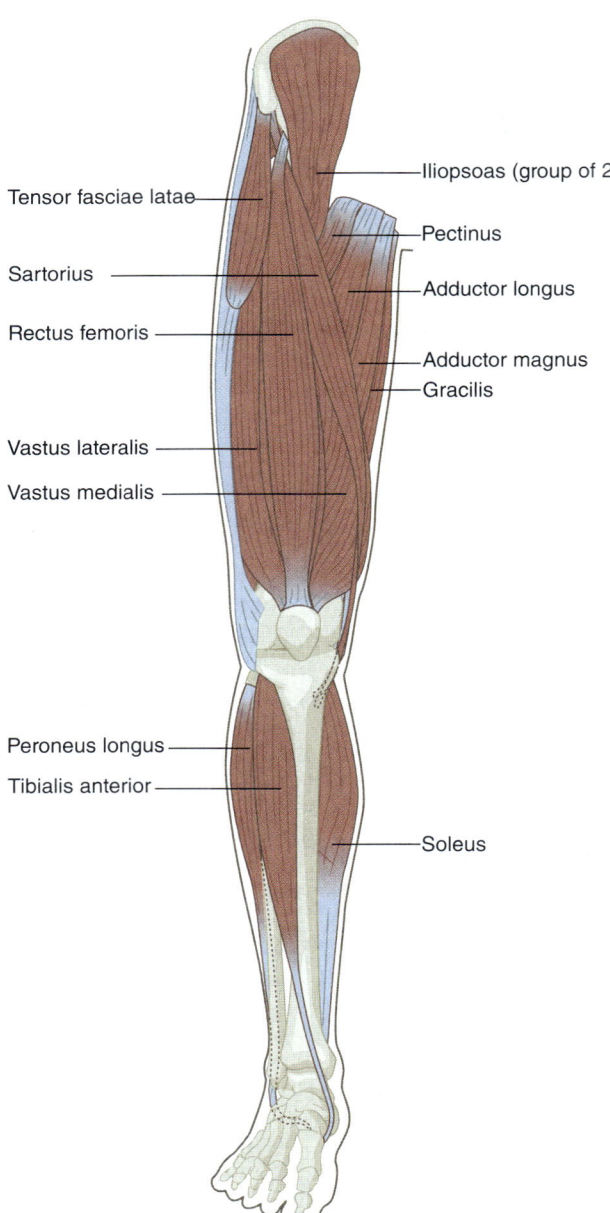

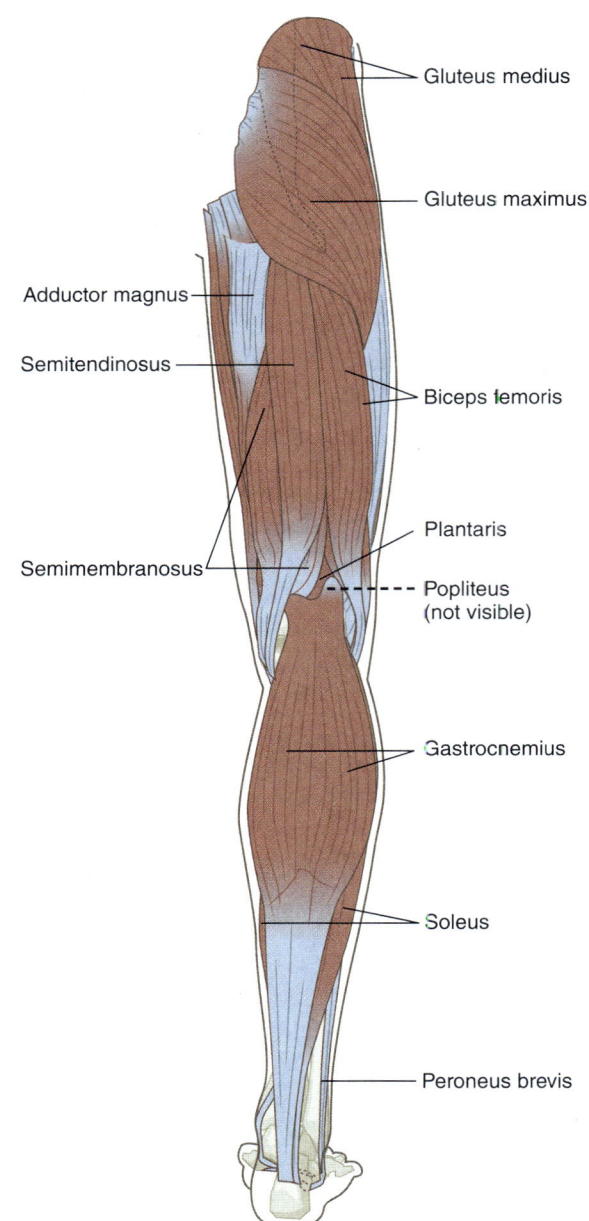

Figure 14.4 Hip flexors and anterior leg muscles.

Figure 14.5 Hip extensors and posterior leg muscles.

the anterior thigh and attaches to the anterior medial aspect of the tibia. The sartorius becomes one of the muscles of the pes anserinus group.

The main muscles of hip extension are the gluteals and the hamstrings (Figure 14.5). The gluteus maximus is the main hip extensor of the gluteals. The gluteus maximus attaches on the posterior surface of the ilium and runs inferiorly to the femur. The hamstrings attach mainly on the ischial tuberosity; then, two of the muscles, the semitendinosus and semimembranosus, run more medially on the posterior leg and attach near the sartorius and on the

posterior/medial condyle of the tibia, respectively. The biceps femoris runs more laterally on the posterior leg and attaches to the lateral aspect of the tibia and the head of the fibula.

The muscles that adduct the hip are located on the medial portion of the leg commonly called the groin area. The main muscles included in this group are the three adductors (brevis, longus, and magnus) and the pectineus and gracilis. The adductors attach on the pubis and run to the femur. The pectineus also attaches at the pubis and runs to the femur. The gracilis attaches on the inferior portion of the pubis and runs medially down the leg to the anterior medial portion of the tibia. The gracilis, sartorius, and semitendinosus compose the pes anserinus group.

Common Sports Injuries

The hip and pelvic regions are well designed anatomically: Sports-related injuries to the skeletal structures of the hip and pelvis are not common. Injuries to the soft tissues in the region are more common and can be quite debilitating to the athlete. Sports-related injuries to this area commonly involve collision sports or forceful movements pursuant to an activity that requires power and speed of the lower extremities. However, one must remember that overuse injuries can also be associated with the hip and pelvis.

Skeletal Injuries

Fractures of the Pelvis

One of the most devastating injuries to the pelvic region is the fracture of one of the pelvic bones. Typically, a great deal of force is necessary to cause a fracture of this type. This is not a common injury related to sports participation. Still, it can occur in sports, such as hockey, pole-vaulting, or football, in which there is the possibility of direct compression from another athlete, a fall from a height, or being twisted and hit by another player. Skeletal injuries to the pelvis in the adolescent population can be extremely serious, especially if the injury involves an open epiphysis (Patsiogiannis & Giannoudis, 2021). Any suspected skeletal injury to this area should be referred to a physician as quickly as possible.

Signs and symptoms of a fractured pelvis include the following:

- Abnormal pain in the pelvic region after the injury.
- There might be swelling at the site, with the rare occurrence of a visual or palpable deformity at the injury.
- Pain is elicited when the iliac crests are pressed together by the examiner.
- Associated injuries to internal organs, such as the bladder, are possible and should be ruled out only by the proper medical personnel. Blood in the urine (hematuria) must be immediately reported.

First aid care of a fractured pelvis involves the following:

1. Treat for possible shock and internal bleeding.
2. Monitor the athlete's vital signs regularly.
3. Transport the athlete to the hospital on a long spine board with the foot of the board elevated to eliminate pooling of blood in the lower extremities.

A fracture of the pelvis is a serious injury and should be evaluated by a physician as soon as possible. Treatment depends on the severity of the injury and should be complete before the athlete returns to practice or competition. Under no circumstances should an athlete with a suspected fracture of the pelvis return to competition before seeing a physician.

Other Adolescent Fractures

Femoral Neck Stress Fracture

This injury occurs more commonly in the thin amenorrheic athlete involved in running or an endurance sport. A **femoral neck stress fracture** is generally the result of a loss in shock-absorbing capacity of the fatigued muscles in the hip area over time. In the athlete, this problem can also result from improper or worn-out footwear, hard running surfaces, hip deformities, or other kinetic chain problems resulting in excess stresses in the legs. Athletes can complain of severe anterior thigh or groin pain when there is the possibility of a femoral neck stress fracture (Dutton, 2021; Harris et al., 2020). The athlete will be able to walk but will experience significant pain during ambulation. Seeing a physician is necessary to get radiographs, which help to diagnose the problem. As with other stress fractures, initial conventional radiographs may be normal, and the athlete will need to return to the physician at a later date if the symptoms persist (Dutton, 2021). The treatment for most lower extremity stress fractures, regardless of area, is to remove weight bearing and outside forces, which entails no activity and crutches for several weeks.

Slipped Capital Femoral Epiphysis

A **slipped capital femoral epiphysis** occurs most commonly in 10- to 15-year-old boys. Typically, it occurs in boys who are tall and have recently

---

Femoral neck stress fracture A rare stress injury to the bony matrix in the femoral neck of the femur usually due to repetitive stress or overload.

Slipped capital femoral epiphysis Head of femur displaces relative to neck of femur.

experienced a rapid growth period or are overweight (Aprato et al., 2019; Fatakhov & Miranda-Comas, 2021; Fedorak et al., 2018; Mathew & Larson, 2019) and in whom the secondary sex characteristics are late in appearing. In this condition, the head of the femur displaces from the neck of the femur, similar to an ice cream scoop not adequately centered on the ice cream cone. The athlete experiencing this problem will exhibit a flexed hip; lack of hip motion; and pain in the anterior groin, hip, thigh, or knee. Children younger than the age of 12 experiencing significant chronic knee pain should definitely be referred to their physician to rule out the existence of a pathology that may exist. The treatment for this condition is usually surgery to fix the bony problem.

Hip Pointer

Probably the most common injury to the hip region is a contusion to the superior/anterior portion of the iliac crest, which is commonly referred to as a **hip pointer**. Typically, with this injury, the athlete receives a direct blow to the area from an opponent's helmet or falls to the ground with great force (Vázquez-Galliano & Miranda-Comas, 2021). A hip pointer injury can be extremely painful and debilitating for the athlete, but it does not require emergency attention or cause major complications if further activity is necessary.

Signs and symptoms of a hip pointer include the following:

- Swelling at the site of injury.
- Discoloration at the site of injury.
- Pain and discomfort at the site of injury.
- The athlete may walk with a slight limp on the affected side. Coughing, sneezing, and laughing may also produce pain at the site of injury.

First aid care of a hip pointer involves the following:

1. Immediately apply ice to the injured area.
2. Have the athlete rest and avoid activity that involves the lower extremities.

Hip pointer Contusion and associated hematoma to the superior/anterior portion of the iliac crest.

Osteitis pubis Inflammation of the pubis symphysis joint, causing pain, possible dysfunction, and degeneration.

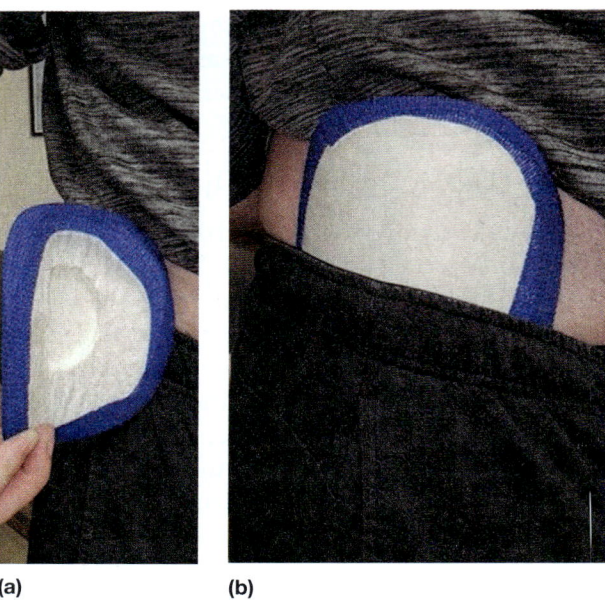

(a) (b)

Figure 14.6 An athlete inserts a hip-pointer pad.
Courtesy of Cindy Trowbridge.

3. If the injury is severe, walking with crutches may be necessary for a few days.

Long-term care for this type of injury is rather simple. The contusion has in most cases caused minimal damage to an area where several muscles attach directly to bone tissue. The muscular attachments in the abdominal region are the cause of pain when the athlete coughs, sneezes, or laughs. The player will usually be able to participate on a limited basis within 1–2 weeks, depending on the severity of the injury. It is important to note that, if an athlete wishes to continue participating in sports while recovering from a hip pointer, the area should be padded well so that further damage cannot occur if a similar incident happens before recovery is complete. Padding this area can be easily accomplished by securing a doughnut-shaped piece of foam padding over the area (Figure 14.6). Additionally, it is helpful to place hard plastic over the doughnut pad to provide even more protection to the area.

Osteitis Pubis

Another type of skeletal injury to the pelvic area is **osteitis pubis**, a condition resulting from continued stress and possibly some degeneration in the symphysis pubis joint (Figure 14.7). This injury is commonly a result of overuse and chronic strain on the joint.

The Pelvic Girdle

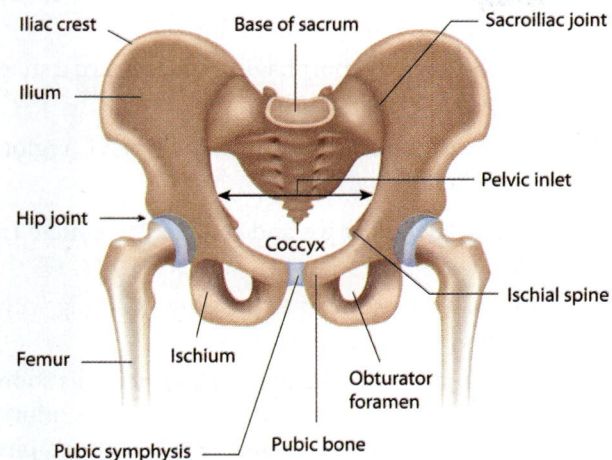

Figure 14.7 Common sites of hip injuries.
© Alila Medical Media/Shutterstock.

Sports in which the participant is required to kick, twist the upper body, or have frequent lateral movements during participation produce a greater number of these injuries. The largest numbers of osteitis pubis injuries are reported in soccer, rugby, football, and ice hockey players (Classie & Best, 2022). Osteitis pubis is a difficult injury to diagnose because of the many muscles and structures in the pelvic area, resulting in a delayed diagnosis or an undiagnosed problem (Gomella & Mufarrij, 2017; Via et al., 2019).

The athlete will complain of an insidious onset of pain that worsens progressively. The athlete may indicate that the pain is in the groin area (unilateral or bilateral) and complain of testicular or scrotal pain along with anterior pubic, suprapubic, or even hip pain when experiencing osteitis pubis (Gomella & Mufarrij, 2017; Via et al., 2019). An athlete complaining of these symptoms should be referred to the appropriate doctor for complete evaluation. Because this is a chronic problem, first aid is typically not necessary, but the athlete benefits from rest, ice, and anti-inflammatory medications, such as ibuprofen. This disorder typically responds well to therapy, with very few if any long-term side effects. An athlete may take anywhere from 3 months to a year to return to preinjury functioning levels. If osteitis pubis is diagnosed by the physician at early onset, the time frame for full return to activity may be reduced because treatment is initiated early. Athletes who do not respond to conservative therapy may be candidates for surgery.

Injury of the Sacroiliac Joint

The sacroiliac (SI) joint, which is the articulation between the sacrum and the pelvis (Figure 14.7), is a common site of pain in the posterior aspect of the pelvis. Movement at this joint is limited because of the configuration of the bones and numerous ligaments. This joint can present problems for the athlete if it becomes completely immobile or inflamed from an injury or other problem (Schnebel, 2018). Injuries resulting in an immobile SI joint require specific movement techniques by an educated professional to restore the normal motion in the joint.

Hip Dislocation

Infinitely more serious is a **hip dislocation**. This injury is actually quite rare in athletic events; however, it may occur to an athlete participating in contact sports (Patsiogiannis & Giannoudis, 2021). If a violent collision occurs between two players or a player and another object (e.g., the boards surrounding a hockey rink), this type of injury can happen. Typically, when this injury occurs, the hip joint is in flexion, and the force is applied through the femur. Most often, the hip dislocates posteriorly, and the athlete experiences extreme pain and loss of movement in the affected extremity.

Signs and symptoms of a dislocated hip include the following:

- Abnormal pain at the site of injury.
- Swelling at the site of injury, with a palpable defect.
- Knee of the involved extremity is angled toward the opposite leg.
- This injury is typically quite visible to the observer.

First aid care of a dislocated hip involves the following:

1. Treat for possible shock.
2. Immobilize the athlete and transport to the nearest medical center.
3. Care should be given to monitor blood flow to the leg at all times.

Hip dislocation Head of the femur fully displaces from the acetabulum.

Soft-Tissue Injuries

Because of the size and functions of the musculature in the hip and pelvic region, soft-tissue injuries are not very common in sports. The ligamentous support of the hip, sacrum, and other structures in the area is very strong; as a result, sprains rarely occur here. However, several muscles attach in the area of the pelvis, including the musculature on both the anterior and posterior aspects of the thigh, and these are subject to avulsion.

Avulsion Fractures

The possibility of muscle avulsions during forceful activity always exists. Skeletally immature athletes are more prone to **avulsion fractures** around the hip because their tendons are stronger than their cartilaginous growth centers. The mechanism of this type of injury is a sudden near-maximal muscle contraction, which results in the tendon pulling off a piece of bone at the attachment site. In a skeletally mature adult, this action usually results in a torn muscle or tendon because the bone is stronger than the tendon. In the adolescent, the tendon is stronger than the bone, so the result is an avulsion fracture. Avulsion fractures occur more commonly in adolescents who participate in sports requiring short bursts of maximal muscle contraction, such as soccer, tennis, sprinting, or jumping (Fatakhov & Miranda-Comas, 2021; Vázquez-Galliano & Miranda-Comas, 2021). The injured athlete will complain of severe, localized pain and bruising (ecchymosis) at the site of the injury. Common sites of injury in the adolescent are the anterior inferior iliac spine where the rectus femoris attaches and the ischial tuberosities where the hamstrings attach.

Signs and symptoms of avulsion fractures in the pelvic region include the following:

- Pain and swelling at the site of injury.
- Inability to produce a specific movement that is usually accomplished easily.
- Point tenderness over the affected area.
- Movement of the muscle closer to its opposite attachment when contracted. This is not easily detected in many avulsion injuries.
- The athlete may report having felt or heard a snap or pop at the time of injury.

First aid care of avulsion fractures in the pelvic region involves the following:

1. Immediately apply ice and require the athlete to rest.
2. Limit motion as much as possible. Walking with crutches may be necessary.
3. Have the athlete evaluated by a physician as soon as possible to determine the extent of the injury if an avulsion fracture is suspected. Radiographs done by the physician will document the avulsion fracture.

Avulsion fractures are debilitating and should be treated conservatively to reduce the amount of scar tissue that can result. It is very wise to allow an athletic trainer or physical therapist to rehabilitate the athlete according to the recommendations of a physician. Without proper treatment and rehabilitation, this type of injury can be a problem in an athlete's future career.

Other Hip Problems

Hip problems such as labral tears and impingement syndromes are becoming more common among all types and ages of athletes. Radiographic studies have shown that athletes participating in soccer and hockey are more likely to have bony deformities to the femoral head, which can lead to labral and impingement injuries (Knapik et al., 2019). Now that we are aware of the potential for hip injury in athletes, this information will assist the medical community in becoming more progressive in the prevention and treatment of these injuries in all populations. **Labral tears** of the hip occur in both the athletic and the general population. In the athletic population, most labral tears result from trauma; repetitive, excessive hip motions (e.g., soccer, hockey, basketball, and dance); and/or femoroacetabular impingement (Vázquez-Galliano & Miranda-Comas, 2021). Athletes experiencing this injury generally complain of anterior hip or groin pain, and some may indicate buttock or leg pain (Chahla et al., 2018). Cianci and

---

Avulsion fracture Piece of bone is pulled off by tendons or ligaments likely due to strong forces.

Labral tear Tear in cartilage surrounding hip or shoulder joint.

colleagues (2019) suggested that a strain injury of the rectus femoris muscle may result in a concomitant tear of the acetabular labrum (particularly in highly active pediatric patients). Treatment for labrum tears consists of rehabilitation and/or surgery depending on the tear. If a tear of the labrum exists, the physician will want to follow the progress of the athlete closely to ensure a safe return to sports participation (Cianci et al., 2019).

Femoroacetabular impingement (FAI) can be a major cause of hip pain in an athlete (DiSilvestro et al., 2020; Gwathmey & Lewis, 2019). The FAI injury is a result of the femoral head not being congruent with the acetabulum. When the hip is being heavily utilized in sports participation, the resulting trauma to the noncongruent bony structures results in hip pain and loss of movement. It is postulated that this problem not only causes immediate pain and loss of movement but can also result in osteoarthritis in populations such as ballet dancers and ice hockey goalies (Charbonnier et al., 2011; Gwathmey & Lewis, 2019). Signs and symptoms of FAI include generalized anterolateral hip pain, either unilaterally or bilaterally (depending on the activity); sharp pain when turning (especially toward the affected side); and pain from prolonged sitting or rising from a sitting position and entering or exiting a car. The athlete will need to be referred to the team physician or their personal physician, who will start with a physical examination, radiographs, and other diagnostic testing (Gwathmey & Lewis, 2019; Vázquez-Galliano & Miranda-Comas, 2021). Treatment for FAI is rehabilitation and/or surgery.

Athletes who participate in excessive running as a part of their sport can experience what is known as **snapping hip syndrome.** Snapping hip is an abnormal sensation around the lateral hip area that occurs when the athlete moves the hip in a specific direction (Vázquez-Galliano & Miranda-Comas, 2021). Usually, there is little if any pain associated with a snapping hip. This problem is attributed to one of the muscles in the lateral hip riding over the top of the greater trochanter of the femur. The structures that could be involved include the iliotibial band, tensor fasciae latae, and gluteus medius. There could be subluxation of the hip or labral tears that induce extra movement of the femur during locomotion. The possibility of a problem occurring in the intra-articular area could produce a snapping hip sensation. Injuries such as labral tears, articular cartilage injury, intra-articular bodies, or other similar problems could be discovered via radiography (Vázquez-Galliano & Miranda-Comas, 2021). Typically, treatment consists of stretching tightened muscles that may contribute to the snapping sensation and correcting any biomechanical deviations of the area (Vázquez-Galliano & Miranda-Comas, 2021). The physician may also recommend anti-inflammatory medications to the athlete.

Some researchers have suggested a surgical release of some of the fibrous bands sliding over the greater trochanter, which can result in some relief for the athlete. This surgical intervention has been shown to have a low recurrence rate and a high rate of patient satisfaction (Randelli et al., 2021). However, most physicians do not view surgical intervention as the first line of treatment for snapping hip syndrome.

Trochanteric bursitis is another rare problem experienced by some athletes. The trochanteric bursa is a fluid-filled sac that covers the trochanter of the femur (lateral side of hip) and prevents irritation during motion from overlying structures, including the gluteus medius muscle and iliotibial band. It is a problem seen most often in middle-aged people, but athletes, especially runners, are becoming more prone to trochantericbursitis. This bursitis is usually a result of either acute trauma to the lateral hip or repeated microtrauma to the musculotendon attachments with secondary inflammation of the trochanteric bursa in the area (Vázquez-Galliano & Miranda-Comas, 2021). The iliotibial band is a likely source of the problem if it is tight and the athlete continues to run even when experiencing signs and symptoms of inflammation. When an athlete is experiencing the onset of trochanteric bursitis, he or she will initially complain of pain over the greater trochanter followed by pain radiating down the anterior or lateral thigh and to the buttock region. Most athletes benefit from stretching the iliotibial band and the low back area in the proximity of the SI joints

---

Femoroacetabular impingement (FAI) Pinching of tissues around the hip joint due to the femoral head not being congruent with the acetabulum.

Snapping hip syndrome A lateral hip pain with only certain motions caused when soft tissue "snaps" over the greater trochanter of the femur.

Trochanteric bursitis Bursitis of the trochanter bursa due to tight lateral soft tissue of the hip.

and taking a nonsteroidal anti-inflammatory drug. For some athletes, it may be necessary to pad the area if there is a chance of external trauma, such as falling or being hit by another athlete in the hip. On rare occurrences, athletes do not respond to conservative treatment and benefit from surgical management (Pianka et al., 2021). Few athletes will need surgery if proper treatment is initiated early in the injury cycle.

Injuries to the Male Genitalia

An injury that is experienced by male athletes and is typically transient in nature is **testicular contusion**. Most male athletes competing in contact sports considered high-risk activities for testicular trauma wear a cup protector. However, this device does not always provide complete protection, nor do athletes always wear one. When the athlete receives a contusion to the testicular region, there is extreme pain and usually a complete loss of mobility for a short period of time. Typically, this pain and the resulting partial loss of movement are transitory; however, severe damage, such as a ruptured testicle, can be caused by extreme trauma to the testicles (Chen et al., 2019; Fitch & D'Souza, 2021; Wang et al., 2016).

Signs and symptoms of testicular contusions include the following:

- Extreme pain and point tenderness.
- The athlete may get into the fetal position and grasp his testicles.
- The athlete will report a direct blow to the testicles.

First aid care of testicular contusions involves the following:

1. Allow the athlete to rest on the sideline until he is ready to return to activity.
2. In severe cases, apply ice, and allow the athlete to remain lying down in the locker room or athletic training facility when possible.
3. If there is swelling or lasting pain, refer the athlete to a physician as soon as possible.

Testicular contusion Bruise to the testicles from direct trauma.

Testicular torsion Twisting of the testicles from traumatic or nontraumatic events.

Hernia Protrusion of a part of an organ or tissue through an abnormal opening.

> ### WHAT IF ?
>
> You are coaching a high school sophomore in the high hurdles on a cool, rainy afternoon in early spring. As the young man completes a start and five consecutive high hurdles, he grabs the back of his right leg, just below the buttock, and falls to the ground in obvious pain. You go to his aid immediately, and, on examination, you note that he is extremely tender in the region of the ischial tuberosity (origin of the hamstring muscles). He reports that he felt something tear and heard a pop while crossing the last hurdle, with immediate sharp pain. He has no history of a previous injury to this region. However, he has been complaining of tight hamstrings for the past several weeks. What type of injury may be present? What should be done for first aid? Should this athlete be referred to a physician?

The pain and debilitation associated with injuries to the testicles are transitory and should resolve without much intervention in a relatively short period of time (typically a few minutes). If the pain and debilitating effects last much longer than a few minutes, the athlete must see a physician to determine whether severe damage has been sustained by the testicles at the time of injury.

Testicular torsion, or twisting of the testicles, can occur and should be recognized quickly; if this happens, the athlete should be referred to a physician immediately. One of the testicles may, for any number of reasons, get twisted; as a result, the blood supply is compromised to or from the area, causing swelling to occur in the testicular area. The swelling may become quite uncomfortable, and the athlete needs to be transported to a medical facility as quickly as possible for treatment. Swelling in the testicular area can have serious side effects if not cared for immediately (Hyun, 2018; Laher et al., 2020).

Hernias

A **hernia** is the protrusion of abdominal viscera (large intestines) through the abdominal wall, typically occurring in the groin area. Inguinal hernias are more common among males and femoral hernias among females (Reisner & Reisner, 2022) because of anatomical differences. Powerful movements associated with sport motion or weight training are often the cause of abdominal wall stress that can lead to hernias. Most hernias are detected during a preparticipation physical examination. However, an athlete who is suffering from a hernia most likely has an abnormal protrusion in the groin area and experiences pain in the groin. Males will often also experience pain in the testicles. Surgical repair of hernias is usually necessary because the abdominal wall viscera can suffer necrosis (death) if the hernia is left untreated. The athlete should seek proper medical advice promptly to discern how soon the hernia will have to be repaired.

Athletes can experience groin pain, athletic pubalgia, or "sports hernias" in which the posterior inguinal wall and **pubic aponeurosis** (neurovascular fascial sheath) are weakened without any protrusion of abdominal contents through the abdominal wall (Choi et al., 2016; Vázquez-Galliano & Miranda-Comas, 2021). The neurovascular fascial sheath often experiences minor tears in athletes competing in sports with high velocity accelerations and direction changes resulting in inflammation. In this situation, no palpable hernia is discovered during a routine physical examination, yet the athlete complains of continuing pain in the groin and lower abdominal regions. The athletic pubalgia/sports hernia is difficult to diagnose for the physician and usually exhibits diffuse, deep groin pain that does not have a specific onset and gradually gets worse as the days pass (Figure 14.8). The athlete may complain of pain along the inguinal ligament and into the rectus abdominus muscles.

It has been suggested that athletic pubalgia/sports hernias may be a common cause of chronic groin pain in athletes; however, there is now conflicting evidence relative to the exact cause of long-standing groin pain in athletes (Dempsey et al., 2021; Drager et al., 2020; Zuckerbraun et al., 2020). Athletic groin pain can come from multiple pathologies, including tendinopathies, osteitis pubis, nerve entrapment, sports hernia, and "undiagnosed chronic groin pain." Other researchers indicate that the sports hernia is one piece of a more complex syndrome sometimes referred to as groin disruption injury (Garvey et al., 2010). If, after a reasonable time period of conservative treatment, the groin pain is not resolved, medical advice should be sought. Athletic pubalgia/ sports hernia can respond to active rehabilitation (Abouelnaga & Aboelnour, 2019), but often require surgical

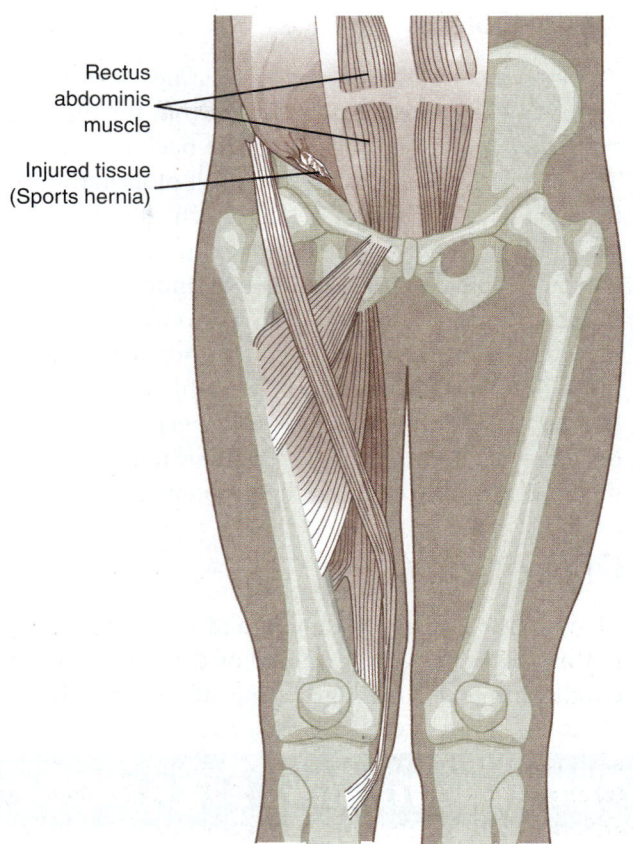

Figure 14.8 Sports hernia is generally damage to the deep muscle tissue under the rectus abdominis.

intervention; other coexisting conditions, such as femoral acetabular impingement or labral tears, should be ruled out (Drager et al., 2020).

In any case, groin pain must be addressed with proper treatment, and the course of action taken needs to follow a predetermined timeline. For example, conservative treatment of rest, ice, and stretching and a change in kicking biomechanics may be all that are needed to relieve groin pain in a soccer player. If the symptoms do not resolve over a 2-week period, it is time to have the team physician attend to the athlete. Athletes need to understand that many techniques for rehabilitation or surgical repair exist and new ideas are being reported in the literature every year (Zuckerbraun et al., 2020).

Pubic aponeurosis Complex fascial layer formed by a confluence of fibers from the rectus abdominus, adductor longus, gracilis, transversus abdominus and internal oblique (conjoint tendon), and external oblique.

Nerve Problems

A common complaint among many athletes is a burning or tingling sensation radiating from the hip and buttocks area and going down the back of the leg. These symptoms are often the result of irritation of the sciatic nerve (Petron & Makovitch, 2018). There are many reasons this nerve becomes inflamed or painful. Typically, if an athlete continues to pursue the activity that has caused the irritation, the pain will radiate farther down the leg to the foot and become more debilitating over time. The athlete must seek the advice of a physician and will need to rest and perform stretching and strengthening exercises, depending on the cause of the problem.

Prevention

Many of the injuries to the hip and pelvis discussed in this chapter can be prevented by the use of proper conditioning and strengthening of the associated musculature. Adequate and appropriate conditioning of athletes decreases the amount of stress placed on specific muscle groups and results in fewer soft-tissue types of injury. Groin strains, osteitis pubis, and some of the stress types of fractures can be avoided by conditioning and strengthening techniques that follow a planned protocol that includes proper rest periods. Rest is important for the body to repair micro damages incurred by the stresses of training.

Prevention of the hip pointer injury is generally a function of protective equipment as part of the uniform. Specifically, football pants include a hip pad, but other uniforms do not typically provide protection for injury to the anterior hip region. Athletes may ask the certified athletic trainer to custom-make a protective device if they have a tendency to experience constant external trauma to the area of the hip-pointer injury to reduce injury recurrence and long-term problems.

The use of proper shoes for each activity can be helpful in preventing slipping or sliding by the

Athletic Trainers SPEAK OUT

Why is it so important for athletic trainers to use evidence-based practice?

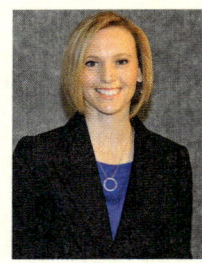

Courtesy of Sarah A. Manspeaker.

As an athletic trainer, the benefits to using evidence-based practice (EBP) include improving patient outcomes through relevant clinical practice and accurate decision-making, and contributing to the evidence base of our profession. Athletic trainers who are most successful typically incorporate the most up-to-date evidence to achieve the highest quality patient care. EBP has gained traction in health care over the past few decades within the athletic training profession and clinical practice. It has become a focus of educational programs at the professional and postprofessional levels and now resides in the requirements for continuing education and maintenance of the ATC® professional practice credential. The most widely accepted process of EBP includes the identification of a clinical question and then attempting to answer that question through evaluation of the available literature and research, referencing personal clinical experience, and consideration of the individual needs of your patients.

Unfortunately, even though there is wide acceptance of evidence-based athletic training practice, the profession is still viewed as having a clinical practice that is largely based on anecdotal evidence when compared with other health professions. Therefore, it is important for athletic trainers to learn, embrace, and apply evidence in clinical practice to achieve the best possible patient outcomes. More succinctly, athletic trainers should have the ability to utilize EBP to *connect theory to practice*. Translating evidence-based knowledge into clinical practice and creating a culture of clinical practice that uses evidence is very important for athletic trainers no matter what their job setting. Practicing with the best evidence can be done during real-time patient care by using clinical prediction rules, practice briefs, consensus statements, and position statements. The fusion of evidence with clinical practice should lead to improved patient outcomes and will help athletic trainers to solidify their place within a dynamic healthcare team.

—**Sarah Manspeaker, PhD, ATC**

Sarah Manspeaker is an Associate Professor in the Department of Athletic Training at Duquesne University in Pittsburgh, Pennsylvania.

athlete that might result in overstretching or tearing of muscles. Soccer players or similar types of athletes slipping on a wet field can sustain severe groin injury. Baseball players typically elect to wear a protective cup in an attempt to reduce trauma to the testicles from a hit by a baseball, and catcher's masks now include a throat protector to deflect the shock of a foul-tipped ball away from the throat. Other sports also have equipment specific to that sport that has been developed for protection from potential injury.

Even though injuries to the hip and pelvis are relatively uncommon as a result of sports participation, it is important to realize that injuries to this area do occur and that they can be debilitating to the athlete. Always consider the possibility of a severe injury when counseling an athlete about an injury to the hip and pelvis. First aid emergency care is important when treating these injuries. With most athletes, rehabilitation is also important if they are to continue the enjoyment of specific sports.

Review Questions

1. What type of joint is the hip joint?
2. Name the bones that make up the hip joint.
3. Explain the actions of the gluteal muscles.
4. Outline the location of the muscles that cause flexion, extension, adduction, and abduction of the hip.
5. List the bones in the hip area that are susceptible to fracture.
6. What structures are injured when an athlete suffers a hip pointer?
7. List the symptoms of osteitis pubis.
8. Explain the difference between testicular contusion and testicular torsion.
9. Define *hernia*, and outline what a coach should do if one is suspected.
10. What should be done if an athlete is experiencing pain radiating down the back of the leg?

References

Abouelnaga, W. A., & Aboelnour, N. H. (2019). Effectiveness of active rehabilitation program on sports hernia: Randomized control trial. *Annals of Rehabilitation Medicine, 43*(3), 305–313.

Aprato, A., Conti, A., Bertolo, F., & Massè, A. (2019). Slipped capital femoral epiphysis: Current management strategies. *Orthopedic Research and Reviews, 11*, 47.

Chahla, J., Kraeutler, M. J., & Garrido-Pascuai, C. (2018). Pelvis, hip, and thigh injuries. In C. C. Madden, M. Putukian, E. C. McCarty, & C. C. Young (Eds.), *Netter's sports medicine* (2nd ed., pp. 425–433). Philadelphia, PA: Elsevier.

Charbonnier, C., Kolo, F. C., Duthon, V. B., Magnenat-Thalmann, N., Becker, C. D., Hoffmeyer, P., & Menetrey, J. (2011). Assessment of congruence and impingement of the hip joint in professional ballet dancers. *American Journal of Sports Medicine, 39*(3), 557–566.

Chen, A. W., Archbold, C. S., Hutchinson, M., & Domb, B. G. (2019). Sideline management of nonmusculoskeletal injuries by the orthopaedic team physician. *Journal of the American Academy of Orthopaedic Surgeons, 27*(4), e146–e155.

Choi, H. R., Elattar, O., Dills, V. D., & Busconi, B. (2016). Return to play after sports hernia surgery. *Clinics in Sports Medicine, 35*(4), 621–636.

Cianci, A., Sugimoto, D., Stracciolini, A., Yen, Y. M., Kocher, M. S., & d'Hemecourt, P. A. (2019). Nonoperative management of labral tears of the hip in adolescent athletes: Description of sports participation, interventions, comorbidity, and outcomes. *Clinical Journal of Sport Medicine, 29*(1), 24–28.

Classie, J. A., & Best, T. M. (2022). Osteitis pubis. *UpToDate*. Retrieved from https://www.uptodate.com/contents/osteitis-pubis#

Dempsey, P. J., Power, J. W., MacMahon, P. J., Eustace, S., & Kavanagh, E. C. (2021). Nomenclature for groin pain in athletes. *British Journal of Radiology, 94*(1126), 20201333.

DiSilvestro, K., Quinn, M., & Tabaddor, R. R. (2020). A clinician's guide to femoacetabular impingement in athletes. *Rhode Island Medical Journal, 103*(7), 41–48.

Drager, J., Rasio, J., & Newhouse, A. (2020). Athletic pubalgia (sports hernia): Presentation and treatment. *Arthroscopy, 36*(12), 2952–2953.

Dutton, R. A. (2021). Stress fractures of the hip and pelvis. *Clinics in Sports Medicine, 40*(2), 363–374.

Fatakhov, E., & Miranda-Comas, G. (2021). The pediatric athlete. In G. Miranda-Comas, G. Cooper, J. Herrera, & S. Curtis (Eds.), *Essential sports medicine* (pp. 421–434). New York, NY: Springer, Cham.

Fedorak, G. T., Brough, A. K., Miyamoto, R. H., & Raney, E. M. (2018). The epidemiology of slipped capital femoral epiphysis in American Samoa. *Hawai'i Journal of Medicine & Public Health, 77*(9), 215–219.

Fitch, R. W., & D'Souza, D. (2021). Chest and abdominal injuries in football. In K. W. Farmer (Ed.), *Football injuries* (pp. 385–399). New York, NY: Springer, Cham.

Garvey, J. F. W., Read, J. W., & Turner, A. (2010). Sportsman hernia: What can we do? *Hernia, 14*(1), 17–25.

Gomella, P., & Mufarrij, P. (2017). Osteitis pubis: A rare cause of suprapubic pain. *Reviews in Urology, 19*(3), 156.

Gwathmey, F. W., & Lewis, D. (2019). Femoroacetabular impingement in the adolescent athlete. *Operative Techniques in Sports Medicine, 27*(3), 152–158.

Harris, J. D., Le, J., & Jotwani, V. (2020). Stress fractures of the hip and femur. In T. L. Miller & C. C. Kaeding (Eds.), *Stress fractures in athletes* (pp. 217–227). New York, NY: Springer, Cham.

Hyun, G. S. (2018). Testicular torsion. *Reviews in Urology, 20*(2), 104–106.

Knapik, D. M., Gaudiani, M. A., Camilleri, B. E., Nho, S. J., Voos, J. E., & Salata, M. J. (2019). Reported prevalence of radiographic cam deformity based on sport: A systematic review of the current literature. *Orthopaedic Journal of Sports Medicine, 7*(3), 1–8.

Laher, A., Ragavan, S., Mehta, P., & Adam, A. (2020). Testicular torsion in the emergency room: A review of detection and management strategies. *Open Access Emergency Medicine, 12*, 237–246.

Mathew, S. E., & Larson, A. N. (2019). Natural history of slipped capital femoral epiphysis. *Journal of Pediatric Orthopaedics, 39*, S23–S27.

Moini, J. (2020). *Anatomy and physiology for health professionals* (3rd ed.). Burlington, MA: Jones & Bartlett Learning.

Patsiogiannis, N., & Giannoudis, P. V. (2021). Acute fractures in sport: Pelvis and acetabulum. In G. A. J. Robertson & N. Maffuli (Eds.), *Fractures in sport* (pp. 339–359). New York, NY: Springer, Cham.

Petron, D. J., & Makovitch, S. A. (2018). Neurologic problems in the athlete. In C. C. Madden, M. Putukian, E. C. McCarty, & C. C. Young (Eds.), *Netter's sports medicine* (2nd ed., pp. 265–279). Philadelphia, PA: Elsevier.

Pianka, M. A., Serino, J., DeFroda, S. F., & Bodendorfer, B. M. (2021). Greater trochanteric pain syndrome: Evaluation and management of a wide spectrum of pathology. *SAGE Open Medicine, 9*, 1–12.

Randelli, F., Mazzoleni, M. G., Fioruzzi, A., Giai Via, A., Calvisi, V., & Ayeni, O. R. (2021). Surgical interventions for external snapping hip syndrome. *Knee Surgery, Sports Traumatology, Arthroscopy, 29*(8), 2386–2393.

Reisner, H., & Reisner, E. (2022). *Crowley's an introduction to human disease* (11th ed.). Burlington, MA: Jones & Bartlett Learning.

Schnebel, B. (2018). Thoracic and lumbosacral injuries. In C. C. Madden, M. Putukian, E. C. McCarty, & C. C. Young (Eds.), *Netter's sports medicine* (2nd ed., pp. 415–424). Philadelphia, PA: Elsevier.

Vázquez-Galliano, J., & Miranda-Comas, G. (2021). Pelvis, hip, and thigh injuries. In G. Miranda-Comas, G. Cooper, J. Herrera, & S. Curtis (Eds.), *Essential sports medicine* (pp. 293–313). New York, NY: Springer, Cham.

Via, A. G., Frizziero, A., Finotti, P., Oliva, F., Randelli, F., & Maffulli, N. (2019). Management of osteitis pubis in athletes: Rehabilitation and return to training: A review of the most recent literature. *Open Access Journal of Sports Medicine, 10*, 1–10.

Wang, Z., Yang, J. R., Huang, Y. M., Wang, L., Liu, L. F., Wei, Y. B., Huang, L., Zhu, Q., Zeng, M. Q., & Tang, Z. Y. (2016). Diagnosis and management of testicular rupture after blunt scrotal trauma: A literature review. *International Urology and Nephrology, 48*(12), 1967–1976.

Zuckerbraun, B. S., Cyr, A. R., & Mauro, C. S. (2020). Groin pain syndrome known as sports hernia: A review. *JAMA Surgery, 155*(4), 340–348.

CHAPTER 15
Injuries to the Thigh, Leg, and Knee

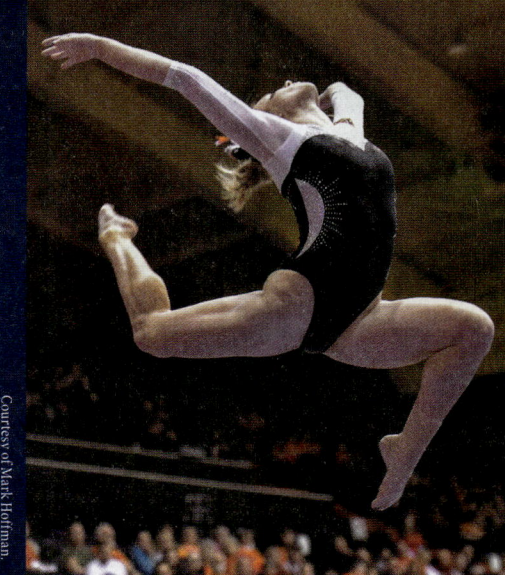

MAJOR CONCEPTS

Numerous injuries to the thighs and knees of male and female participants occur in a variety of sports. Because this area is difficult to protect and a major location of body contact between opponents, it can experience repeated trauma in contact and collision sports, thereby compounding earlier injuries. Knowledge about potential injuries to the thigh and knee is important for people working with young athletes. Untreated or poorly treated injuries to the thigh and knee, like any other injury, can have long-term consequences on the health of the athlete.

This chapter begins with a brief anatomy overview that covers the bones, ligaments, tendons, muscles, nerves, and blood vessels of the region; it goes on to describe the kinesiology of movements created by the muscles through the major joints.

The chapter continues with a description of soft-tissue injuries to the thigh that can become debilitating if not cared for properly, including contusions, strains, and various joint-related injuries. The knee joint, much like the foot and ankle, is required to provide maximum stability and mobility, thereby increasing the possibility of injury to this joint. The chapter covers problems such as osteochondritis dissecans, inflamed bursae, and patellar dislocation, along with injuries caused by chronic exercise. The knee joint is a complex configuration of bones, ligaments, and muscle tendons, any of which may be injured during sports participation. The chapter describes the four major ligaments of the knee and injuries to those ligaments; it also discusses the menisci (i.e., cartilage) within the knee joint, which can be injured during sports participation. The chapter concludes with a discussion of prophylactic and functional knee bracing.

Anatomy Review

The lower extremity is an area where many athletes experience some type of injury during their sports career. Injuries can occur to the thigh, knee, lower leg, ankle, and foot. The bones of this extremity include the femur, tibia, fibula, patella, and those of the foot (Moini, 2020). The femur, or thigh bone, is the longest, strongest, and heaviest bone in the body. It has a rounded, ball-like head that attaches to the hip bone with the help of a very strong network of ligaments. The head of the femur is attached to the shaft of the femur by a region known as the neck, which is susceptible to fractures. The femur becomes flatter and wider as it proceeds toward the knee joint, where it articulates with the tibia.

The thigh has a great deal of blood and nerve tissue going through it, both anteriorly and posteriorly. The anterior portion of the thigh contains the long saphenous vein and several branches of the femoral nerve. In the posterior section of the thigh are the deep femoral artery and the major nerve to the leg, the sciatic nerve. Most of the blood vessels and nerves are quite well protected by the musculature of the thigh.

The muscles of the thigh can be broken down into three basic regions. First, the anterior muscles of the thigh, commonly called the **quadriceps** (Figure 15.1), have two functions. The vastus lateralis, vastus intermedius, vastus medialis, and rectus femoris work together to extend the leg at the knee joint. Three of these muscles—vastus medialis, intermedius, and lateralis—attach on the femur and run down the thigh to the quadriceps tendon. The rectus femoris is the main working muscle of this group; it helps the hip flexors to flex the hip and assists in steadying the hip joint in this position. The rectus femoris attaches on the hip at the anterior inferior iliac spine and runs down the leg to the quadriceps tendon. The other muscle in the anterior portion of the thigh is the sartorius; it also attaches on the hip and runs somewhat diagonally down the thigh to the anterior medial portion of the tibial condyle. This muscle is

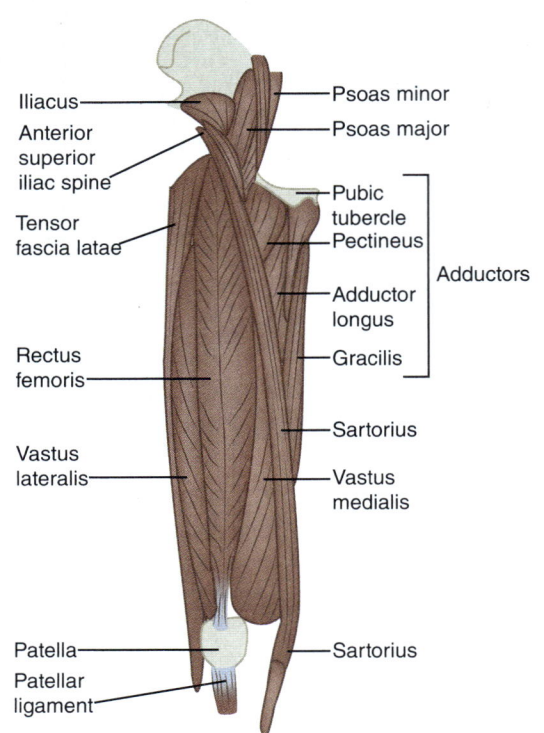

Figure 15.1 The quadriceps muscles of the anterior thigh serve two functions.

Quadriceps Group of four muscles (vastus medialis, vastus intermedius, vastus lateralis, and rectus femoris) of the anterior thigh that perform knee extension.

Hip adductors Group of three main muscles on the medial thigh that perform hip adduction (i.e., adductor magnus, adductor longus, adductor brevis).

Hamstrings Group of three muscles on the posterior thigh that perform knee flexion (i.e., semimembranosis, semitendinosis, and biceps femoris).

Tibiofemoral joint Articulation of the tibia and femur, or "knee" joint, specifically the articulation between both femoral condyles and both tibial condyles.

Patellofemoral joint Articulation of the patella and femur, specifically the posterior surface of the patella and the anterior surface of the femoral condyles.

responsible for flexing, abducting, and laterally rotating the thigh at the hip.

Next, the main muscles of the medial aspect of the thigh include the **hip adductors**—adductor longus, adductor brevis, and adductor magnus—and the gracilis (Moini, 2020). These muscles attach on the anterior aspect of the pelvis and run to the femur. The main function of these muscles is to adduct and help with flexion of the hip. The third group of muscles in the thigh are in the posterior aspect of the thigh and are commonly known as the **hamstrings**. The hamstrings include the semitendinosus, semimembranosus, and biceps femoris (Moini, 2020). All these muscles attach on the posterior aspect of the pelvis and run down the leg to the tibia. The main function of this group of muscles is to flex the leg at the knee. Table 15.1 lists the thigh's muscle groups, actions, and innervations.

The knee is a very complex joint; it can be damaged through any number of accidents occurring during sports participation. The femur and the tibia articulate with each other here (**tibiofemoral joint**), and the patella and the femur also have an articulation (**patellofemoral joint**). The patella is a sesamoid bone,

Table 15.1
Main Muscle Groups, Actions, and Innervations of the Thigh

Muscle Group	Action(s)	Innervation
Quadriceps		
Rectus femoris	Knee extension	Femoral
	Hip flexion	
Vastus medialis	Knee extension	Femoral
Vastus lateralis	Knee extension	Femoral
Vastus intermedius	Knee extension	Femoral
Hamstrings		
Semitendinosus	Knee flexion	Tibial
	Knee internal rotation	
Semimembranosus	Knee flexion	Tibial
	Knee internal rotation	
Biceps femoris	Knee flexion	Long head—Tibial
	Knee external rotation	Short head—Common peroneal
Adductors		
Adductor longus	Adduction	Obturator
	Hip flexion	
Adductor magnus	Adduction	Obturator
	Hip flexion (adductor portion)	
	Hip extension (hamstring portion)	
Adductor brevis	Adduction	Obturator
Gracilis	Adduction	Obturator
	Hip flexion, internal rotation	
Abductors		
Gluteus medius	Abduction	Superior gluteal
	Hip internal rotation, flexion (anterior portion)	
	Hip external rotation, extension (posterior)	
Gluteus minimus	Abduction	Superior gluteal
	Hip internal rotation	

(continues)

Table 15.1 (continued)
Main Muscle Groups, Actions, and Innervations of the Thigh

Muscle Group	Action(s)	Innervation
Others		
Gluteus maximus	Hip extension	Inferior gluteal
	Hip external rotation	
Sartorius	Knee flexion	Femoral
	Hip abduction, external rotation, flexion	
Tensor fasciae latae	Hip flexion, internal rotation	Superior gluteal
	Knee extension	

which means that it is totally enclosed within a tendon, in this case the quadriceps tendon. The patella does not articulate with the tibia. Many ligaments support the knee joint; however, four major ligaments serve as the primary stabilizers. They include the tibial, or medial, collateral ligament; the fibular, or lateral, collateral ligament; the anterior cruciate ligament; and the posterior cruciate ligament (Figure 15.2).

The tibial (or medial) collateral ligament extends from the medial epicondyle of the femur down to the medial condyle of the tibia. The fibular (or lateral) collateral ligament begins at the lateral epicondyle of the femur and extends to the head of the fibula. The fibular collateral ligament is the stronger of the two. Both ligaments help limit motion and disruption of the knee joint when movement at the joint is in a side-to-side direction, which is medically termed *valgus* (i.e., knock-knees) and *varus* (i.e., bowlegs).

The cruciate ligaments, unlike the collateral ligaments (which are located on the medial and lateral aspects of the knee joint proper), are situated on the inside of the joint.

The anterior cruciate ligament attaches on the anterior portion of the intercondylar area of the tibia and runs superiorly and posteriorly to the internal aspect of the lateral femoral condyle. The posterior cruciate ligament attaches on the posterior aspect of the intercondylar area of the tibia and runs superiorly and anteriorly, passing the anterior cruciate ligament on the medial side and attaching to the internal aspect of the medial femoral condyle. The function of these two ligaments is primarily to reduce or prevent anterior and posterior displacement of the femur or the tibia.

Two semicircular fibrocartilaginous disks, commonly called cartilage and more scientifically termed the **menisci**, are located within the space between the tibia and femur. The menisci assist with the lubrication and nourishment of the knee joint, aid in the

Menisci Fibrocartilaginous structures within the knee joint for protection of the condyles.

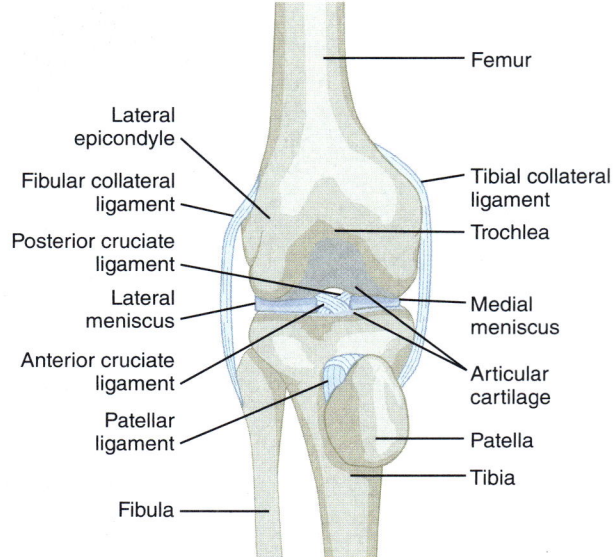

Figure 15.2 Major ligaments of the knee joint.

distribution of weight and stress applied to the joint surfaces, and help with the biomechanics of the joint (Markes et al., 2020). Serious injuries to these disks, specifically the medial and lateral menisci, have caused the demise of many athletic careers. Orthopedic surgeons can repair some meniscus tears, and other tears they will carefully trim to maintain as much healthy tissue as possible. Thus, athletes can and do continue to participate in athletics after meniscus injury, surgery, and rehabilitation.

Tendons of the muscles mentioned earlier in the description of the thigh run across the knee. Between the tendons and bone are several bursae, which reduce the friction of muscle tendons rubbing over a prominent area of bone, thereby adding some padding for the exposed bony areas of the knee.

Common Sports Injuries

Injuries to the thigh and knee can occur in almost any sport. In addition, this area can sustain injuries that are a result of overuse, trauma caused by an opponent, or trauma produced by the power and explosive movements required in some sports. Because of the structure and function of the knee, it can be an often-injured joint, and knee problems, not properly treated, have caused a great many athletes to shorten their athletic careers.

Because the knee is part of a complex mechanical system that includes the foot, ankle, lower leg, hip, and pelvis, there are times when another part of this system causes problems that can eventually be exhibited in the knee. For this reason, it is wise to obtain competent medical advice when athletes are experiencing knee pain or chronic problems with the joint.

Skeletal Injuries

Femoral Fractures

The femur is the longest bone in the body and is therefore subject to being fractured; however, **femoral fractures** require a great deal of force and are not common occurrences in sports. If a fracture does occur to the shaft of the femur as a result of sports participation, the injury is quite obvious; the athlete is in a great deal of pain, and ambulation will be difficult with the affected leg (see Figure 15.3). The athlete should not attempt to walk on a femoral fracture. In such instances, the athlete must be immediately transported

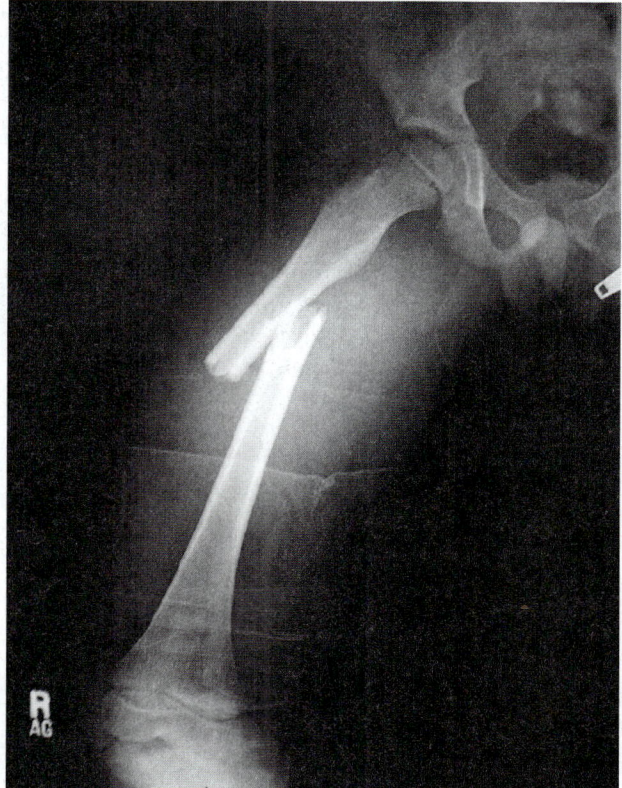

Figure 15.3 Femoral fracture of the right leg.

to the nearest medical facility with the leg splinted and without bearing any weight on the affected limb. A femoral fracture requires urgent medical attention because the initial trauma can lead to multiple problems, including a lack of circulation, blocked nervous innervation, the potential of shock, and other urgent medical issues (Schultz & Egol, 2021).

The neck of the femur can also be fractured. This can occur more often in sports than a fracture of the shaft, although neither happens frequently in healthy athletes. Older children and teenagers are at greater risk because a fracture in the area of the femoral neck can potentially affect a growth plate. Among younger athletes these fractures can be the result of direct trauma or overuse (Schultz & Egol, 2021). If direct trauma is the cause, the athlete typically had a foot planted and then got hit in the hip or upper thigh with a great deal

Femoral fracture Fracture of the femur, which can be in several different areas of the bone.

of force. When this injury does occur, it needs to be evaluated by a physician as soon as possible. In any athlete, one complication of a fracture in the neck of the femur is **avascular necrosis** (i.e., tissue death) of the femoral head; this is caused by a decrease in the blood supply to the bony portion of the femoral head. Avascular necrosis can present 6 months to 2 years after a femoral neck fracture. Although rare, avascular necrosis can become a severe, complex pathological condition that may include severe deformity and chronic hip subluxation (Li et al., 2021; Schultz & Egol, 2021).

Signs and symptoms of a fracture of the femur include the following:

- Pain at the site of injury.
- Difficulty ambulating on the affected leg.
- Swelling and/or deformity may occur.
- The athlete may report a traumatic event as the cause.
- The athlete may report having heard or felt a severe pop or snap at the time of injury.

First aid care of a femoral fracture involves the following:

1. Be prepared to treat the athlete for shock if necessary.
2. Splint the injured leg, preferably with a traction splint.
3. Apply sterile dressings to any related open wounds.
4. Monitor vital signs and circulation to the lower leg.
5. Arrange for transport to the nearest medical facility.

Patellar Fractures

Other skeletal problems that may arise include **patellar fractures** and dislocation of the knee or tibiofemoral joint. Although the patella can be fractured, this is not a common occurrence in sports participation.

Avascular necrosis Tissue death due to lack of blood supply.

Patellar fracture Fracture of the patella, which can be in several areas of the bone.

Dislocation of the tibiofemoral joint Complete separation of the tibia and femur joint ("knee joint"), which is usually visually obvious and a medical emergency.

In most cases, a patellar fracture is caused by violent trauma, and the athlete is incapacitated for a short period of time following the trauma. There is a great deal of pain associated with this injury, and the athlete will need to see a physician as soon as possible (Aitken, 2021). Because the patella is a sesamoid bone, the blood supply is limited, resulting in a longer healing time for such an injury. It is also possible to fracture the growth cartilage of the patella during the adolescent years. This may not be as obvious as a patellar fracture in an older individual because the young athlete may have no obvious deformity and maybe able to walk relatively normally and without pain. However, this injury may have repercussions later if it is not treated appropriately by an orthopedic physician as soon as possible after the injury (Aitken, 2021).

Dislocation of the Tibiofemoral Joint

Dislocation of the tibiofemoral joint is possible and, in some instances, can compromise the blood flow to the lower leg. If there is a dislocation of the tibiofemoral joint, it would be outwardly apparent, and the athlete would experience marked pain. This injury must be splinted, and the athlete referred to the nearest medical facility without delay. Circulation and nerve innervations to the knee and lower leg must not be compromised for even a brief period of time, or significant tissue damage will ensue (Herickhoff & Safran, 2019).

Soft-Tissue Injuries to the Thigh

Most of the soft-tissue injuries to the thigh are either the result of contact with an opponent or explosive movement by the athlete causing a self-inflicted muscle strain. Many sports, such as football and hockey, use some type of protective padding to prevent contact with an opponent to the thigh region. However, complete prevention is not always possible, and injuries do occur.

Myositis Ossificans

When an athlete receives a blow to the quadriceps muscle group from an opponent's knee, hip, or other body part or there is a contusion to the musculature from some other violent force (internally or externally), bleeding and damage often occur within the muscle fibers. Depending on the force of impact and the muscles involved, the contusion may be of varying degrees of severity. In any case, the athlete must be counseled about the care of this injury and the long-term complications of improper care of a muscular contusion, which can result in a condition called **myositis ossificans**. The initial muscular contusion causes bleeding within the muscle; if not cared for properly or further damage occurs, there is an increase in the amount of blood that collects in the same area. The body utilizes a natural process to remove the extra blood in the muscle; however, continued insult and bleeding in the area can result in calcification within the muscle and abnormal bone growth, possibly leading to further disability (Vázquez-Galliano & Miranda-Comas, 2021).

Signs and symptoms of a muscular contusion include the following:

- The athlete will report a forceful impact to the area.
- Muscular tightness and swelling may be present.
- The athlete has decreased ability to forcefully contract the muscle.
- The athlete has difficulties in ambulating with the affected leg.

First aid care of a muscular contusion involves the following:

1. Apply ice and compression immediately.
2. If the injury is severe, place the athlete on crutches.
3. Have the athlete rest and avoid any contact with the area.

With this type of injury, the athlete must be allowed plenty of rest and time to permit the natural bodily processes to remove blood from the area so that healing will be complete. Early controlled movement of the contused muscle assists in regenerating the muscle when the athlete is ready to return to participation. The early mobilization in this case must be well controlled, and the athlete should not be allowed to participate in full-contact practice or competition until complete healing has occurred. Because further direct contact to the area may increase the risk of myositis ossificans, the area should be padded if the athlete continues to participate. Moreover, the player should be well aware of the long-term consequences of continued trauma to the area and should initiate treatment quickly if additional insult occurs.

Muscular Strains to the Thigh

Almost any of the muscles in the thigh region are susceptible to strains. Most of the strains to athletes, however, are to the hamstrings and adductor muscles (Palermi et al., 2021; Vázquez-Galliano & Miranda-Comas, 2021). Strains to the adductor muscles are commonly known as groin pulls. Most strains occur to the muscle itself and not to the tendon. Such strains are usually the result of muscles being stretched too far, which generally occurs in the adductor muscles. However, strains can be the result of miscommunication or an imbalance of strength between **agonist muscles** and **antagonist muscles**, which is the case with many muscle strains involving the hamstrings.

If the muscle is stretched too far, the fibers of the muscle will be damaged and bleeding will occur; the result is loss of contractibility, stiffness, and impaired movement. Because both the quadriceps and hamstring muscles cross both the hip and knee joint, there is more chance for miscommunication between agonist and antagonist muscles during running and jumping. For example during a vertical jump or a sprint, the quadriceps musculature is contracting causing the knee to extend while the hamstrings are also contracting causing the hip to extend. Unfortunately, this combined motion puts the hamstring a risk because it is the weaker muscle. The hamstring musculature can be strained and damaged as it is overloaded when it contracts from an elongated position. The quadriceps musculature can also suffer damage as an athlete tries to control their landing from a jump because the knee will flex, thereby stretching the quadriceps in an effort to absorb the shock of the landing, and the hamstrings will contract at the hip to help maintain an upright trunk position; however, the quadriceps will eventually contract again to prevent a collapse to the ground. The overloading of the elongated quadricep muscle will often result in a strain to the musculature. Typically, the hamstrings are the weaker of the

> **Myositis ossificans** The abnormal calcification or ossification of bone within muscle tissue after an injury.
>
> **Agonist muscles** Muscles that are considered the prime movers of a joint.
>
> **Antagonist muscles** Muscles that counteract the action of the agonist muscles.

two groups; therefore, this is the musculature that is usually strained resulting in subsequent bleeding and hematoma formation.

Many athletes experience chronic tightness and repetitive strains to the muscles of the thigh adductor (groin) region. Specifically, the adductor brevis, longus, and magnus muscles can exhibit problems, especially in athletes participating in activities requiring multiple changes in speed and/or direction. It is not uncommon for a track, soccer, football, or volleyball athlete to complain of tight, sore, or strained muscles in the groin region. The groin muscles are critical movers in speed and change-of-direction movements and can require extra time to warm up and prepare for competition. Athletes must give special attention to these muscles as they prepare for practice or competition.

These thigh injuries can be debilitating if not cared for properly and quickly (see **Time Out 15.1**). Typically, when a strain to one or more of the thigh muscles occurs, the athlete feels a sharp pain in anterior

TIME OUT 15.1

Case Study of a Ruptured Rectus Femoris Muscle

There is always a chance that a muscle injury can be more severe than first expected. The soccer player in this case study thought he had severely contused and strained his quadriceps muscle group during a soccer match when an opponent stepped on his thigh. There was abnormal swelling and a great deal of pain associated with the initial injury. Standard first aid procedures included ice, compression, and rest until the athlete attempted to play again on a wet field; at one point, when he planted his leg to start running, he felt something tear. At that point, he decided to take some time off to let the injury heal. Months later, when the athlete was still having problems with pain and a lack of contractile ability, it was discovered that the injury to the quadriceps muscle was much more severe than thought during the initial evaluation.

In this case, the rectus femoris muscle had torn from its attachment at the patellar tendon and had not been repaired in time to salvage the muscle attachment. As shown in Figure 15.4, the muscle belly of the rectus femoris muscle draws up the leg when the athlete forcefully extends the lower leg. This athlete now must deal with a weak quadriceps mechanism and a strange feeling in his thigh each time he contracts his quadriceps muscles in that leg. This injury has ended his participation in collegiate soccer.

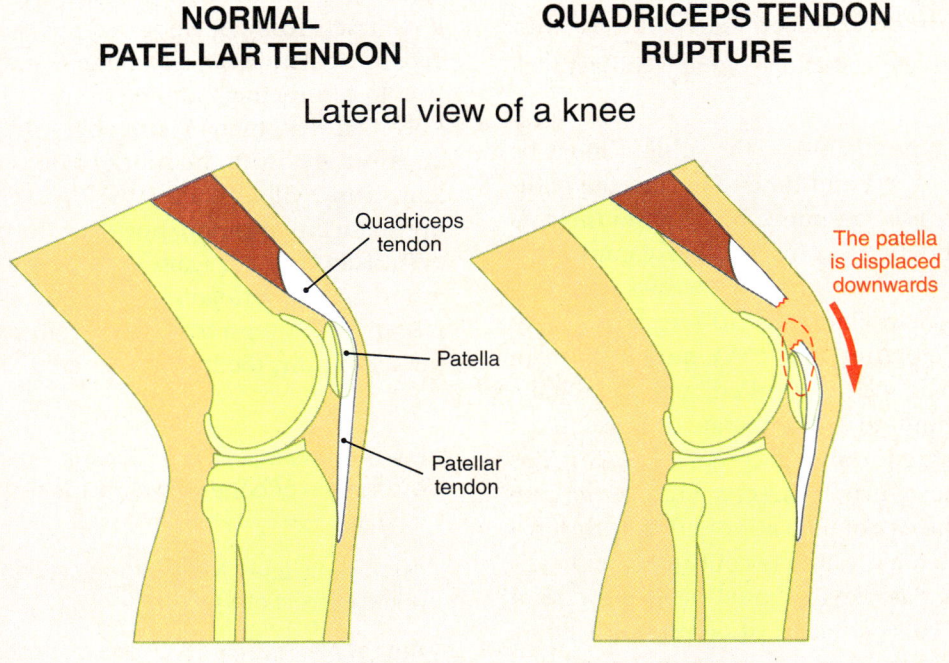

Figure 15.4 Ruptured quadricep tendon.

(quadriceps), posterior (hamstrings), or medial (groin) aspects of the thigh, they may also report a "tearing" feeling. Not long after this incident, the athlete will complain of soreness, stiffness, and a lack of movement in the area. At times, even with continued use in even the most restricted situation, the muscle or muscles take a long time to heal completely. Healing takes so long because the muscles affected are being used unconsciously for many daily activities in movements that cause small microtraumas, which do not allow the damaged muscle to heal. To this end, constant adherence to the proper treatment regimen is necessary until a complete recovery is made.

During and after recovery, athletes need to implement a stretching program that specifically targets the quadriceps, hamstrings, and adductor muscles. To reduce scarring of the affected muscles, stretching must be an integral part of the recovery from this and any other muscle strain injuries.

Signs and symptoms of muscle strains to the thigh include the following:

- A sharp pain in the affected muscle.
- Swelling and inflammation in the immediate area.
- Weakness and inability of the muscle to contract forcefully.
- After a few days, there may be discoloration of the area.
- In severe cases, a visible defect is noted in the muscle.

First aid care of muscle strains to the thigh involves the following:

1. Apply ice and compression immediately.
2. Have the athlete rest and use crutches if necessary.
3. Have the athlete evaluated by a member of the medical team.

Proper care and rehabilitation for any injury to the thigh is important. Because a strain to the hamstrings, quadriceps, or groin muscles is not considered serious, these injuries sometimes are not rehabilitated properly. The result can be a shortened career for the athlete because of repeated injuries and an inability to return to high levels of sport function. Therefore, it is essential to follow a structured rehabilitation program

WHAT IF ❓

You are coaching a junior high school basketball game. During the first half, your starting guard drives in for a layup, colliding with an opponent. The point of contact was her left thigh, which was struck severely by her opponent's knee. On further examination, you note tightness and swelling in the quadriceps muscles and an unwillingness by the athlete to put weight on her leg. Based on this history and the signs and symptoms, what would you conclude? What would be the appropriate first aid in this situation?

Athletic Trainers SPEAK OUT

How have residency programs enhanced the preparation of athletic trainers?

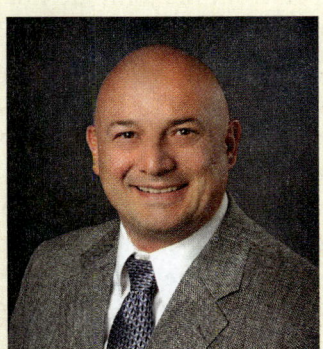

Courtesy of Forrest Pecha.

To better understand how residency programs have enhanced the preparation of athletic trainers, we must first understand what a residency program is and what it is supposed to do. The breadth of entry-level athletic training educational knowledge is wide; however, the depth is shallow. Residency programs are developed to create depth of knowledge and advanced skill sets to advance the preparation of athletic trainers through a planned clinical and didactic educational program. They should be focused on patient-based specialization preparing the resident as an advanced practice healthcare provider. They are not and should not be intended as an alternative to graduate assistant programs, provide a labor source for an institution, or an employer-based on-the-job training program. *Residency* is defined as advanced medical training in a specialty area of medicine.

In following the existing medical education model our healthcare colleagues already incorporate, the Commission on Accreditation of Athletic Training Education (CAATE) has developed accreditation standards for postprofessional athletic training residencies. For physicians, The Accreditation Council for Graduate Medical Education (ACGME) sets standards for accreditation of medical residencies and fellowships. Only those programs that meet ACGME standards become accredited, bringing credibility and validity to their educational programming, and graduate the next generations of physician specialists. This post-professional education and training can also be found in pharmacy, physical therapy, nursing, and other allied healthcare professions.

The CAATE, consistent with the ACGME and the Institute of Medicine (IOM), developed six core competencies required for accreditation of athletic training residency programming: (1) Patient-Centered Care, (2) Interdisciplinary Collaboration, (3) Evidence-Based Practice, (4) Quality Improvement, (5) Healthcare Informatics, and (6) Professionalism. The CAATE has also identified eight focused areas of clinical practice as approved residency specialty areas: (1) Prevention and Wellness, (2) Urgent and Emergent Care, (3) Primary Care, (4) Orthopedics, (5) Rehabilitation, (6) Behavioral Health, (7) Pediatrics, and (8) Performance Enhancement. These may look familiar to other healthcare professionals; however, these specialty areas are and have been imbedded within athletic training education for decades.

Residency programs have enhanced the preparation of athletic trainers though their development and comprehensive educational programming. An athletic trainer who graduates from a CAATE-accredited postprofessional residency program is identified and considered a content specialist and advanced practice healthcare provider in the focused area of clinical practice from which they graduated. Although athletic training is in the early stages of postprofessional education, as compared to healthcare colleagues, we have been able to demonstrate evidence of advanced knowledge for those athletic trainers graduating from a residency program. Employers are seeking residency-trained athletic trainers, and placement rates for those athletic trainers graduating residency programs is nearly 100%. Through postprofessional residency programs, athletic training education is creating clinical specialists, aligning athletic training with other healthcare professions.

—**Forrest Pecha, MS, LAT, ATC, OTC, CSCS**

Forrest Pecha serves as the Director of Clinic and Outreach at Steamboat Orthopedic and Spine Institute in Steamboat Springs, Colorado.

---

individualized to the athlete and their injury (Palermi et al., 2021).

Patellofemoral Joint Injuries

Several injuries to the patellofemoral joint, both chronic and acute, can become debilitating if appropriate treatment is not instituted early. Early treatment and intervention are required if the athlete is to return to participation at peak level. Some of the problems causing injury are the result of faulty mechanics or growth in adolescents and are not caused by anything that could be prevented initially. Many of the injuries to the patellofemoral joint, however, can be helped via intervention by the athletic trainer or physician, and the

Osteochondritis dissecans (OCD) Condition in which a fragment of cartilage and underlying bone are detached from the articular surface; also called "joint mice."

athlete can participate at peak level when recovery is complete.

Osteochondritis Dissecans

Osteochondritis dissecans (OCD) has also been called "joint mice" because small pieces of bone that have been dislodged or chipped from the joint are floating within the joint capsule. In adolescents, OCD is a common cause of a loose body in the joint space. Damage to the joint surfaces caused by these osteochondral fragments can be a serious problem. When the joint surfaces are damaged and no longer make smooth contact with each other, further pain and joint damage are almost always inevitable. The piece of bone does not always have to be freely floating within the joint space; it may be partially dislodged yet still attached to the original bone and causing painful movement. If the piece of bone is freely floating within the joint space, it can cause a blocking or locking action that limits the movement at the knee joint. The causes of OCD are not fully understood, although most experts believe it is a direct result of some type of trauma (Fatakhov & Miranda-Comas, 2021). When OCD occurs in juvenile athletes, the athlete should be referred to a physician for diagnosis and determination of the course of treatment. Many juvenile athletes respond to conservative treatment, whereas others may require surgical intervention.

Signs and symptoms of OCD include the following:

- Chronic knee pain with exertion that is generalized.
- There may be chronic swelling present.
- The knee may lock if there is a loose body within the joint. The athlete may be unable to fully extend the extremity.
- The quadriceps group may atrophy.
- One or both femoral condyles may be tender to palpation when the knee is flexed.

First aid care of OCD involves the following:

1. Apply ice and compression.
2. If the athlete has difficulty walking or the knee is locking, have him or her use crutches.
3. Have the athlete see a physician for proper treatment.

Inflamed Bursae

A bursa is a small fluid-filled sac located at a strategic point in the body that assists in the prevention of friction between bony surfaces, tendons, muscles, or skin. There are numerous bursae in the knee joint; however, only a few are commonly irritated (Figure 15.5). A bursa can become inflamed as a result of trauma or infection. The inflammation of the bursa, or **bursitis**, can also be the result of chronic overuse and irritation of the bursa (McCarty et al., 2018). The prepatellar bursa is located just under the skin and above the patella and can be susceptible to direct trauma. In the case of trauma, a football player may hit a knee quite hard on another player's helmet or on the playing surface, thereby causing the prepatellar bursa to become swollen and enlarged (Figure 15.6).

Most of the other bursae—suprapatellar, superficial, and deep infrapatellar; pes anserine; and semimembranosus—located throughout the knee complex are also susceptible to chronic insult. The constant use of the legs and knees in some exercises or kneeling for long periods creates excessive friction in the area, and the bursae respond by becoming inflamed. It is also possible for these bursae to become inflamed from direct trauma, although this is not as common.

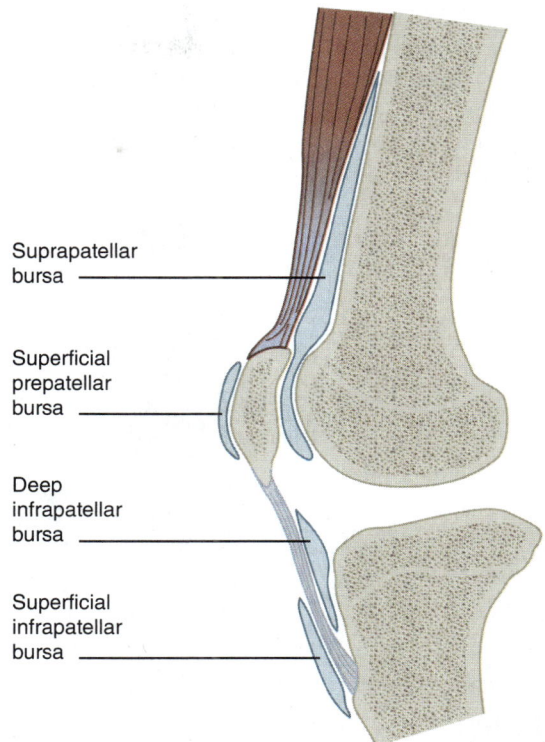

Figure 15.5 Commonly irritated bursae of the knee.

Signs and symptoms of an inflamed bursa include the following:

- Swelling and tenderness at the site.
- Increased pressure externally typically causes pain.
- The athlete may report direct trauma or a chronic buildup of swelling.

First aid care of an inflamed bursa involves the following:

1. Apply ice and compression.
2. Reduce activity for a short period of time.
3. In chronic cases, anti-inflammatory agents may be helpful.

Bursitis Inflammation of a bursa.

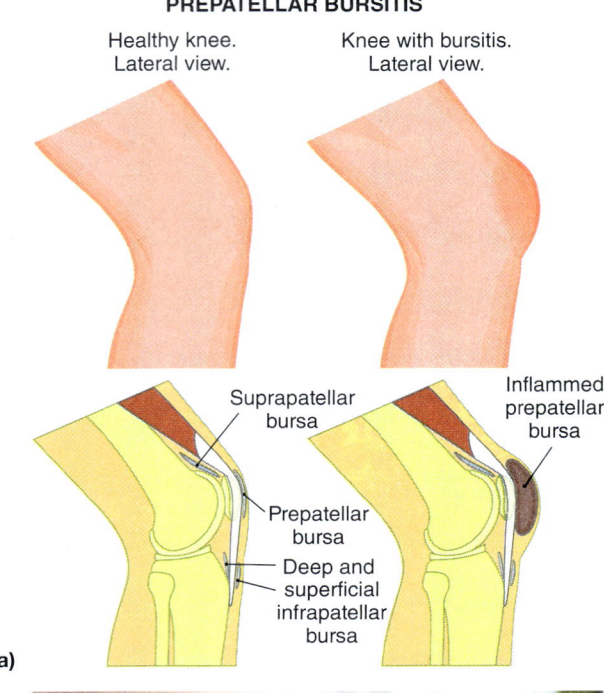

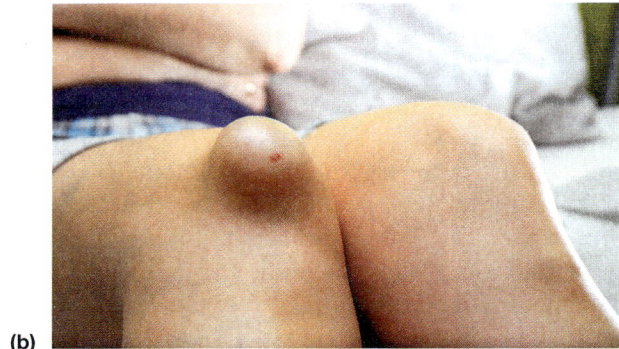

Figure 15.6 Prepatellar bursitis. **(a)** Illustration of prepatellar bursa and inflammation. **(b)** Young athlete with prepatellar bursitis.
(a) © Aksanaku/Shutterstock; (b) © Dziewul/Shutterstock.

Patellar Subluxation/Dislocation

When an athlete makes a quick, cutting motion to either side, a great deal of force is generated within the knee. If the sudden force is abnormal in nature, the patella can move laterally outside of the femoral groove, which can result in a

Patellar subluxation/dislocation Patella moves partially (subluxation) or completely (dislocation) out of its groove with the femur.

patellar subluxation/dislocation. In a subluxation, the patella will partially move laterally outside the femoral groove and may return by itself to the femoral groove while a patellar dislocation is when the patella is completely outside of the patellar groove and remains there (McCarty et al., 2018). Whether the patella remains dislocated or returns to its normal position spontaneously tends to be related to the distance it travels outside of its normal groove and the number of times this type of incident has occurred in the past. In some cases, if the athlete is a chronic subluxor, the patella will reduce (i.e., return to a normal position) without intervention. If it is the first time the patella has dislocated, it may or may not reduce spontaneously. In most instances of patellar dislocation, the athlete knows that the patella has moved out of its normal position, the knee will be flexed, and the athlete will experience pain and anxiety and will not want to move the leg or foot.

Signs and symptoms of a subluxation/dislocation of the patella include the following:

- Athlete will report a great deal of pain and an abnormal movement of the patella when the injury occurred.
- There will be associated swelling.
- The knee and patella will be extremely tender, and, on visual inspection, the patella will appear to be moved laterally to the normal position.

First aid care of a subluxation/dislocation of the patella involves the following:

1. Apply ice immediately.
2. Compression and elevation will also be helpful.
3. Splint the entire leg.
4. Arrange for transport to the nearest medical facility.

When a patellar dislocation occurs, the patella most often moves laterally. In addition, when an athlete experiences a patellar dislocation, soft-tissue damage to the medial aspect of the knee will most likely accompany it. If not cared for properly, this injury can become a chronic problem.

Osgood–Schlatter Disease and Jumper's Knee

The attachment of the patellar tendon at the tibial tubercle can be the site of two similar problems associated with athletes who do a great deal of jumping, although jumping is not a prerequisite to experiencing either Osgood–Schlatter disease or jumper's knee. These two injuries can be confused with one another if the athletic trainer does not look carefully at the age of the athlete and the signs and symptoms the athlete is experiencing. The main difference in these two conditions is the exact location of the injury. Osgood–Schlatter disease is typically a problem at the junction of the patellar tendon and the tibial tuberosity in the adolescent athlete. On the other hand, jumper's knee can exhibit itself at multiple sites within the patellar tendon along the entire tendon down to the tibial tuberosity attachment (Micheo, 2021).

Osgood–Schlatter disease is technically defined as an osteochondritis of the epiphysis of the tibial tuberosity. For this disease to occur, there must be a growth plate at the site of the tibial tubercle; consequently, this condition is unique to children and adolescents. Constant jumping creates a pull on the patellar tendon and its attachment at the tibial tuberosity. During the growth phase, there is an epiphyseal plate that is being pulled on simultaneously by the attachment of the patellar tendon at the tibia. This irritation causes inflammation and swelling to occur around the tibial tuberosity and may result in a bump (Figure 15.7). Usually this condition is managed by decreasing activity to manage pain as well as wearing a brace if determined helpful by the athlete. Pain and discomfort may persist for months until growth slows (Micheo, 2021).

Signs and symptoms of Osgood–Schlatter disease include the following:

- Pain and tenderness about the patellar tendon complex.
- Swelling in the associated area. This swelling may be more localized to the tibial tuberosity.
- Decreased ability to use the quadriceps for running or jumping.
- If the inflammation continues, the area over the tibial tuberosity may become more solid when palpated.
- Symptoms seem to be exacerbated by activity.

First aid care of Osgood–Schlatter disease involves the following:

1. Apply ice and compression to the area.
2. Have the athlete see a physician as soon as possible.
3. Rest is important until the inflammation subsides.

Jumper's knee is also an irritation of the patellar tendon complex between its attachments on the tibia and the patella. This problem is common to the athlete who must jump a great deal as part of sports participation. Typically, the athlete experiences pain at one of three sites within this complex. The pain may be localized over the superior or inferior pole of the patella or at the tibial tuberosity. Regardless of the exact location of this condition, the athlete complains greatly of pain associated with jumping (Micheo, 2021).

Signs and symptoms of jumper's knee include the following:

- Pain and tenderness about the patellar tendon complex.
- Swelling in the associated area, which may spread from the patella to the tibial tuberosity.
- Decreased ability to use the quadriceps for running or jumping.
- Symptoms seem to be exacerbated by activity.

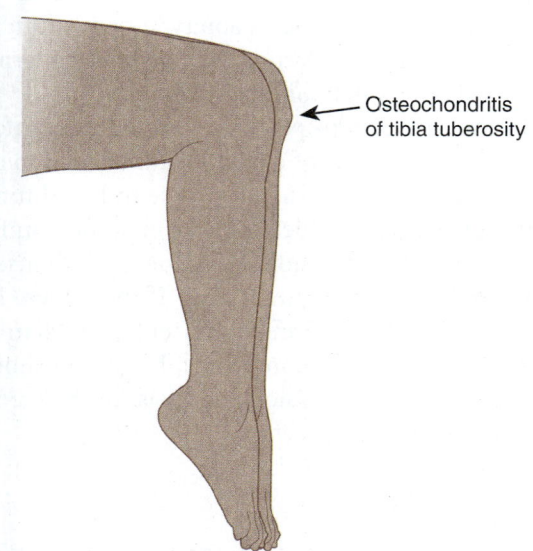

Figure 15.7 Osgood-Schlatter disease of the adolescent knee.

Osgood–Schlatter disease Epiphyseal inflammation of the tibial tubercle or apophysitis of the tibial tubercle.

Jumper's knee Irritation anywhere within the patellar tendon complex.

First aid care of jumper's knee involves the following:

1. Apply ice and compression to the area.
2. Have the athlete see a physician, who might prescribe anti-inflammatory medications.
3. Rest is helpful to the ailing athlete.

Patellofemoral Conditions

At times, athletes complain of nonspecific pain behind the patella. Patellofemoral syndrome is a fairly common injury, especially in runners, females, and adolescents, comprising 25–40% of all knee injuries evaluated in sports medicine clinics (Micheo, 2021). Sometimes, this pain is caused by an increased quadriceps angle, known as the Q angle, or the pain can be caused by any one of a number of other problems.

As shown in Figure 15.8, the **Q angle** is the difference between a straight line drawn from the anterior superior iliac spine and the center of the patella and one drawn from the center of the patella through the center of the tibia. This angle represents the vector of action between the quadriceps muscles and the patellar tendon. The larger this angle, the greater the chance of the patella being pulled too far laterally during extension of the knee; consequently, the patella rubs on the condyle of the femur, causing pain and irritation. It is generally accepted that this angle is larger in females because of the width of their pelvis (Sener & Durmaz, 2019). Most authorities report that a Q angle of 15–20° is acceptable. However, this is highly individual because there are often associated problems with patellar tracking, such as weak musculature or an abnormal patellofemoral skeletal configuration.

If there is abnormal patellofemoral configuration as a result of some skeletal, muscular, or mechanical dysfunction, it, too, can create retropatellar (i.e., behind the patella) pain of an **idiopathic** nature. A mechanical dysfunction may result in an abnormal amount of friction between the patella and the femur (Micheo, 2021).

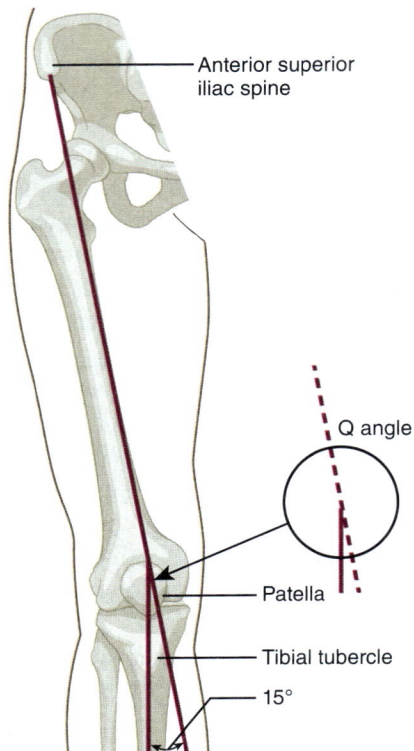

Figure 15.8 Measuring the Q angle at the knee.

This typically occurs in athletes, such as runners or gymnasts, who perform a great deal of repetitive movements in their sports activities. If this problem is allowed to continue, the possibility of chondromalacia exists. **Chondromalacia** is a softening and wearing out of the posterior cartilage surface of the patella. This condition is detrimental to the athlete's ability to perform in the future because there is associated pain and tenderness with this disorder that inhibit movement.

In the case of retropatellar pain and discomfort, the athlete complains of chronic pain and disability. There is no immediate first aid care to be administered; however, the athlete may gain some comfort from rest, ice, compression, elevation, and the use of nonsteroidal anti-inflammatories. If the athlete has an abnormally large Q angle, muscular imbalances, or other predisposing conditions, he or she should seek the advice of a physician to assist in the care of retropatellar pain disorder.

Menisci Injuries

Injury to the menisci in the active population is a fairly common episode, and, as people age, this injury appears to be more common. A population

---

Q angle Angle made by a line from the anterior superior iliac spine and the center of the patella and a line from the center of the patella to the center of the tibia.

Idiopathic Cause of the condition is unknown.

Chondromalacia Abnormal softening of cartilage between the patella and the femur.

> **WHAT IF** ❓
>
> You are teaching a junior high school weight-training class. One of the young boys in your class comes to you complaining of a chronic aching he has had for several days in the anterior knee, inferior to the patella, at the insertion of the patellar tendon. The boy reports the pain is worse in the mornings, especially when walking up and down stairs. Based on this history, what is the likely cause of this pain? What do you recommend for this child?

based study of active U.S. service members determined that age was a significant factor as those service members older than 40 years of age experienced injuries more than 4 times as often as those under 20 years of age (Jones et al., 2012). As mentioned earlier, the menisci have partial attachments to other structures about the knee joint, such as the cruciate ligaments, the tibial tubercles, and others; these partial attachments create problems when either the menisci or various other structures are damaged. If a violent force injures the medial collateral ligament, there is also the possibility of damage to the medial meniscus because of a partial attachment between the two structures.

More commonly, a meniscus is damaged by being torn as a result of quick, sharp, cutting movements that occur when the foot is stabilized so that the body does not turn (McCarty et al., 2021). This movement and others that cause excessive stress in abnormal planes can tear the meniscus at different points. A torn meniscus can affect the athlete in a variety of ways. Some athletes can function normally; others cannot completely extend the leg at the knee joint because of a tear in the meniscus that causes a blocking or locking effect.

Signs and symptoms of a suspected torn meniscus include the following:

- The athlete reports that a pop or snap was heard when the knee twisted.
- The athlete may not have any swelling, depending on the structures involved in the injury.
- The athlete may not complain of any pain.
- Depending on the severity of the injury, there may be a loss of range of motion and/or movement with a blocking or locking effect.
- The athlete may be able to continue participation with the injury.
- The athlete may report a feeling of the knee "giving out" at times.

First aid care of a suspected torn meniscus involves the following:

1. Apply ice and compression.
2. If the athlete has a blocked or locked knee, crutches should be used to aid in walking.
3. Encourage the athlete to see a physician as soon as possible.

Meniscus injuries do not necessarily have to end an athlete's playing season or career. New methods of surgery enable many athletes to return to participation relatively quickly (3-6 months). However, athletes should not be encouraged to finish the season with a suspected meniscus injury without first seeking the advice of a physician.

Knee Ligament Injuries

Several ligaments can be damaged through trauma; however, only four of the main ligaments are discussed here. The four that are most commonly injured are the medial (i.e., tibial) collateral ligament (MCL), the lateral (i.e., fibular) collateral ligament (LCL), the anterior cruciate ligament (ACL), and the posterior cruciate ligament (PCL). These ligaments are important stabilizers of the knee joint and are subject to many stresses, both internal and external. These ligaments, like any others in the body, can be traumatized and suffer first-, second-, or third-degree sprains (Micheo, 2021).

The mechanisms by which ligaments can be injured include a broad range of maneuvers, from the athlete making a quick, sharp, cutting step and twisting the knee excessively to having an opposing player hit the knee from one side. Athletes also may be kicked in the tibia or attempt to stop an opponent and forcefully drive the tibia anteriorly or posteriorly. All of these movements can damage one or more of the major supporting knee ligaments. It is important to remember that the knee can be injured by all types of forces, both internal and external, even when it does not appear that the athlete is in danger during an activity, such as running.

Collateral Ligament Injuries

One of the more common injuries to knee ligaments in athletics is a sprain to the MCL (Figure 15.9). This sprain occurs when an opponent is blocked or hits the athlete's leg and knee from the outside. The opponent lands forcefully on the lateral side of the knee, resulting in the joint being pushed medially (i.e., valgus stress); this force creates stress on the MCL beyond what it can withstand (Figure 15.10).

If just the opposite mechanism occurs and an opponent lands on the inside of a player's knee and pushes the joint laterally (i.e., varus stress), then the LCL is stressed beyond the normal level and sprained.

Both of these ligament injuries render the knee unstable in side-to-side movements. Because the knee is a hinge joint and little sideways movement occurs there, this would seem to create very few problems for the athlete. Although this may make logical sense, biomechanically, the collateral ligaments are important in assisting the knee with overall stability, and injury to either of these structures does result in significant instability in the knee (Grawe et al., 2018; Wierer et al., 2021). The more severe the ligament injury, the more unstable the knee is during movement and activity.

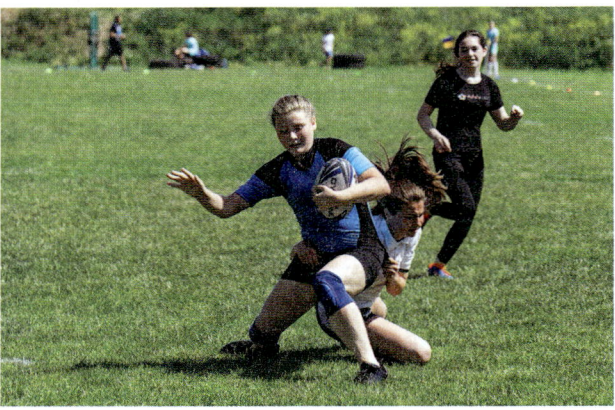

Figure 15.10 Excessive stress on the MCL.
© A_Lesik/Shutterstock.

Cruciate Ligament Injuries

The ACL can be injured by the tibia's forceful movement in an anterior direction (Figure 15.11). This injury can occur when an athlete is making a very

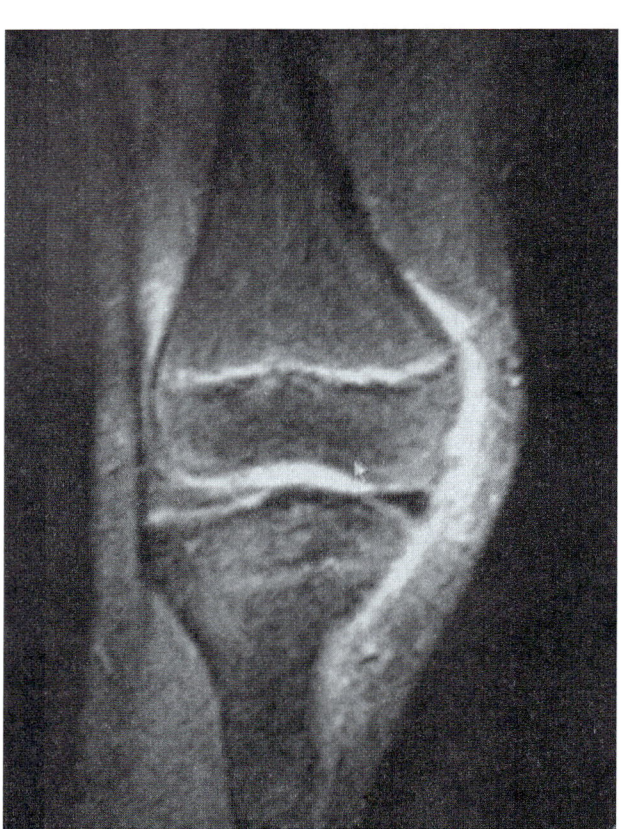

Figure 15.9 Coronal plane MRI image of a torn MCL. Note the brightly colored region along the medial side of the knee indicating damage to the MCL rather than other structures that appear darker in the image.
Courtesy of Kevin G. Shea, MD, Intermountain Orthopaedics, Boise, Idaho.

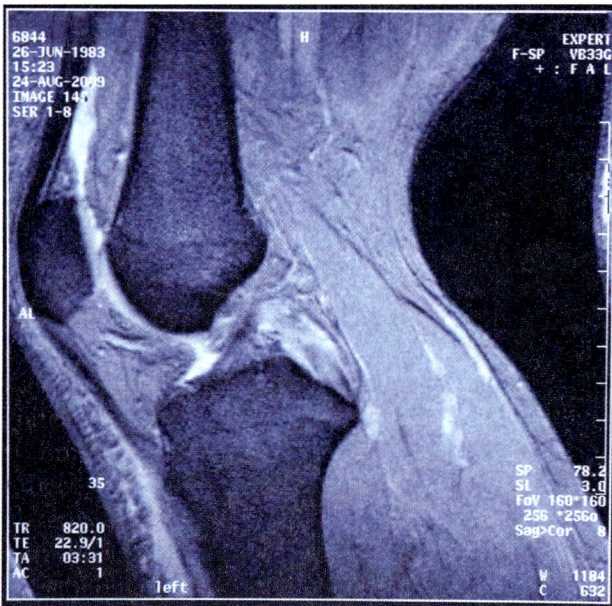

Figure 15.11 Sagittal plane MRI of a torn ACL in the right knee. Note the bright white region within the knee indicating damage to the ACL.
© Kondor83/Shutterstock.

quick, cutting motion on a hard surface; when an athlete gets hit from behind in the lower leg; or when the femur gets pushed backward while the tibia is held in place, as happens in contact sports. If the opposite occurs and the tibia is forced posteriorly, the PCL can be disrupted and injured. The main function of these two ligaments is to stabilize the knee in anterior and/or posterior directions (Micheo, 2021). In addition, quick rotational forces can injure the ACL. A rotational injury can result from a noncontact mechanism. For example, a football or basketball player may make a very quick change in direction with a firmly planted foot, and, if the upper body goes off balance and twists, the knee must absorb potentially abnormal forces built up by the twisting motion. If the circumstances are such that the soft-tissue structures in the knee cannot withstand the extra forces, they can be damaged.

The cruciate ligaments work in conjunction with the collateral ligaments to create a stable knee; any time one or more of these ligaments are injured, the knee becomes unstable. A large majority of ACL injuries are from noncontact mechanisms. It is now generally accepted that ACL injuries are multifactorial in nature. There are neuromuscular, biomechanical, anatomic, genetic, hormonal, environmental, and other factors that can be additive, which result in an ACL injury. Over the years, there has been a great deal of research into the basis for these noncontact ACL injuries. Much of the research has focused on the sport of soccer and specifically the female athlete. It appears that female soccer athletes are at a much higher risk for ACL injury compared to males, as recent research suggests that females have a three times greater rate ratio across both competition and practice, and that they also have a larger proportion of noncontact ACL injuries than their male counterparts (Gupta et al., 2020). Overall, ball sports such as basketball, volleyball, soccer, and handball exhibit more noncontact ACL injuries than sports such as judo where the mechanism of injury is contact related (Takahashi et al., 2019). And when similar high school sports are compared across genders, female softball, basketball, soccer, and volleyball players all experience more knee ligament sprains than males (Brant et al., 2019).

Each year, the amount of sports injury data increases due to a number of organizations' efforts. High school sports injury data are collected by the National High School Sports-Related Injury Surveillance Study Group (Datalys, n.d.), college sports injury information is available through the National Collegiate Athletic Association (NCAA), and each professional sports organization maintains injury data specific for that professional sport. The NCAA maintains an injury database on its website to assist with an understanding of injury epidemiology of NCAA athletes. For the years 2004–2005 through 2012–2013, the NCAA determined that most ACL injuries occurred to women via a noncontact mechanism as compared to a contact mechanism for males. The greatest annual rate of ACL injury for males occurred in football and, for females, occurred in lacrosse (Agel et al., 2016). In the NCAA and the National Football League, injury rates to the ACL appear to increase when the athlete is participating on an artificial surface (Loughran et al., 2019; Mack et al., 2019). Recurrent or rerupture of a primary ACL injury occurs in 1–11% of all athletes; however, recent research has noted that male football players, female gymnasts, and female soccer players have the highest reoccurrence rate across all sports (Gans et al., 2018). It should be noted that, in almost every study being published, the authors are calling for more research on ACL injuries.

Female athletes experience three to six times more noncontact ACL injuries, but researchers have been unable to discern the exact reasons for this phenomenon (Parsons et al., 2021). Parsons and colleagues (2021) wrote an excellent review of the literature regarding this question. The authors note that the risk factors for ACL injury need to be more fluid and integrated rather than binary (i.e., intrinsic or extrinsic factors). Typical intrinsic factors are anatomy, genetics, strength, and neuromuscular system qualities; extrinsic factors often include weather, facilities, opponents, and playing surface. However, Parsons and colleagues (2021) present that these factors interact and may influence the gender disparity in ACL injury, as oftentimes women's sports have lacked access to equipment and facilities that would allow for the development of strength and neuromuscular control. Therefore, risk factors should be considered modifiable and nonmodifiable. There are **environmental** bases for these injuries, including the surface, weather, footwear, and

> **Environmental** The aggregate of surrounding things, conditions, or influences related to one's surroundings.

shoe–surface interface research reports, and these are both modifiable and nonmodifiable. The **anatomic** rationale that has been and is currently being studied includes mass, joint laxity, pelvis and trunk actions, Q angle, posterior tibial slope, notch width, and foot pronation, which are typically considered nonmodifiable. The effect of sex **hormones** during the monthly menstrual cycle has received increased attention as both a modifiable and a nonmodifiable risk factor. The **neuromuscular** activity that continually occurs during movement, including strength and recruitment of muscle fibers, joint stiffness, and muscular fatigue, and the biomechanical rationale for noncontact ACL injury with an analysis of the planes of movement are modifiable and are often the focus of prevention programs. Looking at the overall picture of ACL injuries, a group of researchers and scholars gather regularly to review the results and discuss the direction of future research opportunities. The ACL Research Retreat VIII in 2019, produced recommendations regarding ACL injuries that focus on primary, secondary, and tertiary prevention of ACL injuries (Shultz et al., 2019). The attendees at the meeting divided into interest groups and provided updates relative to the most recent research findings. Some of the relevant information from this meeting includes the following:

1. **Risk factor assessment.** Risk factors for ACL injury can be divided into modifiable and nonmodifiable risk factors. Namely, the modifiable risk factors—those that are **neuromechanical** (neuromuscular and biomechanical), which help control movement of the trunk and lower extremity—have received much research attention. Cutting and landing with rapid deceleration, possibly in an upright position and especially when fatigue is present, increases the strain on the ACL due to anterior tibial forces, tibial femoral compression, and/or a combination of knee abduction and internal rotation moments. The research involving nonmodifiable risk factors—anatomy, genetics, hormones, and maturation—found that a smaller ACL and femoral notch and width, less collagen fiber density, genetics, and/or hormones that affect collagen metabolism and, thus, the structural intrinsic integrity of the ACL, may also be involved in ACL injury rates. Specifically, there appears to be a greater chance of ACL injury in the female athlete in the preovulatory as opposed to the postovulatory phase of the menstrual cycle. Finally, a portion of the retreat discussion involved **neurocognitive insufficiency** in which the suggestion was made that slower reaction time and cognitive processing and less spatial awareness may affect ACL injury.

2. **Screening.** Research has shown that ACL injury is more common in game situations as opposed to practices. Clinical screening for abnormal movement and addressing those deficits in a prevention program have been done in the past and proved to be helpful. Even though clinical screening tools, such as the Landing Error Scoring System, are found to be good indicators of possible future issues, they may be population specific to identifying risk.

3. **ACL injury prevention programs.** Neuromechanical characteristics can be positively affected by improved hip, core, and upper body mechanics. Multidynamic, warm-up–style prevention programs, which include balance, plyometrics, strength, education, technique/agility, and feedback training, appear to be effective in reducing ACL injury provided they are conducted two or three times per week for a minimum of 10–15 minutes. Compliance with these programs has been associated with a reduction in ACL injuries (Padua et al., 2018; Sugimoto et al., 2012).

Athletic trainers and coaches are interested in the prevention of noncontact ACL injury, and

Anatomic Pertaining to anatomy.

Hormones Various internally secreted compounds formed in endocrine glands that affect the functions of specifically receptive organs or tissues.

Neuromuscular Having characteristics of both nervous and muscular tissue.

Neuromechanical The interaction of the nervous system with mechanical activity that creates movement.

Neurocognitive insufficiency Slower reaction time and cognitive processing of movement patterns.

there has been a great deal of progress made in this arena since the early 2000s. Many researchers are now proposing that players, parents, coaches, administrators, and others responsible for any of the parameters of sports programs be well-versed in the types of and need for ACL injury–prevention programs (Padua et al., 2014; Shultz et al., 2019; Sugimoto et al., 2012). Most of the prevention programs target the female soccer player, but some programs encourage both male and female players to become involved in these prevention programs. It appears evident that the prevention programs targeted at enhancing the neuromuscular training are beneficial in reducing the number of noncontact ACL injuries in both female and male athletes, as a review of the literature indicates that prevention programs allow for a 50% reduction in the risk of all ACL injuries in all athletes and a 67% reduction in females (Webster & Hewett, 2018). Although there are barriers to the development of an effective ACL prevention program, it is important to engage an interdisciplinary team so long-term viability can be maintained (Padua et al., 2014).

Athletic trainers, coaches, athletes, and researchers are also interested in the increasing incidence of posttraumatic osteoarthritis (OA) in patients suffering from ACL injuries. Bodkin, Werner, Slater, and Hart (2019) noted that almost 1 in 8 patients undergoing ACL reconstruction seek further medical care within 5 years and are diagnosed with knee OA. Research in this area is growing regarding the causes, prevention, and treatment of posttraumatic OA because a patient with a knee injury is more likely to get a knee replacement and be younger when getting it than someone without a history of knee ligament injury (Khan et al., 2018).

Signs and symptoms of an injury to the knee ligaments include the following:

- Athlete reports that the knee was forced beyond its normal range.
- Athlete complains of pain at the site of injury.
- Swelling may occur in and around the knee.
- Athlete may complain of an unstable feeling in the knee.
- Athlete may report having felt a pop or tear or having heard a snapping sound.

First aid care of an injury to the knee ligaments involves the following:

1. Apply ice and compression immediately.
2. If the knee is unstable, have the athlete walk with crutches.
3. Have the athlete seek proper medical advice.

At times, an athlete will receive a blow from the lateral side that injures the MCL and ACL along with the medial meniscus or will experience a rotary injury that compromises the LCL, ACL, and lateral meniscus. These injuries have sometimes been called the "unhappy triad" or the "terrible-triad injury." Obviously, injuring all these structures creates a very unstable knee. Anytime an athlete has a suspected injury to knee ligaments, caution must be exercised, and care by the proper medical personnel is critical. Knee ligament injuries with or without surgery can take anywhere from 3–18 months to completely rehabilitate and are all very individual to the mechanism of the injury, any surgery, and the athlete.

There are so many types of knee injuries, and each of those injuries can be significantly different in severity. It is important to always work with the physician of the team or encourage the athlete and his or her parents to ensure that proper care and level of activity are followed. Table 15.2 provides a general outline of the type of care and possible activity level for athletes with knee injuries. This table is provided to assist the athletic trainer or coach in discussions with the physician caring

WHAT IF ❓

You are coaching a high school basketball game. It is late in the game; your team is on the defense, with their opponent's guard driving to the basket. Suddenly, your post player, who was attempting to block the opponent's jump shot, falls to the floor, grabbing her left knee. On further examination she states that, when she landed from jumping up to block the shot, her knee twisted, and she felt something snap inside. You note that she also states that her knee feels very unstable. Given this information, what would you conclude? What would be the appropriate first aid for this injury?

Table 15.2
General Suggestions for Participation of Athletes with Knee Injuries

Common Locations		Severity	Possible Implications for Participation*
Ligament	MCL	1st	Limit movements of knee to flexion and extension with hinge brace—avoid valgus stresses and extremes of flexion and extension.
		2nd	May need crutches; physician will determine length of time on crutches.
		3rd	Physician to determine course of action.
	LCL	1st	Hinge brace for protection and avoid extremes of flexion and extension.
		2nd	Brace and immobilization; physician will determine further treatment.
		3rd	Brace and immobilization surgery required for repair of ligament.
	ACL	1st	Immobilization and brace required initially; physician will determine activity levels.
		2nd	Immobilization followed by hinge brace to limit movement; surgery may be necessary.
		3rd	Immobilization followed by hinge brace to limit movement; surgery required for repair of ligament.
	PCL	1st	Limit movement of knee to flexion and extension.
		2nd	Limit movement of knee totally.
		3rd	Surgery required for repair of ligament.
Cartilage	Meniscus		Early surgical intervention recommended; physician should explain the rationale for early or delayed treatment of meniscus injury.
			Participation will depend on activity and pain tolerance; non-weight-bearing activities recommended.
	Hyaline		Early surgical intervention recommended; participation will depend on activity and pain tolerance; non-weight-bearing activities.
	Osteochondritis		Participation limited to activities that have reduced impact on the knee.
Tendon	Patellar/jumper's knee		Participation based on pain tolerance of the athlete and physician treatment options.
	Osgood–Schlatter Disease		Participation based on pain tolerance of the athlete and physician treatment options.
	Tendinopathies		Limited participation depending on activity and level of pain experienced; repetitive activity should be avoided.
Bursa	Bursitis		Participation based on pain tolerance and activity level. Repetitive activity should be avoided.

Patella	Dislocation	All participation contraindicated until physician clearance.
	Tracking	Participation allowed based on pain, inflammation, and treatment to correct problem
	Chondromalacia	Participation in repetitive activity movements limited—other activity based on pain tolerance—and weight lifting restricted.
Fracture	Tibia	No participation.
	Femur	No participation.
	Patella	No participation.

*Implications may vary greatly depending on the attending physician's diagnosis and standard of care philosophy.

for the injured athlete so that an activity level can be determined for the future participation of the athlete.

Prevention

The quest to prevent injuries to the leg and knee continues for athletes, coaches, and athletic trainers. As discussed earlier, the increase in female ACL injuries has resulted in many research teams looking for an answer or model for prevention of such injuries. In the future, research will continue to outline techniques that can prevent the various injuries to the thigh, leg, and knee.

The prevention of strain injuries to the musculature of the thigh and leg is very similar to the techniques used to prevent injury in other areas of the body that contain a great deal of muscle tissue. To many athletes, proper warm-up and stretching of the muscles to be used are important in preparing for activity. Not all athletes require stretching before an activity, but some find it beneficial to their overall participation. Correcting muscle imbalances is also important in preventing strains as a weaker muscle can be negatively dominated by a stronger muscle and experience injury easier.

Preventing knee injuries has become much more of a focus of the medical and allied health professionals. For many years and into the present day, a variety of bracing options purport to provide peripheral mechanical stabilization for the ligaments of the knee when forces are applied externally. Today, some football coaches require interior linemen and linebackers to wear bilateral prophylactic knee braces during practice and games. Knee bracing should be an individual choice for athletes. If athletes believe prophylactic knee bracing can benefit them, they should be provided the opportunity to use these devices. Knee braces continue to evolve and have been through many prototype tests and marketed units. Initially, the braces were designed to minimize medial and lateral stresses to the knee. As materials became available that were lighter and stronger than metal hinges taped to the athletes' legs, more options for knee protection became available.

The newest trend in prevention of ACL injuries is in using specific jumping and landing training techniques. Some authors suggest that specialized proprioceptive training programs can decrease the number of ACL injuries in athletes (Padua et al., 2018; Schultz et al., 2019; Webster & Hewett, 2018). Numerous jumping and landing training programs are being promoted by certified athletic trainers, strength and conditioning specialists, physical therapists, and other healthcare professionals. These programs are designed to enhance the dynamic function of the leg musculature. The concept of this type of training is to train the appropriate muscles in the legs to contract or relax at appropriate moments, with the idea that the muscles will assist the function of the ACL during activity. Many of the people promoting these programs claim that athletes (especially females) can benefit from this type of training and can reduce the chance of an ACL tear when they are participating in sports. The *Journal of Athletic Training* (Padua et al., 2018) recently published a position statement entitled "Prevention of anterior cruciate ligament injury." Padua et al. (2018) concluded that prevention training programs that protect the knee from excessive loading by improving biomechanics and neuromuscular control represent the best opportunity to reduce risk of ACL injury.

Prevention programs with multiple components, including strength, plyometrics, agility, flexibility, and balance performed regularly (2–3 times/week for 15–10 minutes) can reduce ACL injury rates up to 75% in females in high-risk sports like soccer and basketball (Padua et al., 2018).

Knee Bracing

There are several types of knee braces for various stages of knee protection – before injury, during injury recovery, and after surgery through the rehabilitation process. In terms of prevention of knee injury, there are well-known positions in certain sports that are more prone to knee ligament injury and for those reasons, some suggest preventative knee bracing is appropriate. While recovering from knee injuries such as tendinitis, there are braces that will support the knee. These can be worn during injury recovery and after the athlete returns to activity. Lastly, there are braces athletes wear immediately after surgery, called postoperative braces, which can limit range of motion to various degrees and protect the surgical repair. As the athlete progresses through rehabilitation after surgery, the brace will also be progressed to allow more motion yet provide stability. Finally, as the athlete is ready to return to sport, many will wear a functional knee brace, which controls transverse plane motion (i.e., twisting) often used in many athletic maneuvers.

One of the biggest controversies in sports medicine literature and in many athletic departments across the country is the use of prophylactic knee bracing with athletes. A **prophylactic knee brace** has two attachments: one above the knee and one below the knee, with either unilateral or bilateral supports running vertically on the medial and/or lateral sides. These braces are typically constructed of a lightweight material. The bracing is meant to augment the stabilizing effect on each side of the knee joint (Figure 15.12).

Reports of epidemiological and biomechanical studies on knee bracing have been published since

Prophylactic knee brace Braces used to prevent collateral ligament injuries or stabilize the knee, usually for linemen in football.

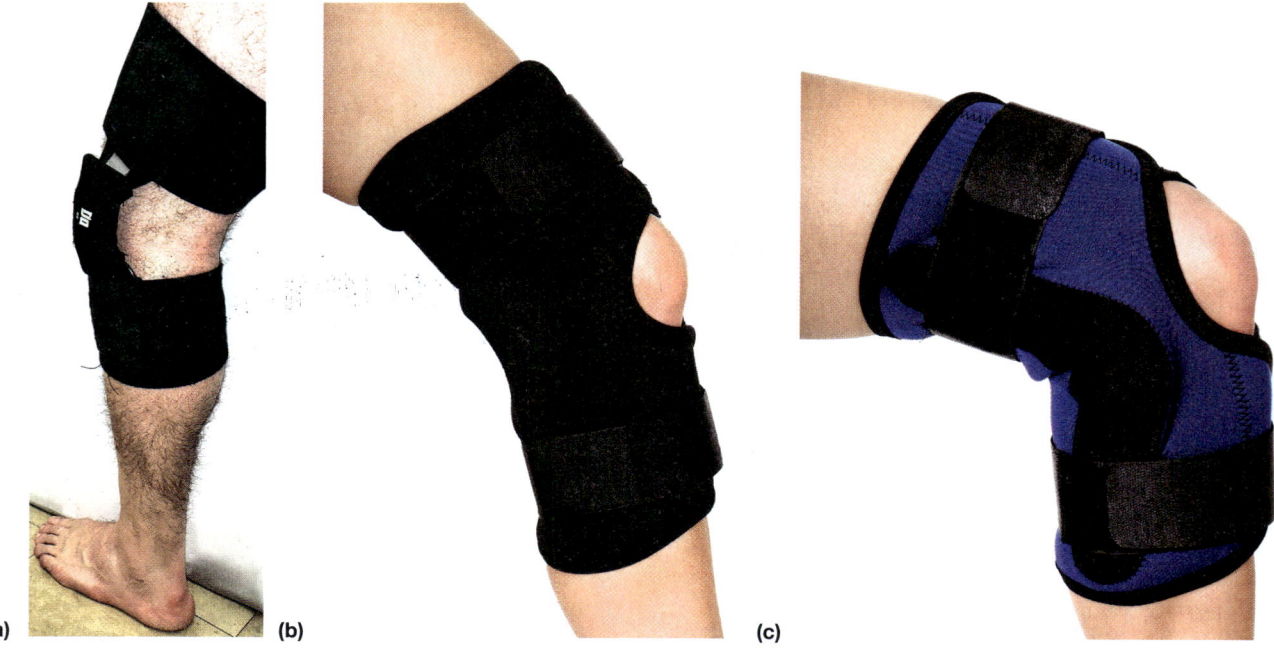

Figure 15.12 **(a)** An example of a prophylactic knee brace. **(b)** General neoprene knee sleeve. **(c)** Neoprene knee sleeve with medial and lateral bracing. The neoprene is useful in keeping the joint warm during exercise.
(a) Courtesy of Cindy Trowbridge; (b) and (c) © Poznyakov/Shutterstock.

the 1970s. Pietrosimone, Grindstaff, Linens, Uczekaj, and Hertel (2008) performed a systematic review of the knee brace literature spanning the years 1970–2006. In that 36-year time frame, they determined there were only seven published studies that met their criteria for scientific rigor. One part of their scientific rigor criteria was a direct comparison of braced to nonbraced collegiate football players. They concluded that there was insufficient evidence for or against the use of prophylactic knee bracing in college football. Many of the epidemiological studies have been criticized for lacking proper methods of study design. The biomechanical studies are criticized for not incorporating proper mechanisms and forces to study the effects of prophylactic braces.

Additionally, Rishiraj, Grindstaff, Linens, Uczekaj, and Hertel (2009) conducted a review of knee-bracing studies on the prophylactic and functional roles of injury prevention. They reviewed more than 200 published studies and came to a similar conclusion that there is a general lack of consistency in determining the effectiveness of either functional or prophylactic knee bracing (Rishiraj et al., 2009). One area of ongoing prophylactic knee brace research concerns the movement of the brace on the leg while the athlete is participating. In early studies, it was demonstrated that prophylactic braces can move up or down the leg, some more than others, and this movement can sometimes lead to negative changes in the muscle activity, biomechanics, speed, and overall agility of the athlete (Greene et al., 2000; Osternig & Robertson, 1993). This has led to poor compliance in wearing the braces by the athletes, and thus a lack of well conducted and published research in documenting the effectiveness of prophylactic knee bracing in athletes. More recent studies indicate some prophylactic braces and knee sleeves are better fitting and do not have a negative effect on athletes' performance (Baltaci et al., 2011; Mortaza et al., 2012).

The general consensus regarding prophylactic knee braces indicates that these braces are not completely successful in preventing knee ligament injury (Rishiraj et al., 2009; Salata et al., 2010). Therefore, the specific brace design and fit, plus the ideal situations for use, need to be determined by the athletic trainers and team physicians who are in direct contact with the athlete (Blecha et al., 2022).

Functional knee braces (i.e., braces specially constructed to assist an athlete who is returning to

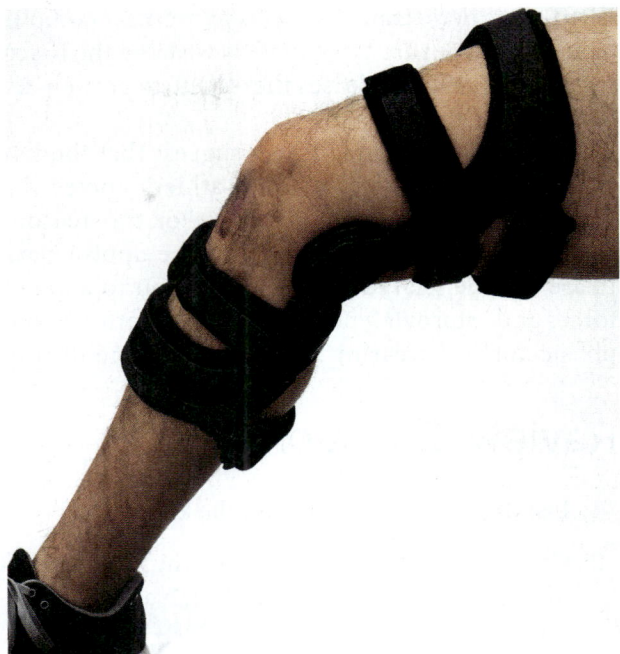

Figure 15.13 An example of a functional knee brace used after ligament surgery or later in the healing/rehabilitation process.
© W. Scott McGill/Shutterstock.

participation after a knee injury) appear to have a better record for assisting the athlete after surgical reconstructionas functional knee brace has been found to be beneficial in providing stability to the ACL repaired knee (Rishiraj et al., 2009). The functional brace (Figure 15.13) may initially slightly alter the biomechanics of the athlete's running, jumping, or landing, but the brace is constructed so that it provides some protection for the knee and minimizes future injury. After wearing the functional brace in practice for a week or more, the athlete will adapt to the feel of the functional brace and return to close to normal playing levels (Rishiraj et al., 2011). The athlete may be required by a physician to wear a functional knee brace after ACL reconstruction; therefore, the coach or athletic trainer will not be responsible for deciding whether the athlete should wear a knee brace. When the athlete is required to wear the brace during participation, the coach's or

Functional knee brace Braces used after a rehabilitation program while the athlete returns to sport.

certified athletic trainer's role is to monitor compliance and make sure the athlete is wearing the brace until the physician releases the athlete to participate without the brace.

On the other hand, others suggest that the tissues of the body won't adapt to athletic forces if a knee brace acts as a stress-shield. For this reason, rehabilitation without a brace at the appropriate phase is beneficial for tissue adaptation to applied forces and improving neuromuscular control. Some physicians feel wearing a functional brace during activity for only a year is warranted as more focus should be on regaining efficient neuromuscular control rather than potentially contributing to lower extremity compensation patterns by wearing a brace.

In summary, knee braces need to match the athlete's needs at various points in their activity or return to activity (Blecha et al., 2022), and ideally, but not in every case, athletes should be progressively weaned off of braces to re-instate tissue integrity and adaptability as well as neuromuscular control. (Nyland et al., 2016).

Review Questions

1. List the bones that comprise the knee joint.
2. Give the common name for the muscles located on the anterior portion of the thigh and list these muscles.
3. Give the common name for the muscles located on the posterior thigh region and list these muscles.
4. Give the common name for the muscles located on the medial aspect of the thigh and list these muscles.
5. Where do the quadriceps attach on the lower leg?
6. Define a *sesamoid bone* using the patella as an example.
7. Explain the articulation of the knee joint, including the involvement of the patella.
8. List and explain the attachments of the four main ligaments of the knee.
9. True or false? There are two menisci located in the knee joint.
10. Explain the first aid care for a severe contusion of the thigh.
11. Explain which muscles of the thigh can experience strains through athletic participation.
12. True or false? If the patella dislocates, it will not return to its proper position without surgical intervention.
13. Define *joint mice*.
14. What age group is most susceptible to Osgood–Schlatter disease?
15. Describe how to care for an athlete with jumper's knee.
16. What population is more susceptible to Q-angle alignment problems?
17. True or false? An athlete with a torn meniscus will always have a great deal of swelling in the knee joint after the injury.
18. Explain the mechanism by which the MCL and LCL are damaged.
19. Define and list the structures damaged if an athlete experiences a terrible-triad injury.
20. Explain why an athlete should or should not choose to use a prophylactic knee brace.

References

Agel, J., Rockwood, T., & Klossner, D. (2016). Collegiate ACL injury rates across 15 sports: National Collegiate Athletic Association injury surveillance system data update (2004–2005 Through 2012–2013). *Clinical Journal of Sport Medicine, 26*(6), 518–523.

Aitken, S. (2021). Acute fractures in sport: Knee. In G. A. J. Robertson & N. Maffuli (Eds.), *Fractures in sport* (pp. 227–244). New York, NY: Springer, Cham.

Baltaci, G., Aktas, G., Camci, E., Oksuz, S., Yildiz, S., & Kalaycioglu, T. (2011). The effect of prophylactic knee bracing on performance: Balance, proprioception, coordination, and muscular power. *Knee Surgery, Sports Traumatology, Arthroscopy, 19*(10), 1722–1728.

Blecha, K., Nuelle, C. W., Smith, P. A., Stannard, J. P., & Ma, R. (2022). Efficacy of prophylactic knee bracing in sports. *Journal of Knee Surgery, 35*(3), 242–248.

Bodkin, S. G., Werner, B. C., Slater, L. V., & Hart, J. M. (2019). Post-traumatic osteoarthritis diagnosed within 5 years following ACL reconstruction. *Knee Surgery, Sports Traumatology, Arthroscopy, 28*(3), 790–796.

Brant, J. A., Johnson, B., Brou, L., Comstock, R. D., & Vu, T. (2019). Rates and patterns of lower extremity sports injuries in all gender-comparable US high school sports. *Orthopaedic Journal of Sports Medicine, 7*(10), 2–7.

Datalys Center. (n.d.). High School Reporting Information Online (High School RIO™). Retrieved from https://www.datalyscenter.org/rio/

Fatakhov, E., & Miranda-Comas, G. (2021). The pediatric athlete. In G. Miranda-Comas, G. Cooper, J. Herrera, & S. Curtis (Eds.), *Essential sports medicine* (pp. 421–434). New York, NY: Springer, Cham.

Gans, I., Retzky, J. S., Jones, L. C., & Tanaka, M. J. (2018). Epidemiology of recurrent anterior cruciate ligament injuries in National Collegiate Athletic Association Sports: The Injury Surveillance Program, 2004–2014. *Orthopaedic Journal of Sports Medicine, 6*(6), 1–7.

Grawe, B., Schroeder, A. J., Kakazu, R., & Messer, M. S. (2018). Lateral collateral ligament injury about the knee: Anatomy, evaluation, and management. *Journal of the American Academy of Orthopaedic Surgeons, 26*(6), e120–e127.

Greene, D. L., Hamson, K. R., Bay, R. C., & Bryce, C. D. (2000). Effects of protective knee bracing on speed and agility. *American Journal of Sports Medicine, 28*(4), 453–459.

Gupta, A. S., Pierpoint, L. A., Comstock, R. D., & Saper, M. G. (2020). Sex-based differences in anterior cruciate ligament injuries among United States high school soccer players: An epidemiological study. *Orthopaedic Journal of Sports Medicine, 8*(5), 2325967120919178.

Herickhoff, P., & Safran, M. (2019). Knee dislocation in athletes. In F. Margheritini, J. Espregueira-Mendes, & A. Gobbi (Eds.), *Complex knee ligament injuries* (pp. 181–194). Berlin, Heidelberg: Springer.

Jones, J. C., Burks, R., Owens, B. D., Sturdivant, R. X., Svoboda, S. J., & Cameron, K. L. (2012). Incidence and risk factors associated with meniscal injuries among active-duty US military service members. *Journal of Athletic Training, 47*(1), 67–73.

Khan, T., Alvand, A., Prieto-Alhambra, D., Culliford, D. J., Judge, A., Jackson, W. F., Scammell. B. E., Arden, N. K., Price, A. J. (2018). ACL and meniscal injuries increase the risk of primary total knee replacement for osteoarthritis: a matched case–control study using the Clinical Practice Research Datalink (CPRD). *British Journal of Sports Medicine, 53*(15), 965–968.

Li, Z., Zhuang, Z., Hong, Z., Chen, L., He, W., & Wei, Q. (2021). Avascular necrosis after femoral neck fracture in children and adolescents: Poor prognosis and risk factors. *International Orthopaedics, 45*(11), 2899–2907.

Loughran, G. J., Vulpis, C. T., Murphy, J. P., Weiner, D. A., Svoboda, S. J., Hinton, R. Y., & Milzman, D. P. (2019). Incidence of knee injuries on artificial turf versus natural grass in National Collegiate Athletic Association American Football: 2004–2005 through 2013–2014 seasons. *American Journal of Sports Medicine, 47*(6), 1294–1301.

Mack, C. D., Hershman, E. B., Anderson, R. B., Coughlin, M. J., McNitt, A. S., Sendor, R. R., & Kent, R. W. (2019). Higher rates of lower extremity injury on synthetic turf compared with natural turf among National Football League athletes: Epidemiologic confirmation of a biomechanical hypothesis. *American Journal of Sports Medicine, 47*(1), 189–196.

Markes, A. R., Hodax, J. D., & Ma, C. B. (2020). Meniscus form and function. *Clinics in Sports Medicine, 39*(1), 1–12.

McCarty, E. C., Walsh, W. M., & Madden, C. C. (2018). Knee injuries. In C. C. Madden, M. Putukian, E. C. McCarty, & C. C. Young (Eds.), *Netter's sports medicine* (2nd ed., pp. 434–445). Philadelphia, PA: Elsevier.

Micheo, W. (2021). Knee injuries. In G. Miranda-Comas, G. Cooper, J. Herrera, & S. Curtis (Eds.), *Essential sports medicine* (pp. 315–340). New York, NY: Springer, Cham.

Moini, J. (2020). *Anatomy and physiology for health professionals* (3rd ed.). Burlington, MA: Jones & Bartlett Learning.

Mortaza, N., Ebrahimi, I., Jamshidi, A. A., Abdollah, V., Kamali, M., Abas, W. A., & Osman, N. A. (2012). The effects of a prophylactic knee brace and two neoprene knee sleeves on the performance of healthy athletes: A crossover randomized controlled trial. *PLOS One, 11*(7), 1–6.

Nyland, J., Mattocks, A., Kibbe, S., Kalloub, A., Greene, J. W., & Caborn, D. N. (2016). Anterior cruciate ligament reconstruction, rehabilitation, and return to play: 2015 update. *Open Access Journal of Sports Medicine, 7*, 21.

Osternig, L. R., & Robertson, R. N. (1993). Effects of prophylactic knee bracing on lower extremity joint position and muscle activation during running. *American Journal of Sports Medicine, 21*(5), 733–738.

Padua, D. A., DiStefano, L. J., Hewett, T. E., Garrett, W. E., Marshall, S. W., Golden, G. M., Schultz, S. J., & Sigward, S. M. (2018). National Athletic Trainers' Association position statement: Prevention of Anterior Cruciate Ligament Injury. *Journal of Athletic Training, 53*(1), 5–19.

Padua, D. A., Frank, B., Donaldson, A., de la Motte, S., Cameron, K. L., Beutler, A. I., DiStefano, L. J., & Marshall, S. W. (2014). Seven steps for developing and implementing a preventive training program: Lessons learned from JUMP-ACL and beyond. *Clinics in Sports Medicine, 33*(4), 615–632.

Palermi, S., Massa, B., Vecchiato, M., Mazza, F., De Blasiis, P., Romano, A. M., Di Salvatore, G. D., Della Valle, E., Tarantino, D., Ruosi, C., & Sirico, F. (2021). Indirect structural muscle injuries of lower limb: Rehabilitation and therapeutic exercise. *Journal of Functional Morphology and Kinesiology, 6*(3), 75.

Parsons, J. L., Coen, S. E., & Bekker, S. (2021). Anterior cruciate ligament injury: Towards a gendered environmental approach. *British Journal of Sports Medicine, 55*(17), 984–990.

Pietrosimone, B. G., Grindstaff, T. L., Linens, S. W., Uczekaj, E., & Hertel, J. (2008). A systematic review of prophylactic braces in the prevention of knee ligament injuries in collegiate football players. *Journal of Athletic Training, 43*(4), 409–415.

Rishiraj, N., Grindstaff, T. L., Linens, S. W., Uczekaj, E., & Hertel, J. (2009). The potential role of prophylactic/functional knee bracing in preventing knee ligament injury. *Sports Medicine, 39*(11), 937–960.

Rishiraj, N., Taunton, J. E., Lloyd-Smith, R., Regan, W., Niven, B., & Woollard, R. (2011). Effect of functional knee brace use on acceleration, agility, leg power and speed performance in healthy athletes. *British Journal of Sports Medicine, 45*(15), 1230–1237.

Salata, M. J., Gibbs, A. E., & Sekiya, J. K. (2010). The effectiveness of prophylactic knee bracing in American football: A systematic review. *Sports Health, 2*(5), 375–379.

Schultz, B. J., & Egol, K. A. (2021). Acute fractures in sport: Hip. In G. A. J. Robertson & N. Maffuli (Eds.), *Fractures in sport* (pp. 197–221). New York, NY: Springer, Cham.

Sener, O. A., & Durmaz, M. (2019). Effect of sport training and education on Q angle in young males and females. *Journal of Education and Training Studies, 7*(7), 17–21.

Shultz, S. J., Schmitz, R. J., Cameron, K. L., Ford, K. R., Grooms, D. R., Lepley, L. K., Myer, G. D., & Pietrosimone, B. (2019). Anterior Cruciate Ligament Research Retreat VIII summary statement: An update on injury risk identification and prevention across the anterior cruciate ligament injury continuum, March 14–16, 2019, Greensboro, NC. *Journal of Athletic Training, 54*(9), 970–984.

Sugimoto, D., Myer, G. D., Bush, H. M., Klugman, M. F., Medina McKeon, J. M., & Hewett, T. E. (2012). Compliance with neuromuscular training and anterior cruciate ligament injury risk reduction in female athletes: A meta-analysis. *Journal of Athletic Training, 47*(6), 714–723.

Takahashi, S., Nagano, Y., Ito, W., Kido, Y., & Okuwaki, T. (2019). A retrospective study of mechanisms of anterior cruciate ligament injuries in high school basketball, handball, judo, soccer, and volleyball. *Medicine, 98*(26).

Vázquez-Galliano, J., & Miranda-Comas, G. (2021). Pelvis, hip, and thigh injuries. In G. Miranda-Comas, G. Cooper, J. Herrera, & S. Curtis (Eds.), *Essential sports medicine* (pp. 293–313). New York, NY: Springer, Cham.

Webster, K. E., & Hewett, T. E. (2018). Meta-analysis of meta-analyses of anterior cruciate ligament injury reduction training programs. *Journal of Orthopaedic Research, 36*(10), 2696–2708.

Wierer, G., Milinkovic, D., Robinson, J. R., Raschke, M. J., Weiler, A., Fink, C., Herbort, M., & Kittl, C. (2021). The superficial medial collateral ligament is the major restraint to anteromedial instability of the knee. *Knee Surgery, Sports Traumatology, Arthroscopy, 29*(2), 405–416.

CHAPTER 16
Injuries to the Lower Leg, Ankle, and Foot

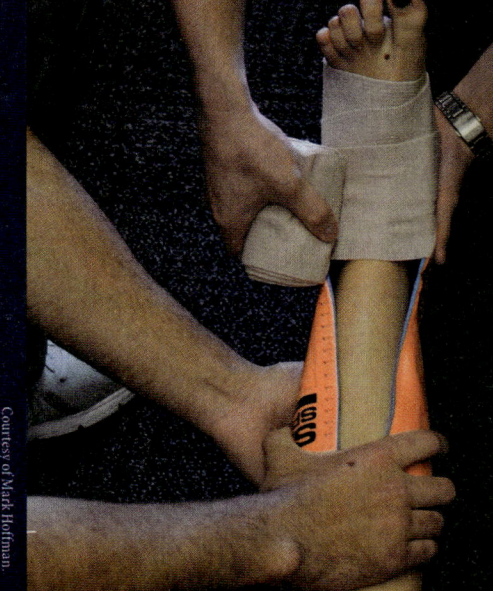

MAJOR CONCEPTS

For an athlete to move well, there must be excellent functioning of the lower leg, ankle, and foot. The foot must provide a stable base of support and be flexible and extremely mobile. This chapter discusses the skeletal and muscular anatomy of the foot and lower leg, with emphasis on the ligaments of the ankle; it also covers the compartments of the lower leg, with an overview of the muscular actions of each compartment. Sports participation can cause fractures of the bones of the lower leg and foot as a result of acute trauma and chronic overuse. This chapter discusses such fractures and common sprains of ankle ligaments. Treatment of ankle sprains and control of possible future sprains are controversial issues, and potential solutions should be studied, weighed, and considered carefully when determining whether an athlete will be able to participate.

Injuries to the tendons that cross the ankle joint are also quite common among athletes. This chapter reports on the recognition, care, and treatment of tendon injuries along with compartment problems and considers the immediate and long-term effects of these disorders. It also focuses on the treatment and care of athletes with shin splints and considers ways to enhance the participation options of these athletes. Finally, the chapter discusses foot disorders, such as plantar fasciitis, heel spurs, Morton's neuroma, arch problems, bunions, blisters, and calluses, and provides guidelines for recognition, first aid treatment, and long-term care. It is critical to remember the importance of the lower leg, ankle, and foot when assisting the athlete to perform at peak levels; even small, seemingly insignificant injuries to these areas can affect an athlete's performance.

Anatomy Review

The normal foot contains 26 bones (Figures 16.1 and 16.2), which are interconnected and supported by numerous ligaments. Many joints within the foot also assist with support and movement. The **talocrural**, or **ankle**, **joint**, where the tibia, fibula, and talus join, provides mainly **plantar flexion** and **dorsiflexion** of the foot. The **subtalar joint**, which

> **Talocrural (ankle) joint** Articulation formed by the distal tibia and fibula with the superior surface (dome) of the talus.

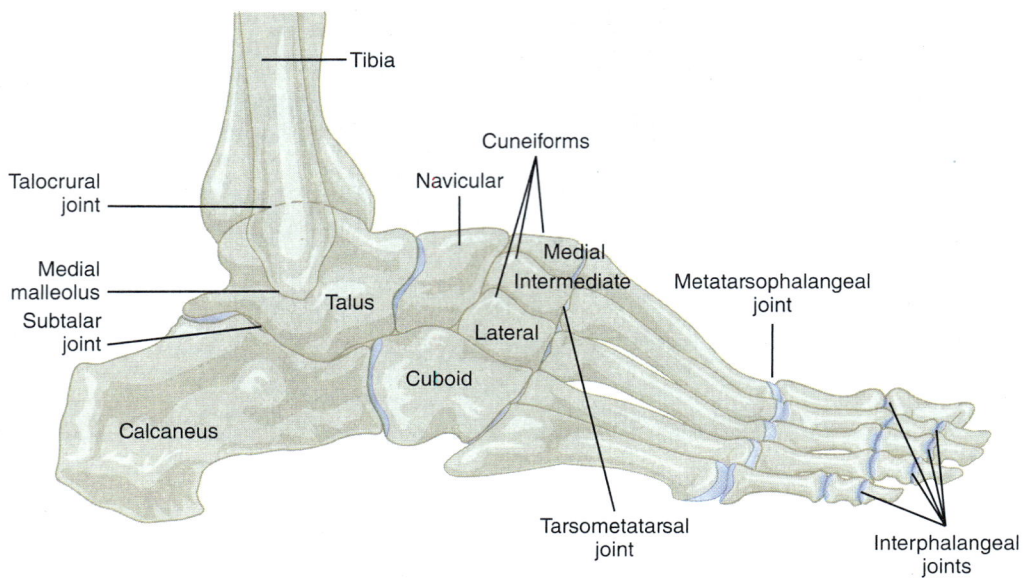

Figure 16.1 Major bones, joints, and arches of the foot (lateral view).

Plantar flexion Moving the top of the foot away from the shin, as in pointing the foot and ankle in dance.

Dorsiflexion Bending the foot toward the dorsum, or shin; the opposite of plantar flexion.

Subtalar joint Articulation (arthrodial) formed by the inferior surface of the talus and the superior surface of the calcaneus.

Inversion Movement that entails turning the sole of the foot inward; inner border of the foot lifts.

Eversion Movement that entails turning the sole of the foot outward.

is the articulation of the talus and the calcaneus, is primarily responsible for the foot's **inversion** and **eversion** movements. Both of these joints are synovial, which means they are surrounded by a capsule and supported by ligaments.

The lower leg, ankle, and foot work together to provide a stable base of support and a dynamic system for movement. The skeleton of the lower leg consists of the tibia and fibula. The tibia is the larger and stronger of the two bones and is commonly called the shin bone; it typically supports about 98% of body weight. The fibula is a smaller bone that supports about

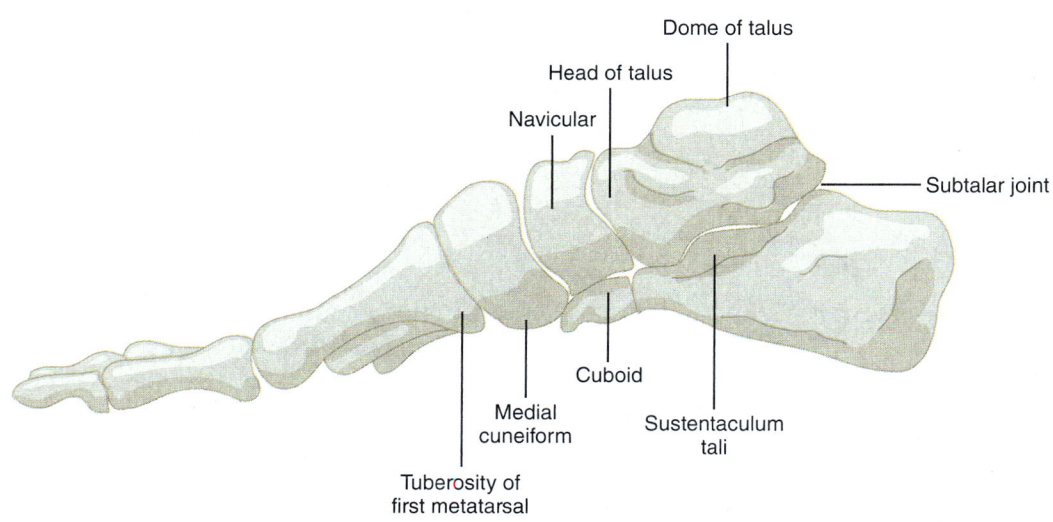

Figure 16.2 Major bones, joints, and arches of the foot (medial view).

2% of body weight; in addition, it acts as an attachment for various muscles and helps to provide a mechanical advantage for some of them.

The ankle (talocrural) joint is supported on the medial side by the large and strong deltoid ligament (Figures 16.3). On the lateral side of the ankle, the joint is supported by the anterior talofibular, the posterior talofibular, and the calcaneofibular ligaments (Figures 16.4). These ligaments are not as large or as strong as the deltoid ligament. Additional lateral stability for the ankle joint is provided by the length of the fibula on the lateral side of the ankle. The ankle joint is stronger when it is placed in dorsiflexion, as opposed to plantar flexion, because the talus fits much tighter between the tibia and fibula in this position.

The joints, ligaments, and muscles help to create and maintain the two arches in the foot (Moini, 2020). The longitudinal arch has medial and lateral divisions running posterior to anterior along the plantar aspect of the foot. There is one transverse arch running from medial to lateral under the distal metatarsal area. These arches assist the foot as shock absorbers; they also provide propulsion assistance during movement.

As shown in **Time Out 16.1**, the muscles of the lower leg are divided into anterior, posterior, and lateral compartments. The muscles of the anterior compartment essentially produce dorsiflexion and extension of the toes. The muscles in this compartment include the tibialis anterior, extensor digitorum longus, extensor hallucis longus, and peroneus tertius. The anterior compartment is a very compact area, with little room for any extra tissue or fluid.

The posterior compartment of the lower leg mainly functions to produce plantar flexion of the

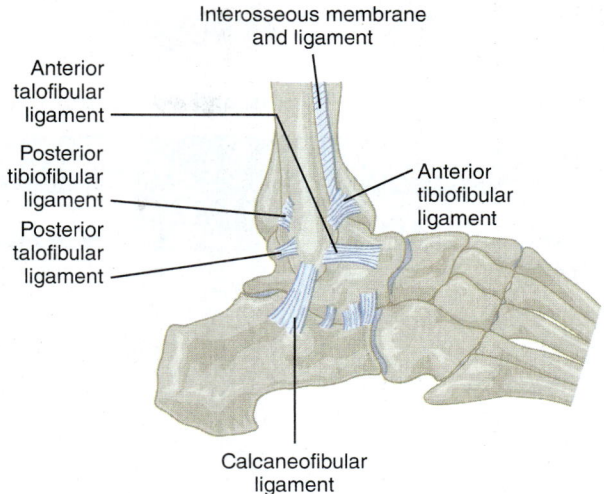

Figure 16.4 Major ligaments of the ankle joint (lateral view).

foot. This compartment is commonly referred to as the calf muscles.

Many anatomy books subdivide this compartment into superficial and deep sections. In the superficial section are the gastrocnemius, soleus, and plantaris muscles. The gastrocnemius and soleus muscles have a common attachment on the calcaneus via the Achilles tendon. The plantaris muscle is small and insignificant in action and may be absent in some individuals. The deep section of this compartment houses the tibialis posterior, flexor digitorum longus, flexor hallucis longus, and popliteus muscles. With the exception of the popliteus, these muscles course behind the medial malleolus of the tibia and along the bottom of the foot. They assist with plantar flexion as well as flexion of the toes. The popliteus muscle is important in knee flexion—it actually initiates knee flexion by unlocking the knee. The lateral compartment of the lower leg contains the peroneus longus and peroneus brevis muscles. These muscles are mainly evertors of the foot but do assist with some plantar flexion. Both of these muscles course behind the lateral malleolus of the fibula, which provides a mechanical advantage for these muscles. The peroneus longus courses under the lateral side of the foot and runs across the bottom to the first metatarsal and cuneiform bones. The peroneus brevis attaches at the base of the fifth metatarsal. Also, in this compartment is the peroneal nerve, a superficial nerve that is susceptible to injury. The posterior tibial artery supplies blood to the peroneal muscles. The arteries

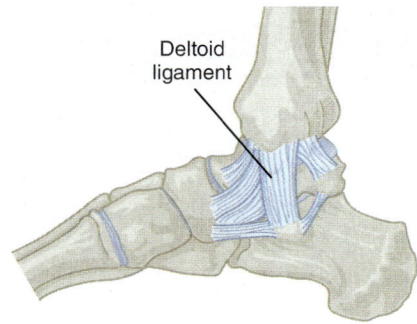

Figure 16.3 Major ligaments of the ankle joint (medial view).

TIME OUT 16.1

Main Muscle Groups, Actions, and Innervations of the Foot and Ankle

Muscle Group	Action(s)	Innervation
Posterior Compartment		
Flexor digitorum longus	Flexion of 2–5 PIP and DIP Flexion of 2–5 MTP joints Assists in plantar flexion Assists in inversion	Tibial
Flexor hallucis longus	Flexion of first MTP and IP Assists in flexion of first MTP Assists with inversion Assists with plantar flexion	Tibial
Gastrocnemius	Ankle plantar flexion Assists with knee flexion	Tibial
Soleus	Ankle plantar flexion	Tibial
Plantaris	Assists with knee flexion	
Popliteus	Tibial rotation Assists with knee flexion	Tibial

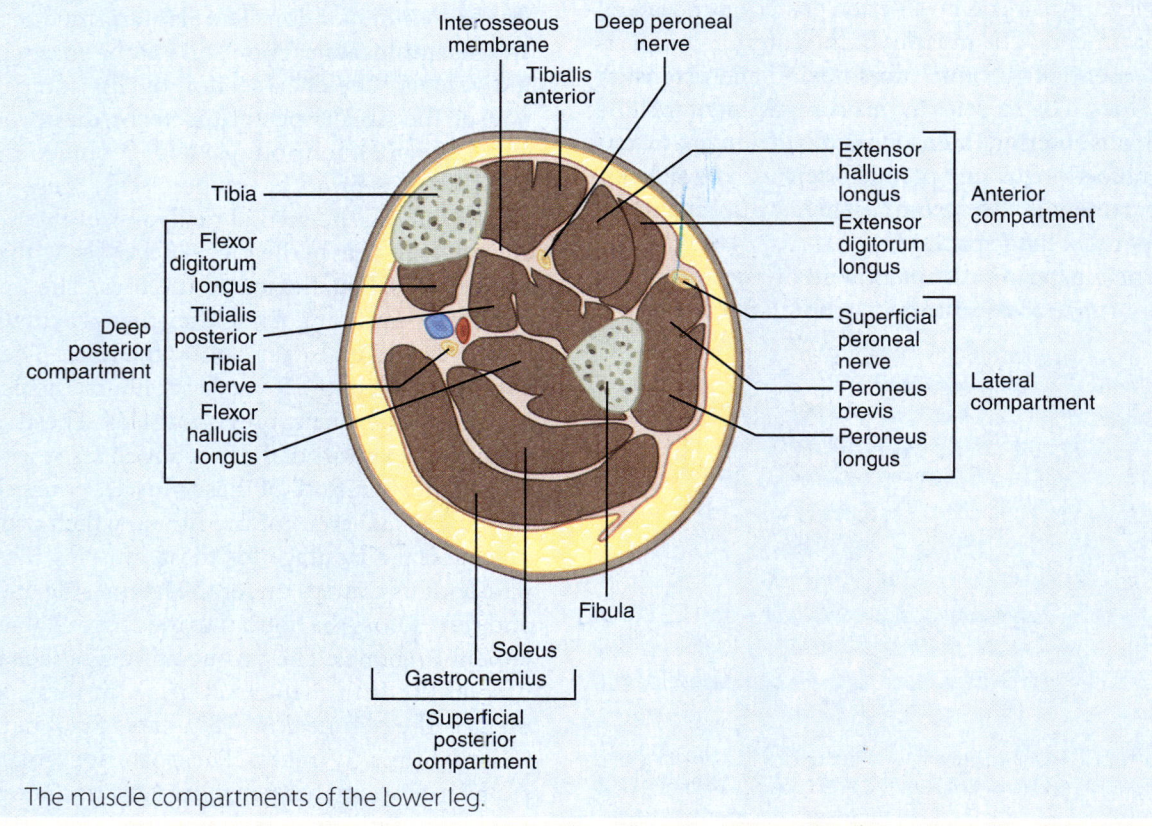

The muscle compartments of the lower leg.

Anterior Compartment		
Extensor digitorum longus	Extension of 2–5 MTP Assists with extension of 2–5 DIP and PIP Assists with eversion Assists with dorsiflexion	Deep peroneal
Extensor hallucis longus	Extension of first MTP and IP Assists in ankle dorsiflexion	Deep peroneal
Peroneus tertius	Assists with dorsiflexion of ankle Assists with eversion of foot	Deep peroneal
Tibialis anterior	Dorsiflexion of ankle Inversion of ankle	Deep peroneal
Lateral Compartment		
Peroneus brevis	Eversion Assists with plantar flexion	Superficial peroneal
Peroneus longus	Eversion Assists with plantar flexion	Superficial peroneal

PIP, proximal interphalageal joint; IP, interphalangeal joint; DIP, distal interphalangeal joint; MTP, metatarsal phalangeal joint.

of the leg can be compromised after trauma below the knee. It is important to always check the pulses of the foot to ensure there is blood flow to the area (discussed later in this chapter).

Common Sports Injuries

Many sports-related injuries occur to the lower leg, ankle, and foot; some can be classified as traumatic, and others are chronic in nature. Traumatic injuries typically involve skeletal structures; chronic injuries usually involve damage to soft tissues in the area. However, there are definitely exceptions to this rule. There are times when overuse can be a factor in fractures and other times when trauma can be the cause of soft-tissue damage, resulting in severe complications.

Skeletal Injuries

Fractures

Direct trauma through contact causes most fractures to the lower leg. The magnitude of contact necessary to fracture a bone, such as the tibia or fibula, can vary (Figure 16.5). A fracture can be caused by being kicked by an opponent in a soccer match or having a 300-pound lineman land on a leg in a professional football game. Fractures to the foot can also occur from trauma, for example, when an opponent lands forcefully on a player's foot. However, violent trauma is not always required in fractures of the bones of the leg and foot (Patel et al., 2021; Porter et al., 2021). Stress fractures can occur from overuse or **microtrauma**. In running, for example, each time the foot strikes the ground it produces a small amount of trauma to the bone. This trauma damages a few bone cells, which the body must repair as quickly as possible. When the body cannot maintain the repair process and keep up with repeated microtrauma to a specific bone, a stress fracture results (Kasitinon & Argo, 2020). Additionally, an **avulsion** fracture of the fifth metatarsal can occur in association with a lateral ankle sprain; therefore, the possibility of such a fracture should be examined

Microtrauma Injury from overuse or repetitive stress.

Avulsions Forcible tearing away or separation.

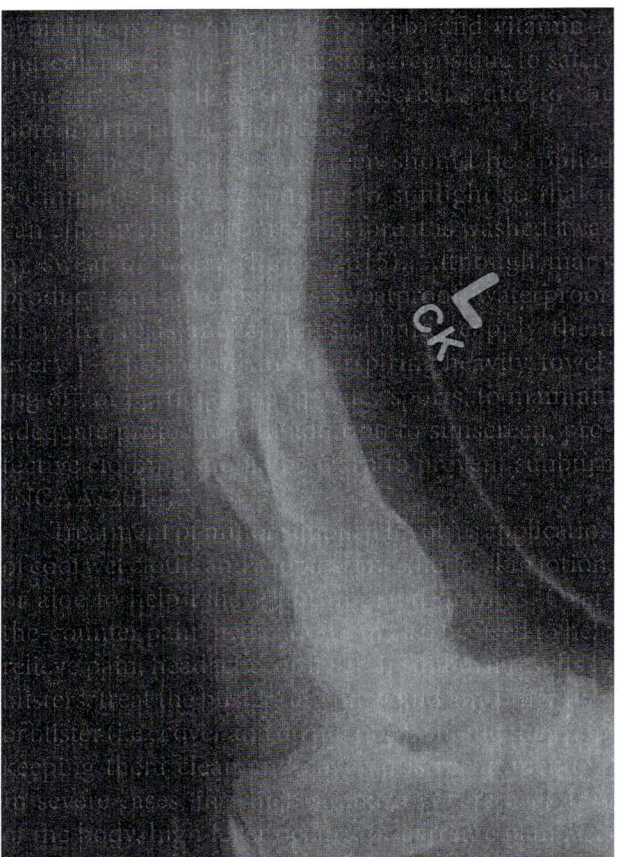

Figure 16.5 Fracture of the tibia and fibula in the left leg.
Courtesy of Brent Mangus.

when an athlete sprains his or her ankle (Quirolgico & Townsend, 2021). Patel and colleagues (2021) noted that a fracture in the fifth metatarsal is considered high risk due to the poor blood supply to the bone, and therefore these fractures have an increased incidence of nonunion. If there is any question about the viability of the bone after an injury to this area, have the athlete consult with a physician.

Signs and symptoms of a fracture in the lower leg or foot include the following:

- Swelling and/or deformity at the location of the trauma.
- Discoloration at the site of the trauma.
- Possible broken bone end projecting through the skin.
- The athlete reports that a snap or a pop was heard or felt.
- The athlete may not be able to bear weight on the affected extremity.

- In the case of a stress fracture or a growth plate fracture that did not result from a traumatic event, the athlete complains of extreme point tenderness and pain at the site of suspected injury.

First aid care of a fracture in the lower leg or foot involves the following:

1. Watch and treat for shock if necessary.
2. Apply sterile dressings to any related wounds (i.e., an open fracture).
3. Carefully immobilize the foot and leg using a splint.
4. Arrange for transport to a medical facility.

In the event that bones are fractured, the physician will either apply a cast to the foot and ankle or have the athlete immobilized in a walking boot for a specified time. When the fracture has healed properly, the physician will release the athlete for rehabilitation, practice, and competition, in that order. There are extreme cases of athletes participating in sporting events with a broken bone in the lower leg or foot. This may happen in professional sports in which athletes get paid for participation in the activity. Participation while a fracture is healing is not recommended because it may slow the healing process. As noted earlier, it is also important to note that there is a possibility of nonunion of a fracture, especially in the fifth metatarsal of the foot, as a result of diminished blood supply. Careful attention must be paid to the healing process of any broken bone.

Soft-Tissue Injuries

Ankle Injuries

One of the most common sports injuries to the lower leg and ankle is a sprained ankle (Figure 16.6a and b). Sprains are abnormal stresses placed on ligamentous structures and cause various levels of damage. Sprains can occur to the lateral or medial ligaments of the ankle, depending on which direction the foot moves when abnormal stress is placed on the ligaments as the foot rolls to one side (Quirolgico & Townsend, 2021).

By analyzing the anatomic relationships of the components of the ankle, it can be seen that the noncontractile structures on the lateral aspect of

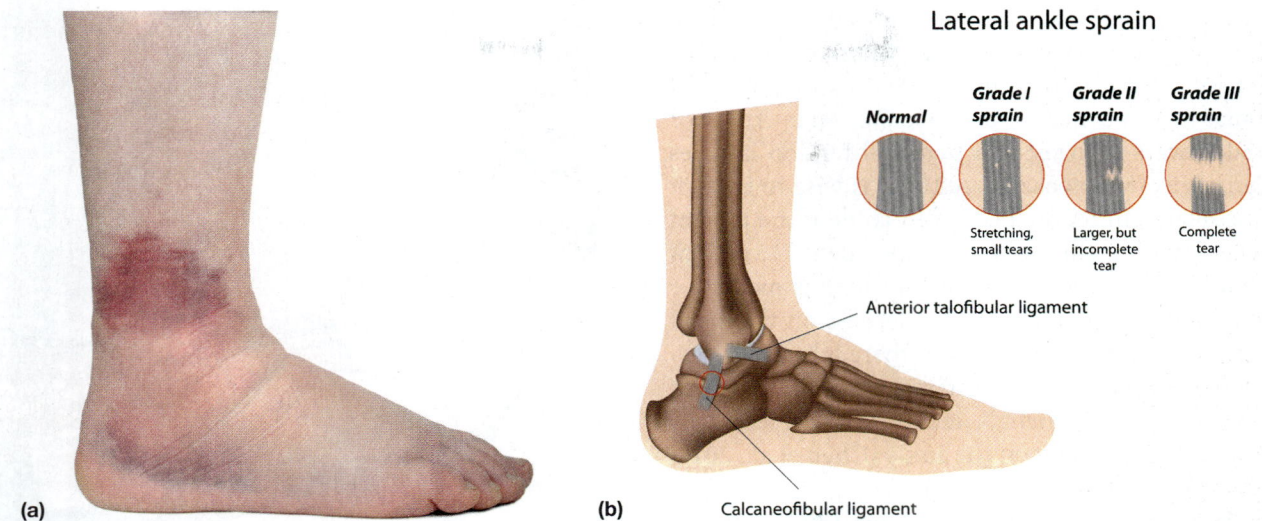

Figure 16.6 (a) Acute swelling after a second-degree ankle sprain. (b) The damage done to the lateral ligaments of the ankle from different grades of ankle sprain.
(a) © SeDmi/Shutterstock; (b) © Alila Medical Media/Shutterstock.

the ankle are most susceptible to injury. The formation of the bones of the ankle helps to stabilize it; the fibula extends inferiorly, approximating the lateral talus completely. Also, the ligaments on the lateral side—the anterior talofibular, the posterior talofibular, and the calcaneofibular ligaments—are not as large or as strong as the deltoid ligament on the medial side of the ankle joint. With the wide anterior superior aspect of the talus being securely wedged in the mortise formed by the inferior surfaces of the tibia and fibula, the joint is more stable in a dorsiflexed position and weaker in a position of plantar flexion. Therefore, when comparing the typical movements of the foot with the anatomic structure of the ankle joint, it becomes clear that the lateral ligaments are more prone to damage via excessive movement than is the deltoid ligament on the medial aspect of the ankle. Most ankle sprains occur to the lateral ligaments (Herzog et al., 2019; Quirolgico & Townsend, 2021). A scoping review by Herzog and colleagues (2019) reported that an estimated 2 million acute ankle sprains occur each year in the United States. It is the most common musculoskeletal injury in college sports, especially those that are characterized by running, cutting, and jumping. In adolescents, the peak incidence is from 10 to 14 years of age in females versus 15 to 19 years of age in males. Even though ankle injuries are often seen as minor, up to 70% of those affected may develop residual physical disability after an ankle sprain (Herzog et al., 2019).

Ankle sprains, overstretching any of the ligaments of the ankle, can occur in virtually any sport and can limit the abilities of the athlete in performance until resolution of the injury is complete. As the severity of the ankle sprain increases, so does the instability of the ankle. It is generally accepted that an **eversion**, or **medial, ankle sprain**, which affects the deltoid ligaments, is more severe compared to a lateral ankle sprain, as a medial ankle sprain is associated with greater instability, or unsteadiness with walking, and should be cared for more conservatively. As mentioned earlier, the **inversion**, or **lateral, ankle sprain**, which affects the lateral ankle ligaments, involves over 70% of the ankle sprains in athletes, and its evaluation becomes a very important part of the treatment and rehabilitation processes. It is in the best interest of the athlete to have a competent healthcare provider evaluate this injury because concomitant injuries do occur

Ankle sprain Injury to any of the ligaments of the ankle.

Eversion (medial) ankle sprain Injury to the medial ligaments due to excessive eversion.

Inversion (lateral) ankle sprain Injury to the lateral ligaments due to excessive inversion.

and can be overlooked (Simon et al., 2019). There are times when an ankle sprain can also have associated injuries, such as a fracture of the proximal or distal fibula, fifth metatarsal, or navicular, talar dome, or syndesmosis injuries, and peroneal tendon injuries (Quirolgico & Townsend, 2021). It is wise to request a medical opinion on a sprained ankle if the patient meets any of the three Ottawa ankle rules: (1) a patient should be referred for an x-ray if there is medial or lateral ankle pain and bony tenderness on the distal or posterior tibia or fibula; (2) if there is bony tenderness over the navicular or fifth metatarsal and midfoot pain; or (3) if the patient is unable to take at least four steps and bear weight on the ankle (Chen et al., 2019; Quirolgico & Townsend, 2021).

Signs and symptoms of a lateral ankle sprain include the following:

- First-degree sprain: Pain, mild disability, point tenderness, little laxity, little or no swelling.
- Second-degree sprain: Pain, mild to moderate disability, point tenderness, loss of function, some laxity (abnormal movement), swelling (mild to moderate).
- Third-degree sprain: Pain and severe disability, point tenderness, loss of function, laxity (abnormal movement), swelling (moderate to severe).

First aid care of a lateral ankle sprain involves the following:

1. Immediately apply ice, compression, and elevation. A horseshoe- or doughnut-shaped pad kept in place by an elastic bandage aids at this stage in the compression and reduction of fluid (Figure 16.7).
2. Have the athlete rest and use crutches to ambulate with a three- or four-point gait if a second-or third-degree sprain has occurred. Physical rehabilitation should begin immediately to reduce atrophy and complications associated with ligament laxity and poor neuromuscular control (Vuurberg et al., 2021). Ultimately, those who did not seek rehabilitative treatment had worse subjective function and more incidents of the ankle giving way or recurrent sprains (Hubbard-Turner, 2019).
3. If there is any question concerning the severity of the sprain, splint and transport the athlete to a medical facility for further evaluation by a physician.

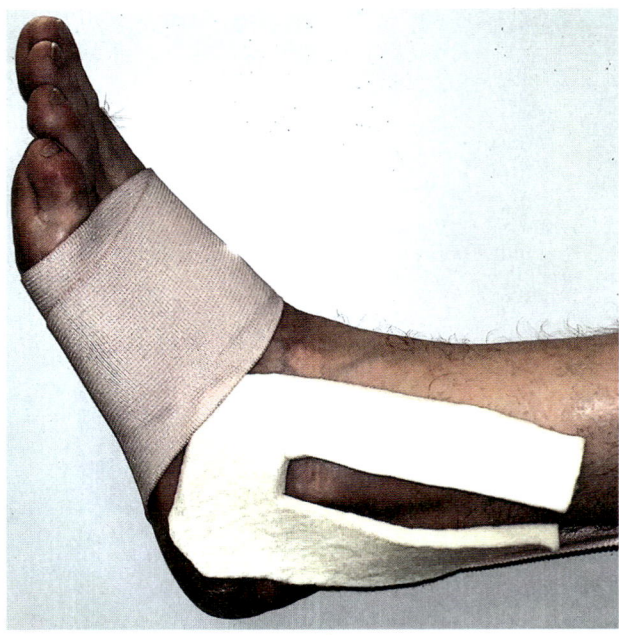

Figure 16.7 A horseshoe-shaped pad is used to ease inflammation after an ankle sprain.
Courtesy of Cindy Trowbridge.

It is important to recognize the possibility of a **tibiofibular (tib/fib) syndesmosis sprain** in conjunction with or masquerading as a lateral ankle sprain. At times, a tib/fib syndesmosis sprain is treated as a lateral ankle sprain, which is inappropriate and will not allow the athlete to progress in the healing process as quickly as if the tib/fib syndesmosis sprain had been treated properly. To discern the difference between the sprains, it is important to note that there is a significant difference in the etiology and specific location of the injuries. With the lateral ankle sprain, there is an inversion mechanism, which includes supination. In the tib/fib syndesmosis sprain, the mechanism is dorsiflexion, followed by axial loading of the lower leg, with external rotation of the foot and internal rotation of the lower leg (Prakash, 2020). Typically, athletes have their foot

---

Tibiofibular syndesmosis sprain Injury to the distal tibiofibular ligament, also known as a high ankle sprain.

planted firmly with the foot in external rotation, and the lower leg twists medially, forcing the talus into the ankle mortise; the axial load forces the tibia and fibula to separate slightly and sprain the syndesmosis. The syndesmosis sprain affects the interosseous membrane that connects the distal sections of the tibia and fibula. This area is immediately superior to the joint mortise, which is why this is often referred to as a "high ankle sprain" in the media. The location of the lateral ankle sprain is generally distal, with point tenderness and swelling occurring at or about the joint mortise area. U.S. football, wrestling, and ice hockey are sports with the highest risk (Chen et al., 2019).

Signs and symptoms of a tib/fib syndesmosis sprain include the following:

- The mechanism of injury is different from a lateral ankle sprain; ankle dorsiflexion and foot external rotation are combined with internal rotation of the lower leg.
- The typical ankle sprain tests may be positive, but the athlete will complain of a great deal of pain and point tenderness in the area of the tib/fib syndesmosis.
- Performing the "squeeze" test (squeezing the tibia and fibula together superior to the syndesmosis; Figure 16.8) elicits pain in the syndesmosis area.

First aid care of a tib/fib syndesmosis sprain involves the following:

1. Immediately apply ice, compression, and elevation. A horseshoe- or doughnut-shaped pad kept in place by an elastic bandage aids at this stage in the compression and reduction of fluid accumulation in the local area (see Figure 16.7).
2. After the athlete has been diagnosed with a syndesmosis sprain by the physician, the athlete will be counseled to rest and use crutches to ambulate for the first 72 hours, followed by the use of a walking boot for a minimum of 3 days and preferably for 7 days following the initial injury (Knapik et al., 2018).
3. If there is any question concerning the severity of the sprain, splint and transport the athlete to a medical facility for further evaluation by a physician. Unfortunately there is no consensus on standard management preoperatively,

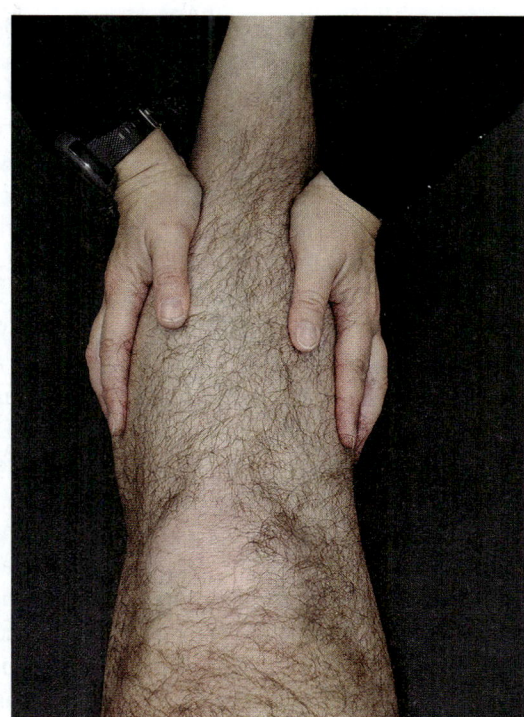

Figure 16.8 The "squeeze" test to determine whether the tib/fib syndesmosis is involved in an injury.
Courtesy of Cindy Trowbridge.

intraoperatively, or postoperatively of these types of ankle sprains. However, it is clear that poor functional outcomes develop when the acute injury is not managed appropriately (Yuen & Lui, 2017).

The control of subsequent ankle sprains is a source of a great deal of research and debate in sports medicine literature. Preventive exercise programs

WHAT IF ❓

One of your high school soccer players has just injured his ankle, apparently while moving the ball downfield. He has fallen to the ground and is in obvious pain, holding his right ankle. During your examination, you note swelling and discoloration in the region of the lateral malleolus and point tenderness over the area of the lateral ankle ligaments. Based on this history and the signs and symptoms, what is the likely injury? What is the appropriate first aid for such injuries?

and external supports (i.e., braces and athletic tape) are effective for ankle sprain risk reduction in both uninjured and previously injured populations (Kaminski et al., 2019). Although it is recognized that taping or bracing can reduce the number of ankle sprains (Verhagen & Bay, 2010), ankle bracing may provide better risk reduction and tends to cost less over the long term (Kaminski et al., 2019). The standard ankle-taping procedure is also often used as a prophylactic treatment for ankles with no history of previous injury. However, well-designed prospective randomized controlled trials investigating prevention of lateral ankle sprains across a range of sport settings do not exist (Kaminski et al., 2019). Thus, the decision of whether to brace or tape is typically up to the athlete or coach (Zwiers et al., 2016). In published research studies, ankle taping has been demonstrated to help with the neuromuscular response of the muscles (Lohrer et al., 1999) and to provide stability if done in a specific manner (Alt et al., 1999). Both of these factors can contribute to a reduction in ankle sprains.

Most researchers agree that the best-known method of ankle support, the prophylactic adhesive-taping procedure, supports the ankle for only a short period of time after exercise begins (Lohkamp et al., 2009). It is suggested that the reason ankle taping loses its prophylactic effect over time is that the soft tissues of the ankle region become more mobile as the athlete utilizes them and more flexible as the practice or game progresses (Ricard et al., 2000).

Some researchers now maintain that bracing is better than taping for the prevention of ankle injuries, owing to the reduction in range of motion, either at excessive points or within normal ranges (Babins, 2012; Kaplan, 2011; McGuire et al., 2011; McGuire et al., 2012). A recent systematic review revealed that ankle bracing effectively reduced ankle injuries in both athletes without a previous injury (risk reduction = 47%) and athletes with previous injury (risk reduction = 63%; Barelds et al., 2018). Very good ankle braces are now on the market (Figures 16.9 through 16.11) that provide the necessary protection at a low overall cost. It has also been suggested that some high-top shoes may reduce the number of lateral ankle sprains (Ricard et al., 2000). The combination of high-top shoes and taping or bracing can be helpful to athletes in reducing the number of ankle sprains they experience. Although there have been mixed results regarding the effectiveness of different types of taping and bracing in chronic ankle instability patients, two recent studies determined that a variety of taping techniques (e.g., complex, simple, Kinesiotape™) and bracing (e.g., elastic, soft, rigid) all improved static and dynamic balance, proprioception, and vertical jump performance (Alawna & Mohamed, 2020; Hadadi et al., 2020).

Recent research has been focusing on the prevention of lower extremity injury through proper warm-up progressions or specific training techniques. Longo and colleagues (2012) demonstrated how a specific warm-up program reduced injuries in basketball players over a 9-month season. Another area of research in injury prevention is through proprioception training. Proprioception training exercises can be helpful in reducing chronic ankle instability (Verhagen & Bay, 2010). Proprioception training can also be an important part of preventive and rehabilitative aspects of ankle functioning (Hubscher et al., 2010). An interesting analysis of ankle sprain and fracture injuries was conducted by the U.S. Army on paratroopers,

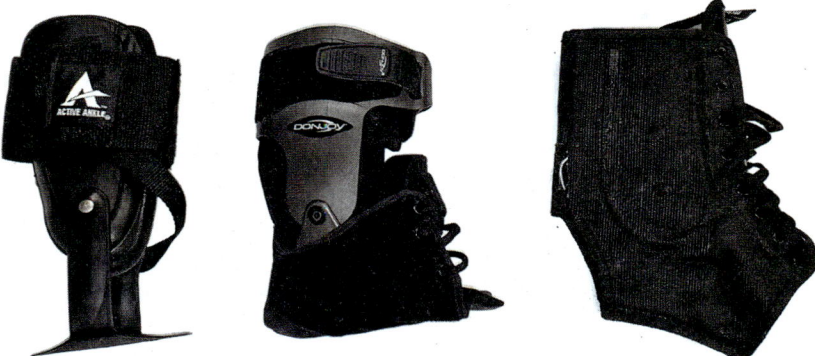

Figure 16.9 Prophylactic ankle braces come in a variety of styles.
Courtesy of Cindy Trowbridge.

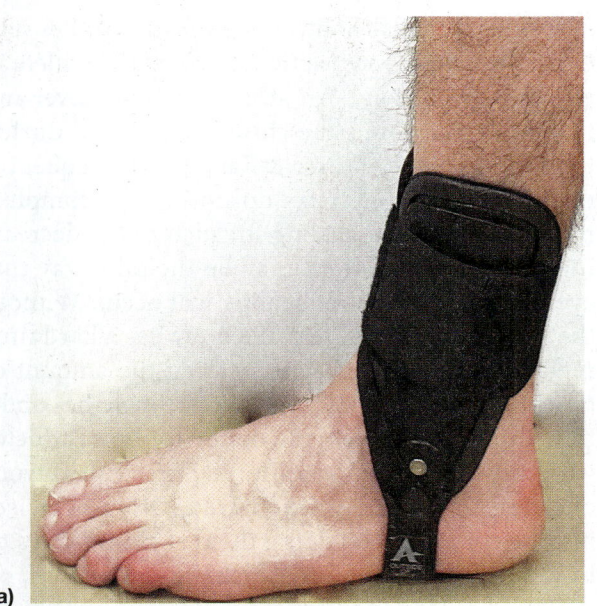 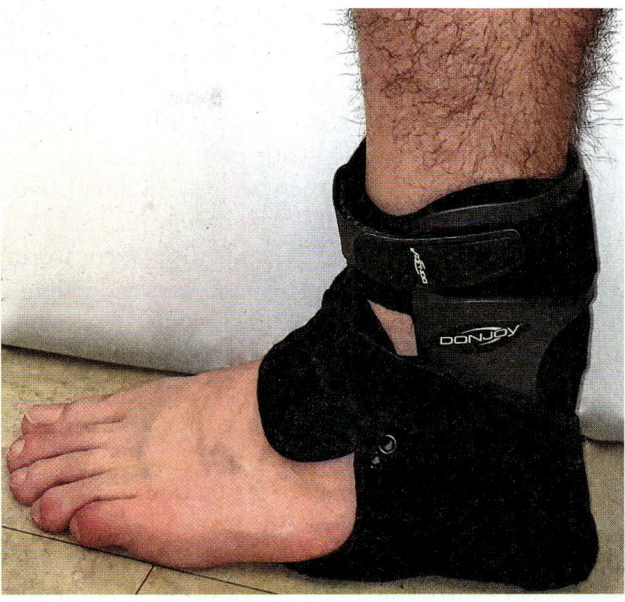

Figure 16.10 **(a)** A medial and lateral rigid ankle brace is used for protection after an ankle has been sprained. **(b)** A more encompassing rigid ankle brace is used for extra protection after an ankle has been sprained.
Courtesy of Cindy Trowbridge.

documenting that ankle injuries were the most common injury in these soldiers. The army reported that up to 43% of all soldiers' injuries involved the ankle. The use of braces in paratroopers was implemented, and the injury rate among these soldiers was significantly decreased. The army medical staff calculated the use of ankle braces saved between $7 and $9 for every dollar spent on the purchase of the braces (Knapik et al., 2010).

Whatever the choice of the coach or athlete, many factors must be considered in preventing ankle sprains. These factors include the type of activity, the compliance of the athlete in wearing braces or prophylactic taping, the cost to the school or athlete, and the effectiveness of the brace as reported in research studies. Even though most coaches believe that adhesive taping is effective in reducing ankle-related injuries, there are some serious consequences of poorly applied adhesive tape, including blisters, tape cuts, and loss of circulation. If ankle taping is to be part of an athlete's protective equipment, then it must be applied properly to perform correctly (see the section titled Preventive Ankle Taping later in this chapter).

Tendon-Related Injuries

The Achilles tendon is commonly injured in long-distance runners, basketball players, and tennis players. The onset of tendinitis may be slow among runners but much more rapid among basketball or tennis players, who make a great many short-burst movements requiring jumping or rapid motion from side to side.

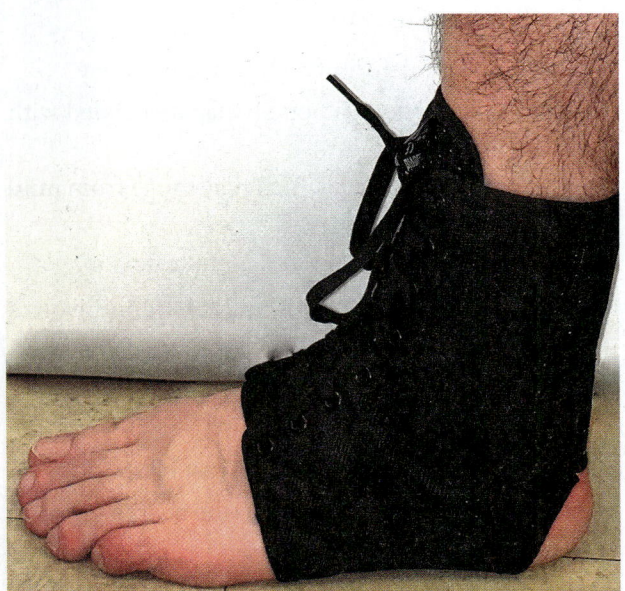

Figure 16.11 This socklike brace is also helpful in the prevention of ankle sprains.
Courtesy of Cindy Trowbridge.

Some controversy exists about the actual injury that constitutes **Achilles tendinitis**. The Achilles tendon itself, which attaches the gastrocnemius and soleus muscles to the calcaneus, can become inflamed. However, either the tendon sheath or the subcutaneous bursa dorsal to the tendon can become inflamed, both of which can be part of Achilles tendinitis. Athletes who dramatically increase their running distance or workout times and do so running on hard, uneven, or uphill surfaces are prone to Achilles tendinitis (Quirolgico & Townsend, 2021). Achilles tendinopathy represents between 55% and 65% of disorders of the Achilles tendon and is a common overuse injury in running sports (Pearce & Tan, 2016).

Achilles tendinitis causes the tendon to be warm and painful upon touch, and the tendon will also appear thickened. The pain associated with this condition is localized to a small area of the tendon and typically intensifies when movement is initiated after rest. These signs and symptoms can be seen over an extended period of time (days to weeks), or, in some athletes, over a shorter time period (days). Early detection of this problem usually enhances resolution of the symptoms and assists the athlete in returning earlier to practice and competition (Pearce & Tan, 2016). Referring the athlete with an unresolved Achilles tendon problem to the team physician will put the athlete on the right track for treatment, rehabilitation, and avoidance of this problem in the future. The physician will outline a treatment plan that will contain some or all of the components explained in the following paragraphs.

Treatment for chronic Achilles tendinitis is immediate rest until the swelling subsides. Usually the application of ice, nonsteroidal anti-inflammatory drugs (e.g., aspirin or ibuprofen), and a small heel lift assist in the reduction of swelling and the return to practice and competition. Stretching can be beneficial to athletes with Achilles tendinitis. Controlled stretching on a slant board or against a wall each day will aid in a return to participation. Additionally, if an athlete must exercise or run, it is advised that this be done in a controlled environment, perhaps in a swimming pool. Controlled, gradual stretching exercises using the eccentric contraction of the Achilles tendon, common to most activities, assist the athlete in returning to activity. An athlete's activity level and type of exercise must be closely monitored during the healing phase (Pearce & Tan, 2016). Frequently, runners or other athletes do not accept complete rest as the route to healing. In such cases, decreasing the amount of work may be the only way that even a small amount of healing will occur. Without the proper amount of rest, the body has a hard time repairing injury, thereby increasing the amount of time the athlete experiences difficulty with the condition. Running in water is an option for those athletes who must maintain conditioning or want to work out even though they are injured. Other exercises may be completed by doing them at slower rates or in controlled situations in which the stress placed on the Achilles tendon is limited.

Explosive jumping or direct trauma from some type of impact can cause traumatic injury to the Achilles tendon by tearing, or rupturing, it; such an injury is called an **Achilles tendon rupture**. This type of injury has been known to occur in athletes participating in many different sports, and risk for this injury increases with age, as well as if the athlete has a previous history of Achilles tendonitis (Tarantino et al., 2020; Yasui et al., 2017).

Signs and symptoms of a ruptured Achilles tendon include the following:

- Swelling and deformity at the site of injury.
- The athlete reports a pop or snap associated with the injury.
- Pain in the lower leg, which may range from mild to extreme.
- Loss of function, mainly in plantar flexion.

First aid care of a ruptured Achilles tendon involves the following:

1. Immediately apply ice and compression to the area.
2. Immobilize the foot by an air cast or splint.
3. Arrange for transportation to the nearest medical facility.

During the acute phase of the healing process, try to minimize active dorsiflexion and eliminate forced dorsiflexion because these movements can produce more damage and inflammation to the area (Tarantino et al., 2020).

Achilles tendonitis Inflammation of the Achilles tendon.

Achilles tendon rupture Complete tear of the Achilles tendon.

The long-term effects of a ruptured Achilles tendon depend on the severity or completeness of the rupture. If surgery is necessary, the athlete will most likely be out of athletic participation for the rest of the season. In any case, the athlete will need to be careful and aware of the value of stretching and warming up in any future sports activity (Tarantino et al., 2020).

Other tendon problems typically occur with the tendons on the lateral side of the ankle, including those of the peroneus longus and peroneus brevis muscles. These muscles originate on the lateral aspect of the tibia and fibula; the tendons then run an inferior course behind the lateral malleolus in the peroneal groove and attach on the lateral and posterior aspects of the foot. There is a small retinaculum band attaching on the fibula and running posteriorly to the calcaneus, which assists in holding the tendons in place. As these tendons run their course behind the lateral malleolus, there is a possibility of their dislocating and/or subluxating as a result of trauma or extreme force and actually popping across the lateral malleolus. This can be very painful and is an unusual athletic injury. In fact, a review of the literature found that 23% to 77% of patients with lateral ankle instability are at risk for peroneal tendon pathology (van Dijk et al., 2019).

The athlete with tendon problems should be seen by a member of the medical team, and a course of action should be outlined. Sometimes, these problems can be controlled by taping or bracing and strengthening the musculature in the area. Recurrent problems warrant further investigation by the physician; other modes of controlling recurrent subluxation are possible.

Compartment Syndrome

Another possible problem that can result from chronic or acute conditions is **compartment syndrome**. This syndrome is associated with the lower leg, which is divided into four distinct compartments (see Time Out 16.1). The majority of compartment syndrome problems occur in the anterior compartment, which has very little room to expand if there is swelling or effusion into this compact space.

Some athletes may chronically overuse the muscles in the anterior compartment, leading to an inflammatory process in the musculature and an overall increase in the pressure within the compartment. This may be followed by extreme pressure on the blood vessels and nerves in the compartment, thereby compromising their functions. Trauma to the anterior portion of the leg (e.g., by being kicked or hit with a ball) can result in internal bleeding and swelling in the compartment (Buerba et al., 2019). A similar scenario can cause the same results in the other compartments of the lower leg, which are so tightly packed with muscles, nerves, and blood vessels that there is little room for expansion when extra fluid is present. Any scenario that results in a pressure increase in the compartment requires immediate attention. The "Five Ps" of pain, pallor, pulselessness, paresthesias, and paralysis comprise the classic lower extremity compartment syndrome symptoms (Lloyd & Lueders, 2021). Compartment injuries require early intervention and detection of any compromise in the dorsalis pedis and the posterior tibial arteries. Checking the pulses of both arteries is of critical importance in an athlete's experiencing a lower leg problem (Figure 16.12). If either or both of the pulses are diminished or nonexistent, the athlete must immediately be evaluated by a physician.

Many soccer athletes tend to want to wear small shin guards (Figure 16.13) because they contend that large shin guards inhibit their play. When athletes wear shin guards that are too small, however, they run the risk of not having appropriate preventive padding if they are kicked in the lower leg. Fortunately for the athlete shown in Figure 16.14, the kick was to the medial side of the leg, which allowed the hematoma to be controlled and reduced in a short time. Being kicked on the lateral side of the leg could have resulted in excessive anterior compartment pressure and loss of blood flow and/or function requiring immediate medical attention.

Signs and symptoms of compartment syndrome include the following:

- Pain and swelling in the lower leg.
- Athlete's complaint of chronic or acute injury to the area.
- Loss of sensation or motor control to the lower leg and/or foot.
- Loss of pulse to the foot.
- Athlete's inability to extend the great toe or dorsiflex the foot.

Compartment syndrome Inflammation of one of the lower leg compartments leading to increased pressure within the compartment and diminished sensation, blood flow, and function of the foot and ankle.

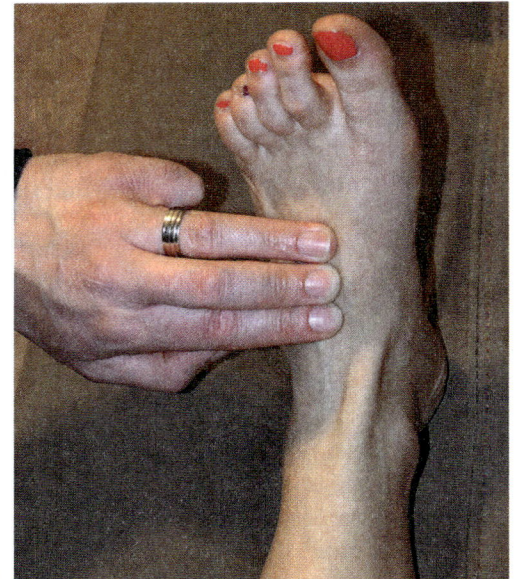

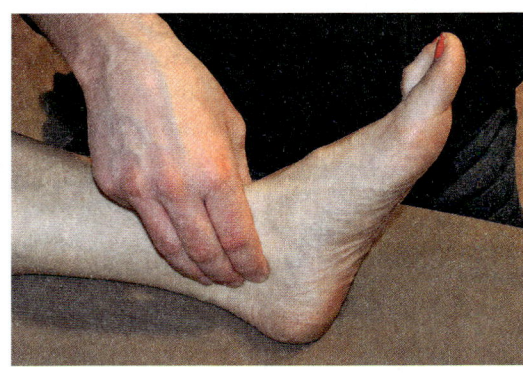

Figure 16.12 Checking the pulse of **(a)** the dorsalis pedis and **(b)** the posterior tibial arteries.
Courtesy of Brent Mangus.

First aid care of compartment syndrome involves the following:

1. Apply ice and elevate. Do not apply compression because the area is already compromised with too much pressure.
2. If the foot becomes numb or there is loss of movement or pulse to the foot, seek medical help immediately.
3. Seek proper medical advice early because these problems can worsen very quickly.

Shin splints Exercise-induced tibia pain; also called medial tibial stress syndrome, tibial stress injury, or chronic exertional compartment syndrome.

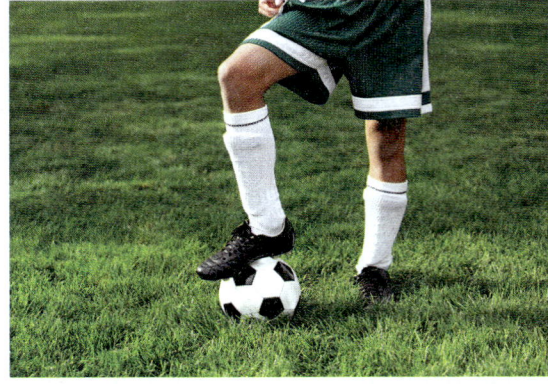

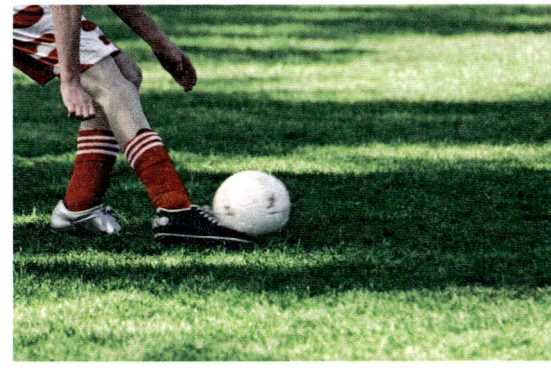

Figure 16.13 (a) Shin guards protect the front of the lower leg and help prevent contusions and hematomas. **(b)** Some soccer players wear shin guards that are too small.
(a) © Le Do/Shutterstock; (b) © Corepics VOF/Shutterstock.

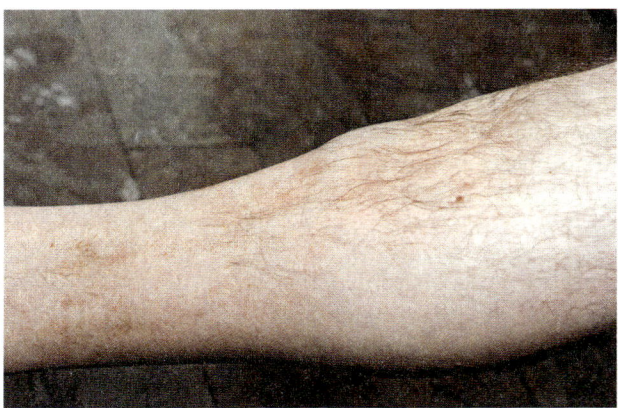

Figure 16.14 Contusion with hematoma formation on the anterior aspect of the lower leg, which might have been prevented by the athlete's wearing larger shin guards.
© Lapis2380/Shutterstock.

Shin Splints

Another very common disorder of the lower leg is "shin splints," a term used to describe exercise-induced leg pain. **Shin splints** are also called medial tibial stress syndrome (MTSS), tibial stress injury (TSI), or chronic exertional compartment syndrome (CECS), all of which can describe a wide variety of exercise-induced lower leg disorders. This disorder is dubious in that it does not have definite parameters to follow for determining the exact problem that is causing pain in the lower leg. Over time, medical professionals have attempted to rename this problem using the descriptive terms (i.e., MTSS, TSI, and CECS) rather than shin splints, but they are merely a description rather than a diagnosis of the problem (Brewer & Gregory, 2012; Hubbard et al., 2009; Moen et al., 2012). The types of activities that produce this problem and the manifestations of the injury vary depending on the athlete. However, to date there has not been a positive link between any one specific cause and the resulting leg pain (Becker et al., 2020). Moreover, it is generally accepted that with rest the pain will subside and the athlete will be able once again to participate.

Signs and symptoms of shin splints include the following:

- Lower leg pain either medially or posteromedially.
- Typically, the athlete reports a chronic problem that gets progressively worse.
- The pain and discomfort can be bilateral or unilateral.

First aid care of shin splints involves the following:

1. Apply ice and have the athlete rest.
2. Nonsteroidal anti-inflammatory medications may help.

To help the athlete work through shin splints, suggest a change in workout routine (Menéndez et al., 2020). Recommend that the athlete run in water, reduce running, or eliminate the irritating stimulus altogether and use another type of exercise until there is an improvement. The athlete may also want to have his or her gait analyzed to look for biomechanical deficiencies, such as overpronation. Myriad related problems can exacerbate the pain and discomfort associated with shin splints. If the problem worsens, the athlete must seek professional medical advice so that long-term complications do not arise. An athletic

WHAT IF ?

A high school gymnast has just struck the front of her lower left leg on the lower bar of the uneven bars. She immediately grabs her leg and complains loudly of extreme pain. On further examination, you note that she has swelling and discoloration directly over the muscles of the anterior compartment. In addition, she states that she is unable to extend her big toe. What is the likely cause of these signs and symptoms? What would be the most appropriate first aid for this injury?

Athletic Trainers SPEAK OUT

How have athletic trainers advanced the health care of our police and firefighters?

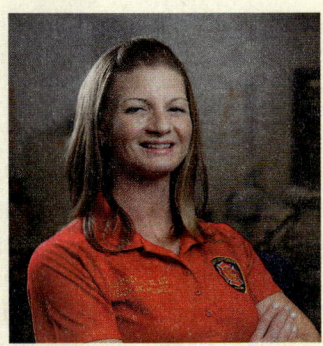

Courtesy of Deena Kilpatrick, MS, LAT, ATC.

When people think about athletic training, they traditionally associate the profession with organized sports and the medical professionals found on the sidelines. The individuals that comprise law enforcement, emergency medical services (EMS), and fire and rescue professionals make up one of the emerging settings in the field of athletic training: the public safety setting. The individuals within this setting, termed *tactical athletes*, must perform tasks that require speed, strength, stamina, and flexibility.

Research proves that more than 50% of injuries incurred by tactical athletes are sprains and strains. Athletic trainers provide immediate care of injuries and the subsequent case management to see these injuries through the entire treatment, rehabilitation, and reconditioning process. Public safety agencies employing athletic trainers have recorded reductions in healthcare costs, decreases in the number and severity of injuries, and increases in productivity. Unlike the traditional setting, athletic trainers within the public safety setting work with tactical athletes for the entirety of their career, which could span more than 20 years. Athletic trainers employed in-house by an agency become more familiar with the job demands for these tactical athletes and provide injury prevention plans as well as functional return-to-duty testing.

Although public safety is still an emerging setting for the athletic training profession, agencies have begun to recognize the worth and value of adding an athletic trainer to their workforce. Prior to 2015, there was one athletic trainer employed by a public safety agency. In the last 4 years, 10 more agencies have employed athletic trainers through various methods and models, with additional agencies diligently working to create positions in the near future.

—**Deena Kilpatrick, MS, LAT, ATC**

Deena Kilpatrick is an Athletic Trainer for the San Antonio Fire Department in San Antonio, Texas.

trainer can assist the athlete with shin splints through preventive taping procedures and some therapies. However, long-term treatment with adhesive tape is not advised: The skin of the lower leg will become irritated, and, often, this does not alleviate the initial problem causing the pain and discomfort. Each athlete responds differently to taping and therapy; therefore, a controlled progression of alternative taping procedures and a well-planned and implemented approach to the rehabilitation program are important in determining which factor the athlete is responding to during the healing process.

Foot Disorders

The foot contains many bones, joints, ligaments, muscles, and other tissues. It is important to remember that some injuries are more common to specific sports.

Plantar Fasciitis

The plantar fascia is a dense collection of tissues, including muscles and tendons, that traverses from the plantar aspect of the metatarsal heads to the calcaneal tuberosity. If this collection of tissues becomes tight or inflamed by overuse or trauma, it can produce pain and disability in the bottom of the foot, known as **plantar fasciitis**. A change in shoes, training technique, activity, or other factors may be precipitating factors to this injury. People who spend most of the week at a desk and then try to get in as much exercise as possible on the weekend are more susceptible to this problem than are full-time athletes. Plantar fasciitis in the young athlete typically is a combined problem with calcaneal apophysitis (Sever's disease;

Plantar fasciitis Inflammation of the plantar tissues of the foot.

Heel spur Bony formation on calcaneus as a result of plantar fasciitis.

Ramponi & Baker, 2019). It is important to remember that, in the adolescent athlete, this condition may also include medial arch and/or heel pain (Quirolgico & Townsend, 2021). To determine whether the condition is plantar fasciitis, the examiner must take a thorough history. Ask the athlete whether he or she experiences almost unbearable pain in the plantar aspect of the foot with the first steps taken on getting out of bed in the morning and the pain eases with each of the following steps. Also, inquire whether there is point tenderness on the plantar aspect of the calcaneal tuberosity or along the longitudinal arch. If both of these symptoms exist, there is a high probability that plantar fasciitis is the problem.

Treatment of plantar fasciitis is typically conservative; it includes rest, anti-inflammatory drugs, and the use of alternating cold and heat to enhance healing (Trojian & Tucker, 2019). A heel pad and stretching the Achilles tendon complex can assist in recovery and resolution. The use of semirigid orthoses has also been shown to be effective in recovering from plantar fasciitis; however, many athletes find it difficult to participate in sports with such an orthotic in their shoes. Athletes will be tempted to continue exercising with this injury. However, the more the injury is aggravated by further insult to the same area, the longer it will take to heal, even when the healing process is being augmented with assorted therapeutic agents.

Heel Spurs

Heel spurs can also be related to plantar fasciitis; sometimes, with chronic cases of inflammation, ossifications occur at the site of the muscular attachment on the plantar aspect of the calcaneus. They result in long-term disability for many athletes because they can become problematic at any time during the exercise or activity program. Additionally, these small ossifications can occur on the posterior aspect of the calcaneus, just below the attachment of the Achilles tendon. These ossifications can also become disabling to an athlete. The athlete needs to consult a physician to determine the proper treatment plan if these spurs become too incapacitating. Doughnut-shaped pads placed beneath the heel and some therapeutic interventions may assist the athlete to participate fully, but rarely do they ameliorate the problem.

Morton's Foot

Morton's foot typically involves either a shortened first metatarsal bone or an elongated second metatarsal bone. The result is that the majority of weight bearing is done on the second metatarsal instead of along the first metatarsal and spreading out to the remainder of the foot. This problem can result in pain throughout the foot and difficulty in ambulation. The use of padding can help the athlete, but, to have the problem correctly addressed, the athlete should see a physician so that the proper treatment can be prescribed.

Also associated with this area is a condition called **Morton's neuroma**. This is a problem with the nerve, usually between the third and fourth metatarsal heads. As a result, pain radiates to the third and fourth toes. A neuroma is an abnormal growth on the nerve itself. Tight-fitting shoes have been blamed for irritation of the nerve in many cases of Morton's neuroma. Consequently, going barefoot is one of the best methods of pain relief for this problem. This condition is most often taken care of by a medical doctor, who should always be consulted regarding the early detection of foot problems (Thomson et al., 2020).

Arch Problems

Athletes can experience several problems associated with the arches of the foot (Figures 16.1 and 16.2). Essentially, arch problems can be classified into two categories: **pes planus** (an abnormally flat foot) and **pes cavus** (an abnormally high arch in the foot). Both problems present difficulties to some athletes. Other athletes with similar foot conditions may never complain of problems associated with arches.

Athletes with flat feet may have too much foot pronation, causing difficulties with or around the navicular bone, which leads to generalized discomfort around the foot and ankle. A low-cost alternative and potential method of determining whether the athlete could benefit from an orthotic (Figure 16.15) or some other type of augmentation for flat feet is to begin with an arch-taping procedure. Several taping

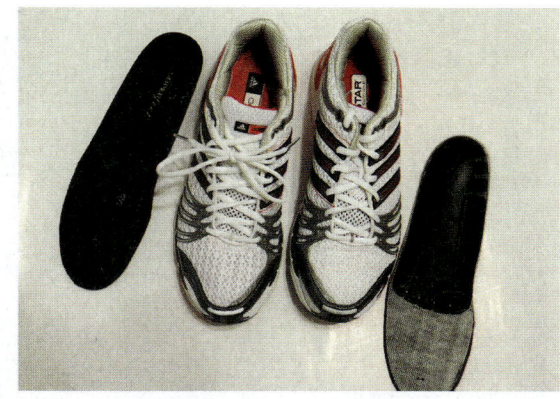

(a)

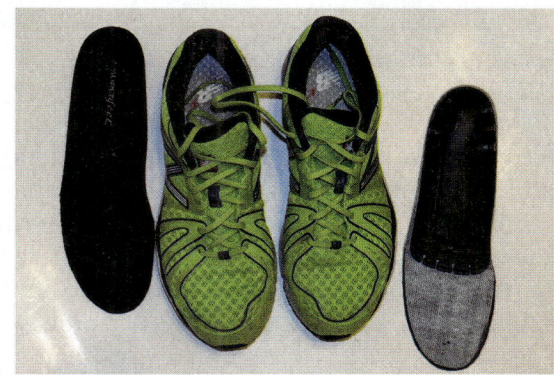

(b)

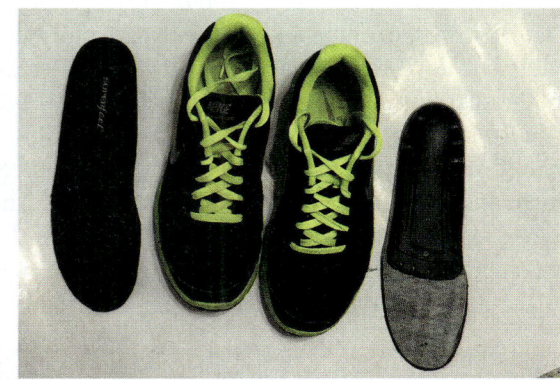

(c)

Figure 16.15 Soft orthotics can be placed in athletes' shoes to assist with some foot problems.
Courtesy of Brent Mangus.

Morton's foot Shortened first metatarsal or elongated second metatarsal bone that causes most of the weight bearing to be on the second metatarsal.

Morton's neuroma Abnormal growth on nerves between the metatarsal heads.

Pes planus Abnormally flat foot or loss of the longitudinal arch which may lead to compensation patterns.

Pes cavus Abnormally high longitudinal arch which may lead to compensation patterns.

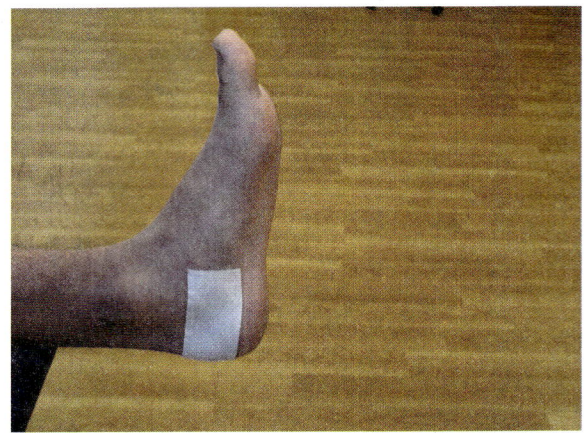 (a)

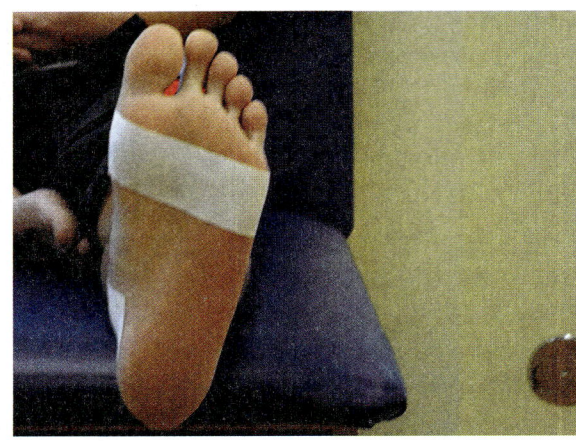 (b)

Figure 16.16 After an adhesive is applied, begin with anchor strips on the heel and base of the toes.
Courtesy of Brent Mangus.

procedures have been developed to augment the arch in athletes. How long the effects of taping enhance the arch has been evaluated by at least one research team, whose findings were consistent with those for ankle-taping procedures. There seems to be limited effectiveness in adhesive-strapping techniques for the person who walks for a minimum of 10 minutes continuously (Lohkamp et al., 2009). However, it may be worth trying to tape the arch(es) with the intent to determine whether the application provides any benefit for the athlete during practice (Figures 16.16 through 16.18). A Board of Certification (BOC)–certified athletic trainer can assist in providing direction in this taping procedure. Coaches should not attempt to apply adhesive tape to an athlete until they have received the proper training. Many athletes with flat feet can be helped in the long term by orthotics and proper shoe selection. It should be noted, however, that there is no evidence that the flat-footed athlete is a slower runner or has less motor ability than the athlete with a regular or high arch.

Occasionally, an athlete may feel one or both feet experiencing a generalized soreness or weakness due to fatigue. As mentioned earlier, orthotics may be necessary to assist the athlete on a long-term basis, but, for the short term, arch-support taping may assist the athlete to get through a practice or game. In some athletes, support taping for one or both arches can help reduce this feeling of sore or weak feet during participation.

In many cases, the athlete with an excessively high arch also has foot problems. There are research reports outlining the abnormal forces placed on the high-arch foot suggesting a potential for injury (Buldt et al., 2018). A foot with too much arch is often associated with

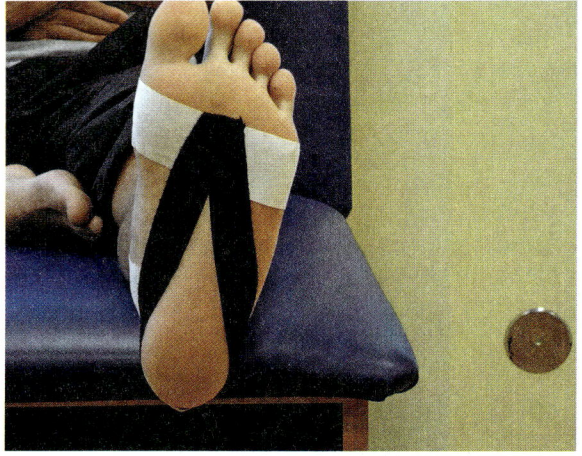 (a)

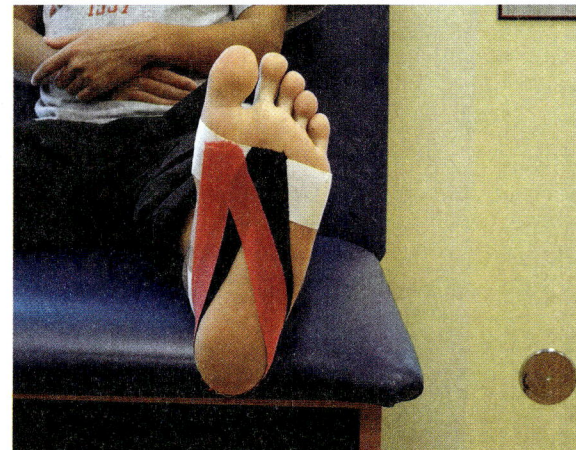 (b)

Figure 16.17 Apply support strips starting from medial moving to lateral, as demonstrated.
Courtesy of Brent Mangus.

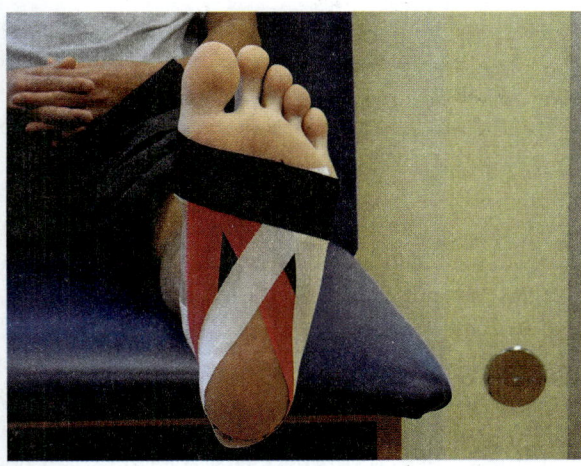
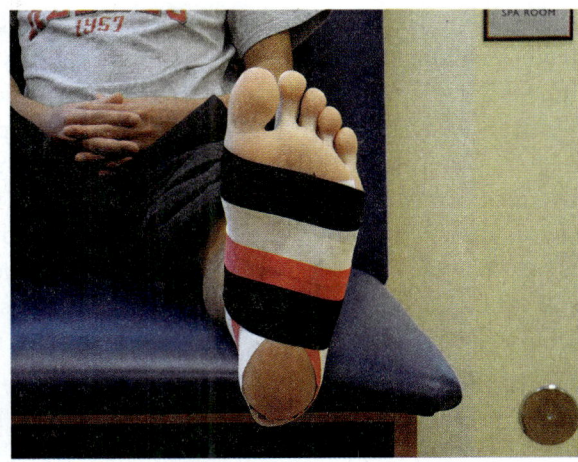

(a) (b)

Figure 16.18 Finish by alternating strips around the foot to maintain and stabilize the arch tape.
Courtesy of Brent Mangus.

plantar fasciitis and clawing of the toes. There have also been cases of athletes with too much arch having generalized discomfort about the foot and ankle because of the inability of the foot to absorb forces owing to the tightness of joints there. These athletes can also benefit from some orthotic help and proper shoe selection. As with the athlete with flat feet, the height of an athlete's arch need not hinder athletic performance.

Bunions

Bunions (Figure 16.19) are not very common in athletes at the high school and college levels. They can simply be a matter of inflamed bursae, or they can involve complicated bone and joint deformities such as severe hallux valgus and rotation of the first metatarsal phalangeal joint. Many times, bunions are caused by improperly fitting footwear. By getting the athlete into correctly fitting shoes, the early signs of a bunion should resolve. If an athlete has had a bunion for an extended period of time (weeks to months), then the athlete should seek the advice of a physician in the care of this condition.

Blisters and Calluses

Blisters and **calluses** are very common formations on athletes' feet. Excessive amounts of movement can produce a great deal of friction between the layers of skin in the foot and the shoe, resulting in the formation of either a blister or a callus. When the athlete starts to experience this abnormal friction (termed a "hot spot"), the application of padding or lubricant to the localized spot will avert the formation of a blister. If a blister forms, the layers of skin have been separated, and the friction has built up a fluid deposit. Always observe the color of the fluid within a blister. Most often, the fluid is clear, but on occasion it will be dark, which means there is blood in this small cavity. Frequently, the pain and discomfort from a blister prevent the athlete from participating in sports. If the blister is large, the fluid should be drained and the area padded well to prevent further friction and blister formation. When a blister is drained, it is best

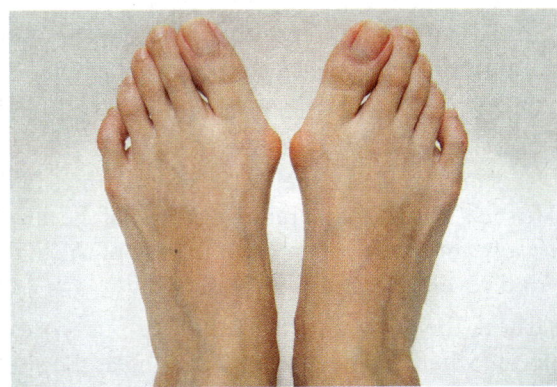

Figure 16.19 Bunions of the first MTP joint.
© kohide/Shutterstock.

Bunion Inflammation and joint deformity of the first metatarsal phalangeal joint usually accompanied by pain and dysfunction.

Blister Excessive friction causing a buildup of fluid between the tissues of the skin.

Callus Rough, raised, and thickened area of skin due to friction.

to leave the top layer of skin in place until a new layer develops, thereby reducing the possibility of introducing infection into the area. In addition, place a doughnut-shaped pad made of felt or a large pad of thin adhesive directly over the blister to reduce friction. In case the blister opens inadvertently (the top flap tears off for some reason), care needs to be taken to ensure that the area is clean and the possibility of infection is reduced. Anytime the blister opens there is a possibility of infection entering the body. If the skin over the top of the blister tears, it is important to try to maintain the torn flap and keep it in contact with the blister if possible. This maintains a little protection for the area. Apply an antibacterial ointment to the area and cover it as necessary.

When draining a blister, be sure to follow the recommended precautions regarding blood-borne pathogens:

1. Always use sterile instruments and keep the environment sterile.
2. Use latex gloves or some other barrier so that body fluids are not contacted.

The following procedure should be followed when draining a blister:

1. Initially, wash the area with soap and warm water, and sterilize the area with rubbing alcohol.
2. Using a sterile needle, puncture the base of the blister and gently drain by applying light pressure. This may need to be repeated several times in the first 24 hours. Do not remove the top of the blister; apply antibiotic ointment to the top of the blister and cover with a sterile dressing.
3. Check the area daily for redness or pus to determine whether infection is occurring at the site.
4. After 3–7 days, gently remove the top of the blister, apply an antibiotic ointment, and cover with a sterile dressing.
5. Watch the area closely for signs of infection, such as redness or pus, and pad the area well with hydrocolloid blister bandages, foam pads, and light tape. This allows for healing to occur without further irritation.

Subungual hematoma Blood formation under a nail.

If the blister is small, padding the area to prevent further friction usually suffices until the blister heals. Athletes should be encouraged to report the formation of any new hot spots or blisters as soon as possible so that padding and protection can be provided. It is definitely best to help prevent blisters by having properly fitting footwear and giving new shoes a short break-in period before using them in practice or competition.

In addition to blisters, excessive tissue can build up on the bottom of the feet, which is commonly known as a callus. Calluses tend to build up over a bony area of the foot and should not be allowed to become large and extremely thick. If this happens, the callus can begin to move with the shoe and not with the foot. This creates an area of friction between the callus and layers of skin, causing a blister to form between the callus and the next lower layer of skin. This can cause problems because the blister is difficult to drain and can be very painful to the athlete. To prevent this from happening, a callus should be shaved regularly to allow for only a small amount of buildup, which then acts as a padding for the area. If a callus gets too large, the athlete will begin to complain of pain and discomfort in the area.

Toe Injuries

The toes can also be injured during sports participation. In some sports, the toes can be stepped on, resulting in torn-off nails or **subungual hematoma** formation under the nail (Figure 16.20). This collection of blood under a nail needs to be released. Numerous techniques to remove this blood exist. Commercially available nail drills bore a small hole in the nail and allow the trapped blood to be released. Releasing this blood provides a great deal of relief to the athlete because this injury can produce a great deal

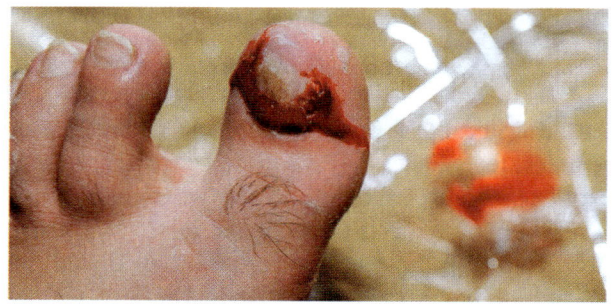

Figure 16.20 Players' toes can be stepped on, resulting in bleeding and significant toenail damage.
© ungvar/Shutterstock.

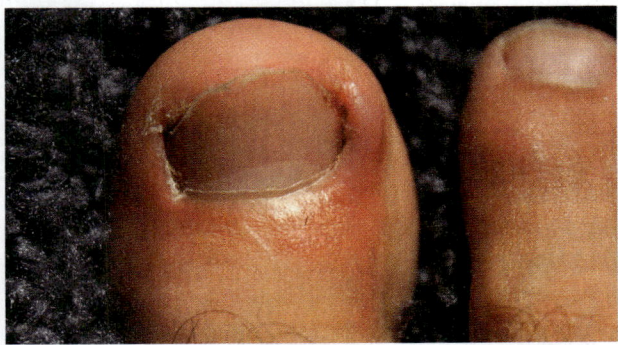

Figure 16.21 Shoes that are too tight can lead to ingrown toenails in the athlete.
© EF Photography/Shutterstock.

of pain. If an athlete wears shoes that are too tight or too small, this can also create a situation in which a toenail is smashed and blood collects under the nail. Shoes that are too small or too tight can also result in an **ingrown toenail** (Figure 16.21). Ingrown toenails need to be treated early because delaying care can result in infection and serious problems. The ingrown nail can produce an open sore on the toe; when the foot is placed in the sport shoe, bacteria can enter this open sore and result in further problems. Ingrown toenails should be treated by soaking them in a warm antibacterial solution. The nail needs to be elevated so that it will grow in a normal direction. This can be done by placing a small cotton roll under the affected part and leaving it there as the nail grows. It is important to address the situation that led up to the ingrown toenail. If the athlete is wearing shoes that are too small or too tight, he or she needs to get a shoe that has a more comfortable fit. Another prevention technique for ingrown toenails is to have the athlete trim the nail straight across, which will encourage the nail to grow out normally.

With the advent of artificial playing surfaces, there has been in increase in the number of injuries to the toe, which has been termed "turf toe" in the athletic population. **Turf toe** is essentially a hyperextension sprain to the ligaments of the great toe and can include an inflammatory process to the sesamoid bones, located just under the first metatarsal joint. Athletes will either push off in an explosive move or be tackled; the foot moves, but the great toe, for some reason, remains on the turf (Najefi et al., 2018). In the case of an immediate-onset injury, athletes will report they heard a pop and felt a sharp pain in their great toe. In chronic cases, the symptoms of pain and inflammation in the big toe area are progressive over time. This is an injury that typically occurs on artificial turf but can occur on other surfaces. Care for turf toe is similar to other sprains: Ice, compression, and elevation should be implemented. Often, athletes do not want to rest this injury, and, in some cases, turf-toe taping is helpful to allow the athlete to continue to participate during the recovery period (Figures 16.22 through 16.25).

> **Ingrown toenail** Partial toenail growth laterally into the skin around the nail causing pain and inflammation.
>
> **Turf toe** Hyperextension of the first metatarsal phalangeal joint causing a sprain to the ligaments and inflammation.

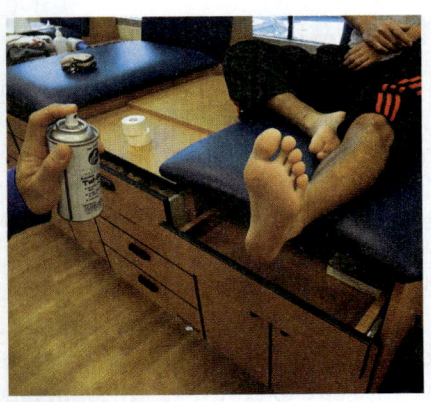
(a)

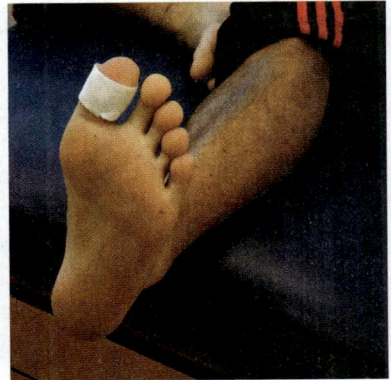
(b)

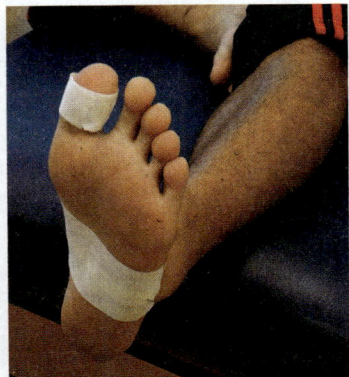
(c)

Figure 16.22 After an adhesive is applied, begin with a toe and foot anchor strip.
Courtesy of Brent Mangus.

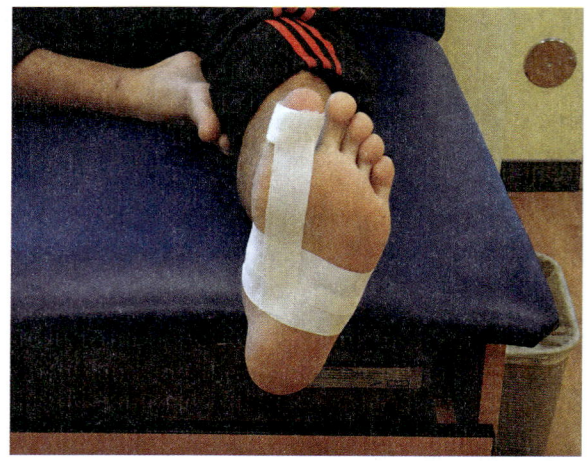
(a)

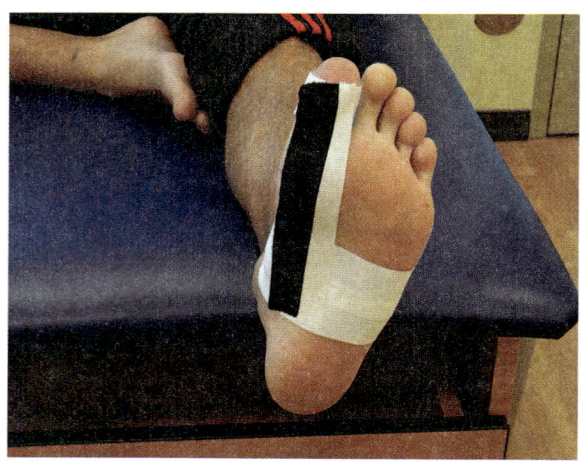
(b)

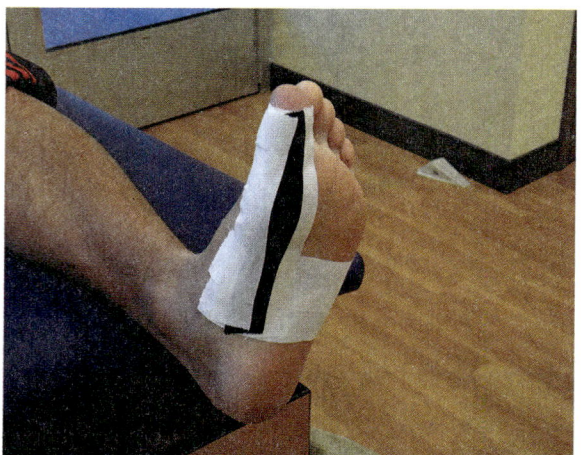
(c)

Figure 16.23 Apply stabilizing strips as demonstrated.
Courtesy of Brent Mangus.

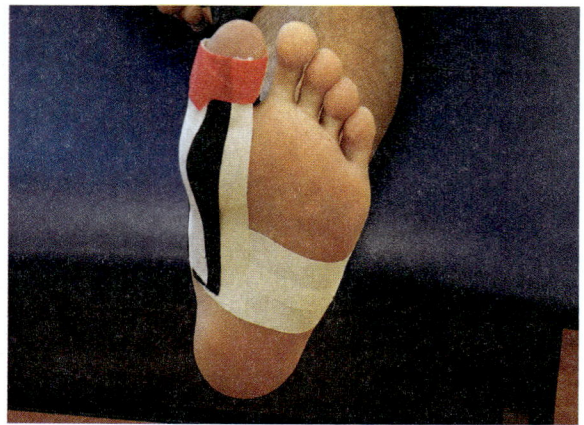
Figure 16.24 Lock down the stabilizing strips at the toe.
Courtesy of Brent Mangus.

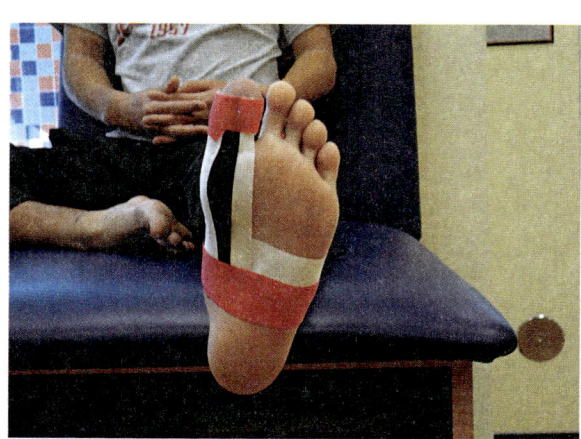
Figure 16.25 Lock down the stabilizing strips at the foot.
Courtesy of Brent Mangus.

Preventive Ankle Taping

Applying preventive ankle taping to athletes is a popular practice among many high school, collegiate, and professional athletic trainers. Athletes commonly have their ankles taped as a routine procedure before practice or competition to prevent or reduce ankle injuries.

The advantages and disadvantages of preventive ankle taping have been discussed widely, and a continuum of recommendations—from not using taping as a preventive measure to always taping both ankles when participating in any sport—is advocated by various athletic trainers.

Some athletic trainers promote the use of lace-up and other rigid braces rather than preventive taping. Recent research concludes that ankle braces are just as effective, if not more so, as preventive taping in reducing inversion ankle sprains (Kaminski et al., 2019; McGuire et al., 2011; McGuire et al., 2012). This concept has been verified by research demonstrating that ankle bracing can reduce inversion ankle sprains in soccer, football, basketball, and volleyball players (Barelds et al., 2018) and assists in the stabilization of the lower extremity (Kaminski et al., 2019). It has also been demonstrated that ankle braces do not detract from an athlete's ability to run, jump, or perform other skills as necessary during athletic competition.

Such information creates an interesting decision matrix for coaches and athletic trainers when determining which preventive measures should be implemented to reduce inversion ankle sprains in athletes. Realizing the probability that preventive ankle taping can result in a reduction in efficacy of the tape reducing inversion movement over time (Fleet et al., 2009), the athletic training and coaching staff need to determine the most efficient means of preventing ankle sprains in the athletic population of their school. There is a time- and cost-benefit analysis that should be evaluated by the staff personnel in making this decision. Some coaches believe that taping the ankles is more efficient when it is done on a semiregular basis, for example, once or twice a week. From a cost analysis, if a player is going to be taped multiple times a day or week, it may be less expensive to use prophylactic braces that the athlete can put on himself or herself before each practice or game.

There are many factors—for example, athlete comfort—that must be analyzed when deciding to use tape or braces for the athletes. Some athletes feel like the braces are bulky and do not let them move normally. Some athletes contend that the ability to wear them with the proper shoes for practice and games is compromised by the size of the brace. Some sports require shoes that are tight and not conducive to fitting the foot and the brace in the shoe. Braces are hardware; they do wear out, and their effectiveness diminishes over time. The cost of the braces is an up-front cost and, sometimes, is expensive for the athlete or the school to purchase. These issues are just some of several other issues that must considered when deciding how to prevent inversion ankle injuries in athletes at a specific location.

Preventive ankle taping is an important skill that must be learned properly, practiced until a level of mastery is gained, and then applied in an athletic team setting. Taping is an art and a science, and each strip of tape has its own function. The following preventive taping outline is intended to provide the beginning student with the theoretical basis for the reasons the tape is applied. If students are interested in developing taping skills, it is recommended that they work under the direct supervision of a BOC-certified athletic trainer to learn and practice the art of taping.

As shown in Figure 16.26, the use of prewrap and anchoring strips is important in starting the taping procedure correctly. An adherent is used to help the prewrap stay in place. If an adherent is not used, the tape will, in most situations, loosen and slide, thus diminishing the effectiveness of the taping procedure. The use of stirrups (Figures 16.27 through 16.29 a and b) is intended to maintain the foot in a normal or slightly everted position. Stirrups are combined with horseshoe strips (Figures 16.28 a and b), which help to hold the stirrups in place and reduce the gaps in the tape on the posterior portion of the foot. Figures 16.30 through 16.32 demonstrate the use of heel locks, which assist in stabilizing the subtalar joint. Heel locks are followed by the use of another figure eight (Figures 16.33 a and b),

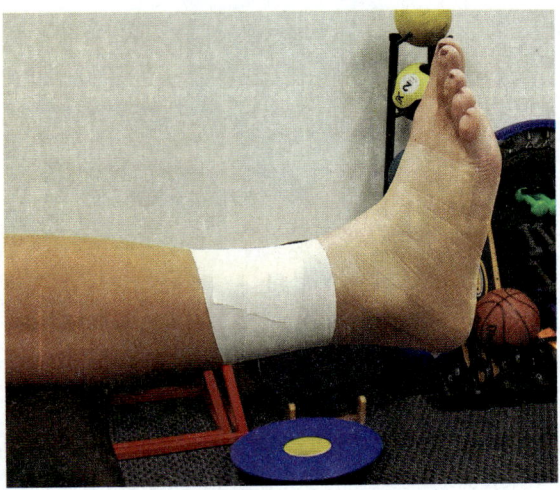

Figure 16.26 Prewrap and tape anchors are used to start a preventative ankle taping job.
Courtesy of Cindy Trowbridge.

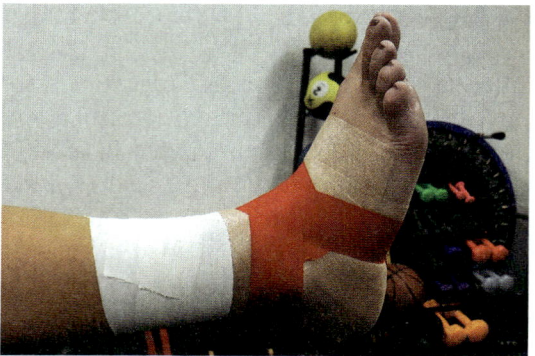

Figure 16.27 A figure eight is completed around the arch and above the malleoli. A figure eight takes practice in order to get the proper placement and direction of pull on the tape.
Courtesy of Cindy Trowbridge.

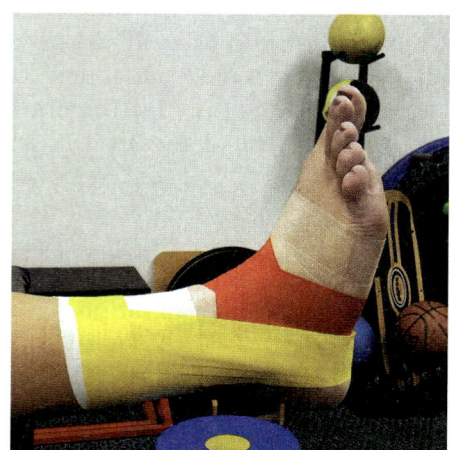

(a)

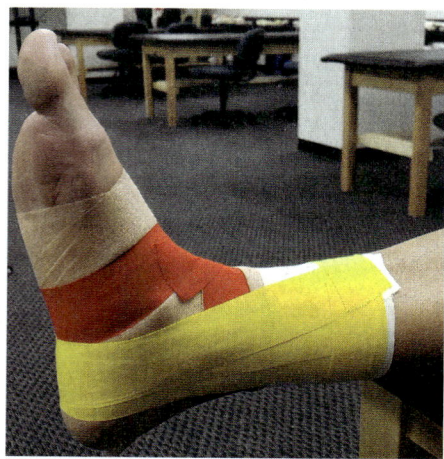

(b)

Figure 16.28 A minimum of three stirrups are applied from medial side to lateral side and are anchored proximally. Tape should cover malleolus and provide an eversion force. Stirrups are used to maintain a normal or slightly elevated foot position. **(a)** Lateral view. **(b)** Medial view.
Courtesy of Cindy Trowbridge.

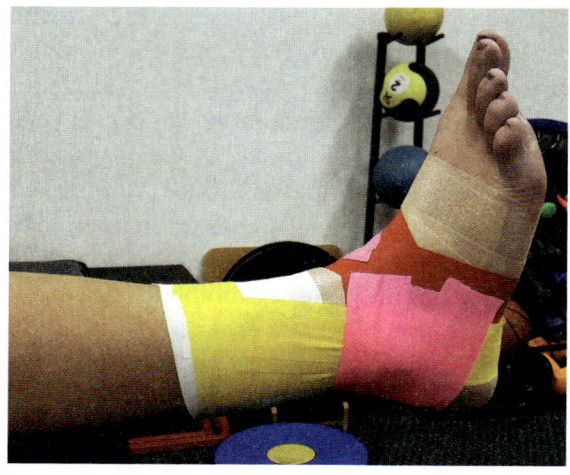

(a)

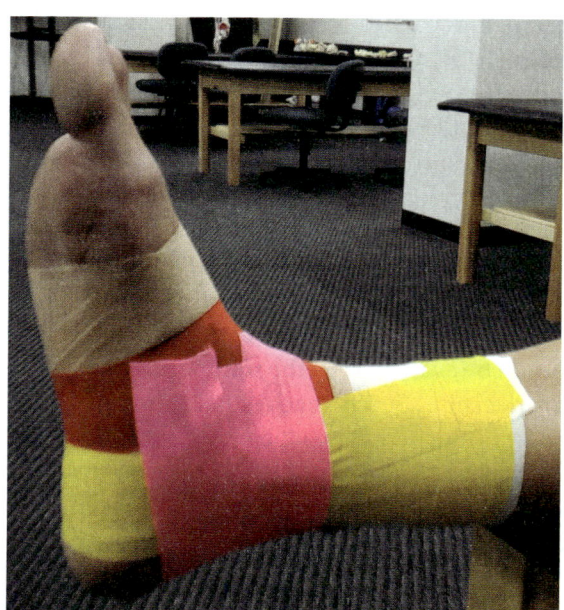

(b)

Figure 16.29 A minimum of three horseshoes are applied above and below the malleoli, moving proximal to distal to provide a tibiofibular compression force. **(a)** Lateral view. **(b)** Medial view.
Courtesy of Cindy Trowbridge.

which are intended to help stabilize the talocrural joint and the transverse tarsal joint. From this point on, the procedure involves using finishing strips to make sure there are no gaps or holes between strips of tape, securing the tape at the bottom, and using a final covering to ensure that tape ends do not get rolled or wrinkled as the athlete puts on socks and shoes (Figures 16.34 a, b, and c).

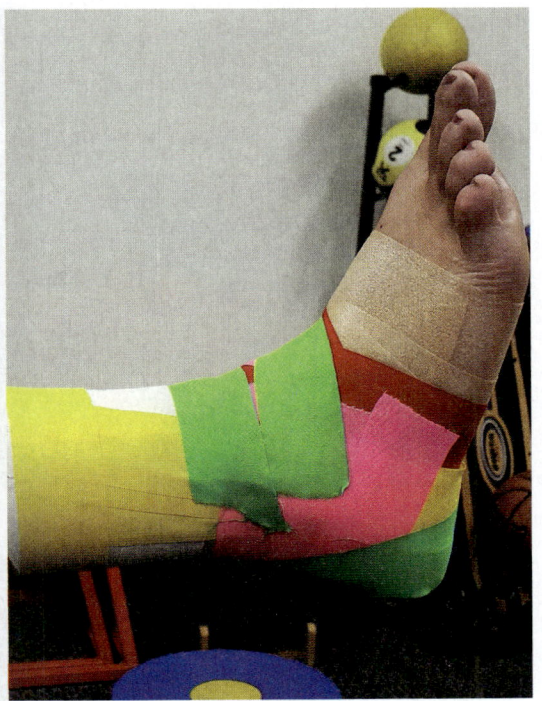

(a)

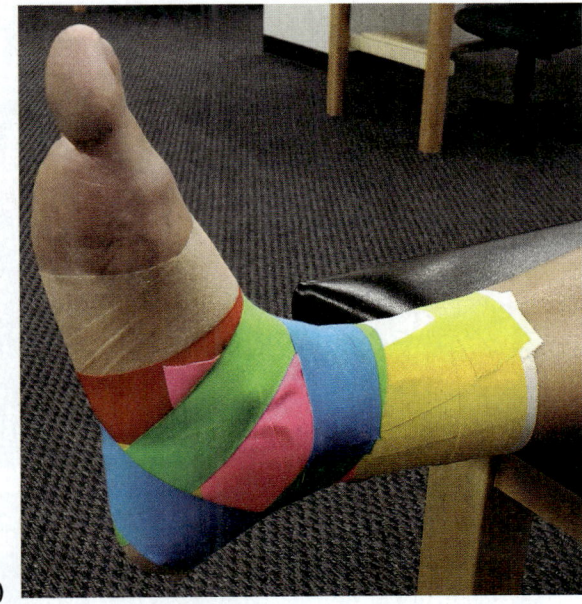

(a)

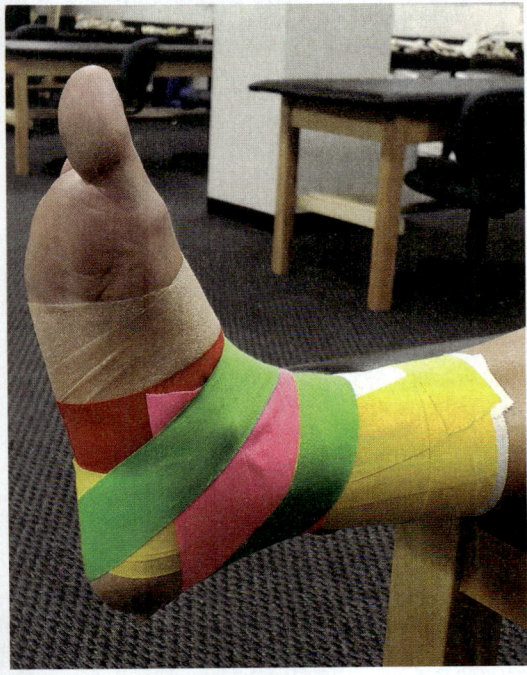

(b)

Figure 16.30 A lateral heel lock is applied to secure the subtalar joint and position the ankle in a neutral to everted position in an effort to restrict inversion and plantarflexion. Lateral heel lock can be applied in an upward or downward direction as it crosses the heel near the subtalar joint. **(a)** Lateral view. **(b)** Medial view.
Courtesy of Cindy Trowbridge.

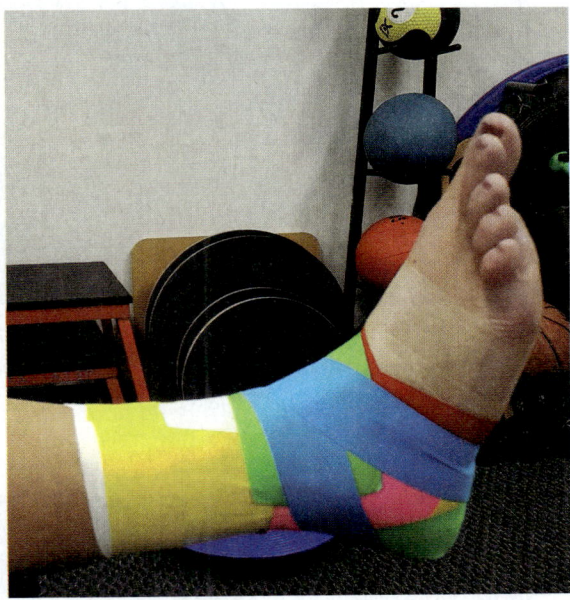

(b)

Figure 16.31 A medial heel lock is applied to secure the subtalar joint and position the ankle in a neutral to everted position in an effort to restrict inversion and plantarflexion. Medial heel lock can be applied in an upward or downward direction as it crosses the heel near the subtalar joint. **(a)** Medial view. **(b)** Lateral view.
Courtesy of Cindy Trowbridge.

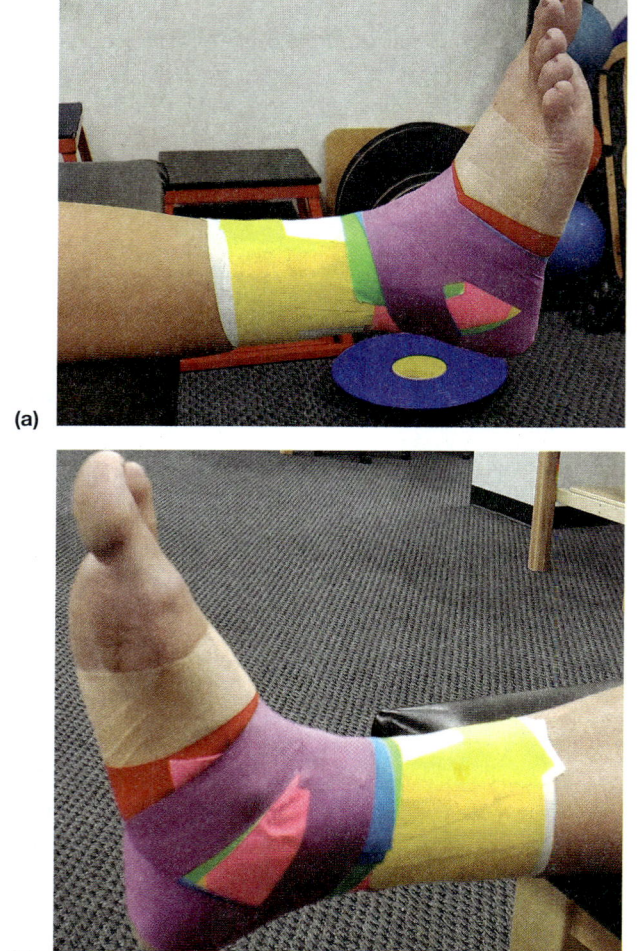

(a)

(b)

Figure 16.32 A combined lateral and medial heel lock is applied to secure the subtalar joint and provide increased stability. (a) Lateral view. (b) Medial view.
Courtesy of Cindy Trowbridge.

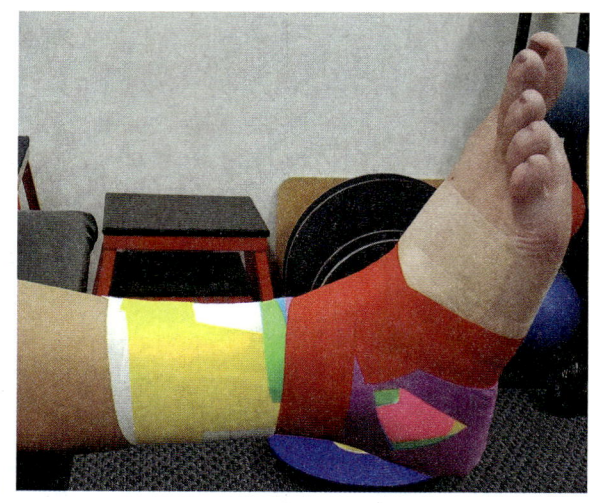

(a)

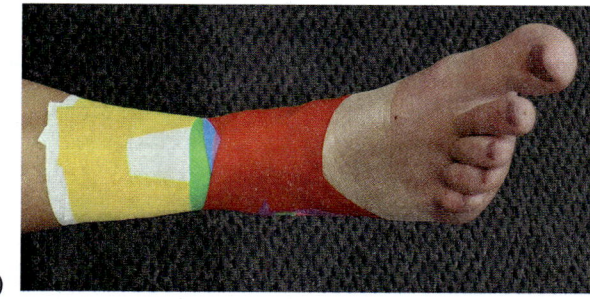

(b)

Figure 16.33 A second figure eight is completed around the arch and above the malleoli to provide increased stability. (a) Lateral view. (b) Top view.
Courtesy of Cindy Trowbridge.

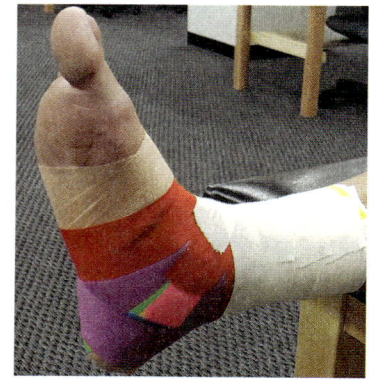

(a)

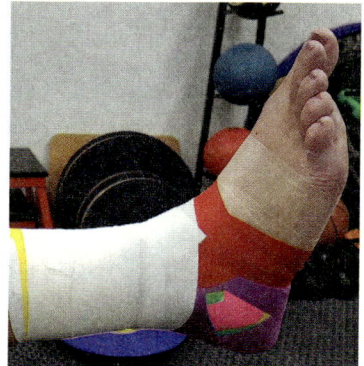

(b)

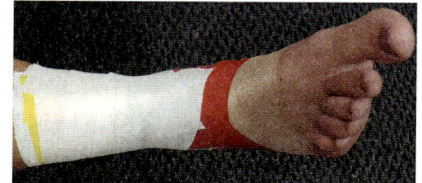

(c)

Figure 16.34 The completed ankle taping procedure. (a) Lateral view. (b) Medial view. (c) Top view.
Courtesy of Cindy Trowbridge.

Review Questions

1. Name the two bones located in the lower leg.
2. Explain where the fibula is located and approximately how much body weight is supported by this bone.
3. What is the technical name for the ankle joint?
4. Name the strongest and largest of the ankle ligaments.
5. Draw or outline the compartments of the lower leg, and describe the actions that the muscles in each compartment have on the foot.
6. Which compartment of the lower leg presents the most problems with fluid accumulation?
7. Outline the signs and symptoms of a fracture of the lower leg.
8. True or false? An inversion ankle sprain is more common than an eversion ankle sprain.
9. Explain which type of ankle sprain is more severe.
10. Describe where the Achilles tendon attaches, and describe the signs, symptoms, and treatment of Achilles tendinitis.
11. Explain the possible long-term complications if problems with anterior compartment syndrome are left untreated.
12. Explain what types of changes (e.g., biomechanical and training) an athlete may need to make to alleviate and prevent further episodes of shin splints.
13. Outline the key signs and symptoms of plantar fasciitis, and explain how heel spurs are associated with this condition.
14. What structures are involved in Morton's foot?
15. Explain the difference between pes cavus and pes planus.
16. Explain the difference between a blister and a callus.
17. Outline how a blister should be cared for when it is drained.
18. Explain how blisters can be prevented.
19. True or false? It is not possible for a callus to form over a blister.
20. True or false? Callus formation on the plantar aspect of the foot should be trimmed regularly to reduce friction.

References

Alawna, M., & Mohamed, A. A. (2020). Short-term and long-term effects of ankle joint taping and bandaging on balance, proprioception and vertical jump among volleyball players with chronic ankle instability. *Physical Therapy in Sport, 46*, 145–154.

Alt, W., Lohrer, H., & Gollhofer, A. (1999). Functional properties of adhesive ankle taping: Neuromuscular and mechanical effects before and after exercise. *Foot & Ankle International, 20*(4), 238–245.

Babins, E. M. (2012). Lace-up ankle braces reduced acute ankle injuries in high school basketball players. *Clinical Journal of Sports Medicine, 22*(4), 377–380.

Barelds, I., van den Broek, A. G., & Huisstede, B. (2018). Ankle bracing is effective for primary and secondary prevention of acute ankle injuries in athletes: A systematic review and meta-analyses. *Sports Medicine, 48*(12), 2775–2784.

Becker, J., Nakajima, M., & Wu, W. F. (2018). Factors contributing to medial tibial stress syndrome in runners: A prospective study. *Medicine & Science in Sports & Exercise, 50*(10), 2092–2100.

Brewer, R. B., & Gregory, A. J. M. (2012). Chronic lower leg pain in athletes: A guide for the differential diagnosis, evaluation, and treatment. *Sports Health, 4*(2), 121–127.

Buerba, R. A., Fretes, N. F., Devana, S. K., & Beck, J. J. (2019). Chronic exertional compartment syndrome: Current management strategies. *Open Access Journal of Sports Medicine, 10*, 71–79.

Buldt, A. K., Allan, J. J., Landorf, K. B., & Menz, H. B. (2018). The relationship between foot posture and plantar pressure during walking in adults: A systematic review. *Gait & Posture, 62*, 56–67.

Carson, D. W., Myer, G. D., Hewett, T. E., Heidt Jr., R. S., & Ford, K. R. (2012). Increased plantar force and impulse in American football players with high arch compared to normal arch. *Foot, 22*(4), 310–314.

Chen, E. T., McInnis, K. C., & Borg-Stein, J. (2019). Ankle sprains: Evaluation, rehabilitation, and prevention. *Current Sports Medicine Reports, 18*(6), 217–223.

Fleet, K., Galen, S., & Moore, C. (2009). Duration of strength retention of ankle taping during activities of daily living. *Injury, 40*(3), 333–336.

Hadadi, M., Haghighat, F., Mohammadpour, N., & Sobhani, S. (2020). Effects of kinesiotape vs soft and semirigid ankle orthoses on balance in patients with chronic ankle instability: A randomized controlled trial. *Foot & Ankle International, 41*(7), 793–802.

Herzog, M. M., Kerr, Z. Y., Marshall, S. W., & Wikstrom, E. A. (2019). Epidemiology of ankle sprains and chronic ankle instability. *Journal of Athletic Training, 54*(6), 603–610.

Hubbard, T. J., Carpenter, E. M., & Cordova, M. L. (2009). Contributing factors to medial tibial stress syndrome: A perspective investigation. *Medicine & Science in Sports & Exercise, 41*(3), 490–496.

Hubbard-Turner, T. (2019). Lack of medical treatment from a medical professional after an ankle sprain. *Journal of Athletic Training, 54*(6), 671–675.

Hubscher, M., Zech, A., Pfeifer, K., Hänsel, F., Vogt, L., & Banzer, W. (2010). Neuromuscular training for sports injury prevention: A systematic review. *Medicine & Science in Sports & Exercise, 42*(3), 413–421.

Kaminski, T. W., Needle, A. R., & Delahunt, E. (2019). Prevention of lateral ankle sprains. *Journal of Athletic Training, 54*(6), 650–661.

Kaplan, Y. (2011). Prevention of ankle sprains in sport: A systematic literature review. *British Journal of Sports Medicine, 45*(4), 355.

Kasitinon, D., & Argo, L. R. (2020). Risk factors for developing stress fractures. In T. L. Miller & C. C. Kaeding (Eds.), *Stress fractures in athletes* (pp. 3–20). New York, NY: Springer, Cham.

Knapik, D. M., Trem, A., Sheehan, J., Salata, M. J., & Voos, J. E. (2018). Conservative management for stable high ankle injuries in professional football players. *Sports Health, 10*(1), 80–84.

Knapik, J. J., Spiess, A., Swedler, D. I., Grier, T. L., Darakjy, S. S., & Jones, B. H. (2010). Systematic review of the parachute ankle brace: Injury risk reduction and cost effectiveness. *American Journal of Preventive Medicine, 38*(1S), S182–S188.

Lloyd, A., & Lueders, D. (2021). Leg injuries. In G. Miranda-Comas, G. Cooper, J. Herrera, & S. Curtis (Eds.), *Essential sports medicine* (pp. 341–366). New York, NY: Springer, Cham.

Lohkamp, M., Craven, S., Walker-Johnson, C., & Greig, M. (2009). The influence of ankle taping on changes in postural stability during soccer specific activity. *Journal of Sport Rehabilitation, 18*(2), 482–492.

Lohrer, H., Alt, W., & Gollhofer, A. (1999). Neuromuscular properties and functional aspects of taped ankles. *American Journal of Sports Medicine, 27*(1), 69–75.

Longo, U. G., Loppini, M., Berton, A., Marinozzi, A., Maffulli, N., & Denaro, V. (2012). The FIFA 111 program is effective in preventing injuries in elite male basketball players. *American Journal of Sports Medicine, 40*(6), 996–1005.

McGuire, T. A., Brooks, A., & Hetzel, S. (2011). The effect of lace-up ankle braces on injury rates in high school basketball players. *American Journal of Sports Medicine, 39*(9), 1840–1848.

McGuire, T. A., Hetzel, S., Wilson, J., & Brooks, A. (2012). The effect of lace-up ankle braces on injury rates in high school football players. *American Journal of Sports Medicine, 40*(1), 49–57.

Menéndez, C., Batalla, L., Prieto, A., Rodríguez, M. Á., Crespo, I., & Olmedillas, H. (2020). Medial tibial stress syndrome in novice and recreational runners: A systematic review. *International Journal of Environmental Research and Public Health, 17*(20), 7457–7470.

Moen, M. H., Holtslag, L., Bakker, E., Barten, C., Weir, A., Tol, J. L., & Backx, F. (2012). The treatment of medial tibial stress syndrome in athletes: A randomized clinical trial. *Sports Medicine, Arthroscopy, Rehabilitation Therapy & Technology, 4*(12), 1–8.

Moini, J. (2020). *Anatomy and physiology for health professionals* (3rd ed.). Burlington, MA: Jones & Bartlett Learning.

Najefi, A. A., Jeyaseelan, L., & Welck, M. (2018). Turf toe: A clinical update. *EFORT Open Reviews, 3*(9), 501–506.

Patel, K. A., Richards, S. M., Day, J., & Drakos, M. C. (2021). Acute fractures in sport: Foot. In G. A. J. Robertson & N. Maffuli (Eds.), *Fractures in sport* (pp. 283–307). New York, NY: Springer, Cham.

Pearce, C. J., & Tan, A. (2016). Non-insertional Achilles tendinopathy. *EFORT Open Reviews, 1*(11), 383–390.

Porter, D. A., Hurst, K., & Walrod, M. (2021). Acute fractures in sport: Ankle. In G. A. J. Robertson & N. Maffuli (Eds.), *Fractures in sport* (pp. 245–282). New York, NY: Springer, Cham.

Prakash, A. A. (2020). Epidemiology of high ankle sprains: A systematic review. *Foot & Ankle Specialist, 13*(5), 420–430.

Quirolgico, K., & Townsend, C. (2021). Ankle and foot injuries. In G. Miranda-Comas, G. Cooper, J. Herrera, & S. Curtis (Eds.), *Essential sports medicine* (pp. 367–390). New York, NY: Springer, Cham.

Ramponi, D. R., & Baker, C. (2019). Sever's disease (calcaneal apophysitis). *Advanced Emergency Nursing Journal, 41*(1), 10–14.

Ricard, M. D., Schulthies, S. S., & Saret, J. J. (2000a). Effects of high-top and low-top shoes on ankle inversion. *Journal of Athletic Training, 35*(1), 38–43.

Ricard, M. D., Schulthies, S. S., & Saret, J. J. (2000b). Effects of tape and exercise on dynamic ankle inversion. *Journal of Athletic Training, 35*(1), 31–37.

Scheer, R. C., Newman, J. M., Zhou, J. J., Oommen, A. J., Naziri, Q., Shah, N. V., Pascal, S. C., Penny, G. S., McKean, J. M., Tsai, J., & Uribe, J. A. (2020). Ankle fracture epidemiology in the United States: Patient-related trends and mechanisms of injury. *Journal of Foot and Ankle Surgery, 59*(3), 479–483.

Simon, J. E., Wikstrom, E. A., Grooms, D. R., Docherty, C. L., Dompier, T. P., & Kerr, Z. Y. (2019). Athletic training service characteristics for patients with ankle sprains sustained during high school athletics. *Journal of Athletic Training, 54*(6), 676–683.

Tarantino, D., Palermi, S., Sirico, F., & Corrado, B. (2020). Achilles tendon rupture: Mechanisms of injury, principles of rehabilitation and return to play. *Journal of Functional Morphology and Kinesiology, 5*(4), 95.

Thomson, L., Aujla, R. S., Divall, P., & Bhatia, M. (2020). Non-surgical treatments for Morton's neuroma: A systematic review. *Foot and Ankle Surgery, 26*(7), 736–743.

Trojian, T., & Tucker, A. K. (2019). Plantar fasciitis. *American Family Physician, 99*(12), 744–750.

van Dijk, P. A., Kerkhoffs, G. M., Chiodo, C., & DiGiovanni, C. W. (2019). Chronic disorders of the peroneal tendons: Current concepts review of the literature. *Journal of the American Academy of Orthopaedic Surgeons, 27*(16), 590–598.

Verhagen, E. A. L. M., & Bay, K. (2010). Optimizing ankle sprain prevention: A critical review and practical appraisal of the literature. *British Journal of Sports Medicine, 44*(15), 1082–1088.

Vuurberg, G., Spennacchio, P., Laver, L., Pereira, J. P., Diniz, P., & Kerkhoffs, G. M. M. J. (2021). Current concepts in ankle sprain treatment. In H. Pereira, S. Guillo, M. Glazebrook, M. Takao, J. Calder, N. Van Dijk, & J. Karlsson (Eds.), *Lateral ankle instability* (pp. 93–104). Berlin, Heidelberg: Springer.

Yasui, Y., Tonogai, I., Rosenbaum, A. J., Shimozono, Y., Kawano, H., & Kennedy, J. G. (2017). The risk of Achilles tendon rupture in the patients with Achilles tendinopathy: Healthcare database analysis in the United States. *BioMed Research International, 2017*(4), 1–4. doi:10.1155/2017/7021862

Yuen, C. P., & Lui, T. H. (2017). Distal tibiofibular syndesmosis: Anatomy, biomechanics, injury and management. *Open Orthopaedics Journal,* 11, 670–677. doi:10.2174/1874325001711010670

Zwiers, R., Vuurberg, G., Blankevoort, L., & Kerkhoffs, G. M. M. J. (2016). Taping and bracing in the prevention of ankle sprains: Current concepts. *Journal of ISAKOS, 1*(6), 304–310.

CHAPTER 17
Skin Conditions in Sports

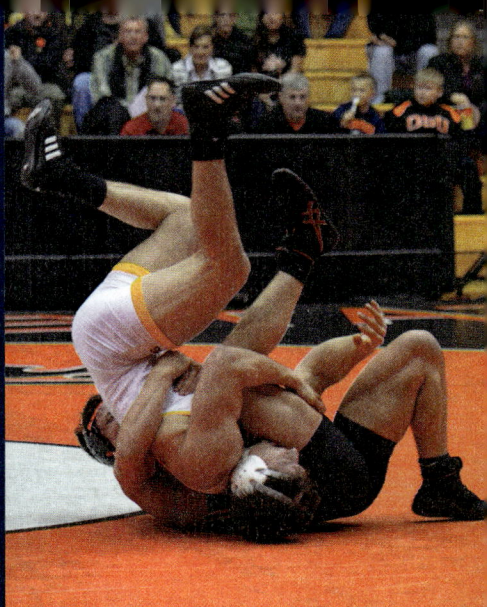

MAJOR CONCEPTS

The skin, the largest organ of the human body, is often involved in sports injuries, which range from simple wounds to a variety of bacterial, fungal, and viral infections to allergic reactions and parasitic issues. This chapter discusses the basic anatomy of the skin and describes the categories of wounds and their care. Obviously, the risk of blood-borne pathogen infection must be considered whenever a potential exposure to blood exists. The chapter presents the latest guidelines available for the prevention of accidental exposure to human blood.

Next, the chapter covers traumatic skin conditions; skin inflammatory conditions, such as ultraviolet exposure and poisons; exacerbation conditions; and skin infections from any number of microorganisms, ranging from minute viruses and bacteria to relatively large fungi. The chapter introduces the reader to the common types of skin infections in sports, with descriptions of signs and symptoms and recommended treatment and prevention protocols. The National Collegiate Athletic Association guidelines on wrestling and skin infections are included along with a listing of conditions to be considered. This section also covers a related group of skin conditions resulting from allergic reactions to plant toxins and other materials.

The skin, or common integument, represents the largest organ of the human body. As shown in Figure 17.1, two major layers of tissues, the epidermis and dermis, combine to form this complex organ, which has a total surface area of 3,000 square inches on the average adult. Located immediately beneath the skin is a layer of subcutaneous fat that helps to insulate the body from the external environment. Skin thickness varies regionally on the body: Thicker skin covers areas subject to pressure, such as the soles of the feet and palms of the hands; thinner skin covers areas where joint mobility is essential.

The skin serves a variety of purposes, not the least of which is protecting the body from the environment. It is also essential for controlling fluid balance within the body, protecting the body from disease organisms, and regulating body temperature. Furthermore, it houses nerves of sensation that register touch, temperature, and pressure. In addition, specialized cells within the skin produce vitamin D.

The skin can be damaged in a variety of ways during participation in sports. External trauma can cause wounds, and damage can result from exposure to ultraviolet rays (sunlight) and burning or freezing

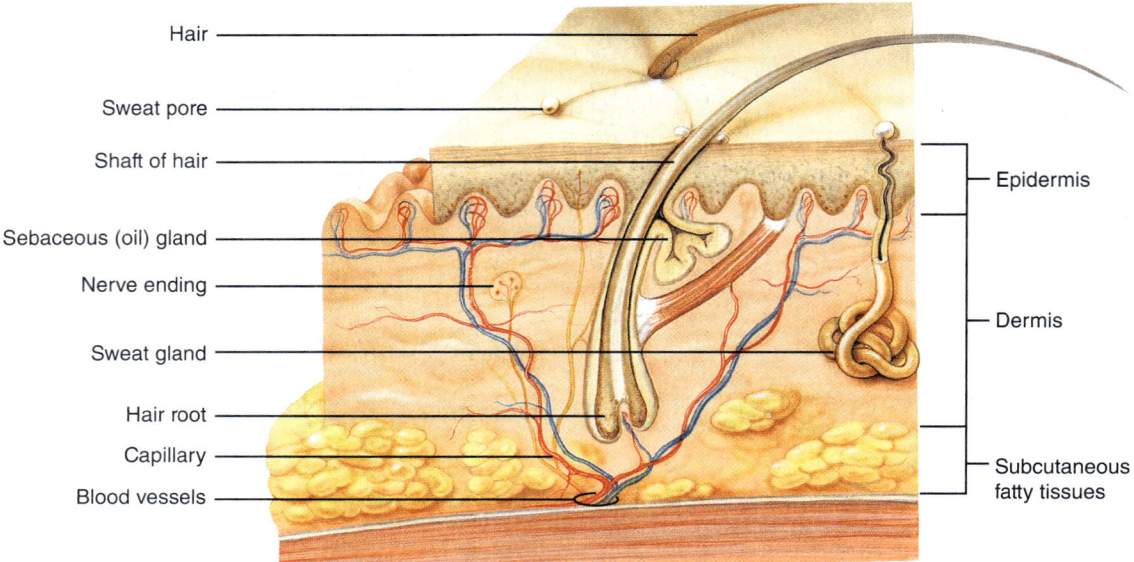

Figure 17.1 A cross section of human skin.

temperatures. Skin infections can arise from a variety of organisms, including **fungi**, **bacteria**, **viruses**, and **parasites**. In addition, allergies can also affect the skin; they may be related to contact with plants or clothing and equipment that contain chemicals to which the athlete is sensitive.

Certain skin conditions can be prevented by practicing good hygiene habits, which include washing hands; showering soon after activity; not sharing items, such as clothing, equipment, braces, towels, and personal items such as brushes and razors; and avoiding direct contact with potentially infected individuals. Additionally, keeping tables and surfaces, locker rooms, and showers clean and disinfected is important for prevention as well. There are several cleaning and disinfecting products on the market. Most manufacturers will list on the label the germs their product destroys. Ideal disinfectants should have a broad spectrum; should not destroy instruments or surfaces; and should be fast acting, nontoxic, odorless, easy to use, soluble in water, and environmentally friendly. Instructions on the label should be followed to ensure proper use (Centers for Disease Control and Prevention [CDC], 2020a).

Fungus (pl. fungi) A eukaryotic organism such as yeasts, molds, and mushrooms.

Bacteria (sing. bacterium) Microorganisms that are usually single-celled and found in most environments on Earth. They are very versatile, can survive in extreme conditions, and can be both harmful and helpful. It is estimated that the human body contains more bacterial cells than human cells.

Virus Infectious agent that lacks cell structure and causes contagious conditions.

Parasite Microscopic organism that lives on or in a host and may cause disease or skin lesions, some of which are contagious.

Abrasions Rubbing or scraping off of skin.

Lacerations Cuts and gashes.

Avulsions Forcible tearing away or separation.

Puncture Wound created when an object punctures the skin and creates a hole.

Incision Wound created when a sharp-edged object cuts through skin.

Traumatic Skin Conditions

Wounds

Sports injuries can cause many types of wounds, including **abrasions** (scrapes), **lacerations** (cuts and gashes), **avulsions** (skin torn from body), **punctures** (object punctures the skin and creates a hole), **incisions** (sharp-edged object cuts through skin), and blisters (patch of raised skin with watery substance underneath), all of which might result in infection and cosmetic complications. The majority of wounds seen in sports are abrasions caused by rubbing, scraping, and burning; lacerations produced by a blunt object tearing the skin; and incisions caused by sharp objects. A special type of abrasion, known as turf burn, has been associated with playing surfaces in stadiums made of artificial turf. Turf burns are the result of falls sustained on artificial turf that produce friction and heat.

Wound Treatment

A primary concern when rendering first aid care for any wound is to avoid contact with whole blood, which may transmit **blood-borne pathogens** or infectious organisms, such as the **human immunodeficiency virus (HIV)**, **hepatitis B virus (HBV)**, or **hepatitis C virus (HCV)**. Although the chance of such an occurrence may be remote, some precautions are necessary, especially in sports in which external bleeding is likely. The **Occupational Safety and Health Administration (OSHA)** developed a comprehensive set of guidelines for healthcare workers regarding prevention of exposure to HIV, HBV, and HCV (U.S. Department of Labor & U.S. Department of Health and Human Services, 1987). These guidelines have subsequently been updated and are available online (U.S. Department of Labor, n.d.). Although coaching personnel are not commonly thought of as healthcare providers, virtually all coaches find themselves dealing on a regular basis with open wounds on some of their athletes. Coaches and athletes are routinely exposed to blood-contaminated towels, water bottles, and playing surfaces and blood-soaked bandaging materials. As a result, the prudent coach should make every effort to follow the basic preventive guidelines for blood-borne pathogen transmission that have been outlined by OSHA and/or other entities, such as the National Federation of State High School Associations (NFHS) or the National Collegiate Athletic Association (NCAA).

Human blood and other bodily fluids, except sweat, can carry infectious organisms; for that reason **universal and standard precautions**, or methods, to protect you and others from human blood pathogens and other potentially infected material are recommended by the Department of Health and Human Services and OSHA. Universal and standard precautions involve the use of hand hygiene, personal protective equipment (e.g., medical gloves, masks/face shields, and gowns), safe injection practices, safe handling practices of contaminated equipment and surfaces, and respiratory hygiene. OSHA also requires employers to supply personal protective equipment for their personnel (CDC, 2016a).

Athletes participating in wrestling, tackle football, and boxing frequently sustain bleeding wounds. It is advised that coaches and officials remove players from participation when excessive bleeding is evident. In addition, a saturated uniform needs to be changed before the athlete is allowed to return to activity, and blood-stained towels should not be shared; instead, they should be placed in an appropriate bag for treatment or disposal (NCAA, 2014). People providing first aid care for such injuries should protect themselves by wearing latex or nonlatex medical gloves and perhaps even eye protection when treating a bleeding wound. Athletes, coaches, and healthcare providers should wash their hands and skin as soon as possible after being exposed to the blood of an injured athlete. Conversely, coaches and healthcare providers with

---

Blister Excessive friction causing a buildup of fluid between the tissues of the skin.

Blood-borne pathogen Infectious organism in human blood that can lead to disease and is spread through direct contact with an infected person's blood.

Human immunodeficiency virus (HIV) A virus that destroys important immune function, making it hard to fight disease and infection.

Hepatitis B virus (HBV) A liver infection that can lead to cirrhosis or liver cancer.

Hepatitis C virus (HCV) A short-term or chronic liver infection.

Occupational Safety and Health Administration (OSHA) Agency of the U.S. Department of Labor that is responsible for establishing and enforcing safety and health standards in the workplace.

Universal and standard precautions The practice of avoiding contact with a person's bodily fluids, by means of the wearing of nonporous articles, such as medical gloves, goggles, and face shields. The practice was expanded and is now known as standard precautions.

open wounds should protect athletes from possible infection by wearing medical gloves or bandages and practicing good personal hygiene.

It should be obvious that hand washing is most important for reducing disease transmission. The CDC (2020b) recommends washing hands with soap and water when they are dirty, before and after touching a patient, and after removing gloves and using the restroom. Hands should be rubbed together with soap and water for at least 15 seconds, rinsed, and dried with a disposable towel.

Even though annual HIV infections and rates decreased 15% in ages 13–24 and remained stable in ages 25–34 from 2015–2019 (CDC, 2019a), education of athletes, coaches, and parents about the transmission and prevention of blood-borne pathogens is essential. While participation in organized sports presents a very low risk for contraction of viruses, prudence dictates that precautions be implemented because sports participation does carry some risk to all parties involved—athletes, coaches, and sports medicine personnel. Virtually anyone who is sexually active, including athletes, is at risk of contracting HIV. Athletes who inject anabolic steroids may also be at risk of infection, especially when they share needles (NCAA, 2014). The virus is spread primarily through intimate sexual contact or blood-to-blood exposure, which can easily occur when sharing needles during intravenous drug use. HIV, HBV, and HCV are carried within the blood of infected persons; therefore, anytime such individuals sustain a bleeding wound, the possibility of transmission exists; this is especially true if another athlete who also has an open wound comes into contact with the blood of an infected person.

The primary goals of initial wound care are control of bleeding followed by prevention of infection through cleaning and dressing. Treatment of open wounds in sports can be considered to be a two-phase process. Initial first aid care is designed to control bleeding to prevent additional blood loss, protect others from exposure, and protect the area from further injury. The initial first aid is later followed with ongoing protection of the area so that return to participation is possible while healing takes place. As previously stated, an important aspect of wound care is protection of fellow athletes, coaches, and other personnel from exposure to whole blood, which can result in the transmission of blood-borne pathogens. Risk of exposure involves not only the wound itself but also blood-soaked clothing and any blood that may be on playing surfaces.

Guidelines for the initial treatment of open bleeding wounds are as follows (National Athletic Trainers' Association [NATA], n.d.b; Ubbinek et al., 2015):

1. Before rendering first aid, precautions should be taken against the possible transmission of blood-borne pathogens. Wear latex gloves (or nonlatex medical gloves for those who are allergic). In cases of profuse bleeding or bleeding involving the airway, such as in the nose and mouth, eye protection is recommended.
2. Remove clothing and/or equipment covering the wound. Clean the wound and the area around the wound with lukewarm saline or potable water as soon as possible. To remove debris, gently squirt water into the area and avoid scrubbing or swabbing the wound or using hydrogen peroxide.
3. Control bleeding with direct pressure over the wound site by applying a sterile dressing. Commercial sterile gauze pads are available in an array of sizes and work well in these situations. By definition, a **dressing** is a sterile material, usually gauze, used to cover a wound to control bleeding and prevent contamination.
4. If the dressing becomes soaked with blood, add more dressing on top. Do not remove blood-soaked dressings.
5. Although rare in sports, severe bleeding may not respond to direct pressure. In such cases, combine direct pressure with elevation.
6. Increased hemorrhage control can be achieved via the application of pressure to a point over either the brachial or femoral artery, depending on the location of the wound. Once pressure is applied to either of these points, it should not be released until the athlete is under the care of a physician.
7. Tourniquets should be applied only as a last resort; they are rarely needed in first aid for sports-related wounds.
8. The following scenarios should be referred to a physician:
   a. Unable to stop bleeding.

Dressing Covering, either protective or supportive, that is applied to an injury or wound.

b. Wounds below the dermal layer more than a centimeter.
c. Wounds on the face due to cosmetic reasons.
d. Debris that will not easily rinse out.
e. If cut by rusty object and the last tetanus shot was over 5 years ago.
9. All materials used to treat the wound—gauze pads, towels, and paper towels—should be stored for later disposal or cleaning in a container properly identified as containing biohazardous materials.

At the time of initial first aid, a decision must be made about whether the athlete will be allowed to participate again. Obviously, the health and safety of the athlete must be the first priority; however, the majority of sports-related wounds are not life-threatening occurrences. Another consideration is protection of other participants, coaches, and personnel from exposure to whole blood from any wound. In contact sports, such as wrestling, tackle football, and basketball, wounds must be dealt with in such a way as to protect other athletes and the coaching staff from incidental exposure. Although research indicates that the risk of transmission of HIV and HBV in such athletic situations is extremely low, the possibility does exist (NCAA, 2014).

Once the initial bleeding is arrested, and assuming 1 and 2 from above are completed, the guidelines for wound treatment are as follows (NATA, n.d.b; Ubbinek et al., 2015):

1. The wound should be covered with a commercially made dressing and/or bandage. A **bandage** is used to hold the dressing in place. Bandages need not be anything more than a folded cravat, strips of cloth, or commercially made elastic adhesive tape that can be directly applied to the skin and holds well even near a moving joint. Small wounds are usually treatable by simply applying a bandage (e.g., a Band-Aid); larger wounds, such as an abrasion on the thigh or arm, may require a large sterile gauze pad that is held in place with an elasticized wrap or elastic adhesive tape. Such bandages should be rechecked periodically during participation to ensure that they remain in proper position and bleeding has not resumed.
2. Once the activity is finished, the athlete should have the wound cleaned again. If there are signs of infection (e.g., pain, edema, warmth, drainage, odor, and redness around wound), a topical antibiotic can be applied before covering with a nonocclusive dressing. Infected wounds need to be checked daily. For noninfected wounds with little drainage, an occlusive (i.e., film, foam, or hydrocolloid) dressing is recommended for the duration of healing. Commercial examples of occlusive dressings are Duo DERM® and Bioclusive® and are available at most pharmacies. These dressings can be left on the wound for 3–7 days, depending on the drainage and manufacturer's guidelines. Also follow manufacturer's guidelines for proper application and removal. Occlusive dressings have been found to allow faster healing with less infection (Beam, 2016; Thomas, 2008).
3. Monitor for signs and symptoms of infection (e.g., fever, delayed would healing, redness around wound, odor, edema, pus, warmth, burning sensation, and rash) during healing. If present, the area should be inspected and, at minimum, cleaned and covered again. If the wound is not healing or is infected, it should be seen by a physician.
4. Educate the athlete about taking care of his or her wound. (Beam, 2016)

Friction Blisters

As the name suggests, friction blisters are caused by repetitive frictional forces on the skin due to heat, moisture, poorly fitted shoes or equipment, and/or excessive exercise. Redness develops first, followed by a stinging or burning sensation that perhaps leads to fluid accumulation under the skin. Treatment for blisters should follow the same principles as those applied to a closed or open wound, and they should be monitored for infection. Preventive strategies include wearing wicking clothing and socks and properly fitted equipment and shoes as well as using an absorbent powder or petroleum jelly (Emer, 2015).

Calluses and Corns

Calluses and **corns** are usually found on the hands and feet; they are essentially areas of thick skin deposits that form as a result of the body's protective reaction to high

Bandage Material used to hold a dressing in place.

Callus Rough, raised, and thickened area of skin due to friction.

Corn Thickened skin similar to a callus that develops in response to friction or pressure.

friction and/or pressure. A normal-sized callus is ideal to prevent further friction; however, it can become too large and rip off. Therefore, calluses should be filed down to a normal size and not completely removed. Corns, on the other hand, usually have a shiny surface and become inflamed and tender. Corns may need specialized treatment from a physician, such as surgery or topical prescription medication.

Talon or Tâche Noir

Talon noir (i.e., calcaneal petechiae, or black heel) and **tâche noir** (i.e., black palm) are trauma-related darkened spots on the foot, heel, or palms that are usually asymptomatic and associated with sports that have a fast stop and start or sheering aspects. They require no treatment other than time but can be confused with malignant melanoma (skin cancer).

Skin Inflammatory Conditions

Contact Dermatitis

For those susceptible, contact with an offending chemical results in a condition known as **contact dermatitis**. Certain types of sports equipment and related clothing may contain compounds that cause allergic reactions. Allergies related to chemicals contained in sports equipment or clothing have been receiving increased attention in sports medicine literature. It has been reported that products containing rubber, topical analgesics (pain relievers), resins found in athletic tape, and epoxy used in face gear are associated with allergic reactions in sensitive athletes. The chemicals initiating the allergic reaction are called **sensitizers**. Interestingly, heat, sweating, or other sources of moisture may make a sensitizer more intense.

Talon noir Trauma-related black spots on the heel.

Tâche noir Trauma-related black spots on the palm.

Contact dermatitis Inflammation or an allergic reaction of the skin caused by direct contact with an irritating substance.

Sensitizer A chemical that initiates an allergic reaction.

Poison ivy, oak, sumac Plant sap that contacts the skin and causes an itchy, irregular rash.

Sensitizers can produce classic symptoms of contact dermatitis—swelling and redness of the skin (erythema) followed by the development of pimple- or blisterlike lesions. The average time period between exposure and development of symptoms is 24 to 48 hours but can also occur approximately 7 days after the initial exposure; the earliest symptoms include itching and redness in the affected area. These symptoms are followed by the development of blisters, which often break open and subsequently become crusted. Healing takes place within 1–2 weeks from the time of the initial reaction.

Major sensitizers include synthetic rubber additives commonly found in certain brands of tennis shoes, swim caps, swim goggles, nose clips, and earplugs as well as topical analgesics containing either salicylates or menthol. Adhesive athletic tapes made with formaldehyde resins and face gear and helmets made with epoxy resins can also initiate allergic reactions; however, many of the rubberlike components have been replaced with plastics in recent years (Kockentiet & Adams, 2007).

For athletes with known allergies to any of these products, it is essential that alternative gear be identified if possible. An athlete suspected of having allergic contact dermatitis should be referred to a dermatologist for specific diagnosis and treatment, which includes identification of the sensitizer and treatment of symptoms with anti-inflammatory options (Carr & Cropley, 2019).

Poison (Plants) Allergy

When **poison ivy**, poison **oak**, and poison **sumac** plants are damaged, they release an oil, which in enough quantity and with direct contact onto the skin, can result in skin reactions in 80–90% of adults (CDC, 2018a). Athletes who know they are allergic to poison ivy, poison oak, or poison sumac should learn to recognize the plants to avoid contact with them when participating in outdoor activities. Organizers of events that may place athletes in areas where these plants grow should alert participants to the potential problem. A good example is cross-country running, a traditional autumn sport in high schools across the nation. It is common for training runs and races to take the runners through areas where plants such as poison ivy flourish. Obviously, these athletes need to be able to recognize such vegetation. Coaches and organizers should also make every effort to keep courses well away from areas where such plants may grow.

Latex Allergy

A latex allergy is when someone is allergic to the protein found in natural latex products. Latex comes from a rubber tree, and natural latex is found in medical and dental products, such as disposable gloves, intravenous tubing, dressings, and bandages, as well as in consumer products, such as balloons, condoms, shoes, and waistbands. It should be noted that there are synthetic latex rubber products that do not cause an allergic reaction. People who develop the allergy may be those with more exposure to latex, such as medical professionals, someone who had multiple surgeries, industry workers, and people with other allergies. Direct contact with latex causes hives, itching, and redness where exposed on the skin, stuffy or runny nose, difficulty breathing, or anaphylaxis. A latex allergy is diagnosed through a blood allergy test; the best treatment is to completely avoid latex. As with any allergy or medical condition, individuals should wear medical alert identification and carry an epinephrine autoinjector for emergencies. Individuals should also notify all medical personnel and friends and family of this allergy.

Ultraviolet Light–Related Skin Problems

Outdoor sports can result in exposure of large areas of the body to harmful rays of the sun. Typically, summer sportswear does not cover the arms and legs; in some sports, such as swimming and diving, major portions of the skin are unprotected. Medical evidence is substantial that even minor **sunburn** can be harmful to the skin; it may lead to serious, even lethal, complications, such as skin-related carcinomas and melanomas (Emer, 2015). Two wavelengths of ultraviolet light are involved in the sunburn process: ultraviolet A (UVA) and ultraviolet B (UVB). UVB is a shorter wavelength than UVA and seems more related to the development of skin problems (Emer, 2015).

Ultraviolet (UV) rays are slightly filtered by clouds, so even on cool and cloudy days sunburn can happen. Exposure to sunlight at any time of day can result in sunburn; however, the most dangerous time is between 10:00 a.m. and 4:00 p.m. daylight saving time, from late spring to early summer in North America (CDC, 2021b; NCAA, 2014). Additionally, the closer to the equator or the sun, as in the case of high altitudes, and to materials that reflect the sun, such as snow, sand, and water, UV exposure will increase. Some individuals are at a higher risk for damage from sunlight exposure, especially those with lighter skin, red hair, and freckles (CDC, 2021a; NCAA, 2014).

Sunburn causes intracellular changes, such as DNA damage, and an inflammatory response, resulting in erythema and increased skin sensitivity to mechanical and thermal stimuli. The inflammation, hyperemia, and hyperalgesia usually peak 24 hours after an exposure (Lopes & McMahon, 2016). Thus, a pink appearance to the skin today can result in a burned appearance tomorrow. Although most cases of sunburn result in mild discomfort, with symptoms diminishing within a day or two, more severe cases can include the formation of blisters associated with chills and gastrointestinal distress.

The primary concern should be on protection of exposed skin when an athlete is participating in outdoor sports. Certain body areas may require special protection with a commercially prepared sunscreen, particularly the outer ear, nose, lips, back of the neck, forehead, and (if not covered by clothing) the forearms and hands. Though many sunscreen products are available, athletes should use only those rated with at least a **sun protection factor (SPF)** of 15 and has both UVA and UVB protection. The SPF rating is determined by the sunscreen's ability to absorb harmful ultraviolet light over time. Thus, athletes using a product with an SPF rating of 15 will receive the same amount of ultraviolet light to the skin in 15 hours outdoors as they would have in 1 hour of unprotected exposure. Sunscreens use mineral or chemical filters for UV protection. Mineral sunscreen products contain zinc oxide or titanium dioxide, whereas chemical sunscreen products may contain a variety of chemicals that either absorb or reflect UVA and UVB light. These chemicals may include oxybenzone, avobenzone, octisalate, octocrylene, homosalate, and octinoxate in addition to other chemicals and inactive ingredients (Environmental Working Group [EWG], n.d.b). The Environmental Working Group suggests

> **Sunburn** Reaction to too much UV exposure whereby the skin turns red and may blister.
>
> **Sun protection factor (SPF)** Rating of a sunscreen is determined by the sunscreen's ability to absorb harmful ultraviolet light over time.

avoiding oxybenzone (EWG, n.d.b) and vitamin A ingredients (EWG, n.d.a) in sunscreens due to safety concerns as well as spray sunscreens due to the potential to inhale chemicals.

For best results, sunscreen should be applied 30 minutes before exposure to sunlight so that it can effectively be absorbed before it is washed away by sweat or water (Emer, 2015). Although many products are advertised as sweatproof, waterproof, or water resistant, athletes should reapply them every 1–2 hours and after perspiring heavily, toweling off, or participating in water sports, to maintain adequate protection. In addition to sunscreen, protective clothing should be worn to prevent sunburn (NCAA, 2014).

Treatment of minor sunburn involves application of cool wet cloths and a topical anesthetic, skin lotion, or aloe to help relieve burning and dryness. Over-the-counter pain medication can also be used to help relieve pain, headache, or fever. If sunburn results in blisters, treat the blisters as you would any other type of blister (i.e., cover and do not pop). Should they pop, keeping them clean and covered is recommended. In severe cases, in which sunburn covers over 15% of the body, high fever occurs, or extreme pain lasts longer than 48 hours, medical attention is warranted (CDC, 2018b).

Exacerbation Skin Conditions

Acne Mechanica

Acne mechanica (sports-induced acne) is an acnelike eruption caused by pressure, friction, or heat. It mostly erupts on the chin, forehead, neck, and shoulders or under protective equipment. Treatment is also similar to treatment for acne by using topical or systemic antibiotics and other medications or modalities. Part of treatment is also prevention, which involves wearing moisture-wicking clothing and frequent cleansing after activity (Emer, 2015).

Acne mechanica Sports acne that results from pressure, heat, or friction.

Urticaria Hives that occur from a change in body temperature during exercise.

Urticaria

Urticaria are hives caused by changes in body temperature, sweating, and a stimulus (e.g., cholinergic, hot, cold, sun, water, or pressure) during exercise. Athletes with hives complain of itching, redness, burning, patches of raised skin, and warmth. Treatment consists of cooling the area or whole body, using systemic antihistamines or other medications, and removing the stimulus (Emer, 2015).

Skin Infections

Skin infections first need an agent, or source, of infection; then a susceptible host; and finally a method of transmission, which can occur by direct contact (i.e., skin to skin), indirect contact (i.e., skin to surface), droplet contact (i.e., infected person sneezes or coughs and agent makes contact with eyes, nose, or mouth of another person), or airborne contact (i.e., dust or air that is inhaled). For an infecting agent to take hold, it must have the right conditions present, such as environmental and host conditions as well as the quantity and strength of the infecting agent. If a skin condition is found, reporting to the care provider immediately for accurate diagnosis and treatment is key (Zinder et al., 2010).

A variety of organisms can cause infections of the skin, including fungi, bacteria, viruses, and parasites. Although a detailed discussion of sports dermatology is beyond the scope of this text, some of the more common afflictions—along with their signs, symptoms, and treatment—are presented. It should also be remembered that many apparent skin infections can be symptoms of more serious infectious and/or allergic conditions, including Lyme disease, herpes, or contact dermatitis, and should be referred to a doctor for evaluation. Skin infections in athletes are a major and persistent concern within the sports medicine community. All stakeholders need to work collectively to prevent and control these infections. Given the nature of athletic participation, the likelihood of passing a skin infection to a fellow athlete is high. In recent years, this topic has taken on a new urgency with the arrival of drug-resistant strains of common bacteria, such as *Staphylococcus aureus* (i.e., staph). This particular organism has become a major health concern because it is now resistant to antibiotics, including methicillin, thus the label

WHAT IF ❓

You are the wrestling coach at Johnson High School. Several of your athletes have reported similar skin lesions on their faces and arms. They appear as superficial, brownish red, circular-shaped lesions. What might be causing these lesions, and what, if any, action would you take?

methicillin-resistant *Staphylococcus aureus* (MRSA). As such, everyone, including the athletes, parents, coaches, athletic trainers, and support personnel (e.g., custodians), must remain vigilant. The NATA has published an extensive position statement on skin diseases, which can be used as an additional resource (Zinder et al., 2010). Also, the NFHS and NCAA have published guidelines to prevent the spread of skin infections.

Fungus

A fungus is a eukaryotic organism (i.e., cells containing a nucleus and organelles within a membrane), such as mushrooms, yeasts, and certain molds, and are more genetically related to animals than to plants but share features of both. These organisms live in soil and on animals and humans, and fungal spores can be airborne as well. Anyone can acquire a fungal infection; however, under certain circumstances, such as a warm and moist environment, taking oral corticosteroids, and/or a weakened immune system, people may be more susceptible to an infection. Some fungal infections can be serious, but the fungal infections discussed here are generally less serious and the most commonly seen skin infections in athletics (CDC, 2019b). It is important to know that fungal skin infections can look similar to bacterial or viral skin infections; therefore, if the condition is not improving with the current medication, it is important to see a physician for more thorough testing and diagnosis (CDC, 2019b). As the characteristics of the infectious agent become more similar to those of the vertebrate host's cells and develop the ability to resist drugs designed to treat the agent, complete selective toxicity (i.e., the ability of the drug to target sites that are specific to the microorganism responsible for infection) becomes more difficult to achieve and more side effects are seen (CDC, 2019b).

Tinea

Tinea, commonly known as ringworm, is an infection of the skin caused by a group of fungi. In athletes, the common locations for tinea include the groin region (i.e., tinea cruris, commonly known as jock itch) and the feet (Figure 17.2) and toes (i.e., tinea pedis). Tinea infections are common in these body areas because moisture and warmth make them ideal for fungal growth. Tinea can affect other parts of the

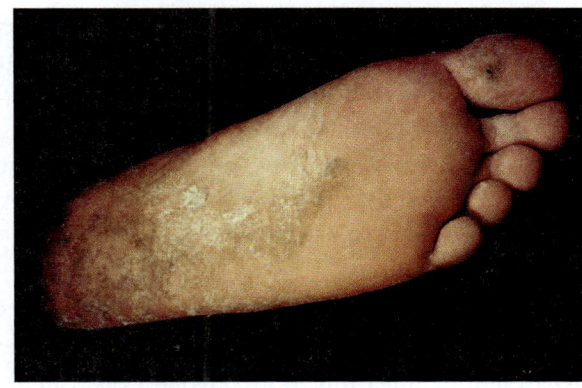

(a)

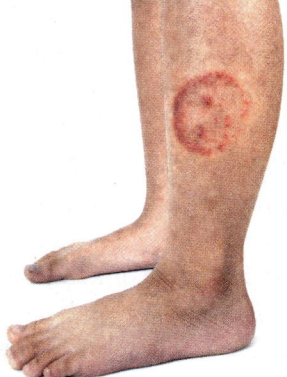

(b)

Figure 17.2 (a) Tinea infection on the foot. **(b)** Tinea corporis (ringworm on the body).
(a) Courtesy of CDC; (b) © Photo Win1/Shutterstock.

Methicillin-resistant *Staphylococcus aureus* (MRSA) A type of staph bacteria that is resistant to several antibiotics.

Tinea Group of fungi-related skin infections, commonly called ringworm, which can affect various parts of the body—groin area (i.e., tinea cruris), feet and toes (i.e., tinea pedis), and scalp (i.e., tinea capitis).

body as well, including the scalp (i.e., tinea capitis) and the extremities. Although tinea infections are not serious, if left untreated they may persist and lead to secondary bacterial infections that can be cosmetically displeasing.

Signs and symptoms of tinea infections include the following:

- Small, superficial, brownish red, elevated lesions that tend to be circular in shape or scaling of the skin over the lesion may be noted.
- When infections involve the foot and toes, thick scaling through the sole of the foot to lateral areas, as if wearing a moccasin, appear and lesions may include maceration, oozing, cracking, and crusting between toes.
- When infections involve the nails, the nails will yellow and become thick, rising up from the nail bed with or without nail debris underneath the nail.
- Itching and pain are associated with tinea pedis and tinea cruris.

Treatment of tinea infections involves the following (Carr & Cropley, 2019; NCAA, 2014; Zinder et al., 2010):

1. Vigilant cleaning of the involved areas, followed by drying with a towel and/or hair dryer.
2. Applying an over-the-counter topical treatment, such as tolnaftate (e.g., Tinactin).
3. Applying a moisture-absorbing powder to the area.
4. Wearing clothing made of natural fibers, such as cotton.
5. Taking systemic medication for more involved cases.
6. Adhering to proper treatment and recommendations for return to activity.
7. Maintaining hygiene practices and prevention methods to reduce reoccurrences.

Tinea versicolor Fungus infection resulting in the formation of circular skin lesions that appear either lighter or darker than adjacent skin.

Antibiotic resistance When bacteria adapt and become resistant to antibiotic medication.

Tinea Versicolor

Tinea versicolor is considered to be the most common warm weather–related skin problem among teenagers and young adults, especially in tropical and subtropical climates. This fungal infection gets its name from the symptoms it produces on the skin of the affected person. It is characterized by the appearance of lesions that are of a different color than the adjacent, normal skin. It is usually confined to the upper trunk, neck, and upper abdomen.

Signs and symptoms of tinea versicolor include the following:

- Circular lesions that appear either lighter or darker than adjacent skin.
- Skin may appear white, in contrast to adjacent, unaffected skin, after exposure to sunlight (i.e., areas of skin that do not tan).
- Lesions are normally found on the trunk.

Treatment of tinea versicolor involves either oral or topical prescription drugs, which may require weeks or even months to be effective, or selenium sulfide shampoo. Prevention strategies include avoiding the sun and wearing loose, dry, wicking clothing (Hudson et al., 2018).

Bacterial Infections

Bacteria are prokaryotic organisms (i.e., cells with a cell wall and membrane). Bacteria live in soil and water, and their biomass outnumbers that of plants and animals. Bacteria also live in the nose, throat, and digestive tract of humans as well as on the skin and hair. There are approximately 10 times as many bacterial cells in the human body than there are human cells, with most of them living in the gut followed by the skin. Many bacteria are beneficial, especially those located in the gut. However, several species of bacteria can cause fatal infections. This chapter focuses on skin infections associated with *Streptococcus* and *Staphylococcus aureus*. Unfortunately, treating bacterial infections can be challenging. Although significant differences in metabolism between bacteria and humans is the target of medication for bacterial infections, bacteria can adapt and become resistant to medication; this is called **antibiotic resistance**, and it is a serious concern (Wright, 2016).

Bacterial infections of the skin are relatively common in sports that involve close physical contact between participants. These infections, known collectively as **pyoderma** (i.e., pus-producing infection of the skin), are normally caused by two common bacteria, *Staphylococcus aureus* and *Streptococcus*. **Folliculitis** (Figure 17.3a), **furuncles**, **carbuncles**, **impetigo** (Figure 17.3b), and **cellulitis** are characterized by infected, **purulent** (i.e., pus-producing) lesions on the skin. For example, in folliculitis the lesions are located at the base of a hair follicle. Furuncles are similar in appearance; however, they form large nodules around the hair follicles and may burst as the infection develops. Carbuncles are larger and deeper infections of groups of hair follicles. Impetigo is similar in appearance but may develop in areas with little or no hair.

Regardless of the specific condition, all pyodermal infections share a common characteristic—the presence of lesions that are obviously infected and associated with drainage and pus formation. Any athlete demonstrating such signs and/or symptoms as described should be removed from participation and referred for medical evaluation. If pyoderma is the diagnosis, the precautions outlined in **Time Out 17.1** should immediately be instituted (Zinder et al., 2010).

Impetigo

Impetigo is caused by both streptococci and staphylococci bacteria and is transmitted by direct contact. Skin lesions are erythematous, yellow, and well defined and may contain crusted plaque most commonly on the extremities, head, and neck. Suspicious lesions should be cultured and tested to ensure accurate diagnosis and proper method of treatment. The treatment of impetigo involves both topical and oral antibiotics as well as removal from activity with direct contact until 3 days of antibiotic treatment has been completed and no new lesions have developed in the previous 2 days (Carr & Cropley, 2019; Zinder et al., 2010).

Signs and symptoms of impetigo and cellulitis include the following:

- The underlying symptom of all forms of pyoderma is a lesion, regardless of location, that is producing pus.
- Often seen on the face, impetigo presents groups of raised skin lesions that are honey colored and crusty in appearance.

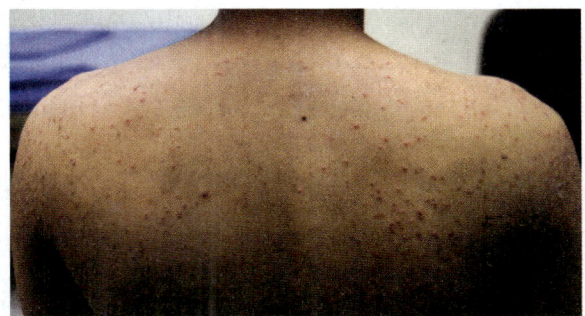

(a)

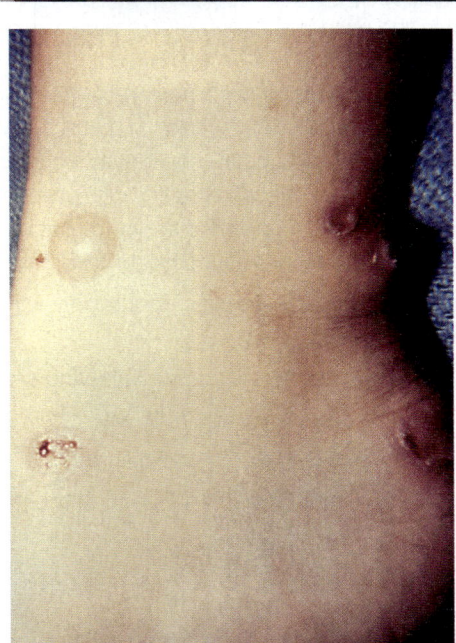

(b)

Figure 17.3 **(a)** Folliculitis. **(b)** Impetigo on the ankle.
(a) © RandomizeTH/Shutterstock; (b) Courtesy of CDC.

Pyoderma Pus-producing infection of the skin.

Folliculitis Inflammation and bacterial infection of a hair follicle.

Furuncle Bacterial infection of a hair follicle that goes into the deeper layers of the skin. A small pocket of pus forms called a boil.

Carbuncle Group of bacterial infected hair follicles with pus. They are larger and deeper than furuncles.

Impetigo Skin infection caused by both streptococci and staphylococci bacteria.

Cellulitis A potentially serious bacterial skin infection. The skin appears red, swollen, and warm and painful to the touch.

Purulent Consisting of, or forming, pus.

TIME OUT 17.1

Official Statement from the National Athletic Trainers' Association on Community-Acquired MRSA Infections (CA-MRSA)

In an effort to educate the public about the potential risks of the emergence of community-acquired methicillin-resistant *Staphylococcus aureus* (CA-MRSA) infection, the National Athletic Trainers' Association (NATA) recommends that healthcare personnel and physically active participants take appropriate precautions with suspicious lesions and talk with a physician.

According to the Centers for Disease Control and Prevention (CDC), approximately 25% to 30% of the population is colonized in the nose with *Staphylococcus aureus*, often referred to as "staph," and approximately 1% of the population is colonized with MRSA.[1]

Cases have developed from person-to-person contact, shared towels, soaps, improperly treated whirlpools, and equipment (mats, pads, surfaces, etc.). Staph or CA-MRSA infections usually manifest as skin infections, such as pimples, pustules, and boils, which initially present as red, swollen, painful, or have pus or other drainage. Without proper referral and care, more serious infections may cause pneumonia, bloodstream infections, or surgical wound infections.

Maintaining good hygiene and avoiding contact with drainage from skin lesions are the best methods for prevention. Proper prevention and management recommendations may include, but are not limited to:

- Keep hands clean by washing thoroughly with soap and warm water or using an alcohol-based hand sanitizer routinely.
- Encourage immediate showering following activity.
- Avoid whirlpools or common tubs with open wounds, scrapes, or scratches.
- Avoid sharing towels, razors, and daily athletic gear.
- Properly wash athletic gear and towels after each use.
- Maintain clean facilities and equipment.
- Inform or refer to appropriate healthcare personnel for all active skin lesions and lesions that do not respond to initial therapy.
- Administer or seek proper first aid.
- Encourage healthcare personnel to seek bacterial cultures to establish a diagnosis.
- Care and cover skin lesions appropriately before participation.

[1]CA-MRSA Information for the Public. Centers for Disease Control and Prevention. Available on-line at: https://www.cdc.gov/mrsa/community/index.html

Reproduction of the Official statement from the National Athletic Trainers' Association on community-acquired MRSA infections. Reprinted with permission.

- Cellulitis is also a skin infection; however, it affects the deeper layer of skin known as the dermis (Figure 17.1). The skin will appear red and warmer than adjacent skin and will be painful to the touch.

Folliculitis, Furuncles, and Carbuncles

These lesions involve infection and inflammation of a hair follicle. They usually occur in occluded areas and are painful (Carr & Cropley, 2019). Signs and symptoms of folliculitis, furuncles, and carbuncles include the following:

- The underlying symptom of all forms of pyoderma is a lesion, regardless of location, that is producing pus.
- Folliculitis involves lesions located at the base of a hair follicle.
- Furuncles, commonly called "boils," are lesions that form large nodules around the base of a hair follicle and may burst as the infection develops.
- Boils can appear anywhere but are more common on the arms, armpits, neck and chest, buttocks, and groin.

Athletic Trainers SPEAK OUT

How has the contracting of athletic trainer services changed the health care of our youth athletes?

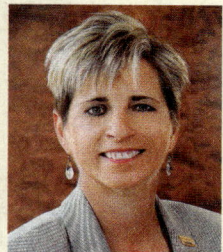

Courtesy of Katherine Dieringer, EdD, LAT, ATC.

Contract athletic trainer (AT) services have definitely had a positive impact on the health care of youth athletes. Prior to this practice, these athletes did not have immediate care of injuries with the exception of an ambulance response to an injury, or a parent in the stands who happened to be a healthcare provider. By contracting AT services at youth events, these athletes experience the health care they deserve, while exposing them to the exceptional skill set of an athletic trainer, often for the first time. Basic tenets of injury prevention and management are introduced early in the athletes' careers. Injury severity can be minimized, and proper management/recovery accelerated due to the presence of an AT.

In addition, those who continue to participate in athletics develop a continued respect for the profession, an important step in establishing our value to our stakeholders. As the practice has become more common, organizing bodies, athletes, and especially parents expect an AT on site for all events, clearly a positive step for the health and safety of the athletes, and for the profession as well.

—**Kathy I. Dieringer, EdD, LAT, ATC**

Kathy Dieringer is the Founder of D & D Sports Medicine in Denton, Texas, and a NATA Hall of Fame Member.

- Carbuncles are essentially a collection of boils that together form a weeping, pus-producing lesion typically found around the posterior neck and upper trunk regions.

MRSA

Methicillin-resistant *Staphylococcus aureus* (MRSA) is a bacterium that is resistant to many antibiotics. About 5% of people in U.S. hospitals have MRSA in their nose or on their skin (CDC, 2019c), and there has been an increase in the prevalence of MRSA found in noses of children and adults over the last decade or more (Zinder et al., 2010). It is transmitted through direct and indirect contact. Most MRSA infections are skin infections that occur at sites of skin trauma, such as cuts and abrasions. They are also common in the groin, armpit, or back of the neck because these areas of the body are covered by hair, making them common sites for hair follicle irritation. An infected site often looks like just a red, swollen, and painful bump; however, if it progresses to a pustule or boil, MRSA can cause complicated secondary infections if it is not recognized and treated correctly.

The first step in protection from MRSA is prevention. The best methods for prevention are teaching and maintaining good hygiene with hand washing (CDC, 2020b) and avoiding contact with drainage from any skin lesions. Specifically, healthcare professionals should encourage athletes to not participate in cosmetic body shaving (e.g., shaving areas other than face or legs) as it has been found to increase MRSA by more than 6-fold (Zinder et al., 2010). In addition, it is important to make sure all staff and administrators are in agreement with standard precautions essential to controlling infectious disease, which means adhering to safe cleaning and disinfecting practices as well as hand hygiene.

Cases of MRSA have developed in athletic populations from sharing towels, soaps, and clothing, person-to-person contact, and improperly cleaned whirlpools or equipment (e.g., mats, surfaces, and protective pads). Cleaning or sanitizing equipment is of the utmost importance, but disinfection is the only way to inactivate germs such as MRSA. Although proper cleaning and sanitizing procedures using typical cleaning agents are great at lifting dirt and germs off the surface, to truly reduce the risk of a MRSA infection, the equipment must be disinfected. Disinfectants effective against *Staphylococcus aureus* are effective against MRSA, and these products are readily available from retail stores. Before using, check the label to determine the germs that the disinfectant can destroy and confirm that the product is registered by the EPA. Registration by EPA is signified with a registration number (CDC, 2019d). Time

Out 17.1 presents a list of recommended actions for the prevention of MRSA in an athletic environment (NATA, 2005).

The next step is appropriate referral and treatment. As a coach or physical educator, referral of athletes with possible infections to a team physician, athletic trainer, school nurse, or primary care doctor should be swift, and, if the athlete is younger than 18 years old, be sure to notify parents or guardians (CDC, 2019e, 2019f). Typical treatment involves incision, drainage, cleaning, and sometimes packing of the wound plus culturing of pus or drainage for confirmation of infectious bacteria. Because MRSA is resistant to typical antibiotics used for other staph infections, antibiotic treatment should be guided by the culture results and the patient's response to immediate treatment. Healthcare providers should also discuss a follow-up plan because MRSA skin infections can develop into more serious infections; therefore, any overall body symptoms (e.g., fever or malaise) or worsening of local skin symptoms (e.g., redness, pus, and swelling) should immediately be referred to a physician. The final step is appropriate return to sport and/or community exposure. Athletes with active infections or open wounds should not use swimming pools or other common-use water facilities, nor should they use therapy pools (whirlpools) that are not cleaned between each athlete's use (Beam, 2016; CDC, 2019e, 2019f; NATA, 2005; Zinder et al., 2010).

Currently, the recommendation for return to sports participation after a bacterial infection is that participation can begin after 72 hours of antibiotic therapy, there is no sign of exudate or drainage, and that no new wounds have developed for at least 48 hours (Zinder et al., 2010). However, for the safety of all concerned, if the activity poses a risk of injury to the infected area, then the athlete should be held from participation, even if the lesion can be properly covered (CDC, 2019e, 2019f; NATA, 2005; Zinder et al., 2010).

Viral Infections

Viruses are infectious agents that lack cell structure yet contain DNA material. Viruses are spread by many means, such as coughing or sneezing or direct contact.

Herpes gladiatorum A common skin condition caused by herpes simplex virus type 1 (HSV-1).

Herpes simplex virus type 1 (HSV-1) Causes the common cold sore, or fever blister.

When a person is infected with a virus, the virus causes an immune response to begin to eliminate the virus, but, when the body cannot handle the virus effectively, infections result. Please note that antibiotic medications have no effect on viruses and the overuse of antibiotic medication for viral infections has contributed to the antibiotic resistance issue. In this chapter, we will discuss only skin viral infections.

Herpes Gladiatorum

Herpes gladiatorum, or "mat herpes" or "wrestler herpes," (Figure 17.4) is the name given to herpes infections among athletes, such as wrestlers. This viral infection is caused by **herpes simplex virus type 1 (HSV-1)**, which is well known as the causative agent of the common cold sore, or fever blister, that typically occurs on the outer lip area. It is transmitted through direct contact, and lesions are often associated with physical trauma, sunburn, emotional disturbances, fatigue, or infection. A unique aspect of herpes infection is its ability to remain dormant for long periods, sometimes months or even years, between active periods when lesions reappear. The infection is most contagious when open lesions are present. Once exposed to the virus, the incubation period may be as long as 2 weeks.

Signs and symptoms of herpes gladiatorum include the following:

- Development of a lesion, on the head, upper extremity, or trunk but commonly on the face, which is characterized by blistering associated with a red, infected area of skin.
- Open, draining lesions may persist for a few days; afterward they become crusted and begin to heal.

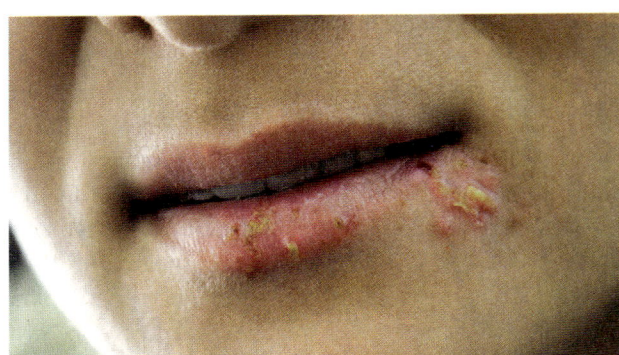

Figure 17.4 Herpes gladiatorum.
© Cherries/Shutterstock.

- General fatigue, body aches, fever, sore throat, and inflammation of lymph glands associated with tenderness.

Outbreaks of herpes must be controlled, or the infection can be devastating in a sport, such as wrestling, in which acute outbreaks can involve many athletes. Coaches and athletes must be educated about the early signs and symptoms of HSV-1 infections. Moreover, any type of open lesion must be evaluated to rule out the possibility of infection. Athletes with active infections must be removed from participation and contact with the team until lesions have healed, no new lesions have surfaced for 72 hours, antiviral medications have been taken for at least 120 hours, and they are free of systemic symptoms. All teammates who were in contact with the affected athlete within 3 days of the appearance of the skin lesion need to be thoroughly evaluated and monitored for 8 days. Antiviral drugs are available for control of the infection; however, they must not be used without the supervision of a physician (Carr & Cropley, 2019; Zinder et al., 2010).

Herpes Simplex Virus

Herpes simplex virus (herpes) is categorized into two types: herpes simplex virus 1 (HSV-1) and herpes simplex virus 2 (HSV-2). Like some other herpes viruses, it will cycle between active disease and remission periods. After the initial infection, the virus moves into the nervous system and resides there for life, resurfacing intermittently. For example, the painful rash of shingles in mostly older individuals is caused by the herpes zoster virus, which is the same virus that causes chickenpox. As the person recovers from chickenpox, the virus lives inactively in the body's nervous system until it reactivates later in life, which causes the rash.

Herpes simplex is transmitted by direct contact. Symptoms of herpes simplex involve illness to flulike symptoms as well as burning or tingling of the skin followed by vesicles on the skin (depending on if it is the initial outbreak or a subsequent outbreak). The skin lesions can be misdiagnosed as folliculitis, and it is important to immediately diagnose these vesicle skin lesions accurately to prevent spread of infection to others. While there is no cure for herpes simplex, antiviral medications can reduce the frequency and severity of the outbreaks.

Molluscum Contagiosum

Molluscum contagiosum is caused by the poxvirus, which manifests as a skin infection (Figure 17.5); it is more common in young children than in teenagers or adults (CDC, 2015b) and is spread by direct contact and sharing items, such as towels, equipment, and clothing. The skin lesions are flesh-colored to light pink raised papules in single formation or in clusters commonly on the trunk or extremities. There is a good chance the lesions will spread to other parts of the body, and secondary infections may result from children picking at the lesions. However, if the skin lesions are close to the genital area, referral to a physician is advised. One of the treatments for molluscum is physical removal of papules, which may include cryotherapy (freezing the lesion with liquid nitrogen), curettage (piercing the core and scraping caseous or cheesy material), and laser therapy. Not only is this painful, but, in young children, scarring may result. The typical course of treatment in young children is keeping them from scratching or picking the lesions; washing towels and bedding frequently; covering the lesions when in close contact with others, such as during school and activities; and not allowing them to share personal items while waiting for the lesions to resolve on their own, which typically takes months to years. Topical treatments are also available

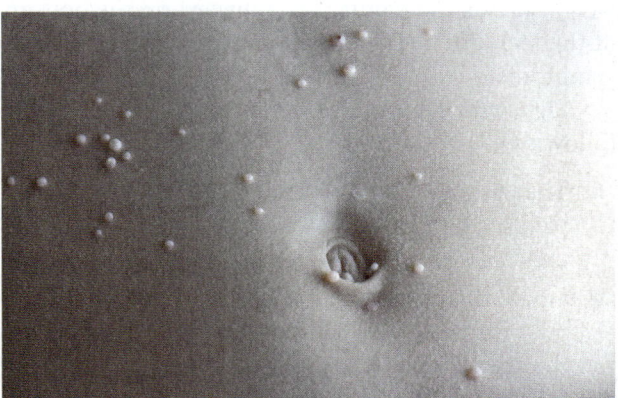

Figure 17.5 Molluscum contagiosum.
© EF Photography/Shutterstock.

Herpes simplex virus (herpes) Categorized into two types: herpes type 1 (HSV-1, or oral herpes) and herpes type 2 (HSV-2, or genital herpes).

Molluscum contagiosum Caused by the poxvirus, which manifests as a skin infection.

but may not be beneficial. If molluscum is found on adults, it is mostly passed through sexual contact. Once the lesions are healed, the virus is also gone and is no longer contagious (Carr & Cropley, 2019).

Warts

Folk beliefs about **warts** suggested that handling a toad or other strange mechanisms caused them. Yet even stranger were the cures for warts, such as rubbing them with beef. As a skin problem, plantar warts (verrucae plantaris) are quite common in the general population and occur as the result of infection by a specific group of viruses known collectively as the **human papillomavirus (HPV)**, of which more than 120 distinct types have been identified. The majority of plantar warts are caused by HPV-1, HPV-2, HPV-27, and HPV-57. The infection is contagious; however, some individuals seem more susceptible, with an **incubation period** ranging from weeks to 12 months (Newton, 2013). The most well-known characteristic of a wart is the abnormal buildup of epidermis around the region of actual infection; warts can vary in size from 1 millimeter in diameter to as large as 1 centimeter or more.

Plantar warts are simply warts that occur on the plantar surfaces of the feet. Although warts elsewhere generally rise up from the skin, the pressure of bearing weight drives the plantar wart inward on the bottom of the feet, often resulting in annoying if not painful symptoms.

Signs and symptoms of plantar warts include the following:

- The warts are usually first noticed when they become painful as an athlete is walking or running because they are located on a weight-bearing surface.
- Small, thickened areas of skin may be noticeable, with tiny black or dark red dots appearing within the area (Newton, 2013).

Wart Circular raised area of skin caused by HPV.

Human papillomavirus (HPV) Over 120 distinct types of these viruses have been identified, at least two of which are related to plantar warts.

Incubation period Time between an exposure to an infectious agent and the appearance of symptoms of that infection.

Scabies Infestation of small mites in the skin that causes intense itching.

- Contrary to popular myth, these small dark spots are not seeds but rather small capillaries that have been destroyed within the wart.
- Sometimes, a group of warts will develop, causing a relatively large involved area. This is referred to as a mosaic wart.

Treatment of plantar warts ranges from the application of chemicals designed to dissolve the wart to surgical removal (although this is not recommended by the medical community), to no treatment. A variety of prescription products are available, most of which contain salicylic, pyruvic, and lactic acids. These compounds soften and erode the wart (the process is known technically as keratolysis); the goal is complete removal of the growth. Sometimes, liquid nitrogen is applied on several occasions to freeze the affected tissue, and then can possibly be followed by surgical removal. Interestingly, in many athletes, plantar warts terminate on their own with no long-term symptoms. Athletes who find plantar warts to be detrimental to participation in sports should consult a doctor to determine the best course of treatment. Coaches and athletes should not attempt treatment because it may result in a worsening of the condition, an infection, and even permanent scarring.

To prevent the spread of warts, they should be covered, and personal items, such as towels, socks, or shoes, should not be shared. Ideally, the feet should be kept as dry as possible by changing socks multiple times a day. Also, appropriate footwear should be worn in and around pool areas (Newton, 2013).

Parasites

Organisms that live in or on another organism can cause skin conditions, illness, and disease. Often, these organisms are microscopic and cannot be seen with the naked eye.

Scabies

Scabies is caused by small mites infesting the skin. Small red bumps erupt on the skin, and intense itching occurs from the mites burrowing into the skin to lay their eggs. Redness on the skin may look like bite marks or be in nonlinear patterns, such as an S shape. Scabies is highly contagious and is spread by direct or close contact. Treatment consists of prescription creams and/or oral medication to kill the scabies as well as oral antihistamines to help relieve itching, which may persist for weeks after the initial treatment. All members of the family or team are usually treated at the same time. In addition, all clothing and bedding need to be washed in hot water and dried in a hot dryer; nonwashable objects, such as pillows, should be placed in a plastic bag for at least a week.

Lice

Like scabies, lice are tiny bugs that can infest the skin; they feed on the host's blood and cause intense itching, especially at night. There are two kinds of lice—head lice (pediculosis) and pubic lice (phthiriasis)—both of which are very contagious and transmitted through close contact and shared items. Head lice is mostly seen in school-aged children, regardless of how clean their hair is. Eggs can be seen on the hair, behind ears, or on the neck. Treatment may vary depending on the patient's age and severity of the lice, but it usually consists of applying a medicated shampoo and using a fine-tooth comb to comb out wet hair. In addition, brushes and combs should be soaked in hot water for 15 minutes. Similar to scabies, all clothing and bedding should be washed in hot water and dried in a hot dryer; nonwashable items should be sealed in a bag for over 2 weeks. At times, medications may also be necessary to kill off the lice. Usually, children can return to school after the first treatment for head lice (CDC, 2020c).

Pubic lice (called "crabs" for short because of their resemblance to a crab) are insects found in the pubic area. The symptoms and transmission are the same as those of head lice—itching and close contact, such as sexual exposure or bedding used by an infected person, respectively. If crabs are found, the patient should also be examined for sexually transmitted disease. The treatment is the same as that for head lice: applying a lice-killing lotion or shampoo to the affected area followed by using a fine-tooth comb and washing clothing and bedding. It is important to notify sexual partners that the infected person had up to a month before the outbreak as well as avoiding sexual contact until partners have been treated.

Bed Bugs

Insects that feed on blood while people sleep are called bed bugs; infestations are found in living areas, such as homes, hotels, cruise ships, and dorm rooms, and in transportation means, such as buses, trains, and airplanes. Bed bugs hide during the day inside mattresses, cracks, and crevices usually within 8 feet of where people sleep and will then emerge at night to feed. Itching and loss of sleep are the major symptoms, but a secondary skin infection can occur from scratching. Because bed bugs inject an anesthetic and an anticoagulant, it may be hard to tell that you have been bitten. Bite marks may be seen on the skin that look similar to a mosquito or flea bite; at times, serious allergic reactions can occur. If bed bugs are suspected, their exoskeletons will be visible in the fold of mattresses and sheets as well as their rusty colored fecal matter. Treatment consists of resisting the urge to scratch, applying antiseptic creams or lotions, and taking antihistamines. The infestation also needs to be addressed; notify the appropriate supervisor or pest control company to apply an insecticide (CDC, 2022a).

Ticks

Bites from infected blacklegged ticks may transfer bacteria to a human that results in Lyme disease. Usually, a skin rash, called erythem achronicum migrans (Figure 17.6), develops, and the person experiences other symptoms, such as fever, headache, and fatigue. Diagnosis is based on symptoms in combination with exposure to infected ticks, such as outdoor activity in an area known to have cases of Lyme disease and infected ticks, such as the U.S. Northeast. Usually, if identified quickly, Lyme disease can be successfully treated with antibiotics for a few weeks. If left untreated, the disease will become systemic and can affect the joints, heart, and central nervous system. It is important to get an accurate diagnosis as quickly as possible so that posttreatment Lyme disease syndrome, which presents itself as continued symptoms and perhaps damage that occurred to tissues of the body during infection, is avoided (CDC, 2022b). More information on Lyme disease can be found in the chapter titled, *General Medical Concerns for Athletes*, in this textbook.

Lice Infestation of small insects in hair (head or pubic area) that causes intense itching.

Bed bugs Small insects in mattresses and other furniture that come out at night to feed on blood.

Lyme disease Bites from infected blacklegged ticks that transfer bacteria to humans, resulting in a skin rash and other symptoms.

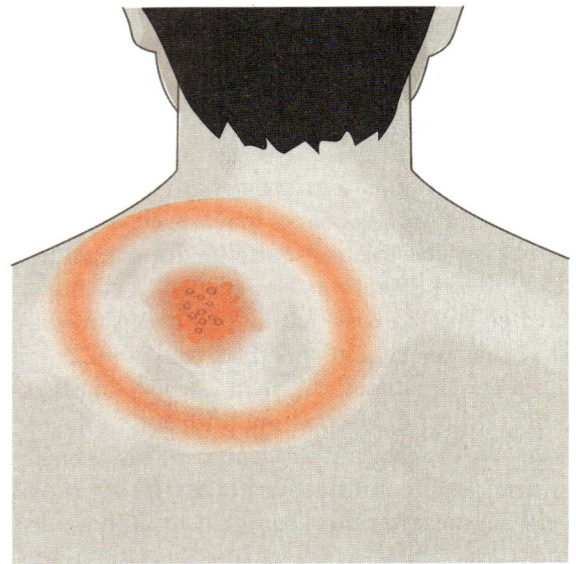

Figure 17.6 Erythema migrans rash caused by Lyme disease.

Wrestling and Skin Infections

Because of the nature of the sport of wrestling, participation with an active skin infection presents special hazards to the athletes involved. At the collegiate level, it has been reported that 17% of practice time–loss injuries are related to skin infections (NCAA, 2014). Common sense should prevail in such situations, and any open sore or skin lesion that cannot be covered adequately should be grounds for removal from participation until the infection subsides. The NCAA has published specific criteria for disqualification because of skin infections among wrestlers (NCAA, 2014). The NCAA recommends that any infected area that cannot be protected adequately should be considered as cause for disqualification from practice and/or competition. The NCAA (2014) has included all of the following infections as worth considering under their recommendations:

- Bacterial skin infections
- Impetigo
- Erysipelas
- Carbuncle
- Staphylococcal disease, MRSA
- Folliculitis (generalized)
- Hidradenitis suppurativa
- Parasitic skin infections
- Pediculosis
- Scabies
- Viral skin infections
- Herpes simplex
- Herpes zoster (chickenpox)
- Molluscum contagiosum
- Fungal skin infections
  - Tinea corporis (ringworm)
  - Tinea pedis (athlete's foot)

Role of the Care Provider

The role of the care provider is crucial when it comes to skin conditions because providers need to quickly and accurately identify skin conditions to prevent the spread of infection to others. Daily skin checks should be performed as well as educating coaches, parents, and athletes about preventing, identifying, and appropriately treating common skin infections. Athletes should be encouraged to practice good nutrition and hygiene by hand washing (CDC, 2020b) and showering soon after activity, maintain clean equipment, and report skin conditions as soon as they are noticed. They should also be directed not to share towels; equipment; water bottles; clothing; and personal items, such as razors and brushes, and to wear proper footwear in locker rooms and community showers. If an athlete has a suspected contagious skin condition, he or she should immediately be isolated from others; have the lesions covered; and referred to a physician, ideally a dermatologist, for accurate diagnosis and treatment. Additionally, the care provider should encourage sampling the lesion to determine an accurate diagnosis. Several of the contagious skin conditions need

WHAT IF ❓

A member of the cross-country team asks you to examine a strange rash he has developed on his legs. He reports that it developed about 12 to 24 hours after he had used a topical analgesic with a wintergreen odor. What is the likely cause of this condition, and what would you recommend to this athlete?

physician approval for return to activity, and the care provider needs to follow return to activity guidelines set by athletic organizations, such as the NFHS and the NCAA (Table 17.1). Beyond these measures, care providers should always protect themselves by wearing gloves when examining and treating skin conditions as well as keeping hands clean through hand washing (CDC, 2020b) and properly cleaning and disinfecting tables and other surfaces, such as whirlpools (NATA, n.d.a; Zinder et al., 2010).

Table 17.1
Skin Conditions, Descriptions, Treatments, and Return-to-Activity Guidelines

	Skin Condition	Description	Treatment	Return to Activity
Fungus	Tinea	Erythemous, scaly patches, itchy	Topical antifungal; systemic antifungal medicine for more widespread fungus	Depends on location and sport; cover lesion
Bacteria	Impetigo	Staph and strep; raised blisters that easily rupture and crust over	Topical antibiotic	No new lesions for at least 48 hours; no further drainage of lesions; minimum of 72 hours of antibiotic medication; cannot participate with covered lesions
	Furuncle, carbuncle	Staph; red swollen area that develops into mass	Systemic antibiotic; refer to MD for incision, drainage, and culture	
	Folliculitis	Staph; papules and pustules at base of hair follicle	Topical antibiotic	
	MRSA	Staph; small pustule that develops into larger ones	Case by case/ individualized; immediate referral	
Viral	Molluscum contagiosum	Poxvirus skin infection; flesh-colored to light pink papules, single or clustered	Topical or physical destruction but may scar	Lesions must be curetted or removed as well as covered
	Herpes simplex	Herpes simplex viral skin infection; localized cluster of vesicles around lip, head, neck, face, upper extremity with or without mild illness symptoms	Oral antiviral medications if lesions are not fully formed, ruptured, or crusted	Free of systemic symptoms; no new lesions for at least 72 hours; minimum of 120 hours of systemic antiviral medication; cannot participate with active lesions
	Herpes gladiatorum	Herpes simplex viral skin infection; tingling followed by clusters of vesicles; may include illness symptoms	Antiviral medication	
	Warts	Human papilloma virus; small, round, elevated lesions with or without small black seed–looking marks inside	May heal on own as immune system reacts; liquid nitrogen, salicylic acid, or dissection	Cover for participation

(*continues*)

Table 17.1 (continued)
Skin Conditions, Descriptions, Treatments, and Return-to-Activity Guidelines

	Skin Condition	Description	Treatment	Return to Activity
Parasites	Scabies	Erythemous marks, raised skin	Topical treatment; address clothing and bedding	Participation after treatment
	Lice, or crabs	Itchy areas; visual eggs in hair	Topical treatment; address clothing and bedding	Participation after treatment and clear of insects
	Lyme disease	Rash; illness symptoms	Systemic antibiotics	Cleared by physician
	Bed bugs	Similar to mosquito or flea bite; itchy, poor sleep	Topical antiseptic; treat infestation with insecticide	Cover for participation

Data sources: CDC references from end of chapter, and Zinder, S. M., Basler, R. S. W., Foley, J., Scarlata, C., & Vasily, D. B. (2010). National Athletic Trainers' Association position statement: Skin diseases. *Journal of Athletic Training, 45*(4), 411–428. Retrieved from http://www.nata.org/sites/default/files/position-statement-skin-disease.pdf

Review Questions

1. Review the primary goals of initial wound care.
2. List the precautions that should be taken when treating an athlete with an open wound to avoid possible transmission of HIV and HBV.
3. Describe and differentiate between a wound dressing and a bandage.
4. True or false? Regarding the types of sunlight that cause sunburn, evidence suggests that UVB is more connected with the development of skin-related problems than are the other types.
5. Discuss the symptoms of sunburn and methods to prevent it.
6. Define the acronym *MRSA*.
7. True or false? The term *pyoderma* implies a pus-producing infection of the skin.
8. Describe the recommended treatment(s) for plantar warts.
9. True or false? There is no evidence that synthetic materials, such as tennis shoes, swim caps, and swim goggles, can cause allergic skin reactions.
10. True or false? An athlete with tinea pedis can continue to participate in soccer while treating the skin lesion.

References

Beam, J. W., Buckley, B., Holcomb, W. R., Ciocca, M. (2016). National Athletic Trainers' Association position statement: Management of acute skin trauma. *Journal of Athletic Training, 51*(12), 1053–1070.

Carr, P. C., & Cropley, T. G. (2019). Sports dermatology: Skin disease in athletes. *Clinics in Sports Medicine, 38*(4), 597–618.

Centers for Disease Control and Prevention (CDC). (2015b). Molluscum contagiosum. Retrieved from https://www.cdc.gov/poxvirus/molluscum-contagiosum/

Centers for Disease Control and Prevention (CDC). (2016a). Guide to infection prevention for outpatient settings: Minimum expectations for safe care. Retrieved from https://www.cdc.gov/infectioncontrol/pdf/outpatient/guide.pdf

Centers for Disease Control and Prevention (CDC). (2018a). Poisonous plants. Retrieved from https://www.cdc.gov/niosh/topics/plants/exposure.html

Centers for Disease Control and Prevention (CDC). (2018b). Sun exposure—sunburn. Retrieved from https://www.cdc.gov/niosh/topics/sunexposure/sunburn.html

Centers for Disease Control and Prevention (CDC). (2019a). *HIV Surveillance Report, 2019* (Volume 32). Retrieved from https://www.cdc.gov/hiv/library/reports/hiv-surveillance/vol-32/index.html

Centers for Disease Control and Prevention (CDC). (2019b). About fungal diseases. Retrieved from https://www.cdc.gov/fungal/about-fungal-diseases.html

Centers for Disease Control and Prevention (CDC). (2019c). Methicillin-resistant *Staphylococcus aureus* (MRSA): General information. Retrieved from https://www.cdc.gov/mrsa/community/index.html

Centers for Disease Control and Prevention (CDC). (2019d). Methicillin-resistant *Staphylococcus aureus* (MRSA): Cleaning and disinfection. Retrieved from https://www.cdc.gov/mrsa/community/environment/index.html

Centers for Disease Control and Prevention (CDC). (2019e). Methicillin-resistant *Staphylococcus aureus* (MRSA): For athletes. Retrieved from https://www.cdc.gov/mrsa/community/team-hc-providers/advice-for-athletes.html

Centers for Disease Control and Prevention (CDC). (2019f). Methicillin-resistant *Staphylococcus aureus* (MRSA): For coaches and athletic directors. Retrieved from https://www.cdc.gov/mrsa/community/team-hc-providers/index.html

Centers for Disease Control and Prevention (CDC). (2020a). Infection control: Guidelines library. Retrieved from https://www.cdc.gov/infectioncontrol/guidelines/index.html

Centers for Disease Control and Prevention (CDC). (2020b). Hand hygiene guidance. Retrieved from https://www.cdc.gov/handhygiene/providers/guideline.html

Centers for Disease Control and Prevention (CDC). (2020c). Lice treatment. Retrieved from https://www.cdc.gov/parasites/lice/head/treatment.html

Centers for Disease Control and Prevention (CDC). (2021a). What are the risk factors for skin cancer? Retrieved from https://www.cdc.gov/cancer/skin/basic_info/risk_factors.htm

Centers for Disease Control and Prevention (CDC). (2021b). What can I do to reduce my risk of skin cancer? Retrieved from https://www.cdc.gov/cancer/skin/basic_info/prevention.htm

Centers for Disease Control and Prevention (CDC). (2022a). Parasites: Bed bugs. Retrieved from https://www.cdc.gov/parasites/az/index.html

Centers for Disease Control and Prevention (CDC). (2022b). Lyme disease. Retrieved from https://www.cdc.gov/lyme/index.html

Emer, J., Sivek, R., & Marciniak, B. (2015). Sports dermatology: Part 1 of 2 traumatic or mechanical injuries, inflammatory conditions, and exacerbations of pre-existing conditions. *Journal of Clinical and Aesthetic Dermatology, 8*(4), 31–43.

Environmental Working Group. (n.d.a). The problem with vitamin A. Retrieved from https://www.ewg.org/sunscreen/report/the-problem-with-vitamin-a/

Environmental Working Group. (n.d.b). The trouble with ingredients in sunscreens. Retrieved from https://www.ewg.org/sunscreen/report/the-trouble-with-sunscreen-chemicals/

Hudson, A., Sturgeon, A., & Peiris, A. (2018). Tinea versicolor. *JAMA, 320*(13), 1396.

Kockentiet, B., & Adams, B.(2007). Contact dermatitis in athletes. *Journal of the American Academy of Dermatology, 56*(6), 1048–1055.

Lopes, D. M., & McMahon, S. B. (2016). Ultraviolet radiation on the skin: A painful experience? *CNS Neuroscience & Therapeutics, 22*(2), 118–126.

National Athletic Trainer's Association (NATA). (n.d.a). Protect yourself: How to avoid common skin conditions in sports. Retrieved from https://www.nata.org/sites/default/files/skin-disease-handout.pdf

National Athletic Trainer's Association (NATA). (n.d.b). Taking the sting out of skin injuries. Retrieved from https://www.nata.org/sites/default/files/skin-injuries-handout.pdf

National Athletic Trainer's Association (NATA). (2005). Official statement from the National Athletic Trainers' Associationon community-acquired MRSA infections (CA-MRSA). Retrieved from https://www.nata.org/sites/default/files/mrsa.pdf

National Collegiate Athletic Association (NCAA). (2014). *2014–15 Sports medicine handbook* (25th ed.). Indianapolis, IN: NCAA. Retrieved from http://www.ncaapublications.com/productdownloads/MD15.pdf

Newton, H. (2013). Viral infections of the skin: Clinical features and treatment options. *Nursing Standard, 27*(52), 43–47.

Thomas, S. (2008). Hydrocolloid dressing in the management of acute wounds: A review of the literature. *International Wound Journal, 5*(5), 602–613.

Tuberville, S. D., Cowan, L. D., & Greenfield, R. A. (2006). Infectious disease outbreaks in competitive sports: A review of the literature. *American Journal of Sports Medicine, 34*(11), 1860–1865.

Ubbink, D. T., Brölmann, F. E., Go, P. M., & Vermeulen, H. (2015). Evidence-based care of acute wounds: A perspective. *Advances in Wound Care, 4*(5), 286–294.

U.S. Department of Labor. (n.d.). Bloodborne pathogens and needlestick prevention. Retrieved from https://www.osha.gov/SLTC/bloodbornepathogens/gen_guidance.html

U.S. Department of Labor, U.S. Department of Health and Human Services. (1987). Joint advisory notice protection against occupational exposure to hepatitis B (HBV) and human immunodeficiency virus (HIV). *Federal Register*, 56:235.

Wright, G. D. (2016). Antibiotic adjuvants: Rescuing antibiotics from resistance. *Trends in Microbiology, 24*(11), 862–871.

Zinder, S. M., Basler, R. S. W., Foley, J., Scarlata, C., & Vasily, D. B. (2010). National Athletic Trainers' Association position statement: Skin diseases. *Journal of Athletic Training, 45*(4), 411–428. Retrieved from http://www.nata.org/sites/default/files/position-statement-skin-disease.pdf

CHAPTER 18
Environmental Injuries and Athletics

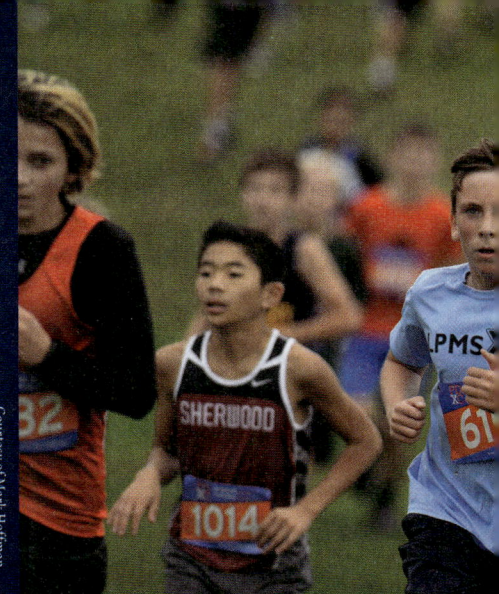

MAJOR CONCEPTS

Sports and athletic events are staged under a wide range of environmental conditions, including indoors, and a nearly infinite variety of outdoor settings. This chapter explores the body's response to extremes of heat, cold, altitude, and lightning, with particular attention given to life-threatening conditions. It is critical to note that a significant percentage of the deaths directly attributable to sports today result from heat-related problems. In addition, the chapter discusses cold-related problems, including hypothermia, frostbite and frostnip, and a relatively unknown condition called cold urticaria, along with conditions due to altitude and lightning.

Heat-Related Conditions

Because of the great range of environmental conditions within which sports, military operations, and occupations take place, a variety of temperature-related health emergencies occur each year; some of those result in death. Those working in hot environmental conditions and/or wearing protective equipment have the greatest risk of developing heat-related illnesses. For example, U.S. football in late summer to early fall has the highest incidence, followed by field hockey and cross country. To emphasize this point, from 1995 to 2010, 35 football players died from heat-related (exertional) illness in the United States (Mueller & Colgate, 2011); from 2008–2012, there was an average of 4.4 deaths from exertional heat illness; and, from 2013–2017, there was an average of 1.6 deaths from exertional heat illness (Kucera et al., 2018). Beyond organized sports, road races and cycling can bring risks as well (Adams & Jardine, 2020).

Normal metabolism can be maintained within only a very narrow range of **core body temperatures**, between 98.0°F and 98.6°F (36.7°C and 37°C) when measured orally. Heat is a natural product of metabolism, but, during exercise, the metabolic rate can increase significantly, resulting in elevations of body temperature over 104°F (40°C) and creating a condition known as **hyperthermia**. Excess heat must be eliminated from the body during exercise, or the body temperature can rise to dangerous levels in a short period of time. The body can rid itself

Core body temperature Internal body temperature usually measured orally or rectally.

Hyperthermia A body temperature above 104°F (40°C).

of excess heat through a complex process known as **thermoregulation**. Thermoregulation is controlled primarily by the temperature-regulating centers within the hypothalamus of the brain (Binkley et al., 2002). A variety of neurological sensors throughout the body, in the deep tissues and the skin, provide information regarding body temperature to the hypothalamus.

Excess heat can be lost through **radiation** (via infrared light), **conduction** (absorbed into surrounding objects), **convection** (moving air currents), and **evaporation** (sweating). Each of these methods is effective, although, during most exercise on dry land, evaporation of sweat from the skin surface is the most efficient. During sweating, the body loses water and that process is called **dehydration**. The body can also dehydrate through respiration, diarrhea, and vomiting. The body's sweating effectiveness as a form of thermoregulation can be severely compromised by extremes in relative humidity (Belval & Morrissey, 2020; Divine et al., 2018).

Relative humidity represents the amount of water vapor suspended in the air; it determines how much water can effectively evaporate from the skin during exercise. The higher the relative humidity, the less ability the surrounding air has to absorb sweat from the skin surface. As a result, the higher the relative humidity, the greater the potential for heat-related problems, regardless of "normal" environmental temperatures (Casa et al., 2015). Relative humidity, ambient air temperature, wind, and solar radiation can be measured with a **wet bulb globe temperature (WBGT)** device. Measurements based on WBGT will determine guidelines for activity modifications, such as time and length of practice, number of water breaks, equipment allowed, and work-to-rest ratios. Therefore, coaches need to make modifications in the demands of the exercise session or consider delaying activity until conditions improve in addition to modifying the equipment needed for practice. These guidelines should be region specific; for example, a football player from Seattle, Washington, would not be comfortable in the same environment as a football player from Orlando, Florida. As shown in Figure 18.1, apparent air temperature can vary significantly, depending on the relative humidity (Casa et al., 2015). If the temperature is 90°F (32.2°C) with 40% relative humidity (heat index of 91°F or 32.8°C), perhaps the football player in Orlando would have fewer activity restrictions than the football player in Seattle (Korey Stringer Institute, n.d.c).

Keep in mind that high exercise intensity can increase core body temperature faster and higher than any other situation and, when high exercise intensity is compounded with high humidity, the body's thermoregulation system can be overwhelmed. Under conditions of high relative humidity, the evaporation process becomes less effective, thereby contributing to increased body temperature.

The greatest risk of exertional heat illnesses is usually the first 2–3 weeks of preseason, when outdoor activity occurs during times of both extremely high temperatures and high humidity. Additionally, athletes who are not accustomed to the heat, are out of shape, wear heavy equipment, become hypohydrated (i.e., deficient in body water) during exercise, and who have illnesses (e.g., viral) or diseases (e.g., sickle cell) are at greater risk for heat illness. Additionally, athletes who have sunburn, certain skin diseases, or participated in drugs or alcohol or take antidepressants are also at greater risk for exertional heat illnesses. Although highly trained and acclimatized athletes have lower risk of developing heat illnesses, they are possible. Furthermore, athletes,

---

Thermoregulation The processes involved in order to maintain an optimal physiological range of core body temperature.

Radiation Emission and diffusion of rays of heat.

Conduction Heating through direct contact with a medium.

Convection Heating through another medium, such as air or liquid.

Evaporation The process of turning liquid into vapor, and the means by which the body cools itself via sweating.

Dehydration Process of losing body water through sweating, diarrhea, respiration, and vomiting.

Relative humidity The moisture content in the air that is expressed as a percentage. The percentage is the percent of moisture in the air that can be retained at a given temperature and pressure.

Wet bulb globe temperature (WBGT) Measure of temperature, humidity, wind speed, and solar radiation to determine heat stress.

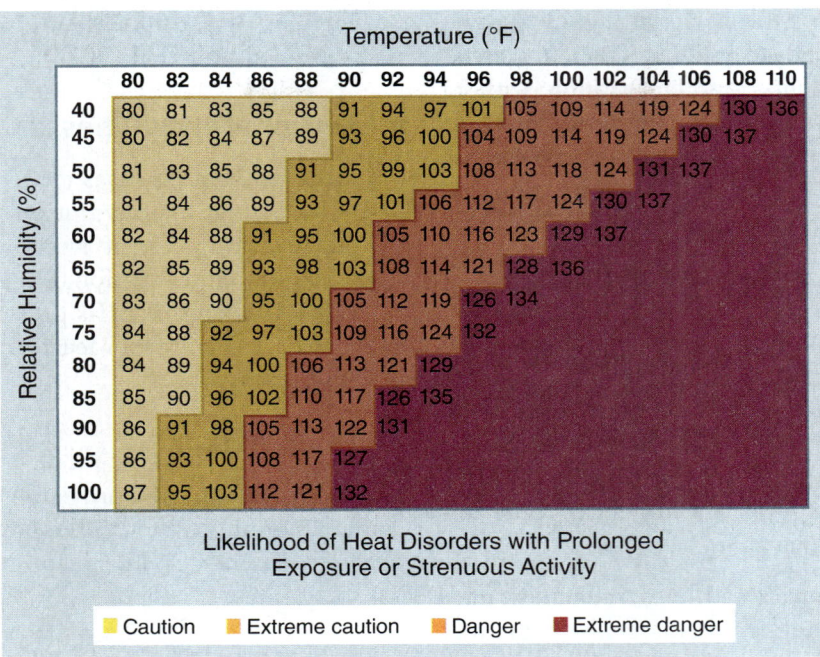

Figure 18.1 Heat index.
Reproduced from the National Weather Service.

regardless of geographic region, can be susceptible to temperature-related conditions even if the environment is cool because the exercise is high intensity or of prolonged duration. Usually, in hot and humid environments, the body physiologically cannot maintain high-intensity exercise for long and will slow down the pace. Some athletes will continue to push through high-intensity exercise in the hot environment and risk collapse (Belval & Morrissey, 2020; Casa et al., 2012; Pryor et al., 2020).

In terms of geographic location and acclimation, athletes living in the Southeastern United States are routinely exposed to the combination of high temperature and high humidity and may tolerate these conditions much easier than athletes living in the Pacific Northwest of the United States. Likewise, athletes who are intensely exercising in the Western United States can be exposed to high temperatures but dry air conditions. A Western U.S. cross-country runner who has not hydrated during the school day will be hypohydrated when he or she begins practice after school in high temperatures. Under these varying environmental conditions, athletes are at an elevated risk for exertional heat illnesses, such as exercise-associated muscle cramps; heat syncope; exertional heat exhaustion; or, in a worst-case scenario, exertional heatstroke (Belval & Morrissey, 2020; Casa et al., 2012; Casa et al., 2015; Divine et al., 2018).

The general prevention of exertional heat illness is as follows:

1. **Preparticipation physical examination.** Athletes with a history of exertional heat illness, sickle cell trait, or other metabolic diseases should be identified as well as monitored for recent illnesses, viruses, or drug or alcohol use.

2. **Euhydration. Euhydration** is the state of being optimally hydrated so body systems can function normally. Athletes should calculate a personal hydration plan, weigh in before and after physical activity, monitor urine color, have fluids and ice tub or towels readily available during activity, maintain proper nutrition, and sleep in a cool environment.

Euhydration The state of being optimally hydrated so body systems can function normally.

3. **Acclimatization.** Athletes should allow 7–14 days or more for the body to gradually adapt to exercise in the environment, or **acclimatization**, without wearing equipment and/or enduring multiple practices a day in the heat. As a general rule, those with a higher level of fitness tend to acclimatize more quickly; adolescents, obese individuals, and those with certain metabolic disorders take longer to readjust their systems (Table 18.1).

4. **Emergency action plan and appropriate medical personnel.** Having an established plan in place before unfortunate events occur is ideal for all medical personnel involved (e.g., certified athletic trainer, school nurse, emergency medical services [EMS], and team physician) to ensure proper and efficient care of exertional heat illnesses.

5. **Education.** Educate athletes, coaches, parents, administrators, and emergency personnel on how to prevent, recognize, and treat heat illnesses (Casa & Csillan, 2009; Casa et al., 2012; McDermott et al., 2017).

Exertional Heat Illnesses

Exertional heat illnesses (EHIs) can involve any of the following: hypohydration, exercise-associated muscle cramps, heat syncope, exertional heat exhaustion, and exertional heatstroke (Casa et al., 2015). All forms of EHIs presented here are in the order of severity from least to greatest, beginning with hypohydration.

Hypohydration

Hypohydration is the provision of less than the normal amount of water to the body to meet its metabolic demands. While respiration, vomiting, and

WHAT IF ❓

During practice in late August, one of your football players, an offensive lineman, suddenly staggers away from the blocking sled, falls to the ground, and is unable to get to his feet. During your initial assessment, you note that he is semiconscious and that his skin is dry, reddish in color, and hot to the touch. He is able to tell you that he is thirsty and that he has not had any water for more than an hour. It is 95°F out, approximately 78% humidity, and there is little wind. Given this scenario, what is most likely the problem? What is the appropriate first aid for this athlete?

Acclimatization The process in which physiology is adapted to suit a new or change in environment (i.e., temperature, altitude, light, etc.).

Exertional heat illnesses (EHIs) A general term given to physical conditions that can occur when exercising in the heat.

Hypohydration The provision of less than the normal amount of water to the body to meet its metabolic demands, creating a shortage of body water (mild, moderate, severe).

Table 18.1

Physiological Responses After Heat Acclimatization Relative to Nonacclimatized State

Physiological Variable	After Acclimatization (10–14 Days) Exposure
Heart rate	Decreases
Stroke volume	Increases
Body core temperature	Decreases
Skin temperature	Decreases
Sweat output/rate	Increases
Onset of sweat	Earlier in training
Evaporation of sweat	Increases
Salt in sweat	Decreases
Work output	Increases
Subjective discomfort (rating of perceived exertion [RPE])	Decreases
Fatigue	Decreases
Capacity for work	Increases
Mental disturbance	Decreases
Syncopal response	Decreases
Extracellular fluid volume	Increases
Plasma volume	Increases

Reproduced from Binkley, H. M., Beckett, J., Casa, D. J., Kleiner, D. M., & Plummer, P. E. (2002). National Athletic Trainers' Association position statement: Exertional heat illnesses. *Journal of Athletic Training, 37*(3), 337. Reprinted with permission.

diarrhea can dehydrate the body, excess **sweat loss** from exercise and inadequate fluid intake can lead to reduced fluid levels in the body. Given the very nature of physical activity and the metabolic processes associated with muscle contraction, a certain amount of dehydration is unavoidable. However, as long as the amount of hypohydration is minimal (i.e., less than 2% body weight lost), the effects usually will not compromise performance or health in general. However, if dehydration is allowed to progress to a point of more than 2% of body weight, performance and thermoregulation can be negatively affected (Casa et al., 2015; McDermott et al., 2017). As fluid loss increases beyond 2% of body weight, the body will decrease sweat production, inhibiting its one mechanism to cool the body.

Signs and symptoms of hypohydration include the following (McDermott et al., 2017):

- Thirst
- Irritability or crankiness
- Headache
- General malaise
- Dizziness
- Nausea or vomiting
- Diarrhea or gastrointestinal cramps
- Excessive fatigue
- Not able to run as fast or play as well as usual
- Heat sensations or chills
- Body mass loss

It is important to recognize these signs and symptoms and treat accordingly because cardiovascular stress and more serious altered thermoregulation can occur if dehydration continues (Belval & Morrissey, 2020; Pryor et al., 2020). Management of dehydration and hypohydration will be discussed later in this chapter.

Heat Syncope

Heat syncope, or dizziness and fainting, happens when an athlete stands for a long time or suddenly changes posture in the heat usually when wearing clothing that does not allow adequate ventilation. This individual is also most likely hypohydrated and has hypotension, which decreases cardiac filling, leading to dizziness and ultimately fainting. Additionally, the individual may have tunnel vision preceding the fainting as well as a weak pulse and sweaty skin. The first 5 days of preseason, when athletes are unaccustomed to the heat, is the most common time for syncope to happen (Casa et al., 2015).

Management of heat syncope involves the individual lying supine with his or her legs in an elevated position above the level of the heart to assist with cardiac filling. However, if the individual has fainted and fallen to the ground, a primary assessment is warranted to ensure that the individual is breathing and has a pulse. A secondary assessment is also warranted to determine whether an extremity fracture was sustained during the fall; if so, then it is important that the individual not be moved while the syncope is being treated. Typically, the individual will regain consciousness soon after fainting; at that time, a more detailed assessment can begin followed by hydration and moving to a cool area (Divine et al., 2018; Giersch et al., 2020).

Exercise-Associated Muscle Cramps (EAMCs)

Unpredictable, sudden, and involuntary muscle twinges may happen before full, very painful muscle contractions during (after 30 minutes) or after activity. These palpable muscle cramps are called **exercise-associated muscle cramps (EAMCs)**; they usually involve exercising muscles that cross two joints, such as the gastrocnemius and hamstrings. EAMCs are common in the preseason when athletes are not properly conditioned, acclimatized to heat, hydrated, and/or have adequate electrolytes.

The cause of the cramping is debated. However, many studies suggest that it maybe not be caused

---

Sweat loss The amount of sweat lost during physical activity calculated by body weight before and after activity.

Heat syncope Orthostatic dizziness or fainting due to heat exposure, hypohydration, and lack of blood flow to the brain; usually occurs during sudden change of position after not moving for a while.

Exercise-associated muscle cramp (EAMC) Involuntary, extremely painful muscle spasm associated with exercise, usually involves the gastrocnemius and hamstrings.

by heat, hypohydration, and electrolyte loss; therefore, "heat cramps" is no longer an appropriate term. Athletes prone to EAMCs are those who have a history of EAMCs, faster performances, and prior soft-tissue injury. Those who experience EAMCs temporarily stop exercising until the cramping has subsided and activity can resume again. Once the cramps dissipate, hydrating with water and/or beverages with carbohydrates and electrolytes may help. Different types of stretching techniques are typically the treatment for EAMCs, and athletes may be sore over the next several days after cramping. If athletes experience frequent EAMCs, they should be directed to a physician for further evaluation (Casa et al., 2015; Divine et al., 2018).

Of particular concern is that sometimes EAMCs may be confused with **exertional sickling**, which is muscle cramps with no palpable muscle contraction and is a very serious medical emergency. Exertional sickling occurs in athletes with **sickle cell trait**, a condition in which red blood cells are shaped like a "sickle," which causes decreased blood flow and eventually leads to breakdown of muscle tissue (i.e., fulminant rhabdomyolysis). Unlike EAMCs, exertional sickling pain is strong and generalized, yet muscles are weak. Athletes usually do not yell like they do when an EAMC occurs; they typically lie still after slumping to the ground. Exertional sickling ordinarily happens within the first 30 minutes of intense workouts. When it happens, these individuals will have trouble catching their breath and will appear weak and fatigued; they may also complain of leg or low back cramps or spasms. It is important to note that not all sickling cases will present the same way. To prevent exertional sickling, athletes should be screened for the trait as part of a preparticipation physical examination when required. Athletes with sickle cell trait should slowly be acclimatized for intense exercise, which includes extended periods of rest between runs. Additionally, sickle cell trait athletes should have water readily available during all exercise sessions and should limit activity if illness, altitude, heat, and asthma are present. Having supplemental oxygen available during workouts may also be helpful (Casa et al., 2012).

To treat someone with exertional sickling, the care provider should stop activity, check the athlete's vital signs, and call 911. Ideally, high-flow oxygen should be delivered by EMS. Medical personnel should be prepared to administer cardiopulmonary resuscitation (CPR) and expect explosive rhabdomyolysis (myoglobin leaking into the bloodstream and causing kidney damage or failure; Korey Stringer Institute, n.d.a; National Athletic Trainers' Association [NATA], n.d.a).

Exertional Heat Exhaustion

Exertional heat exhaustion (EHE), as the term implies, involves generalized fatigue, hypotension, and cardiovascular insufficiency that occurs during exercise when heavy sweating, hypohydration, and elevated core body temperature occur. This type of exhaustion most frequently happens in hot temperatures or high humidity, or both conditions, or with high-intensity exercise, especially in athletes who are not fit and/or not acclimatized to the environment. Though not in itself a life-threatening condition, heat exhaustion can be a precursor to heatstroke, which is a true medical emergency. Prudent coaches should constantly monitor athletes for the signs and symptoms of exertional heat exhaustion when they must practice and compete in climatic conditions of high heat and/or high humidity.

Signs and symptoms of exertional heat exhaustion can include any of the following (Casa et al., 2012, Casa et al., 2015, Korey Stringer Institute, n.d.b):

- Fatigue
- Fainting/collapsing

Exertional sickling A life-threatening condition resulting from many factors that cause lack of blood flow and cell death (e.g., too intense conditioning, heat, hypohydration, high altitude, illness).

Sickle cell trait A condition in which red blood cells are shaped like a "sickle," which causes decreased blood flow and eventually leads to breakdown of muscle tissue (i.e., fulminant rhabdomyolysis).

Exertional heat exhaustion (EHE) Involves generalized fatigue, hypotension, and cardiovascular insufficiency that occurs during exercise when heavy sweating, hypohydration, and elevated core body temperature occur.

- Headache
- Dizziness
- Nausea/vomiting
- Confusion
- Low blood pressure
- Uncoordinated muscle movements

The general management of exertional heat exhaustion entails facility preparation and care for the individual. During times of excessive heat and/or humidity, such as preseason football camp in the Southern and Eastern United States, having hydration stations, ice water baths, and/or cooling stations readily available is ideal (Figure 18.2). If an individual is suspected of having exertional heat exhaustion, a quick assessment for responsiveness and vital signs should occur first. Assuming the individual has a pulse and is breathing, a quick history and intake of signs and symptoms (e.g., Are you nauseated, dizzy?) while moving the individual to a cooler area, such as shade or in an air-conditioned building, and removing excess clothing or equipment should be done. It is recommended to elevate the legs above the heart and obtain a rectal temperature to distinguish exertional heat exhaustion from the more severe scenario of exertional heatstroke. If the rectal temperature is above 104°F (40°C), treatment for exertional heatstroke should begin, which will be discussed in the next section. If the rectal temperature is below 104°F (40°C), the individual can be cooled in a variety of ways, such as applying ice packs or towels, dousing with cold water, and/or fanning while the individual is supine with his or her legs elevated. Also, monitoring for vital signs every 5 minutes is prudent practice as well as continuing to cool the individual. Additionally, if the individual is hypohydrated, which will most likely be the case, and fully conscious and coherent, have the individual consume cool, oral fluids. If the individual is not recovering quickly after beginning treatment, the condition worsens during treatment, or the individual is vomiting or has diarrhea or displays other signs of heat illness, heat stroke should be suspected and a rectal temperature should be obtained (Armstrong, 2020; Casa et al., 2015, McDermott et al., 2017; Korey Stringer Institute, n.d.b).

Exertional Heatstroke

Exertional heatstroke (EHS) happens when metabolic heat production from exercise and environmental heat loads is greater than the body's ability to cool itself and,

> **Exertional heatstroke (EHS)** Excessive heat buildup, with core temperatures exceeding 104°F (40°C) in the body, resulting in the body's inability to cool itself quickly, which may cause organs to malfunction. This is a medical emergency (cool first then transport).

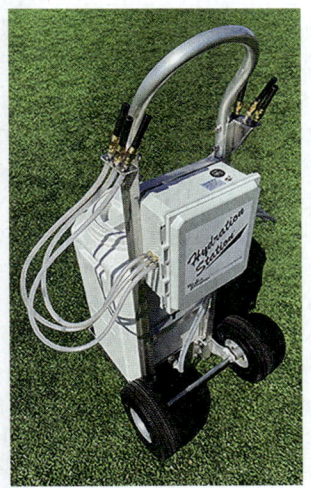
(a)

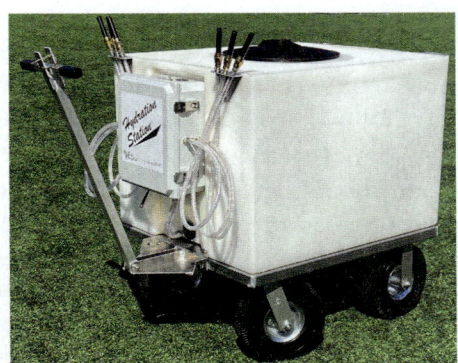
(b)

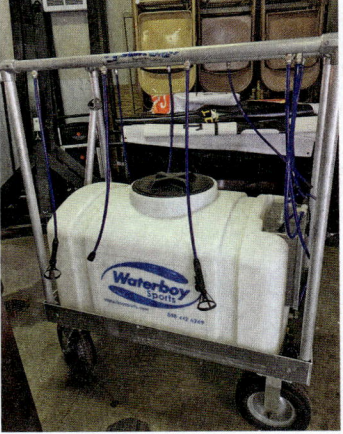
(c)

Figure 18.2 Examples of Hydration Stations. **(a)** Teammate Hydration Station by Wisstech. **(b)** Tanker Hydration Station by Wisstech, **(c)** Waterboy Horizontal Power by Waterboy Sports.
(a) and (b) Courtesy of Bill Wissen; (c) Courtesy of Cheryl Ferris.

as a result, creates a life-threatening condition. Radical elevations in body temperature over 104°F (40°C; Casa et al., 2015) can affect vital organs, such as the heart and brain, and decrease their function. Specifically, when the body can sweat and cool via evaporation and is properly hydrated, it can maintain cardiac filling, blood pressure, and mean arterial pressure. However, without proper hydration, the blood volume lowers, causing low blood pressure and low cardiac filling; without proper cooling, the temperature of the heart is also high and has yet another reason it cannot function properly. Additionally, high body heat can also destroy cell membranes, allowing bacteria to enter the bloodstream from the gut and myoglobin to enter the bloodstream from the muscles, thus causing major complications. EHS is usually related to hot and humid conditions (WBGT > 82°F, or 28°C), when the effectiveness of sweating to carry away heat from the skin surface is reduced. However, it can happen with intense or long-duration exercise in "normal" environmental conditions when there is a lack of evaporative cooling. If unchecked, this condition can degenerate, leading to a loss of thermoregulatory control, which can lead to multiorgan failure and ultimately death (Casa et al., 2015). It is critical to remember that exertional heatstroke is a true medical emergency and must be recognized and treated promptly.

Signs and symptoms of exertional heatstroke can include any of the following (Adams et al., 2020; Casa et al., 2015):

- Hot and wet skin
- Hypohydration
- Hypotension
- Vomiting
- Weakness
- Hyperventilation
- Tachycardia (100–120 heartbeats per minute)
- Body core temperature is higher than 104°F (40°C). The athletic healthcare team should be trained to ascertain **rectal core body temperature** because other methods of assessing body temperature (i.e., ear and mouth) are not reliable for an exercising individual (Casa et al., 2012; Casa et al., 2015; McDermott et al., 2017).

Rectal core body temperature The temperature of the core as measured in the rectal cavity.

- Central nervous system (CNS) dysfunction (e.g., collapse, aggressiveness, irritability, confusion, seizures, altered consciousness, staggering, and hysteria)

It must be emphasized that exertional heatstroke can result in permanent damage to the CNS and other systems in the body. Death can result if the body temperature is not controlled quickly; therefore, correct initial management of heatstroke is critical. Management of exertional heatstroke involves lowering core body temperature to 102°F (38.9°C) within 30 minutes after collapse and then transfer to EMS. If exertional heatstroke is suspected, the individual must be cooled before transferring to EMS.

The most effective way to lower the core body temperature is to quickly remove excess clothing and/or equipment, take vital signs (i.e., heart rate, respiratory rate, blood pressure, and rectal core body temperature), assess CNS function, and then submerge the athlete up to his or her neck in a tub of cold water (35–59°F or 1.7–15°C). A tub can vary in size and shape; for those with limited funds, a plastic baby/kiddie pool may be considered. Ice should cover the surface of the water at all times. If it will take too long to remove excess clothing and equipment, then submerge the athlete immediately and remove equipment while in the tub. Ideally, the water temperature should be monitored and maintained at 59°F (15°C) or below to ensure appropriate cooling rates (Adams et al., 2020; Divine et al., 2018). If full submersion cannot be done because of facility or equipment limitations, partial submersion up to the torso is ideal (Casa et al., 2015; McDermott et al., 2017).

Because the athlete's body temperature will warm the water surrounding his or her body, constantly stirring the water is necessary. While the athlete is submerged, the vital signs should be recorded every 5 minutes. The athlete should be removed when the core body temperature reaches 102°F (38.9°C) and then transported to an emergency department. It has been documented that core body temperature will lower about 1°F every 3 minutes, depending on the length of time from collapse to immersion, the core body temperature, and water temperature. The length of time the core body temperature is above 104°F (40°C) will determine the risk of death (Casa et al., 2012; Casa et al., 2015; McDermott et al., 2017). Refer to Table 18.2 for the steps to take in cold-water immersion.

Table 18.2
Cold-Water Immersion Steps

1. Prepare tub/kiddie pool with water.
2. Add ice to water as soon as EHS is suspected and measure and monitor water temperature.
3. Insert probe for measuring rectal temperature.
4. Lift athlete into tub, immerse as much as possible, and support by looping a towel under armpits.
5. Apply wet, cold towel to the athlete's head every 2–3 minutes.
6. Stir the water, and monitor the athlete's temperature and vitals.
7. Remove the athlete when rectal temperature is 102°F (39°C).
8. Cool for 15 minutes if rectal temperature is not possible.
9. Continue to monitor temperature during recovery because core body temperature may continue to fall. Transport to emergency department.

If full or partial immersion is not possible, then wet ice towels should be used and rotated over the entire body. Cold-water dousing with or without fanning may be used, but it is not as effective as cold-water immersion. Another method of cooling when ideal equipment for cold-water immersion is limited is called tarp-assisted cooling oscillation (TACO). TACO utilizes a tarp and a minimum of three volunteers, two to hold up the tarp's edges and corners and one to add ice and water. First, place the athlete in the middle of the tarp, and then add cold water and ice, thus creating a taco shape in which the athlete can be cooled. It is important to keep the athlete's head and chest above water while in the cold-water taco. Water can be oscillated to prevent it from warming around the athlete (Hosokowa et al., 2017; Luhring et al., 2016).

Over the past several years, much controversy has been generated around acquiring rectal temperature, regardless of its key role in treating exertional heatstroke. In some cases, rectal core temperature cannot be performed for various legal and policy reasons. In the event of this situation, cool for 15 minutes and then transfer. Policies and procedures should be agreed upon and established by medical and administrative personnel before the start of the season (Casa et al., 2012; Casa et al., 2015; McDermott, 2017). Exertional heat illness is survivable if proper recognition and treatment are implemented in a timely manner.

Exercise-Associated Hyponatremia

Unfortunately, there is another life-threatening condition briefly discussed earlier in this book that can present itself during periods of extreme heat and humidity and exercise and often shares the same signs and symptoms of hypohydration, heat exhaustion, and heatstroke. This life-threatening condition is called **exercise-associated hyponatremia (EAH)**. There were two football heatstroke deaths in 2014 as well as in 2015, resulting from overhydrating when trying to prevent heat illness (Kucera et al., 2018). EAH happens when excessive fluid intake (**hyperhydration**) causes the sodium concentration in the blood to be too low. The normal range of serum sodium levels is 135–145 mEq/L; when blood sodium concentrations drop below 130 mEq/L, symptoms, such as dizziness, nausea, muscle cramps, and face or extremity puffiness, can surface. More severe symptoms include altered mental status (e.g., confusion, agitation), seizures, decorticate posture, dyspnea, and frothy sputum. As mentioned previously, EAH signs and symptoms of dizziness, headache, nausea, and muscle twitching are also signs and symptoms of hypohydration. Ideally, serum sodium concentrations should be evaluated as well as taking rectal temperatures because this will determine proper course of treatment. For example, if hypotonic fluids are given to an individual with severely low serum sodium concentrations, it could be deadly. For that reason, if serum sodium concentration is not attainable, and therefore the heat illness cannot be distinguished between EHS and EAH, a hypertonic sodium intravenous treatment (3–5%) will not harm an EHS athlete, and it will be lifesaving to the EAH athlete (McDermott et al., 2017). The treatment for EHS and EAH can be confusing given their

Exercise-associated hyponatremia (EAH) A life-threatening medical condition created when there is a low concentration of sodium in the blood (<135 mEq/L) due to overconsumption of fluids and not enough sodium intake or extreme sodium loss.

Hyperhydration An excess of body water that causes enlarged intracellular and extracellular fluid volume.

similar symptoms. Refer to Figure 18.3 for a flow chart showing how to treat exertional heat illnesses.

In addition to the general prevention methods of heat-related illnesses, it is especially important to pay additional attention to individualized hydration plans and educating athletes about proper hydration and sodium to prevent EAH. Athletes should be encouraged to salt their meals and perhaps consume high-salt foods, such as canned soup or pretzels, especially during times of exercise in the heat and humidity (Casa et al., 2012).

Prevention of Exertional Heat Illnesses

Heat-related illness causing death among athletes is not always preventable. Application of a few simple guidelines and a dose of common sense are all that is needed to avoid possible tragedy. NATA published a position statement titled "Fluid Replacement for the Physically Active" with the objective "to present evidence-based recommendations that promote optimized fluid-maintenance practices for physically active individuals" (McDermott et al., 2017, p. 1, abstract).

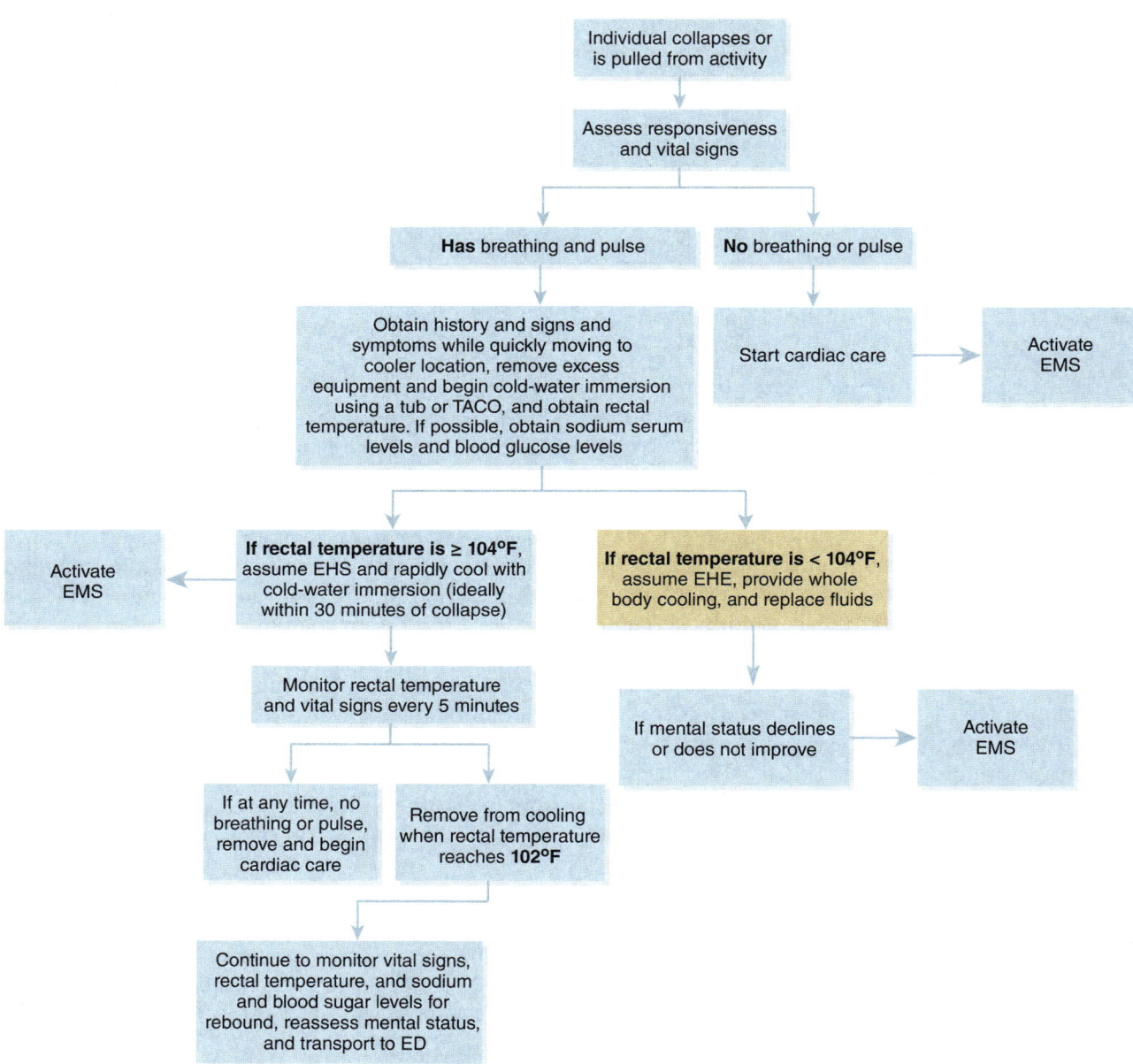

Figure 18.3 Flow chart showing how to treat exertional heat illnesses.

Additional guidelines were published detailing heat-acclimatization recommendations during preseason when activities will be happening in hot environments for secondary school athletes (Casa & Csillan, 2009). These guidelines are based on a 14-day duration model that can be implemented during the typical preseason in late summer for sports such as tackle football and field hockey. The recommendations are listed in Table 18.3. All personnel involved with the supervision of exercising individuals should review the entire NATA document and make every effort to incorporate the recommendations and review Table 18.4.

Heat Illness Prevention

To prevent heat illnesses, athletes, coaches, and parents should comply with the following guidelines:

1. **Preparticipation physical exam.** Determine past medical history for athletes. It is important to gather information regarding past medical history of heat illnesses. Likewise, it is important to know that hypohydration is a predisposing factor for exertional sickling for those who have sickle cell trait as well as for exertional rhabdomyolysis (muscle breakdown due to excessive exercise). Also, other metabolic diseases and recent illnesses/viruses and alcohol/drug use can predispose an athlete to heat-related illnesses.

2. **Euhydration.** Athletes will benefit from adhering to their personal hydration needs to prevent moderate to severe hypohydration (2–5% or more of body mass loss). To determine their needs, they

Table 18.3
Recommendations for the 14-Day Heat-Acclimatization Period

1. Days 1–5 of the heat-acclimatization period consist of the first 5 days of formal practice. During this time, athletes may not participate in more than one practice per day.
2. If a practice is interrupted by inclement weather or heat restrictions, the practice should recommence once conditions are deemed safe. Total practice time should not exceed 3 hours in any 1 day.
3. A 1-hour maximum walkthrough is permitted during days 1–5 of the heat-acclimatization period. However, a 3-hour recovery period should be inserted between the practice and walkthrough (or vice versa).
4. During days 1–2 of the heat-acclimatization period, in sports requiring helmets or shoulder pads, a helmet should be the only protective equipment permitted (goalies, as in the case of field hockey and related sports, should not wear full protective gear or perform activities that would require protective equipment). During days 3–5, only helmets and shoulder pads should be worn. Beginning on day 6, all protective equipment may be worn, and full contact may begin.
    - Football only: On days 3–5, contact with blocking sleds and tackling dummies may be initiated.
    - Full-contact sports: 100% live contact drills should begin no earlier than day 6.
5. Beginning no earlier than day 6 and continuing through day 14, double-practice days must be followed by a single-practice day. On single-practice days, one walkthrough is permitted, separated from the practice by at least 3 hours of continuous rest. When a double-practice day is followed by a rest day, another double-practice day is permitted after the rest day.
6. On a double-practice day, neither practice should exceed 3 hours in duration, and student-athletes should not participate in more than 5 total hours of practice. Warm-up, stretching, cooldown, walkthrough, conditioning, and weight-room activities are included as part of the practice time. The two practices should be separated by at least 3 continuous hours in a cool environment.
7. Because the risk of exertional heat illnesses during the preseason heat-acclimatization period is high, it is strongly recommended that an athletic trainer be onsite before, during, and after all practices.

Reproduced from Casa, D. J., & Csillan, D. (2009). Preseason heat-acclimatization guidelines for secondary school athletics. *Journal of Athletic Training*, 44(3), 332–333. Reprinted with permission.

Table 18.4
Exertional Heat Illness Summary

	EAMC	Heat Syncope	Exertional Heat Exhaustion (Urgent)	Exertional Sickling (Emergent)	Exertional Heat Stroke (Emergent)	Exercise-Associated Hyponatremia (Emergent)
Definition	Painful, involuntary muscle contractions of a specific muscle/s during or after exercise	Fainting in the heat and loss of consciousness	Elevated body heat and inability to exercise because of cardiovascular limitations with or without a collapse	Painful muscles generally throughout the body brought on by intense exercise	Extreme body heat causes overload of thermoregulatory system	Low sodium concentration in the blood (<135 mEq/L)
Physiology	Possibly heat, hypohydration, electrolyte imbalance, and/or fatigue	Standing for a long time in hot environment causing blood to pool in the legs	Heavy sweating, hypohydration, and high skin blood flow causing decreased venous return	Sickle cell trait causes decreased blood flow and cell death under certain circumstances (heat, hypohydration, altitude, extreme conditioning, etc.)	Extreme body heat without heat dissipation	Overconsumption of fluids dilutes sodium concentration in blood causing heat illness symptoms and mental symptoms
Symptoms	Muscle twitches usually followed by palpable and extremely painful muscle contractions; usually occurs during activity in preseason or hot environments	Dizziness, weakness, tunnel vision, fainting, loss of consciousness, weak pulse, sweaty skin	Fatigue, faint/collapse, confusion, weakness, pale, heavy sweating, headache, hyperventilation, nausea, hypotension, dizziness, chills, hypohydrated, core temperature <104°F (40°C)	General muscle pain and weakness with no palpable contraction that causes a person to slump and lie still; usually occurs in the first 30 minutes of intense conditioning	Hot/wet skin, hypohydrated, hypotension, nausea, weakness, hyperventilation, tachycardia, collapse, CNS dysfunction, core temperature ≥104°F (40°C)	Similar to other heat illnesses; sodium loss, disorientation, seizure, coma, death

Treatment	Stop exercise, stretch or massage the contraction, give cold fluids (water and/or sports beverage)	Lie the individual supine and elevate his or her legs, may have to do secondary assessment after fainting, move to cooler area and hydrate after regaining consciousness	Move to cool area; remove excess clothes/equipment; take rectal temperature to rule out EHS; elevate legs; cool individual with ice towels; give fluids to rehydrate; monitor vitals and time to improve; if improvement is not rapid, call 911 and treat as EHS	Remove from exercise, check and monitor vital signs, call 911, have AED accessible, and prepare for high-flow oxygen (15 L/min with nonrebreathing mask) and explosive rhabdomyolysis	Quickly remove excess clothes/equipment, take rectal temperature, call 911, cool ASAP (move to cooler area and ice water immersion to lower to ≤102°F [38.9°C] within 30 minutes), monitor vitals	Depends on severity; DO NOT give normal saline or fluids; mild to moderate: withhold fluids until sodium levels are normal, give salty foods; severe: call 911 (3% hypertonic saline, supplemental oxygen)
Recovery	Usually occurs within minutes to hours; see physician if persistent	Usually occurs within hours	Usually takes a day	As determined by a physician and his or her level of sickling and severity of symptoms	Depends on maximum core body temperature, time to cooling, how cooled; determined by physician and medical tests	Depends on severity and sodium concentration levels; determined by physician

Athletic Trainers SPEAK OUT

What should all coaches and parents know about prevention and treatment of exertional heat illness?

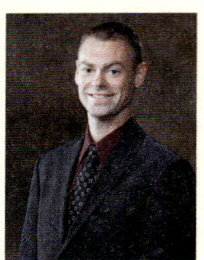

Courtesy of Brendon P. McDermott, PhD, ATC, FACSM.

Exertional heat stroke (EHS) is a potentially fatal condition diagnosed when core body temperature exceeds 104°F (40°C) with simultaneous central nervous system dysfunction (uncoordination, acting out-of-sorts, unconscious, etc.). Athletic trainers are the best-prepared medical professionals to implement and execute prevention, recognition, diagnosis, and treatment for EHS. It is highly recommended that parents and coaches advocate for appropriate medical coverage for athletics at every level to ensure quality care.

Coaches and parents should strive for EHS prevention as much as possible at all levels of athletics. Heat acclimatization is the best protector for an individual against all heat illnesses. This is facilitated by gradually introducing exercise and equipment in hot conditions so that the individual is used to the intensity of exercise in that environment. All sports and coaches should implement an acclimatization plan for athletes. Other documented means of EHS prevention include proper hydration. Athletes typically hydrate well during activity, but are not diligent at maintaining hydration when they're not with coaches. Other daily reminders that help prevent heat illness include adequate sleep, healthy diet, decreased psychological stress, exercise at appropriate intensity based on environmental conditions, and avoiding exercise in the heat when ill.

Once EHS occurs, fatality is 100% preventable provided that efficient recognition and treatment occurs. However, parents and coaches will not have the available knowledge or equipment to distinguish EHS from other conditions that cause redundant signs and symptoms (concussion, low blood sugar, hyponatremia, etc.). Therefore, prevention efforts are paramount in the absence of an onsite athletic trainer.

Parents should advocate for emergency medical personnel to thoroughly assess vital signs if EHS is suspected so that appropriate diagnosis is made. Athletic trainers have established the standard of care for EHS and have developed 100% effective practice guidelines. Patient expectations of standard of care includes appropriate preventive practices and effective emergency action plans that include rectal temperature assessment and immediate cold-water immersion prior to emergency transport for EHS.

—**Brendon P. McDermott, PhD, ATC, FACSM**

Brendon McDermott is an Associate Professor in the Graduate Athletic Training Program in the Department of Health, Human Performance and Recreation at the University of Arkansas in Fayetteville, Arkansas, and a Member, Korey Stringer Institute Medical and Science Advisory Board in Storrs, Connecticut.

---

need to consider their **sweat rate**, acclimatization, environment, body size, gastric emptying rate, daily water intake, exercise duration and intensity, and fluid preferences. These plans need to be recalculated for changing variables. Ideally, fluids should be consumed before, during, and after activity to maintain hydration, and it is important to replace fluids and electrolytes lost in sweat. In addition, it is important to drink fluids with meals as well as be conscious of personal cues, such as thirst, void frequency, and urine color over the course of the day. See Table 18.5 to calculate hydration needs. The following practices are recommended to maintain hydration:

a. **Drink when thirsty.** Easy access to water and frequent water breaks is ideal. However, keep in mind that thirst alone will not prevent dehydration, and some individuals must rehydrate even if they are not thirsty.

b. **Measure body mass.** First morning nude body weight after voiding should fluctuate by less than 1% from day to day. Unfortunately, this

Sweat rate The amount of sweat produced per hour for a given activity.

Table 18.5
Personal Hydration Needs Calculations

Monitor urine color throughout the day and specifically before and after exercise.

Monitor body mass in the morning after the first void and specifically before and after exercise.

Calculate sweat loss:

Sweat loss (L) = Body mass before exercise (kg) − Body mass after exercise (kg) + Volume consumed during exercise (L) − Urine volume during exercise (L)

Calculate sweat rate:

Sweat rate (L/h) = Sweat loss (L)/exercise duration (h)

Based on this information and using hydration guidelines, determine the volume of fluids that need to be consumed throughout the day and, specifically, before, during, and after exercise.

Based on McDermott, B. P., Anderson, S. A., Armstrong, L. E., Casa, D. J., Cheuvront, S. N., Cooper, L., . . . Roberts, W. O. (2017). National Athletic Trainers' Association position statement: Fluid replacement for the physically active. *Journal of Athletic Training, 52*(9), 877–895; American College of Sports Medicine, Sawka, M. N., Burke, L. M., Eichner, E. R., Maughan, R. J., Montain, S. J., & Stachenfeld, N. S. (2007). American College of Sports Medicine position stand. Exercise and fluid replacement. *Medicine & Science in Sports & Exercise, 39*(2), 377–390.

method is mostly at the will of the athlete; however, if the athlete does perform this task, it can provide valuable information to medical personnel. The most common method medical personnel can use to assess hydration is a weight chart. Recording body mass before and after each exercise session and comparing values to the baseline, 3 consecutive days of euhydration, and/or preexercise to preexercise is key to determine whether athletes are dehydrated. Weighing athletes before and after practices should be done with athletes wearing as little clothing as possible to avoid sweat-soaked clothing and shoes adding weight. Preexercise weight is a good indicator of the athlete's rehydration over the past 24 hours, whereas postexercise weight provides an indication of the athlete's ability to drink adequate amounts of fluid during workouts and how much fluid needs to be consumed after exercise to rehydrate adequately. It is important that the same scale be used for all weighing. Coaches and athletic trainers can use a software program, such as Microsoft Excel, to make the calculations of the percentage of body mass lost after exercise and how much fluid the athlete needs to consume to return to an adequate level of hydration.

c. **Monitor urine color.** Documenting urine color is a valuable tool for evaluating hydration status. First-morning urine color is the most valuable indicator of hydration status; any other time of day, urine color may be influenced by diet, exercise, environment, consumed fluid, type of fluid, and fluid volume. However, urine color throughout the day also provides good information. Ideally, urine should be collected in a clear container and then evaluated in adequate lighting because assessing its color in the toilet bowl does not give accurate results. Urine color charts (e.g., hydrationcheck.com) are readily available online, and color data can also be included in the weight chart.

d. **Calculate individual hydration needs before, during, and after activity.** Duration and intensity of exercise, environmental conditions, type of clothing and equipment, body weight, genetic predisposition, gender, age, heat acclimatization state, metabolic efficiency, diet, and sweat rate determine hydration needs. Hydration needs are determined by calculations during trial-and-error exercise sessions and will change based on the variables previously mentioned. In general, total body water ranges from 45–75% of body mass with an average of roughly 60% of total body mass. Usually, athletes have higher total body water values due to having greater muscle mass and lower body fat than other nonactive individuals. A reduction in body weight of 2–5% can result in reduced performance and stress on internal organs, so it is important to be properly hydrated before, during, and after exercise.

   i. **Before exercise.** The goal is to start exercise in a hydrated state with normal electrolyte levels or in a slightly hyperhydrated state if the event or sport and environmental conditions warrant. Usually drinking fluids (water or sports beverages) with meals and adequate recovery time since the last exercise bout will attain proper hydration before exercise begins. However, if hydration is needed before exercise as determined by urine color and volume, slowly drinking about 5–7 mL/kg of body weight (0.07–0.107 fl oz/lb of body weight) of fluid 4 hours before exercise is recommended. If urine color is still dark and urine volume is still reduced, add another 3–5 mL/kg of body weight of fluid 2 hours before exercise to hopefully attain hydration levels (Roy, 2013). Also, consuming beverages with sodium or salty snacks before exercise will help maintain sodium levels. Weighing the athlete before exercise will help determine hydration needs after exercise (Roy, 2013).

ii. **During exercise.** Allowing the athlete to drink as needed is ideal, but, depending on the situation, that may not be possible; therefore, hydrating during time outs, halftime, and water stations during a race is key. If specific trials have been performed under the same circumstances to calculate sweat rate and hydration needs during activity, then that information provides a good guideline and goal for the athlete to consume during activity.

iii. **After exercise.** To calculate the percentage of reduction in body weight due to fluid loss, weigh the athlete before and after practice. Take the number of pounds lost in activity and divide that number by the prepractice weight, and then multiply by 100. For example, if an athlete loses 5 pounds after activity and weighed 150 pounds before activity, this athlete would have lost 3.33% of his or her body weight in fluid, which needs to be replaced. Postexercise rehydration and nutrition should take place within 2–6 hours after the practice or competition, with fluid replacement taking precedence within 2 hours after exercise (McDermott et al., 2017; Roy, 2013; Table 18.6). Lastly, coaches and medical personnel should monitor body weight throughout the season, noting any significant changes. The scale should be located in an easily accessible area, and coaches must require that athletes comply with the daily weight-monitoring protocols.

3. **Acclimatization.** For a period of 7–14 days, it is important to be exposed to heat and humidity during exercise to physiologically adapt (Table 18.4) before adding equipment, multiple practices a day, or other stressors. However, heavy exercise should be avoided during times of extreme environmental conditions, especially when the temperature is above 95°F (35°C) and there is high humidity. Remember that fitness has a positive effect on the ability to function in extreme conditions. The process of developing a tolerance to extremes of

Table 18.6
Hydration Guidelines for Before, During, and After Exercise

Hydration Before Exercise	Rehydration During Exercise	Rehydration After Exercise
5–7 mL/kg 4 hours before activity, OR measure weight and consume as needed throughout the day.	Consume fluid as needed per thirst or based on calculated sweat rate. If exercise is longer than 1 hour in duration, consider fluids with electrolytes and consume 30–60 g of carbohydrates per hour of exercise.	Measure weight and consume as needed; eat and drink within 2 hours after exercise to replace fluids, electrolytes, carbohydrates, and protein; OR consume 1.5 L/kg lost.
Check urine; if dark, increase fluid consumption by 3–5 mL/kg 2 hours before activity. Consider carbohydrates and sodium.	Urine volume and frequency is determined by individualized sweat rate.	Replace fluid and electrolyte balance to ensure urine is light yellow in color and has good volume.

Data from McDermott, B. P., Anderson, S. A., Armstrong, L. E., Casa, D. J., Cheuvront, S. N., Cooper, L., . . . Roberts, W. O. (2017). National Athletic Trainers' Association position statement: Fluid replacement for the physically active. *Journal of Athletic Training, 52*(9), 877–895; Roy, B. A. (2013). Exercise and fluid replacement: Brought to you by the American College of Sports Medicine www.acsm.org. *ACSM's Health & Fitness Journal, 17*(4), 3.

climate, called acclimatization, normally requires a period of weeks. When athletes do exercise in the heat, remember that restrictive garments can impair circulation of air, thus reducing the evaporation of sweat. For example, football equipment can cover 75% of the skin and restrict cooling. Be aware that dark colors on uniforms and helmets may facilitate heat buildup.

4. **Emergency action plan.** An emergency action plan should be developed for handling exertional heat illnesses. This plan should include specifics on how to treat, where to treat, how to transport, and who is involved in these processes. Policies and procedures should be developed according to published guidelines and implemented to prevent, recognize, and effectively treat heat-related illnesses. All that information should be reviewed with the involved personnel, such as the medical staff (e.g., EMS, school nurse, athletic trainers, and team physicians), coaches, parents, and administrators. Some details of the emergency action plan, such as rectal temperature, may need legal guidance as mentioned previously. It is very important to periodically review these policies and procedures with all involved parties as well as practice them to ensure effective and timely treatment.

5. **Education.** Coaches, athletes, parents, medical personnel, and administrators should not only be educated on the prevention, signs and symptoms, and treatment of exertional heat illnesses, but they should also be educated about the policies and procedures. Special attention to educate athletes, coaches, and parents on how to prevent heat illnesses and manage proper daily hydration is of upmost importance.

Prevention of heat illnesses must be a top priority for everyone involved in organized sports. The legal community has shown little tolerance for personnel who are found to be negligent in the implementation of prudent heat-illness prevention procedures. All personnel and athletes should be well versed in the major risk factors for exertional heatstroke (Tables 18.7 and 18.8) as well as the recommended treatment and its associated equipment needs (Table 18.9; Casa et al., 2012; Casa et al., 2015; McDermott et al., 2017).

Table 18.7
Factors That Increase the Risk of Heat Stroke

	Nonenvironmental Risk Factors
Drugs and supplements	Drugs such as cocaine, amphetamines, antihistamines, and antinausea drugs tend to increase physical activity and heat production. Diuretics may cause the loss of electrolytes, and products like caffeine can reduce the awareness of fatigue.
Alcohol	Decreases cardiac output and can cause hyperthermia, electrolyte imbalance, and hypohydration.
Hypohydration and electrolyte imbalance	Hypohydration and electrolyte imbalances prior to exercise and exposure to the environment will increase risk of heat-related illnesses.
Illness	It is particularly dangerous to exercise in the heat when fever is present.
Genetics	Usually males and those with sickle cell trait are at greater risk.
Demeanor	Those with overzealous attitude toward improving fitness level.
Past history of heat illness	Past history may cause individuals to be more susceptible to future illness.
Lack of acclimatization	Usually 10–14 days are needed to physiologically adapt to the environment.

(continues)

Table 18.7 (continued)
Factors That Increase the Risk of Heat Stroke

Lack of physical conditioning	Poor physical condition predisposes an athlete to heat illness because more heat production per unit of work is generated.
Increased BMI	Obesity, or large, heavy physique.
High exercise intensity in the heat	Intense exercise in the heat/humidity will increase risk of heat-related illnesses.
Environmental Risk Factors	
Barriers to heat loss	Being overdressed with clothing and/or equipment prevents the evaporation of sweat from the skin.
Environmental factors	High temperature and/or high humidity or exercising during the hottest part of the day can increase risk of heat illness.

Data from Casa, D. J., & Csillan, D. (2009). Preseason heat-acclimatization guidelines for secondary school athletics. *Journal of Athletic Training, 44*(3), 332–333; Casa, D. J., DeMartini, J. K., Bergeron, M. F., Csillan, D., Eichner, E. F., Lopez, R. M., . . . Yeargin, S. W. (2015). NATA position statement: Exertional heat illness. *Journal of Athletic Training, 50*(9), 986–1000.

Table 18.8
Prevention of Heat Illnesses by Roles of Several Individuals

Athletes	- Hydration: Maintain hydration and electrolytes throughout day and monitor urine color. - Nutrition: Eat nutritious foods. - Sleep: Sleep in cool environment for 6–8 hours a night. - Clothes/equipment: Wear light-colored, lightweight, and wicking clothing if possible and minimize equipment to allow greatest air exchange. - Fitness level: Enter preseason in shape and maintain/improve fitness level as season progresses; no need to push beyond limits during extreme heat conditions. - Illness: Avoid exercising if ill/fever. - Drugs/alcohol: Avoid use of OTC stimulants, OTC cold and allergy medications, caffeine, and alcohol during heat stress; consult physician for risk assessment of prescribed medication and exercising in the heat. - Genetics: Know status of sickle cell trait or other diseases/conditions that increase risk of heat illnesses.
Coaches	- Practice time adjustments: Adhere to WBGT guidelines, avoid activity from 10 a.m. to 5 p.m., decrease warm-up time, allow water and cooling/shade breaks, allow adequate recovery time between practices. - Physical conditioning: Adhere to a slow progression of conditioning and work:rest ratios. - Acclimatization protocols: Adhere to established recommendations for equipment and practice schedules during acclimatization periods. - Monitor athletes: Be on alert for athletes who are showing signs of heat illness.

Athletic trainers	■ PPE: Include exertional heat illness questions on PPE. ■ Policies: Create, maintain, and review emergency action plan with all involved parties (e.g., administration, EMS, coaches, healthcare staff, etc.). ■ Healthcare services: Provide adequate staffing for activities as well as education about management of heat illnesses for staff; provide WBGT measurements and associated recommendations, hydration plans, weigh-ins, access to water for activity. ■ Supplies: Ensure adequate management supplies are available and easily accessible to the activity. ■ Education: Educate coaches, athletes, parents, administrators, EMS personnel, etc. about heat illnesses and the management and prevention of them.

Data from Casa, D. J., & Csillan, D. (2009). Preseason heat-acclimatization guidelines for secondary school athletics. *Journal of Athletic Training, 44*(3), 332–333; and Casa, D. J., DeMartini, J. K., Bergeron, M. F., Csillan, D., Eichner, E. R., Lopez, R. M., . . . Yeargin, S. W. (2015). National Athletic Trainers' Association position statement: Exertional heat illness. *Journal of Athletic Training, 50*(9), 986–1000.

Table 18.9 Recommended Equipment List for Prevention of Heat Illness

Temperature monitoring: Wet bulb globe temperature (WBGT) device, rectal thermometer,* lubricating gel
Cooling materials: Tub or kiddie pool, cooler with ice, towels, and tent/shade
Hydration supplies: Water source and dispenser, hypertonic solution,* IV equipment,* salty food
Emergency supplies: Stethoscope, blood pressure cuff, automatic external defibrillator, portable blood sodium analyzer, glucometer, stretcher, cell phone

*Use of these items should be thoroughly explained in an emergency action plan.

Cold-Related Conditions

Just as extremes in heat and humidity can create problems for athletes, so can cold, wet, and windy environments. Individuals who are physically active and those who participate in winter sports, such as skiing, mountaineering, and snowmobiling; outdoor events; and outdoor team sports that run into colder months; and those employed in outside occupations or in the military are potentially susceptible to cold-related injuries. Maintaining normal body temperature while exposed to the cold depends on heat from metabolic processes (**thermogenesis**) and heat loss to the environment. The body will lose heat down its **thermal gradient**, which is the temperature difference between the core and the extremities and the skin and the environment. Similar to thermoregulation in hot environments, the hypothalamus in the brain is also involved in thermoregulation in cold environments. In the event the body needs heat, it can create it by **shivering**, which are involuntary muscle contractions. The onset and amount a person shivers depends on the intensity and duration of exposure to the cold environment. Usually, shivering begins in the trunk muscles and eventually reaches the extremities. The body will also decrease peripheral blood flow and vasoconstrict to prevent heat loss. This process is controlled neurally, based on skin temperature, core temperature, and baroreceptors. The vasoconstriction response may begin around a skin temperature of 93.2–95°F (34–35°C). However, restricted blood flow to the extremities can cause local cold injuries, so the body will control periodic fluctuations of blood flow to the extremities to limit damage (Cappaert et al., 2008; Madden & Fudge, 2018).

Heat loss in cold environments can happen in the same manner as it does in hot environments, through radiation, convection, conduction, and evaporation. In cold environments, heat loss via radiation can happen when skin, especially the head, face, neck, and hands,

Thermogenesis The creation of heat by various methods.

Thermal gradient The temperature difference and distance between two points, or the change in temperature over a given distance (e.g., difference in temperature between core and extremities).

Shivering A body response to cold temperatures characterized by fast muscle contractions in an effort to increase body heat.

is exposed. Heat loss via convection can happen when the **boundary layer**, or thin layer of warm air around the skin, is removed by air moving across the skin, such as wind, or the person moving, such as when snowmobiling, skiing, or running. To estimate this effect, the **wind chill factor** was created. Figure 18.4 shows the wind chill chart that can be used in a manner similar to how the heat index chart is used. Temperature and wind determine the wind chill, or how cold a person feels in those condition. The wind chill helps predict cooling of exposed skin (frostbite) risk and determine whether outdoor events should be postponed. Keep in mind that the wind chill chart does not account for wind produced by the person's movement, such as when biking or snowmobiling. This additional variable should be included when using the wind chill chart (Cappaert et al., 2008; Madden & Fudge, 2018).

Another way heat is lost is due to conduction, or direct contact with cold surfaces, especially wet surfaces, such as rain- or snow-soaked clothing. Adding rain to cold and windy conditions can lead to significant heat loss because heat transfer via water is up to 70 times greater than via air. Cold, damp days are also likely to be overcast, which does not allow radiant heat through. That's why it is not unusual to feel colder on cold, damp days. In addition, trapped air around the body contains water molecules, as does clothing. Because it takes more heat energy to warm water molecules around the body, an athlete is likely to be chilled faster on a cold, damp day versus a cold, dry day. Wearing proper clothing and footwear will decrease convective and conductive heat loss, which can be up to 15% of overall heat loss. Subcutaneous fat will also help decrease conductive heat loss. Lastly, evaporative heat loss can account for 15–25% as an individual breathes and skin is exposed (Cappaert et al., 2008; Madden & Fudge, 2018).

Certain individuals are at risk for cold-related injuries more so than others. Those with poor nutrition and water intake, who are young or old, are female, of African American race, have greater amounts of body fat and muscle, and are less fit may have a harder time maintaining core body temperature in cold environments. Additionally, those with certain medical conditions, such as exercise-induced bronchospasms, Raynaud syndrome,

Boundary layer Thin layer of warm air around the skin.

Wind chill factor The outdoor temperature after taking wind into account; this is usually lower than the air temperature.

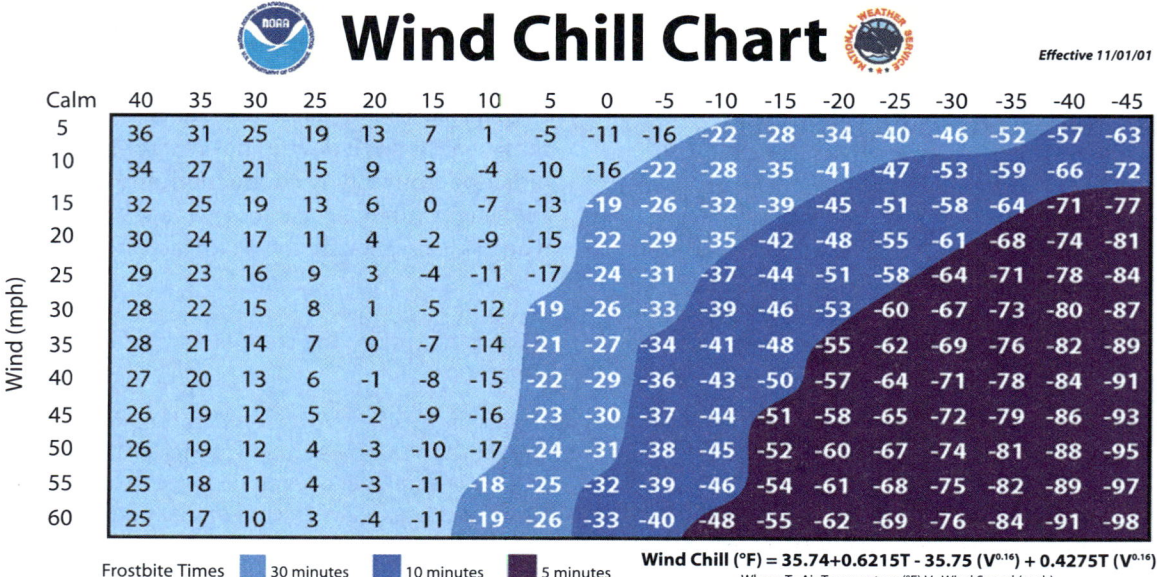

Figure 18.4 Wind chill chart.
Reproduced from the National Weather Service.

anorexia, spinal cord injury with associated paralysis, and cardiovascular disease, are particularly sensitive to the cold and should limit their exposure (Cappaert et al., 2008).

General prevention of cold-related injuries includes the following (Cappaert et al., 2008; Madden & Fudge, 2018):

1. **Preparticipation physical examination.** Identify those with a history of cold-related injuries and those with risk factors that predispose them to cold-related injuries.

2. **Preparation.** Being prepared for cold exposure is ideal to prevent cold-related injuries. The following steps should be taken for prevention.

    a. **Wind chill chart.** Consult the wind chill chart (Figure 18.4) using the temperature, wind speed, and wind speed of activity to assess risk, and make decisions on activity in the cold. Even on days when the temperature is moderate, the wind chill factor can significantly increase the risk of cold-related injuries.

    b. **Supplies.** The ideal situation is having the proper supplies, such as heat packs, blankets, extra dry clothes, rectal thermometer, cell phone or two-way radio, tub for rewarming, designated warming stations both indoors and outdoors for breaks and treatment, and fluids available for hydration.

    c. **Proper attire and preparation.** Wearing proper clothing, head and hand protection, and footwear is prudent practice to decrease heat loss. Specifically, the inside layer, worn closest to the body, should wick sweat and allow for evaporation. Usually, this layer is not made of cotton. The outer layers should be water and wind resistant or proof to reduce conductive heat loss. Bring extra dry clothing, and, when practical, keep your head, hands, and feet protected with extra insulation. Athletes should be well nourished and hydrated before the event or exercise; having fluids available for hydration during and after the event is ideal, especially for generating body heat. Do not drink alcohol, and avoid drugs because they may interfere with the body's ability to generate heat as well as creating an illusion of warmth. Do not embark on a long-duration activity alone. Train with a friend, or, at least, tell someone your plans and when you estimate to return.

    d. **Monitor.** Keep an eye on the athletes who are more at risk of cold-related injuries, and have trained medical personnel onsite.

3. **Education.** Athletes, coaches, parents, and administrators should be educated on the various cold-related injuries and their prevention and care.

4. **Emergency action plan.** Details involving decision-making based on the wind chill chart and proper treatment and care for cold-related injuries should be included in the emergency plan, and everyone involved should be familiar with it.

Exposure to cold can result in several conditions, such as hypothermia, frostbite, frostnip, cold urticaria, trench foot, and chilblain.

Hypothermia

Hypothermia is when the body loses heat too rapidly, resulting in total body cooling. Clinically, hypothermia involves a lowering of the body core temperature significantly below the norm of 98.6°F (37°C). Mild hypothermia begins to occur when core temperature drops to 95°F (35°C). Historically, the study of hypothermia has been limited to military personnel in the North Sea and those taking part in expeditions in extremely cold environments. Recently, however, cases of clinical hypothermia have been documented in athletes involved in outdoor aerobic events, such as long-distance runs. Surprisingly, hypothermia can occur at temperatures well above freezing. The combination of wind and moisture can cause rapid heat loss and the onset of hypothermia, during which the hypothalamus induces shivering in the skeletal muscles to generate heat. If shivering is not successful in generating enough heat, it ceases at around 87–90°F (30.6–32.2°C); then, uncontrolled body cooling occurs (Madden & Fudge, 2018).

Hypothermia A body temperature below 95°F (35°C).

Signs and symptoms of hypothermia, according to the NATA's position statement (Cappaert et al., 2008), include the following:

- In mild cases, the individual will display shivering; loss of fine motor control; slurring of speech; polyuria; rhinorrhea; and mental problems, such as confusion and loss of memory.
- In moderate cases, the individual will have core temperatures of 94–90°F (34–32°C), impaired gross motor control, depressed respiration, cardiac arrhythmias, cyanosis, impaired shivering, slurred speech, loss of consciousness, and dilated pupils.
- In severe cases, the athlete will have a core temperature of less than 90°F (32°C); stiff muscles, giving the appearance of rigor mortis; blue skin; and decreased blood pressure, respiration, and pulse rates. The athlete will be semiconscious or unconscious or comatose.

It is important to know that each athlete is different and will respond differently to cold conditions.

Management of *mild hypothermia* involves the following:

1. Move the athlete to a source of heat and out of the cold environment.
2. Remove any wet clothing.
3. Wrap the athlete in warm, dry clothing or blankets.
4. Use an electric blanket or hot packs placed around the head and neck, armpits, groin, and chest. Avoid rewarming the extremities because doing so may cause vasodilation, resulting in cooled blood from the extremities returning to the core and lowering the core temperature, a condition known as "afterdrop" (Cappaert et al., 2008; Madden & Fudge, 2018).
5. Give warm fluids, such as soup or hot tea.

Management of *moderate or severe hypothermia* (body temperature below 94°F [34°C] or 90°F [32.2°C], respectively) involves the following:

1. Begin with a primary survey, and activate EMS.
2. Quickly move the athlete *gently* to a warmer area free of wind and precipitation. Gentle movement is necessary because cardiac-related problems may result from low body temperatures.
3. Remove cold and/or wet clothing, and insulate with dry, warm clothing or blankets, especially the head. If rewarming is necessary, begin with the trunk, specifically the chest, groin, and axilla.
4. Monitor vital signs, and be prepared to administer artificial respiration or CPR as well as continue to rewarm during transport and at the hospital (Cappaert et al., 2008).

Frostbite and Frostnip

Exposure to extremely cold temperatures can result in skin-related problems, known commonly as frostbite and frostnip. **Frostbite** is the freezing of tissues from excessive exposure to cold. Damage from frostbite is caused by actual freezing of tissues and lack of blood (oxygen) supply to the tissues as a result of clotting. Frostbite also has mild, moderate, and severe categories, based on the depth of frozen tissues. The exposed skin, usually on the face, ears, and hands, is the victim of frostbite. In mild or superficial frostbite, the skin appears dry and waxy as well as blue and gray. There is usually redness, swelling, and tingling or burning sensations. For deeper, or moderate to severe, frostbite, the skin is hard, cold, and white or black/purple and may slough off. There also may be blisters along with burning, throbbing, or shooting pain, neuropraxia, and tissue damage (Madden & Fudge, 2018).

Medical evidence indicates that the most severe damage related to frostbite occurs when the frozen tissue thaws and then refreezes before medical treatment. Fortunately, the risk of frostbite is minimal in most organized outdoor activities, such as team sports. Typically, such activities are held near school or community facilities so that participants can return to a warm environment before any significant freezing takes place.

Frostnip is generally considered less severe than frostbite and involves freezing of only outer layers of skin, without damage to underlying tissue. Both of these conditions can occur when the nose, ears, fingers, and feet are exposed to cold temperatures for a long enough time period for freezing to occur. The probability of frostnip occurring is quite high, however, even under such circumstances because participants may not realize the severity of tissue cooling taking place. During activities in extreme conditions

Frostbite Freezing of tissues from excessive exposure to cold.

Frostnip Less severe form of frostbite.

in which temperatures are below freezing and wind chill is a factor, athletes should be instructed by coaching personnel to watch closely for the early warning signs of frostbite and frostnip. Remember, the early signs of these problems are often noted by someone other than the victim (Cappaert et al., 2008; Madden & Fudge, 2018).

The NATA, in its position statement (Cappaert et al., 2008), has published criteria to aid in the treatment of frostbite and frostnip; its guidelines are listed in **Time Out 18.1**. Tissue freezing can be categorized as either superficial or deep, depending on the duration and extent of exposure.

Chilblain and Immersion (Trench) Foot

Chilblain is an exaggerated inflammatory response to cold exposure for 1–5 hours due to prolonged vasoconstriction of skin blood vessels. It usually occurs on the hands and feet with or without tissue freezing, and edema may be present. There also may be tenderness, itching, and pain. Typically, individuals who spend long time outdoors with wet clothing are at risk.

> **Chilblain** An exaggerated inflammatory response to cold exposure for 1–5 hours due to prolonged vasoconstriction of skin blood vessels.

TIME OUT 18.1

Frostbite and Frostnip Care

CARE FOR A FROSTBITE VICTIM

All frostbite injuries require the same first aid treatment. Seek medical care immediately. Rewarming of frostbite should seldom be attempted outside a medical facility, and hypothermia should be ruled out.

1. Get the victim out of the cold and to a warm place.
2. Remove any wet clothing or constricting items, such as rings, that could impair blood circulation. Rewarming should be done slowly. The affected body part can be pushed against another person's warm skin. Avoid using friction, dry heat, or steam methods to rewarm, and leave blisters intact.
3. Seek immediate medical care.
4. If the affected part is partially thawed or the victim is in a remote or wilderness situation (more than 1 hour from a medical facility) and you have warm water, use the following wet, rapid rewarming method. Place the frostbitten part in warm water, less than 98°F for mild frostbite and 98–104°F (36.7–40°C) for moderate to severe frostbite for 15–30 minutes. If you do not have a thermometer, pour some of the water over the inside of your arm or put your elbow into it to test that it is warm, not hot. Maintain water temperature by adding warm water as needed. For ear or facial injuries, apply warm, moist cloths, changing them frequently.
5. After thawing:
   - If the feet are affected, treat the victim as a stretcher case. The feet will be very difficult to use after they are rewarmed and should be protected.
   - Protect the affected area from contact with clothing and bedding.
   - Place dry, sterile gauze between the toes and the fingers to absorb moisture and keep them from sticking together.
   - Slightly elevate the affected part to reduce pain and swelling.
   - Do not allow the areas to refreeze.
   - If tissue falls off, debridement and infection control are needed.

CARE FOR A FROSTNIP VICTIM

1. Gently warm the affected area by placing it against a warm body part (e.g., put bare hands under the armpits or on the stomach). Rewarming can be painful, so do so slowly. After rewarming, the affected area can be red and tingling.
2. Do not rub the affected area, and do not allow the tissues to refreeze.

Based on Cappaert, T. A., Stone, J. A., Castellani, J. W., Krause, B. A., Smith, D., & Stephens, B. A. (2008). National Athletic Trainers' Association position statement: Environmental cold injuries. *Journal of Athletic Training, 43*(6), 640–658.

The severity of the chilblain is dependent upon the temperature of the wet item (32–60°F or 5.7–15.6°C) and duration of exposure to the wet item. With longer exposure times, such as 12 hours to days, in wet, cold environments, an inflammatory response can develop. This usually occurs on the feet if the socks or footwear are wet and cold for extended periods of time.

The care for chilblain and immersion (trench) foot is to remove wet or constrictive clothing; wash and dry the area carefully; elevate the affected body part; and cover with loose, warm, and dry clothing or blankets. As with frostbite and frostnip care, do not disturb blisters or apply friction, dry heat, or steam methods of rewarming. Soaking in warm water (102–110°F or 38.9–43.3°C) for 5 minutes followed by drying and putting clean, dry, and warm socks on is also an option for treatment of immersion (trench) foot. Also, one should monitor the area for return of circulation and sensation (Cappaert et al., 2008; Madden & Fudge, 2018).

Cold Urticaria

Another related problem of the skin associated with exposure to cold temperatures is **cold urticaria**, which involves a skin reaction of localized **edema** (fluid accumulation) associated with severe itching. The areas involved are usually those directly exposed to the cold or those not well protected by clothing. The exact mechanism of cold urticaria is unknown but appears to be an allergic reaction to cold temperatures. Some individuals are more susceptible, including people with mononucleosis, syphilis, varicella (chickenpox), and hepatitis.

Fortunately, symptoms of cold urticaria tend to be self-limiting, with the acute symptoms resolving within a few hours after rewarming of the affected areas. For athletes who repeatedly suffer such symptoms, medical referral may be warranted. Treatment may include taking drugs, such as antihistamines, to control edema and itching. Athletes may also find certain types of outdoor clothing to be more effective in protecting the skin as well as limiting cold exposure (Madden & Fudge, 2018).

Cold urticaria Condition in which the skin reacts to exposure to cold with localized edema associated with severe itching.

Edema Abnormal accumulation of fluid in the interstitial tissue; disruption of homeostatic fluid balance in the tissues.

Altitude-Related Conditions

At sea level, the atmospheric or barometric pressure, which is the pressure within the atmosphere of earth or the weight of air above a specified point, is 760 mm of mercury (mm Hg) or 14.7 pounds per square inch, and the concentration of oxygen at sea level is approximately 21%. Air pressure also varies depending on temperature, weather, and latitude. In general, as elevation increases, atmospheric pressure decreases because there is less overlying atmospheric mass, and there is a fall in partial pressure of oxygen, or less oxygen pushed from the lungs into the blood. Higher altitude with less air pressure translates to fewer oxygen molecules per breath, causing increased respirations at rest to acquire the oxygen needed to oxygenate the body while at high altitudes. Individuals can adjust to high altitudes through acclimatization (Levine et al., 2018).

To acclimatize to altitude, it is recommended to not ascend more than 1,000 to 1,600 feet (304–487 meters) per day and for every 3,000 feet (915 meters) of elevation gain, a rest day is needed. This means staying overnight, perhaps for several days, at gradually increasing elevations to allow the body to adjust to the new pressure and make cellular changes (e.g., red blood cells). Individuals acclimatize at different rates. When acclimatizing for the first time to high elevation, it is recommended to be cautious. Regardless of experience at high elevations, it is very helpful to stay hydrated since higher elevations also coincide with dryer climates and increased respirations will contribute to hypohydration. As mentioned previously, hydration status can be evaluated by urine color and volume output. It is also helpful to participate in light activity during the day as opposed to napping while acclimatizing since the respiration rate is lower during sleep. It is also recommended to eat a high-carbohydrate diet.

If there is no acclimatization period, altitude illnesses can result. A typical scenario for developing altitude illness is a person from Florida flying into Denver (approximately 5,000 feet or 1,524 meters), then renting a car to drive up to the trailhead at 8,000 feet (2,434 meters). The hike on the next day goes up to 10,500 feet (3,200 meters) and a severe headache, nausea, and weakness sets in. Or, a person from New York flies into Denver, drives to a ski resort (8,000 feet or 2,434 meters), and the next morning takes the ski lift up to 10,000+ feet only to have a headache and dizziness by lunch. Unfortunately, there are no specific characteristics, such as age, gender, fitness level, or ethnic group, that make a person more susceptible to altitude sickness. However, those who have certain conditions, such as sickle cell trait, asthma, COPD, and cardiovascular disease, need to be extremely cautious and conservative when ascending.

Several concepts related to using altitude as a training method have developed over the years. The consensus is to "live high and train low," meaning to live at higher altitudes so the body makes the physical adaptations (e.g., increased red blood cells) and to train at lower altitudes since intensity levels and other physical tasks cannot be performed to maximal effort at higher altitudes. This concept is also applicable to hikers and climbers such that "climb high and sleep low" means to sleep at a lower elevation after climbing high during the day (CDC, 2019).

Altitude Sickness or Acute Mountain Sickness

At approximately 5,000 feet (1,500 m) in elevation, individuals may notice more breathlessness than normal, especially if exercising. At approximately 8,000 feet (2,438 m), most individuals remain well but will experience breathlessness with exercise and physical daily tasks. After a few hours at or over this elevation, symptoms of **altitude sickness** or **acute mountain sickness** may begin, especially for those who are not acclimatized and/or ascended over 1,600 feet (500 m) per day. Symptoms include headache, nausea, vomiting, dizziness, shortness of breath, loss of appetite, general malaise, and poor sleep and depend on the elevation, rate of ascent, and individual characteristics. Symptoms may appear within the first 12 to 24 hours after arrival at altitude, and be more pronounced in the evening, typically decreasing by day 3 at altitude. It is very important that others know if symptoms are being experienced and if symptoms are not relieved by hydration, acclimatization, or over-the-counter medications. Lowering elevation by 1,000 feet (304 meters) for 24 hours can significantly improve symptoms, and the person should remain there until symptoms have subsided (approximately 3 days). Passing a sobriety-like test (e.g., walking heel to toe in a straight line) can help determine if a person is able to ascend. Likewise, it is beneficial to lower elevation before a person cannot walk on their own, which would indicate a more severe form of altitude illness, such as high-altitude pulmonary edema or cerebral edema (Altitude Physiology Expeditions, n.d.; CDC, 2019).

High Altitude Pulmonary Edema

High altitude pulmonary edema (HAPE) occurs when lack of oxygen causes fluid to leak into the lungs. It occurs less frequently than altitude mountain sickness because symptoms are usually treated effectively before this severe condition occurs. As increased fluid accumulates in the lungs, less oxygen is delivered to the tissues of the body, causing shortness of breath at rest, tight chest, fatigue, feeling of suffocation at night, weakness, a productive cough, and eventually cyanosis (e.g., blue skin appearance), impaired cerebral function, and death if not treated immediately. It is easy to confuse this condition with a chest infection due to the productive cough and other symptoms similar to a chest infection. One way to monitor the body at altitude is to check recovery time (e.g., heart rate and breathing rate) after exertion. Recovery time should not be much greater than normal, and this is a sign to proceed with great caution. As mentioned, immediate life-saving treatment is to quickly descend by 2,000–4,000 feet (610–1,220 m) and be transported to a medical facility (Altitude Physiology Expeditions, n.d.; CDC, 2019; Levine et al., 2018).

High Altitude Cerebral Edema

High altitude cerebral edema (HACE), or increased fluid and swelling of the brain due to high altitude, causes headache, loss of coordination, weakness, and a decreased level of consciousness (e.g., disorientation,

---

Altitude sickness Symptoms such as headache, nausea, vomiting, dizziness, and shortness of breath that come on within 24 hours of ascending into altitude; also called acute mountain sickness.

Acute mountain sickness Symptoms such as headache, nausea, vomiting, dizziness, and shortness of breath that come on within 24 hours of ascending into altitude; also called altitude sickness.

High altitude pulmonary edema (HAPE) Fluid and swelling accumulation in the lung due to high altitude exposure.

High altitude cerebral edema (HACE) Fluid and swelling accumulation in the brain due to high altitude exposure.

abnormal behavior, memory loss). Similar to HAPE, it can lead to death if not treated immediately by rapidly descending 2,000–4,000 feet (610–1,220 m) and seeking medical treatment (Altitude Physiology Expeditions, n.d.; CDC, 2019; Levine et al., 2018).

Treatment and Prevention of Altitude Illnesses

The greater and faster the ascent into higher altitude, the higher the risk of altitude illnesses. If signs and symptoms of altitude illness are apparent, do not ascend higher until symptoms decrease. If signs and symptoms increase, descend to lower altitude quickly. Those who experienced altitude illnesses in the past are likely to develop altitude illnesses in the future. It is better to prevent altitude illnesses via acclimatization and hydration than treat it by descending to lower elevation quickly and seeking medical assistance (Figure 18.5).

If you have to ascend quickly and are not acclimatized, there is a prescription drug called Diamox that may decrease the symptoms of altitude illness but will not cure altitude illness. It is advised to start taking Diamox 24 hours before ascending and continuing for 5 days while at altitude. Diamox is classified as a sulfa drug, and those allergic to sulfa should not take it. Interestingly, Diamox can cause a reaction in individuals who are not allergic to sulfa, so for this reason, a medical consult should be attained. Again, proper acclimatization is the best prevention method.

Specialized altitude equipment can assist with altering air pressure and supplying the body with oxygen. A Gamow bag can mimic or create a certain atmosphere of a lower elevation in approximately 10 minutes. Commonly found on most major high altitude excursions, this type of equipment is helpful for immediate treatment while rapidly descending. Other devices used to help with oxygen at altitude are supplemental portable oxygen masks and portable concentrators, recreational oxygen (e.g., canned oxygen), and oxygen "bars"; however, not all are effective. Masks increase the percentage of oxygen in the inspired air and are typically used for high altitude climbing such as Mount Everest. Ideally, supplemental oxygen is most helpful at altitude when sleeping since respiration rates are lower. Recreational oxygen and oxygen bars found in ski resorts may help with breathlessness, energy levels, and reduced headache; however, this effect is only temporary while using the devices and may mask the symptoms of altitude illness or another problem (Altitude Physiology Expeditions, n.d.; CDC, 2019; Levine et al., 2018).

Lightning

Lightning strikes Earth more than 8 million times per day and is the second highest storm related fatality after flooding. Of the people struck by lightning, 10% die, with 90% surviving, usually with long-term devastating effects (Korey Stringer Institute, n.d.d; Walsh, 2013). Approximately 15–30% of lightning strikes occur during summer months, when outdoor activity is most common, and, unfortunately, these fatal strikes often happen when safety options are nearby. Lightning can strike directly (e.g., direct contact) or indirectly through contact (e.g., touching an object that has been struck), side flash (e.g., lightning bounces off a tree), ground current (e.g., lightning passes through ground to person), or through a streamer (e.g., burst of energy coming from objects near the ground) (CDC, 2020).

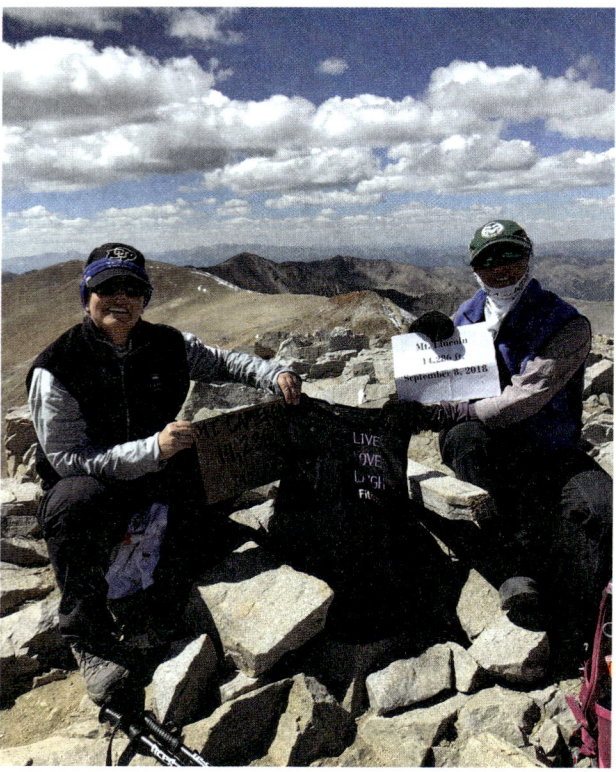

Figure 18.5 Your authors hiked four 14,000-foot mountains in Colorado after acclimatizing to altitude.
Courtesy of Cindy Trowbridge.

Lightning Safety

Lightning can strike without rain and when skies are blue. First and foremost, a lightning policy that is venue specific should be included in the emergency action plan. This policy should include specific criteria for monitoring for lightning (e.g., specific weather watcher, special weather apps, and local weather service phone numbers) and procedures for activity suspension and resumption of activity. There should be signs posted nearby regarding the location of lightning-safe facilities in the event of an evacuation and a plan and announcement system for evacuating athletes and large numbers of spectators. Lastly, educate athletes, parents, coaches, administration, and referees about the dangers of lightning and the appropriate actions to keep everyone safe. Signage stating, "If thunder roars, go indoors," should be posted around the complex and hopefully will serve as a friendly reminder (Walsh, 2013).

More specifically, if a storm is predicted, lightning monitoring should be performed. If the local weather service issues a warning, it is recommended to suspend activity even if lightning or thunder is not observed. After the first sight of lightning or sound of thunder, activity should be suspended, and everyone should seek appropriate shelter until the weather clears. A lightning-safe shelter is a fully enclosed building with plumbing and electrical wires. Tents, pavilions, dugouts, and trees are not lightning-safe options. When indoors, avoid standing close to showers, sinks, appliances, electronics, corded phones, and concrete areas. If a fully enclosed building is not available, vehicles can be used with windows fully closed and doors shut (Korey Stringer Institute, n.d.d). Usually activity can resume if 30 minutes have passed after the last sight of lightning and sound of thunder. This means that after each sight of lightning or sound of thunder the 30-minute clock restarts (Walsh, 2013).

If you find yourself in an open area without shelter, crouch down into a ball-like position with your hands over your ears with minimal contact with the ground, because lightning can travel through the ground over 100 feet away. In the event you have several people in your group, separate from each other to reduce the number of injuries caused by ground transfer. If you are in the mountains, avoid ridges, summits, single trees, power lines, and metal objects. Staying near trees in lower elevations and not continuing to hike/climb for at least 30 minutes after a storm is recommended (CDC, 2020). It is important to educate the community and adminstration about lightning safety in order to assist with compliance to current recommendations (Scarneo-Miller et al., 2021).

Lightning Treatment

If you suspect someone has been struck by lightning, make sure the scene is safe before you assist and call emergency medical services. While no charge will be held in the victim, there may be remaining charges in the area surrounding the victim. After a lightning strike, victims may have severe burns, fractures, shock, or other trauma. Victims may also have a loss of consciousness, blindness, deafness, confusion, and paresthesia. Items to have in preparation of a lightning strike are blankets, a burn treatment kit, splints, and an AED (Korey Stringer Institute, n.d.d).

In terms of return to activity after a lightning strike, the individual needs to be cleared by a medical professional. Due to potential neurological complications, posttraumatic stress disorder, or mental difficulties as a result of the lightning strike, it is important that an individualized, gradual return to activity plan be implemented (Korey Stringer Institute, n.d.d).

Review Questions

1. Describe the normal range for body core temperature.
2. Explain how the body rids itself of excess heat.
3. What is the relationship between relative humidity and the process of evaporation?
4. True or false? Heat exhaustion is potentially more serious than exertional heatstroke is.
5. True or false? EAMCs may be managed with rest, consumption of fluids, and stretching of the affected muscles.
6. What is the recommended fluid intake during physical activity?
7. A fluid loss of what percentage can impair physical performance?

8. At what core temperature does hypothermia begin?

9. At what body temperature does the shivering response cease?

10. What is the relationship between hypothermia and cardiac function?

11. Describe the signs and symptoms of cold urticaria.

12. What is the relationship between hyperthermia and cardiovascular function?

13. What is the best method to acclimatize to altitude?

14. What is the treatment for someone experiencing moderate to severe altitude sickness?

15. How long must activity wait to resume after observance of lightning or thunder?

References

Adams, W. E., Stearns, R. L., Casa, D. J. (2020). Exertional heat stroke. In W. M. Adams & J. F. Jardine (Eds.), *Exertional heat illness: A clinical and evidence-based guide* (pp. 59–80). New York, NY: Springer, Cham.

Adams, W. M., & Jardine, J. F. (2020). Overview of exertional heat illness. In W. M. Adams & J. F. Jardine (Eds.), *Exertional heat illness: A clinical and evidence-based guide* (pp. 1–16). New York, NY: Springer, Cham.

Armstrong, L. E. (2020). Heat exhaustion. In W. M. Adams & J. F. Jardine (Eds.), *Exertional heat illness: A clinical and evidence-based guide* (pp. 81–116). New York, NY: Springer, Cham.

Altitude Physiology Expeditions. (n.d.). Altitude sickness. Retrieved from http://www.altitude.org/altitude_sickness.php

Belval, L. N., & Morrissey, M. C. (2020). Physiological response to heat stress. In W. M. Adams & J. F. Jardine (Eds.), *Exertional heat illness: A clinical and evidence-based guide* (pp. 17–28). New York, NY: Springer, Cham.

Binkley, H. M., Beckett, J., Casa, D. J., Kleiner, D. M., & Plummer, P. E. (2002). National Athletic Trainers' Association position statement: Exertional heat illnesses. *Journal of Athletic Training, 37*(3), 329–343.

Cappaert, T. A., Stone, J. A., Castellani, J. W., Krause, B. A., Smith, D., & Stephens, B. A. (2008). National Athletic Trainers' Association position statement: Environmental cold injuries. *Journal of Athletic Training, 43*(6), 640–658.

Casa, D. J., & Csillan, D. (2009). Preseason heat-acclimatization guidelines for secondary school athletics. *Journal of Athletic Training, 44*(3), 332–333.

Casa, D. J., DeMartini, J. K., Bergeron, M. F., Csillan, D., Eichner, E. R., Lopez, R. M., . . . Yeargin, S. W. (2015). NATA position statement: Exertional heat illness. *Journal of Athletic Training, 50*(9), 986–1000.

Casa, D. J., Guskiewicz, K. M., Courson, R. W., Heck, J. F., Jimenez, C. C., McDermott, B. P., . . . Walsh, K. M. (2012). National Athletic Trainers' Association position statement: Preventing sudden death in sports. *Journal of Athletic Training, 47*(1), 96–118.

Centers for Disease Control and Prevention (CDC). (2010). Heat illness among high school athletes—United States, 2005–2009. *Morbidity and Mortality Weekly Report, 59*(32), 1009–1013.

Centers for Disease Control and Prevention (CDC). (2013). Frequently asked questions (FAQ) about lightning strikes. Retrieved from https://www.cdc.gov/disasters/lightning/faq.html

Centers for Disease Control and Prevention (CDC). (2019). Travel to high altitudes. Retrieved from https://wwwnc.cdc.gov/travel/page/travel-to-high-altitudes

Center for Disease Control and Prevention (CDC). (2020). Lightning: Lightning safety tips. Retrieved from https://www.cdc.gov/disasters/lightning/safetytips.html

Divine, J., Dailey, S., Burley, K. C. (2018). Exercise in the heat and heat illness. In C. C. Madden, M. Putukian, E. C. McCarty, & C. C. Young (Eds.), *Netter's sports medicine* (2nd ed., pp. 143–151). Philadelphia, PA: Elsevier.

Giersch, G. E. W., Belval, L. N., & Lopez, R. M. (2020). Minor heat illnesses. In W. M. Adams & J. F. Jardine (Eds.), *Exertional heat illness: A clinical and evidence-based guide* (pp. 137–148). New York, NY: Springer, Cham.

Hosokowa, Y., Adams, W. M., Belval, L. N., Vandermark, L. W., & Casa, D. J. (2017). Tarp-assisted cooling as a method of whole-body cooling in hyperthermic individuals. *Annals of Emergency Medicine, 69*(3), 347–352.

Korey Stringer Institute. (n.d.a). Exertional sickling. Retrieved from https://ksi.uconn.edu/emergency-conditions/exertional-sickling/

Korey Stringer Institute. (n.d.b). Heat exhaustion. Retrieved from https://ksi.uconn.edu/emergency-conditions/heat-illnesses/heat-exhaustion/

Korey Stringer Institute. (n.d.c). Wet bulb globe temperature monitoring. Retrieved from https://ksi.uconn.edu/prevention/wet-bulb-globe-temperature-monitoring/.

Korey Stringer Institute. (n.d.d). Lightning. Retrieved from https://ksi.uconn.edu/emergency-conditions/lightning/

Kucera, K. L., Klossner, D., Colgate, B. & Cantu, R. C. (2018). Annual Survey of Football Injury Research, 1931–2017. Retrieved from https://nccsir.unc.edu/files/2013/10/Annual-Football-2017-Fatalities-FINAL.pdf

Levine, B. D., Stray-Gundersen, J., & Chapman, R. F. (2018). High altitude training and competition. In C. C. Madden, M. Putukian, E. C. McCarty, & C. C. Young (Eds.), *Netter's sports medicine* (2nd ed., pp. 161–164). Philadelphia, PA: Elsevier.

Luhring, K. E., Butts, C. L., Smith, C. R., Bonacci, J. A., Ylanan, R. C., Ganio, M. S., & McDermott, B. P. (2016). Cooling effectiveness of a modified cold-water immersion method after exercise-induced hyperthermia. *Journal of Athletic Training, 51*(11), 946–951.

Madden, C. C., & Fudge, J. R. (2018). Exercise in the cold and cold injuries. In C. C. Madden, M. Putukian, E. C. McCarty, & C. C. Young (Eds.), *Netter's sports medicine* (2nd ed., pp. 152–160). Philadelphia, PA: Elsevier.

McDermott, B. P., Anderson, S. A., Armstrong, L. E., Casa, D. J., Cheuvront, S. N., Cooper, L., . . . Roberts, W. O. (2017). National Athletic Trainers' Association position statement: Fluid replacement for the physically active. *Journal of Athletic Training, 52*(9), 877–895.

Mueller, F. O., & Colgate, B. (2011). Annual survey of football injury research, 1931–2010. Retrieved from http://nccsir.unc.edu/files/2014/05/2010FBAnnual.pdf

National Athletic Trainers' Association (NATA). (n.d.a). Consensus statement: Sickle cell trait and the athlete. Retrieved from https://www.nata.org/sites/default/files/sicklecelltraitandtheathlete.pdf

Pryor, J. L., Periard, J. D., & Pryor, R. R. (2020). Predisposing factors for exertional heat illness. In W. M. Adams & J. F. Jardine (Eds.), *Exertional heat illness: A clinical and evidence-based guide* (pp. 29–58). New York, NY: Springer, Cham.

Roy, B. A. (2013). Exercise and fluid replacement: Brought to you by the American College of Sports Medicine www.acsm.org. *ACSM's Health & Fitness Journal, 17*(4), 3.

Scarneo-Miller, S. E., Flanagan, K. W., Belval, L. N., Register-Mihalik, J. K., Casa, D. J., & DiStefano, L. J. (2021). Adoption of lightning safety best-practices policies in the secondary school setting. *Journal of Athletic Training, 56*(5), 491–498.

Walsh, K. M., Cooper, M. A., Holle, R., Rakov, V. A., Roederll, W. P., & Ryan, M. (2013). National Athletic Trainers' Association position statement: Lightning safety for athletics and recreation. *Journal of Athletic Training, 48*(2), 258–270.

CHAPTER 19

General Medical Concerns for Athletes

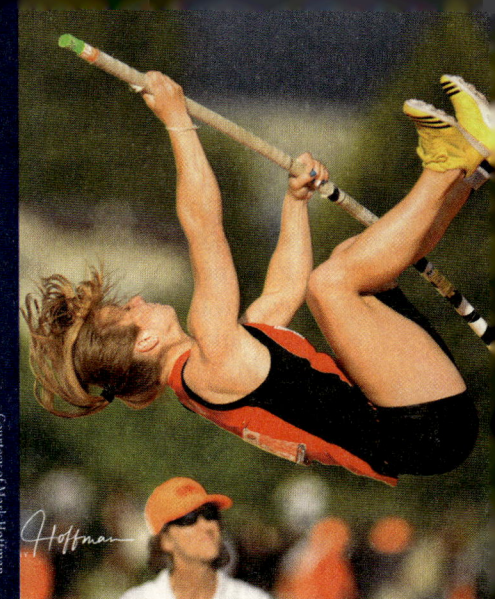

MAJOR CONCEPTS

Athletes, just like everyone else, occasionally become ill with infections that involve the respiratory and/or gastrointestinal systems. This chapter provides participation guidelines along with examples of typical signs and symptoms of the more common types of infections. Increases in cases of Lyme disease within the athletic community have spurred growing concern over the past few years. The chapter outlines early and late signs and symptoms of Lyme disease plus tips on how to avoid exposure. Next, the chapter examines several illnesses caused by viruses, including infectious mononucleosis and infectious strains of hepatitis A and B. All of these conditions pose a serious health risk to athletes; their signs and symptoms can assist the coach in identification. The chapter concludes with a discussion of the current thinking regarding sports participation by athletes suffering from exercise-induced asthma, sickle cell trait, rhabdomyolysis, diabetes, or epilepsy. The emphasis is on identification of the major signs and symptoms of each of these conditions and on management and special precautions related to sports participation.

Exercise and the Immune Response

Physical activity has always been a logical approach to improving health and well-being in addition to improving factors associated with noncommunicable diseases (e.g., cardiovascular disease, diabetes, depression), sports performance, and cognitive abilities. It does not have negative side effects if performed appropriately and is relatively inexpensive. Exercise also has a profound effect on the immune system. Regular exercise is likely to reduce risk of disease due to its anti-inflammatory and immune-boosting effects (Kramer, 2020).

Regular exercise of moderate to vigorous intensity has been shown to be beneficial for the immune system, but it has been suggested that demanding bouts of exercise above and beyond recommendations may be associated with increasing symptoms of upper respiratory tract infections. However, it is difficult to discern if the increased respiratory infection risk is due to exercise, inflammatory stimuli, infectious origin, environmental conditions, or other factors (Simpson et al., 2020). In fact, the decrease in immune cells hours after vigorous and prolonged exercise, which was once interpreted as immune system suppression, actually may represent an increased state of immune surveillance and regulation (Campbell & Turner, 2018; Simpson et al., 2020).

Athletes remain vulnerable to the same illnesses as the general population. Exercise is purported to have modulation effects on stress hormones, immune system dynamics, and possibly immune function; however, the nature of the interactions is very complex and research is ongoing in an effort to better identify the effects of exercise on the immune system (Campbell & Turner, 2018; Simpson et al., 2020; Walsh & Oliver, 2016).

The next discussion focuses on several infectious conditions affecting athletes that involve the respiratory, gastrointestinal, and hepatic systems.

Respiratory Infections

Respiratory infections can be categorized as **upper respiratory infections (URIs)**, which involve the nose, throat, ears and sinuses, tonsils, and associated lymph glands, or **lower respiratory infections (LRIs)**, which involve the lungs, bronchi, and larynx. The majority of URIs and LRIs in athletes are caused by viruses that invade the mucosa linings via inhalation of droplets.

Upper Respiratory Infections

URIs produce classic symptoms of the common cold, sinusitis, and/or pharyngitis. As a rule, these infections are mostly viral in nature and self-limited and last only a few days to a week. The **common cold** causes a stuffy and/or runny nose (i.e., **rhinitis**), sneezing, sore throat, mild fatigue, and perhaps a headache. Colds are usually benign and can be treated symptomatically with over-the-counter medications. Because the infection is most likely related to a virus, antibiotic therapy will have no effect on the organism causing the illness. Athletes with colds should be cautioned not to borrow drugs, such as antibiotics, from a friend or parent because taking a drug that is not specifically prescribed for the athlete could result in drug-related poisoning or allergic reactions.

Athletes with a URI can normally participate in competitive sports when symptoms are mild or there are no specific symptoms that place them at obvious risk. Several symptoms, including fever, **vertigo** (i.e., dizziness and loss of balance), and **myalgia** (i.e., muscle pain), are of particular concern and should restrict an athlete from practice or competition if they exist. Exercise should not occur while an athlete has a fever. Rest is the best medicine during a fever (core temperature >38°C or 100.4°F) because the combination of fever and exercise can increase the load on the heart and alter vascular tone, leading to dysrhythmia (Rice, 2008). Fever impairs concentration, strength, exercise capacity, and coordination (Harris, 2011) and exercising with a fever will also increase heat storage, resulting in decreased heat tolerance and dehydration, thereby increasing the risk of heat illness (Rice, 2008). A fever may also be a sign of **myocarditis** (i.e., inflammation of the heart muscle), which makes usual exercise very dangerous (Rice, 2008). Athletes involved in national or international events must be warned not to treat themselves with over-the-counter medications, such as decongestants or analgesics, because many of these drugs or ingredients within them have been banned by sports regulatory organizations.

A URI may affect any of the areas of the upper respiratory system. **Sinusitis**, or acute inflammation of one or more of the paranasal sinuses, is also a

---

Upper respiratory infection (URI) Infection involving the nose, throat, ears and sinuses, tonsils, and associated lymph glands.

Lower respiratory infection (LRI) Infection that involves the lungs, bronchi, and larynx.

Common cold A viral infectious disease of the upper respiratory tract that primarily affects the nose. The throat, sinuses, and larynx may also be affected.

Rhinitis Irritation and inflammation of the mucous membrane inside the nose. Common symptoms are a stuffy nose, runny nose, sneezing, and postnasal drip.

Vertigo Type of dizziness that causes a perception of motion and includes a loss of balance.

Myalgia General muscle pain.

Myocarditis Infection of the heart with inflammation and damage to the heart muscle.

Sinusitis Acute inflammation of one or more of the paranasal sinuses.

common occurrence, especially after a cold, because the infection moves to other areas of the respiratory tract. Sinusitis can be viral or bacterial in nature. The treatment for sinusitis is analgesics for the pain and/or headache, decongestants for nasal swelling, antibiotics for bacterial infections, and perhaps irrigation for symptom relief.

Pharyngitis, or inflammation of the pharynx or throat, is also possible once an infection is present. Pharyngitis usually occurs from viruses, but it can be bacterial in nature as well. Individuals experience sore, scratchy throats; fever; and headaches. It is usually treated symptomatically with over-the-counter medications. If it is determined to be a bacterial infection, then antibiotics are prescribed.

Lastly, the ears can be infected during a URI. Most often, **otitis media** (i.e., inner ear infection) occurs during or after a common cold. These infections are viral or bacterial and cause ear pain, headache, fever, and temporary hearing loss. They are treated with analgesics for the pain, antibiotics if bacteria are suspected to be the cause of the infection, or surgery (i.e., tubes placed in ear canal) for chronic inner ear infections in children. If an athlete has an ear infection, then the vestibular system is often affected, and vertigo may result. Whenever vertigo occurs, whether due to ear infection or illness, balance is affected, which increases the risk for falls and fractures (Liao et al., 2015), thus making it unwise to allow participation in a sport, especially one demanding a high degree of balance, such as figure skating, gymnastics, or diving. Another type of ear infection, usually not related to URIs, is called **otitis externa** (i.e., external auditory canal infection). Otitis externa, or nicknamed swimmer's ear, may happen due to extended periods of time in the swimming pool or frequent ear cleaning. These infections cause pain, itching, and temporary hearing loss and are usually treated with topical antibiotics or acetic acid solutions.

Infections of the upper respiratory system that persist for more than 1 week might be related to bacterial infections, such as streptococci. There are no key symptoms that determine the difference between a viral and a bacterial infection, but symptoms of bacterial infections are generally more pronounced, with visible lesions in the back of the throat (i.e., strep throat), severe sore throat, extended fever and chills, general discomfort and malaise, and swollen lymph glands in the neck and lower jaw. Medical evaluation is essential; it usually includes a physical assessment; throat culture, to identify the infectious agent; and, in some cases, a prescription for an antibiotic medication. Proper diagnosis is necessary before treatment. Taking antibiotics without a firm diagnosis of a bacterial infection is dangerous and may lower a person's resistance to future infections. Exercising during a URI may cause bronchial hyperactivity and aggravate current symptoms further. URIs are common and do take time to resolve, so athletes demonstrating any symptoms should not be allowed to participate, especially in team sports in which they are in close contact with other athletes because such infections are routinely contagious. The athlete should be advised to rest and drink plenty of nonalcoholic fluids until the major symptoms begin to subside. Return to activity can usually occur within a few days when signs and symptoms reduce and there is no fever or significant fatigue. Return to activity should be based on the individual's symptoms, medical history, and physical exam and worked out among the physician, parent, coach, and care provider.

Lower Respiratory Infections

LRIs can impair performance for periods ranging up to several weeks. Normally related to a viral infection of the bronchi, the symptoms include cough, fever, and **malaise** (i.e., general discomfort). Obviously, athletes involved in aerobic sports, such as running, swimming, cycling, or cross-country skiing, will be directly and negatively affected by such an infection. As is the case with URIs, athletes with LRIs should be isolated from their peers and referred to a physician for complete evaluation and treatment. Such cases are normally treated with rest and medication designed to control coughing and relieve the associated aches and pains. More serious types of infections in the lower respiratory system include bacterial

---

Pharyngitis Inflammation of the pharynx or throat.

Otitis media Inner ear infection.

Otitis externa External auditory canal infection.

Malaise Discomfort and uneasiness caused by an illness.

infections, such as **bronchitis** (i.e., inflammation of the bronchial tree) and **pneumonia** (i.e., inflammation of the lungs), the latter of which can sometimes be life threatening. Symptoms of bronchitis include fever, coughing, chest pain, general feelings of illness, and perhaps headache and nausea. In addition, the cough may yield **sputum** (i.e., bronchial secretions) that appears greenish-yellow in color. The symptoms of pneumonia are more profound and also include coughing up of discolored sputum. A physician must make a diagnosis of either bronchitis or pneumonia, neither of which is determined by the color of the sputum. Treatment includes rest; medication (i.e., antibiotics); and, in severe cases, hospitalization. Decisions regarding when to return to activity should be made on the advice of the attending physician and by the athlete (or parents in the case of a minor). Clearly, there should be no residual signs and symptoms, especially myalgia or malaise, because the stress of exercise might lead to unnecessary musculoskeletal injury.

Gastrointestinal Infections

Illnesses of the **gastrointestinal (GI) system** are typically related to viral, bacterial, or protozoan infections. Known collectively as **gastroenteritis** (i.e., inflammation of the stomach and intestines), these infections produce similar symptoms, which include abdominal cramping, nausea (often associated with vomiting), fever and chills, and diarrhea. When such symptoms occur, the best approach is to remove the athlete from participation, monitor the symptoms for 24 hours, and then make a decision regarding medical referral. Any athlete complaining of severe diarrhea or bloody stools should be referred immediately for a complete medical evaluation. Gastroenteritis, usually self-limiting within 1 to 3 days, is a generic problem that can be the result of a number of causes, including pathogens, such as viruses, bacteria, or protozoa. In addition, such symptoms can be the result of food allergies, food poisoning, and even psychological stress. The athlete should be encouraged to drink plenty of nonalcoholic fluid because dehydration can occur when vomiting and/or diarrhea persist. If symptoms continue for more than a few days, the athlete should consult a physician. Related conditions that may be more serious are caused by bacteria (e.g., typhoid fever) and protozoa (e.g., giardiasis). As a rule, an athlete with GI symptoms that include severe (i.e., explosive or bloody) diarrhea, fever, extreme dehydration, and chills should be referred to a physician for a complete physical evaluation and diagnosis.

A large and diverse number of problems of the gastrointestinal system can produce the symptoms of gastroenteritis. Evidence suggests that, in some athletes, the physical and psychological stress of training and competition may be the causative mechanism behind GI issues. Physiologically, the heat from exercise intensity may cause damage to the intestinal mucosa because blood is pooled away from the intestines to other organs and muscles during exercise. Exercise may also modify gut microbial molecules, which help maintain a healthy gut. Additionally, stress hormones may be produced as a result of exercise, which also leads to an inflammatory response. Not only can physical exercise induce GI disturbances, but the psychological stress of heavy physical demands of training, the pressure to perform, and fatigue influencing one's mood can alter hormones, which may also affect the GI system (Clark & Mach, 2016). Beyond these stressors, athletes' nutritional choices play a crucial role in GI comfort or discomfort. Common GI-related problems include **gastritis** (i.e., inflammation of the stomach lining), **colitis** (i.e., inflammation of the colon), and **colic** (i.e., intra-abdominal pain). As with any recurrent and persistent clinical symptoms, referral to a physician is the prudent choice of action.

Bronchitis Inflammation of the bronchial tree.

Pneumonia Inflammation of the lungs.

Sputum Bronchial secretions.

Gastrointestinal (GI) system The organ system that takes in food, digests it to extract and absorb energy and nutrients, and expels the remaining waste as feces. The mouth, esophagus, stomach, and intestines are part of this organ system.

Gastroenteritis Inflammation of the stomach and intestines.

Gastritis Inflammation of the stomach lining.

Colitis Inflammation of the colon.

Colic Intra-abdominal pain.

Other Infectious Diseases

Several other types of infections can affect athletes, all of which present special problems regarding identification, management, and prevention. Lyme disease has increased in the athletic population but is rarely a life-threatening illness. However, Lyme disease can severely limit an athlete's ability to participate in sports due to symptoms (Centers for Disease Control and Prevention [CDC], n.d.f). Other infectious diseases include infectious mononucleosis and hepatitis A virus (HAV) and hepatitis B virus (HBV), both of which are extremely dangerous conditions.

Lyme Disease

Lyme disease is a bacterial (i.e., *Borrelia burgdorferi*) infection transmitted by an infected blacklegged tick (sometimes called a deer tick in the Midwest or a bear tick in the western United States), which is widespread throughout the United States. Lyme disease derives its name from one of the towns in which the first cases were identified in the 1970s: Lyme, Connecticut (Aronowitz, 1991). Since that time, Lyme disease has surpassed Rocky Mountain spotted fever as the most prevalent tick-borne infectious disease in the United States. In fact, Lyme disease cases have risen in the last several years according to the CDC (CDC, n.d.h), with the highest incidence occurring in the northeastern United States and in Wisconsin and Minnesota (CDC, n.d.g).

The disease is transmitted via a bite from an infected tick. Once a person is infected, initial symptoms may appear as early as 3 days later; however, symptoms may be absent for as long as 1 month or more after the bite. Regardless of the time period, the earliest symptom may be the development of a circular area of reddened skin at the site of the bite, which is technically known as erythema chronicum migrans (ECM; Figure 19.1) and signifies the first stage of the infection. ECM will continue to develop for days and can vary in size from a few inches to a foot or more. Additional symptoms include chills, fever, headache, general aches and pains (i.e., malaise), and general fatigue. Diagnosis is based on symptoms in combination with exposure to infected ticks, such as outdoor activity in an area known to have cases of Lyme disease and infected ticks, such as the northeast United States. Most cases of Lyme disease that are caught early can be treated successfully with a few weeks of antibiotics; however, in prolonged cases, drug therapy has been ineffective (CDC, 2017). Symptoms of untreated Lyme disease can vary but include fever, rash, facial paralysis, swollen lymph nodes, and arthritis up to 30 days after a bite. For months after a bite, severe headaches, neck stiffness, additional rashes, arthritis, facial palsy, heart palpitations, dizziness, nerve pain, brain swelling, and pain in tendons, joints, and bones can occur. In the majority of untreated cases, arthritis will develop, with the knee being the most commonly affected joint. Symptoms may appear together or separately and can be accompanied by a repeated appearance of ECM. It is important to note that untreated Lyme disease can persist for years in the body and produce symptoms of a variety of disorders, thereby making recognition and diagnosis difficult (CDC, 2017).

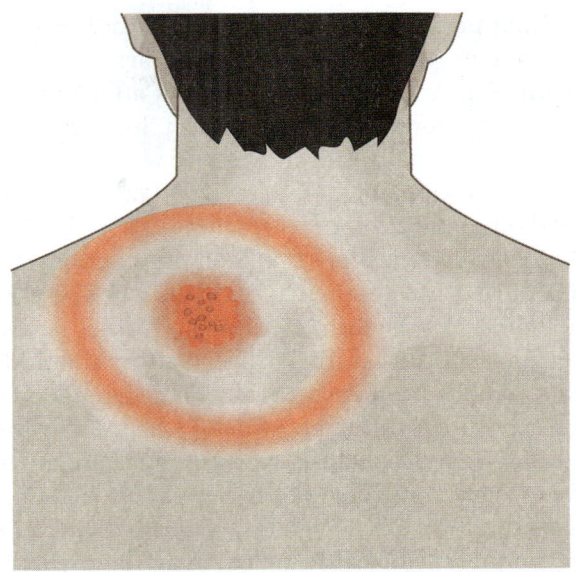

Figure 19.1 Erythema migrans rash caused by Lyme disease.

The best approach is prevention of the disease by avoiding an infectious tick bite. Tick bites can be prevented by walking in the center of trails and avoiding woody and high grassy areas; applying repellants that contain DEET or other chemicals registered with the Environmental Protection Agency; wearing

> **Lyme disease** Bites from infected blacklegged ticks that transfer bacteria to humans, resulting in a skin rash and other symptoms.

clothing pretreated with **permethrin**; and wearing long sleeves, pants, and hats during warmer months (April–September). Within 2 hours after outdoor activity, shower or bathe, and inspect the entire body for ticks, especially ears and hair, as well as inspecting gear, equipment, and pets. Dry clothing can be dried on high heat for 10 minutes to kill ticks.

Sports organizations that promote outdoor activities during the summer months in wooded areas should check with local medical authorities regarding reports of tick activity. Every effort should be made to hold events in areas where the likelihood of tick exposure is minimal. Athletes who are involved in outdoor sports held in wooded areas are at risk of exposure to infected ticks; they should be taught how to perform a thorough inspection of their bodies for the presence of a tick. They may require assistance when inspecting hard-to-see areas, such as the hairline at the back of the neck, behind the ears, and the posterior torso.

Ticks are very small, about the size of a pinhead in the nymph stage, which is the time they are most able to transmit the disease. If a tick is found, it should be removed immediately because it has been found that length of attachment plays a role in likelihood of infection. **Time Out 19.1** outlines recommended procedures for removal of a tick. To dispose of a live tick, submerge it in alcohol, place it in a sealed bag or container, wrap it in tape, or flush it down the toilet. While some areas offer tick testing, it is often not useful because, even if the tick contained the disease, it does not mean that the infection has been transmitted. And, if you are infected, you should not wait until tick testing is completed before starting treatment. Lastly, it should also be noted that ticks in the United States carry pathogens that cause various human diseases, such as Colorado tick fever, Heartland virus, Rocky Mountain spotted fever, and southern tick-associated rash illness (CDC, 2018a; STARI).

Permethrin Broad-spectrum insecticide that can be infused in clothes to prevent insects from approaching and biting.

Infectious mononucleosis Viral infection characterized by general fatigue and enlargement of organs, such as the spleen.

Infectious Mononucleosis

Infectious mononucleosis (IM), also called "mono," is extremely common in the United States among young people and is caused by the Epstein-Barr virus, which

TIME OUT 19.1

Guidelines for Tick Removal

Do not use the following methods of tick removal:

- Petroleum jelly
- Fingernail polish
- Rubbing alcohol
- A hot match

Pull the tick off, employing the following methods:

1. Use tweezers or, if you have to, your fingers; protect your skin by using a paper towel or disposable tissue. Although few people ever encounter ticks infected with a disease, the person removing the tick may become infected by germs entering through breaks in the skin.
2. Grasp the tick as close to the skin surface as possible, and pull away from the skin with a steady pressure or lift the tick slightly upward and pull parallel to the skin until the tick detaches. Do not twist or jerk the tick because doing so may result in incomplete removal.
3. Wash the bite site and your hands well with soap and water. Apply alcohol or iodine to further disinfect the area. Then, apply a cold pack to reduce pain. Calamine lotion might aid in relieving any itching. Keep the area clean.

is in the family of viruses responsible for herpes infections. About 25% of teenagers and young adults will develop mono in the United States, even though most people are infected with Epstein-Barr virus at some point in their lives (Medline Plus, 2021). The initial symptoms of the infection are similar to those of the common cold—sore throat, fever, chills, and enlarged lymph nodes in the neck and jaw region. Infected persons often complain of extreme fatigue as well and may first notice the problem when they find it difficult to participate in sports. As the disease progresses, other organs may become involved, including the liver and spleen.

Transmission of the disease usually occurs via contact with discharge from an infected person's mouth (i.e., airway). Once exposed, the incubation period is variable; however, it usually ranges from 2–6 weeks. Once the illness develops, its duration ranges from 5–15 days, with recovery beginning thereafter. Treatment is essentially symptom control once the diagnosis is made by a physician; the emphasis is on rest and pain control with some type of analgesic drug. Fortunately, infectious mononucleosis is usually a self-limited disease with no long-term effects.

A major concern with infectious mononucleosis, however, is its effect on the spleen. It has been well documented that acute cases may result in enlargement of the spleen (i.e., splenomegaly); in rare cases the spleen will rupture. When the spleen experiences an episode of blunt trauma, as is common in many contact sports, splenomegaly predisposes this organ to rupture. Therefore, the attending physician is faced with the dilemma of determining when it is safe for an athlete to return to participation after recovering from infectious mononucleosis. It has been documented that most spleen ruptures occur within 4 weeks of the illness but have occurred up to 8 weeks after the onset of symptoms; consequently, athletes should not be allowed to participate during this period (Bartlett et al., 2016). The coach, athlete, and parents must rely on the attending physician regarding the best time to resume participation.

Prevention of the spread of infectious mononucleosis is difficult when dealing with athletes involved in team sports in which they are in close contact with one another on a daily basis. Athletes should know that the major mode of transmission of this disease involves coming into contact with an infected person's saliva. Preventive steps include advising athletes not to share water bottles or any other beverage containers and not to engage in kissing with potentially infected individuals. As a general precaution, athletes should not share towels and jerseys because such items may be contaminated with respiratory discharge containing the virus. In addition, athletes should be taught the importance of reporting any symptoms of illness to the coach so that he or she can decide a given athlete's participation status.

Hepatitis Infection

Hepatitis infection, either HAV or HBV, is serious, although HBV, or serum hepatitis, is considered to be the more serious and potentially life-threatening variety. HAV is transmitted via feces and is a serious problem among food handlers who fail to wash their hands after going to the bathroom. Serum hepatitis is transmitted through the blood and sexual fluids of an infected person; it is routinely transmitted among intravenous drug users or accidentally by healthcare workers working with contaminated needles. It is also possible that transmission of HBV may occur during blood transfusions from infected persons.

Once a person is infected, the incubation period for HAV is 15–50 days (CDC, n.d.d; San Francisco Department of Public Health, n.d.a); for HBV it is 45–180 days (CDC, n.d.e; San Francisco Department of Public Health, n.d.b). Symptoms of HAV and HBV infection vary, but symptoms of both strains include nausea, abdominal pain, vomiting, fever, and malaise. If untreated, both strains will begin to affect the liver, resulting in jaundice (i.e., yellowing of the skin). In severe cases, this vital organ may be severely damaged, leading in some cases to death. Treatment for either form of hepatitis infection is limited; thus, prevention is essential. To prevent HBV infection, all athletes should receive hepatitis B vaccinations before participation, any skin lesions should be covered properly, and athletic personnel should use universal precautions when handling blood or body fluids with visible blood (Rice, 2008). To prevent HAV infection, vaccination is available and should be used if teams are traveling to countries that might have low food-quality standards. In treating for HAV, it appears that immediate inoculation with immune serum globulin may confer passive immunity.

There is some evidence that inoculation with immune serum globulin may also be effective in treating cases of HBV exposure. Obviously, an athlete with HAV or HBV infection should be removed from participation and given prompt medical treatment. There is an apparent minimal risk of infection to others when sanitary procedures and universal precautions are followed; therefore, all sports may

Athletic Trainers SPEAK OUT

How do athletic trainers assist those physically active individuals with diabetes?

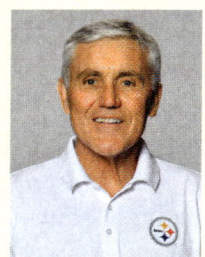

Courtesy of John A. Norwig, MEd, ATC.

As an athletic trainer working in a traditional setting, we are tasked with coordinating the health care of the athletes on our team along with the help of our team physician. On occasion we encounter athletes that are diabetic, and we are asked to oversee their management. The diabetic athlete presents challenges to an athletic trainer. These challenges require us to understand the condition, be prepared for an emergency, and communicate efficiently with all involved.

There are two types of diabetes: type 1 (insulin dependent) and type 2 (non-insulin dependent). Type 1 accounts for about ten percent of all diabetics, and many of these diabetics are diagnosed in their youth. Type 2 is more often diagnosed in adults. However, both type 1 and type 2 diabetes can affect both youth and adults.

In my setting, with a professional football team, I mostly deal with young adults. An athlete in our organization with a type 1 diabetes diagnosis has likely been managing their condition throughout the majority of their young lives, as they have been exposed to youth, high school, and college athletics along with a variety of medical providers. Regardless, my role as an athletic trainer is to assist the athlete in consistently maintaining blood glucose levels in normal or near normal range without provoking undue hypoglycemia (low blood sugar) or hyperglycemia (high blood sugar) conditions.

After a preparticipation physical and in coordination with your team physician, it is important that you have a one-on-one conversation with the athlete so they understand that they will not be treated differently than their teammates; however, you both have responsibilities. The athlete has the responsibility to monitor their blood glucose levels throughout the day and the athlete must follow the diabetic management plan that has been devised by their endocrinologist or physician. But most importantly, the athlete needs to have an open line of communication with you, the athletic trainer. As athletic trainers, it is our responsibility to understand the individual diabetic management plans and how we can assist the athlete in maintaining blood glucose levels. Critical roles include prevention, recognition, and immediate care of hypoglycemia and hyperglycemia, including effective blood glucose and insulin dose monitoring, pre- and post-exercise nutrition, hydration plans, and preparation for emergency management. We also must recognize how the intensity of exercise and the varying conditions of play may effect blood glucose levels. Therefore, we must communicate with the athlete and the other members of the healthcare team to be prepared for changing conditions.

Athletic trainers must be aware of the medications that all athletes under their care are using, but it is extremely important with the diabetic athlete. It is important that blood glucose monitoring equipment and emergency sources of glucose are accessible in both the athletic training facility and on the sidelines in medical kits. Should an emergency situation occur while the athlete is under your care, whether it be at home or on the road, an appropriate plan of action must be well thought out and ready to be implemented.

In addition to assisting our athletes with the management of their diabetes, we as athletic trainers must also be aware that soft tissue trauma affects diabetic athletes differently. Poor glucose control, a result of improper diabetes management, is associated with an increased risk of tissue infection and plays a role in slowing wound and fracture healing. Therefore, an athletic trainer needs to be sure that these athletes are meeting the medical needs of their injury rehabilitation as well as their diabetes.

—**John Norwig, MEd, ATC**

John Norwig is the Head Athletic Trainer for Pittsburgh Steelers NFL Football in Pittsburgh, Pennsylvania.

> **WHAT IF** ❓
>
> You are coaching track at a small college in the Midwest. Your best miler has been suffering from an upper respiratory infection for several days, and, worse, the regional qualifying meet is in 3 days. What would you recommend to this young athlete, and, further, what would you caution regarding over-the-counter medication?

be played as an athlete's state of health allows, but, because of the vulnerability of the liver during hepatitis infection, all decisions regarding return to participation for recovering athletes should be made by the attending physician (Rice, 2008).

Allergies

An **allergy** is an overreaction of the immune system to any substance that initiates an inflammatory response. These substances, called allergens, can be food, mold, medicine, latex, pets, plants, insects, chemicals in products, equipment, or clothes or environmentally related, such as pollution or pollen. Thus, allergens can be inhaled, as with pollen; ingested, as with food; injected, as with insect stings; or absorbed, as with poison ivy. Allergies are quite common because anyone can develop an allergy at any age; more than 50 million Americans currently suffer from allergies (CDC, n.d.b). Allergies are on the rise, and as many as 30% of adults and 40% of children in the United States are affected by allergies (Asthma and Allergy Foundation of America, n.d.a).

Reactions to the allergen can range from watery eyes, sneezing, coughing, rash, redness, itching, gastrointestinal issues, coughing, and swelling to being life threatening. **Anaphylaxis**, which is the most severe reaction, involves symptoms in multiple areas of the body, such as tingling in the palms, soles, and/or lips; dizziness; chest or throat tightness; or respiratory distress. If these symptoms are not treated immediately, they can lead to seizures, cardiac arrhythmia, and even death.

Unfortunately, a person does not always know he or she is allergic to a substance until a reaction occurs, so it is important to accurately diagnose symptoms with the help of a physician and specialized testing, such as skin tests, blood work, X-rays, challenge tests, and/or patch tests (Asthma and Allergy Foundation of America, n.d.b).

After a person discovers he or she is allergic to a certain allergen, he or she should notify medical personnel as well as notify and educate pertinent parties, such as family, coaches, friends, and teachers, of the allergy so that, in the event of a severe reaction, they are able to assist. More serious allergies, such as to bee stings or medications (e.g., penicillin), require strategies for alerting others, such as wearing medical identification bracelets or necklaces at all times, in the event of an emergency situation. Likewise, a person with allergies should input crucial information into his or her mobile devices, designated as ICE (i.e., in case of emergency). Individuals should also make every effort to prevent reactions by avoiding the allergen. There are several strategies for avoiding allergens; following are a few of them:

- Keep windows closed and live in an air-conditioned environment during peak pollen season.
- Eliminate dust mites, dander, and other allergens from the home.
- Avoid certain foods by reading labels and being aware of ingredients.
- Take medication to minimize symptoms or be immunized.

Treatment for an allergy involves avoiding the allergen and using medication as needed. For example, it is common to take antihistamines to control seasonal allergies or need an epinephrine injection to immediately treat an anaphylactic reaction. Persons with allergies should work closely with an allergist physician to appropriately manage the condition.

Asthma

Asthma is a condition in which airways become inflamed and the bronchi become hyperresponsive as a result of various allergens; indoor and outdoor

> **Allergy** An overreaction of the immune system to any substance that initiates an inflammatory response.
>
> **Anaphylaxis** A serious, sudden, and life-threatening allergic reaction that usually presents with throat or tongue swelling, shortness of breath, and other grave symptoms.

pollutants; respiratory infections; aspirin; nonsteroidal anti-inflammatory drugs (NSAIDs); irritants, such as smoke or pool chemicals, as well as cold temperatures; exercise; and other factors (Lalloo et al., 2021). This reaction leads to airway constriction and mucus production, which contributes to the main signs and symptoms of asthma:

- Coughing and tightness in the chest
- Shortness of breath and inability to catch one's breath
- Use of accessory muscles to breathe (abdominal muscles)
- Wheezing

Many of these symptoms will occur at night, in the early morning, during or after exercise, and in cold temperatures. For proper diagnosis, a person should have thorough medical and family histories taken as well as a lung function test performed if they experience more than one symptom of asthma. Vocal cord dysfunction is often confused with asthma due to their sharing similar symptoms; thus, proper diagnosis is essential before medications are prescribed.

Typically, asthma medications include controller medications or rescue medications. Controller medications are those that are used on a daily basis for long-term treatment to control and prevent symptoms from occurring, whereas the rescue medications rapidly treat acute bronchial constriction and the associated symptoms of coughing, wheezing, and chest tightness. A commonly prescribed medication for asthma is housed in a pressurized canister, called an **inhaler**, which propels the medication into the lungs when properly performed. Special education and attention should be focused upon proper inhaler administration because coordinating expelling the medication and inhaling can be difficult. Asthma medications, specifically the rescue inhaler, should be with the individual at all times to be prepared for an acute attack.

Ideally, an emergency plan should be in place once an athlete is known to have asthma. The plan should include checking the athlete's peak flow, administering medications, contacting emergency contacts, and rechecking peak flow after 15 minutes. If no improvement in symptoms occurs after 15 minutes, the athlete has difficulty walking or talking, and his or her lips and nails turn blue in color, emergency medical services (EMS) should be called. While waiting for EMS to arrive, additional quick-relief medicine should be administered.

One concern for athletes with aspirin or NSAID sensitivities or allergies is that they may also have nasal polyps and asthma, which is called triad syndrome. These individuals usually suffer a severe asthma attack when they take NSAIDs. Preventing an asthma attack from occurring can be accomplished by taking prescribed medication as directed, avoiding the allergen (e.g., limiting environmental exposures and eliminating NSAIDs), and exercising to improve respiratory health. In addition to care providers' knowing who the athletes are with asthma, having an emergency plan in place, and being familiar with how to treat someone suffering from an asthma attack, they should be familiar with the different types of asthma medications and how to properly administer them to assist individuals with asthma care (Lalloo et al., 2021). Certain medications for asthma are also on banned drug lists from several sport organizations, so it is important to have proper documentation and physician involvement in asthma cases.

Exercise-Induced Asthma

Asthma may be more difficult to diagnose in athletes than in nonathletes due to inconsistent symptoms, the environment, and the activity performed. **Exercise-induced asthma (EIA)**, or exercise-induced bronchoconstriction (EIB), the term preferred by the American College of Allergy, Asthma, and Immunology (ACAAI), has been defined as a constriction of the airway resulting from participation in strenuous exercise; the typical symptoms associated with asthma (i.e., wheezing, chest tightness, and dyspnea) are also associated with EIA/EIB. The highest incidence of EIA/EIB is found, not surprisingly,

---

Inhaler A pressurized canister in which a prescribed medication for asthma is housed. When used properly, the medication is propelled into the lungs.

Exercise-induced asthma (EIA) A constriction of the airway resulting from participation in exercise. Also known as exercise-induced bronchoconstriction (EIB), the term preferred by the American College of Allergy, Asthma, and Immunology.

among chronic asthmatics: About 90% will develop an attack during exercise (ACAAI, n.d.). Exercise can be the trigger for an asthma attack either during or after exercise in athletes at all levels of competition, regardless of whether the athletes have chronic asthma. However, it is more common in cold-weather sports, such as cross-country skiing, than in warm-weather sports. Although EIA/EIB can impair performance, if it is controlled, it can have no effect (Lalloo et al., 2021).

One pathophysiological theory of EIA/EIB is that, as ventilation increases, airways cool and dehydrate, which leads to bronchoconstriction. The typical scenario for the onset and symptoms of EIA/EIB begins with exercise of sufficient magnitude to be considered intense. Sports, such as basketball, soccer, and distance running, that entail significantly intense activity may elicit an attack (ACAAI, n.d.). Sports that occur in cold air (e.g., hockey, speed skating, and ice skating) or in outdoor arenas with high pollution levels are also likely to elicit attacks, whereas sports that occur in an indoor humid environment are less likely to do so. During exercise, the airway will typically dilate; however, on cessation of exercise, airway restriction or bronchoconstriction will occur within minutes.

In addition to asthma symptoms, the signs and symptoms of EIA/EIB include the following:

- Fatigue and stomachache (in children)
- Alarm and anxiousness in some athletes
- Sore throat
- Decreased exercise tolerance

To diagnose EIA/EIB, the athlete may experience symptoms 5–15 minutes after intense activity. Sometimes, an exercise or general challenge test, where pulmonary function is measured under various conditions, is needed to accurately diagnose EIA/EIB.

To manage EIA/EIB, the athlete generally uses a variety of drugs that prevent airway restriction or bronchoconstriction. Immediate treatment can include opening the airways by encouraging an open-chest position and providing for the inhalation of warm, humid air (e.g., mask and nose breathing or breathing through a scarf, muffler, or hand). Similar to asthma, there are effective drugs for EIA/EIB that can be administered with a rescue inhaler or taken orally (i.e., long-term anti-inflammatory drugs).

As mentioned before, the rescue inhaler is the most important tool in treatment and management of EIA/EIB. The most common drugs used are inhaled beta-2 agonists, which include albuterol, terbutaline sulfate, and salmeterol. The administration of choice is via a rescue inhaler, called a metered-dose inhaler, a device that is held approximately 1.5 inches from the mouth and releases an aerosol form of the drug, which is then inhaled slowly. The same asthma awareness as mentioned before also applies to EIA/EIB; coaches and care providers should be aware of athletes on their roster who suffer from EIA/EIB and use medication to control symptoms; have an asthma action plan for these athletes; and be able to help them retrieve and use medications, including rescue inhalers. If athletes have more than two episodes a week of EIA/EIB and need immediate use of a rescue inhaler to resolve symptoms, their EIA/EIB is not well controlled, and they should be directed to an appropriate healthcare professional. If the athlete is under 18 years of age, then parents or guardians should be notified (Lalloo et al., 2021).

It is important to note that certain drugs have been banned by some major sports-regulating agencies, including the National Collegiate Athletic Association (NCAA) and the International Olympic Committee (IOC). The NCAA continues to allow athletes with diagnosed EIA to self-treat with beta-2 agonists via a metered-dose inhaler. The IOC has prohibited the use of beta-2 agonists, with the exception of inhaled albuterol and salmeterol at certain dosages in a given time frame. In addition, the athlete must have submitted written notification from his or her personal physician to the IOC for therapeutic use exemptions (U.S. Anti-Doping Agency, 2018).

Highly susceptible individuals may be required to avoid certain activities, such as high-intensity and low-rest activities, or at least be cognizant of environmental conditions and avoid such activity on cold, dry, or polluted days. Sports involving short bursts of activity followed by periods of rest are excellent alternatives for high-risk athletes. For outdoor activities on cold, dry days, wearing a mask or scarf has been recommended. Warm-up exercises have also been found to help reduce the likelihood of an attack (ACAAI, n.d.). The National Athletic Trainers' Association (NATA) has published a comprehensive position statement on the management of asthma in athletes.

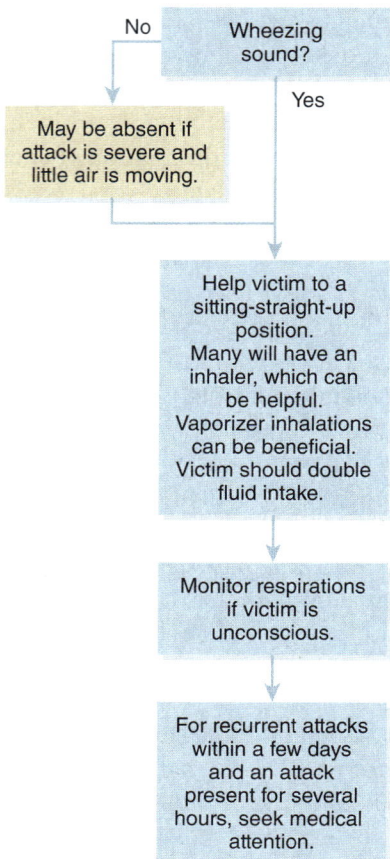

Figure 19.2 First aid procedures for asthma victims.

The appropriate steps in the management of an athlete suffering an acute attack of EIA are shown in Figure 19.2.

Exercise-Induced Bronchospasm

In the past, the terms EIA, exercise-induced bronchoconstriction (EIB), and exercise induced-bronchospasm were used interchangeably. It is hard to determine the incidence of exercise-induced bronchospasm given the confusing history between EIA and exercise-induced bronchoconstriction and exercise-induced bronchospasm. However, these are separate conditions, and the treatment may be different. As mentioned previously, the ACAAI suggests the use of the term exercise-induced bronchoconstriction instead of EIA. Others suggest that there is a distinction between bronchoconstriction and bronchospasm, which is inflammation versus spasm. With EIA/EIB, there is inflammation and the asthmatic signs and symptoms, such as dyspnea, wheezing, and chest tightness, when a person exercises. With exercise-induced bronchospasm, there is an acute bronchospastic component that may present with the same signs and symptoms as EIA; however, the symptoms occur with a specific exercise duration and intensity, and the person may not have asthma in general (Stack & Hakemi, 2011).

Exercise-induced bronchospasm is associated with a transient exercise-induced restriction in the airways during and after strenuous exercise. The bronchospasms may peak 5–10 minutes after stopping exercise and last an additional 20 or more minutes. Athletes may experience isolated exercise-induced bronchospasm or chronic asthma that is triggered by exercise. It is important to make this distinction, but it is often difficult when the signs and symptoms (i.e., coughing, wheezing, and chest tightness) of each one are similar. However, other symptoms of exercise-induced bronchospasm are fatigue and complaints of being out of shape. Symptoms may come on after 6–15 minutes of continuous exercise at 80% or more maximal workload, making endurance sports more likely to have individuals suffering from exercise-induced bronchospasm than other sports (Stack & Hakemi, 2011).

Proper diagnosis can be achieved with a thorough history, pulmonary function tests, and pulmonary stress tests (i.e., exercise challenges) as well as challenges involving hyperventilation and using substances such as saline and mannitol. Athletes with normal physical findings at rest are more likely to have exercise-induced bronchospasms. If a person is found to have isolated exercise-induced bronchospasms, the treatment is usually short-acting bronchodilators before exercise. Other athletes with chronic asthma who suffer an attack that is induced by exercise may need additional treatment, as discussed previously (Stack & Hakemi, 2011).

The Athlete With Sickle Cell Trait

Sickle cell trait (SCT) is not a disease, will not turn into sickle cell anemia, and is not a restriction in sports participation. SCT does not cause anemia, but it is possible to experience symptoms of sickle cell anemia under extreme physical exercise and/or environmental conditions, such as low oxygen levels. It is a genetic trait where the individual has inherited one gene for normal hemoglobin and one gene for sickle hemoglobin (Mitchell, 2018; O'Connor et al., 2021). SCT occurs in about 8% of the African American population and rarely in the Caucasian population. It is also common in individuals with ancestors from Africa, South or Central America, the Caribbean, Mediterranean countries, India, and Saudi Arabia (Mitchell, 2018; O'Connor et al., 2021). Currently, the NCAA mandates SCT testing of all Division I–III athletes because athletes may not be aware they have SCT, even though screening is normally done on all U.S.-born babies. SCT is not a deterrent to outstanding performances, and many athletes compete at the high school, collegiate, and professional levels without any complications. However, the reason that individuals with SCT need to be identified is that intense exercise, especially in hot and humid conditions and/or at high altitudes, can predispose an athlete to a sickling collapse, which can result in death. A sickling collapse can mimic heat illness, asthma, or overall exhaustion, but it must be treated differently, including immediate activation of emergency services by calling 911; if a healthcare provider is present, then supplemental oxygen should be delivered.

A sickling crisis occurs during intense exertion because red blood cells, which deliver oxygen, can change from their typical doughnut-shaped appearance to a "sickle," or a quarter-moon shape (Mitchell, 2018; O'Connor et al., 2021). The change in shape causes less efficiency in oxygen delivery; the sickle cells can also stick together and block blood flow to organs and tissues. Because there is less blood flow and oxygen delivery during a sickling crisis, an athlete can experience intense pain in the legs and low back, weakness, shortness of breath, and swelling of the extremities. Unfortunately, these signs and symptoms can also be seen in other conditions and may be missed initially. However, in athletes with SCT, these signs and symptoms can turn lethal due to the lack of blood flow to the kidneys and spleen (Mitchell, 2018; O'Connor et al., 2021). Gross hematuria (i.e., blood in the urine), splenic infarction (i.e., spleen lesions), and exertional rhabdomyolysis (i.e., skeletal muscle breakdown due to intense physical activity) are constant concerns for individuals with SCT. Splenic infarction may occur at any time but is more likely to occur at high altitudes. Exertional rhabdomyolysis occurs when a person exercises too intensely for his or her current fitness level, causing muscle damage that spills muscle contents into the bloodstream. It can be lethal for anyone, but those with SCT are at an increased risk, up to 200 times greater than a person without SCT (O'Connor et al., 2021). Dehydration, altitude, and uncontrolled asthma can predispose athletes with SCT to experience a crisis situation (Mitchell, 2018; O'Connor et al., 2021).

For coaches and physical educators, prevention and recognition are the primary goals if athletes with SCT are practicing and competing under their supervision. Several training techniques can be used to minimize the possibility of a sickling crisis, such as allowing athletes with SCT to set their own pace, participate in a slow and gradual progression of training during preseason conditioning programs, be excused from all-out exertion drills, and have longer rest periods. Athletes also need to maintain adequate hydration, control asthma symptoms, and stop any activity if signs and symptoms appear (Mitchell, 2018; O'Connor et al., 2021). The common signs and symptoms of a pending sickling crisis in an athlete include the following (Mitchell, 2018; O'Connor et al., 2021):

- Appears dazed or confused
- May experience sudden collapse, but remain conscious
- Appears weak and fatigued and is not keeping up with other team members
- Experiences shortness of breath
- Experiences significant muscle pain and/or cramping that is not easily resolved

A sickling crisis is a medical emergency and must be treated immediately via activation of EMS. Ideally, healthcare providers would be available who can deliver supplemental oxygen. However, when the athlete is conscious, cooling and rehydration are essential. While waiting for EMS, applying basic first aid techniques (e.g., monitoring vitals and preventing shock) is acceptable (Ko & Chiampas, 2021).

Exertional Rhabdomyolysis

When a person appropriately overloads his or her current exercises by gradually increasing weight, repetitions, or distance and experiences delayed muscle soreness the next few days, the body is physiologically adapting to the exercise, which means it is getting stronger. However, when a person exercises too intensely or overloads too much for his or her current fitness level (i.e., suddenly increases intensity or volume or both), skeletal muscle may break down, and its contents, such as creatine kinase, myoglobin, and electrolytes, will enter the bloodstream; myoglobin may also be present in the urine. The leaking of the muscle contents into the bloodstream is called **exertional rhabdomyolysis (ER)**; cases can range from mild to severe (Nye et al., 2021).

The person may experience muscle pain, extreme soreness, weakness, loss of range of motion, and swelling in addition to dark red or brown urine, nausea and vomiting, and malaise (Nye et al., 2021). Individuals who may be at increased risk for ER are those with metabolic disease, illness, sickle cell trait, or sickle cell anemia; those who have endured dehydration and environmental conditions, such as heat and altitude; and those who use medications, alcohol, or drugs.

Immediate medical attention should be obtained if extreme novel exercise has taken place and extreme muscle pain and weakness are present; other risks, such as heat and dehydration, are present; dark red or brown urine is present; or fever, confusion, malaise, or nausea is present. If ER is not recognized and treated quickly, it may lead to acute renal failure. The main method for diagnosing ER is evaluated levels of creatine kinase in the blood and myoglobin in the urine as well as taking a thorough history. However, there is no clear answer as to a minimum level of serum creatine kinase in determining whether someone is experiencing ER or predicting or preventing complications, such as renal pathology, because normal creatine kinase levels vary by gender, ethnicity, muscle fiber type, sport, and stage of training (Kim et al., 2016; Oh et al., 2015). Additionally, the rate of rise in creatine kinase values varies among ER cases, making diagnosis based on these levels more difficult. However, a valued estimate of serum creatine kinase levels of 5-10 times above the upper normal limit (5,000 to over 20,000 units per liter of creatine kinase) should be considered criteria for diagnosis in conjunction with the aforementioned symptoms. Therefore, ER should be treated individually according to symptoms and test results (Cleary et al., 2007; Kim et al., 2016; Manspeaker et al., 2016).

Exertional rhabdomyolysis (ER) Skeletal muscle breaks down, and its contents, such as creatine kinase, myoglobin, and electrolytes, enter the bloodstream; myoglobin may also be present in the urine.

In January 2011, after 3 weeks of winter break, 13 Iowa football players were hospitalized as a result of performing 100 back squats with 50% of the highest weight lifted at the last assessment. It was unclear to some players whether they were allowed water breaks (i.e., to take their hands off the bar). There was no time limit for performing all 100 squats, but players were timed. Because of being timed, the players viewed it as a competition. After a lengthy investigation, the determination was made that the hospitalizations were due to the sudden increase in exercise volume and not due to other potentially contributing factors, such as supplements, drug and alcohol use, or medications ("Report of the Special Presidential Committee," 2011). This is just one of several "rhabdo" clusters that have occurred in college athletics in recent years. It should serve as an important educational example to all athletes, coaches, and medical personnel about ER and how to avoid it.

To prevent ER, workouts should be carefully planned so they do not occur in extreme environmental conditions or, if that is not possible, to at least offer cooling devices, such as fans or misters; proper exercise progressions should be adhered to; and NATA's or other medical professions' guidelines for acclimation should be followed. Also, maintaining proper hydration and electrolytes is important as is wearing the proper attire for the exercise to ensure cooling. The following scenarios are red flags that can increase the risk of ER (Nye et al., 2021):

- Workouts that are not part of a periodized program or are new, especially after a break
- Workouts that are used for punishment or discipline or to build toughness
- Workouts that involve pushing the muscle to failure and often involve eccentric contractions to do so
- Workouts that increase the number of repetitions and decrease the amount of time to perform them or increase the amount of weight as a percentage of body weight
- Workouts that are intense and occur in hot environmental conditions and/or are restricted hydration
- Athletes who give it their all and group workouts that encourage competition
- If one athlete reports ER symptoms (there are likely others with symptoms)

Educating athletes about how this condition is caused, what to look for, how to treat it, and how to avoid it is key. Unfortunately, if ER does occur, there are few guidelines regarding return to activity. In general, the person should be free of muscle pain, fever, illness, and myoglobin in the urine, and serum creatine kinase should be at normal levels for at least 3 days before any activity resumes. It is suggested that a gradual progression of exercise should occur over an average period of 15 weeks before full return to activity. This time frame can be adjusted based on the individual's needs. The athlete should begin with general exercise and avoid eccentric muscle contractions in a well-hydrated state under normal environmental conditions. Aquatic exercise removes many eccentric contractions that would normally occur during land-based training and can be used in the initial stages of rehabilitation for ER. As eccentric contractions are progressed back into rehabilitation, the athletes should be monitored for symptoms of ER. Increases in resistance or weight can be implemented when exercises do not cause delayed muscle soreness the next day. Generally, exercise can be progressed if the athlete can perform the same workout for 2 consecutive days. Jumping and intense eccentric contractions should occur toward the end of the program. Again, going back to the pool to begin jumping exercises is ideal for reducing the load on the body. When jumping exercises can be moved to land, it is recommended that a recovery period of 48–72 hours occur before the next jumping exercise session. Monitoring the athlete's urine color (hydration status) during the rehabilitation time period is beneficial, especially as the athlete is gradually exposed to hot environmental conditions. Proper acclimatization protocols should be followed as well. It is important for this gradual progression of exercise and exposure to hot environments take place before an athlete returns to activity (Cleary et al., 2007). The consensus statement regarding return to strength and conditioning suggests following the 50/30/20/10 rules (volume reduction of 50%, etc.) for a 2–4 week period (Caterisano et al., 2019).

Athletes With Diabetes

The American Diabetes Association (ADA, n.d.a) defines diabetes as "a group of diseases characterized by high **blood glucose** (blood sugar) levels that result from defects in the body's ability to produce and/or use insulin." **Insulin** is a hormone that transports glucose from

Table 19.1
Symptoms of Diabetes Before Diagnosis (Hyperglycemia)

- Lethargy
- Fruity breath
- Weight loss
- Frequent thirst and urination
- Nausea and/or vomiting

Data from Centers for Disease Control and Prevention. (n.d.). Basics: Diabetes. Retrieved from https://www.cdc.gov/diabetes/basics/diabetes.html

the blood into the cells of the body. Without insulin, glucose stays in the blood, creating high levels, which can eventually cause damage to organs, the cardiovascular system, and nerves of the body (CDC, n.d.a).

According to the CDC (n.d.c), 30.3 million people have diabetes. The two most common forms of diabetes are **type 1 diabetes** and **type 2 diabetes**. There are many similarities between the two types yet also many differences. The commonalities between the two types of diabetes are the initial symptoms of the disease (Table 19.1), difficulty controlling blood sugar, the physical complications of long-term uncontrolled blood sugar, constant monitoring of blood sugar, and the importance of diet and exercise for overall wellness and prevention of disease complications. The diseases are physiologically different in that type 1 is an autoimmune condition whereby the body attacks the pancreatic beta cells, rendering them incapable of producing insulin.

Blood glucose The amount of sugar in the blood, measured in milligrams per deciliter (mg/dL) or millimol per liter (mmol/L).

Insulin A hormone that transports glucose from the blood into the cells of the body.

Type 1 diabetes Insulin-dependent type of diabetes mellitus usually diagnosed in children and adolescents, but anyone can be diagnosed at any age. In this autoimmune disease, the body does not produce insulin.

Type 2 diabetes Non-insulin-dependent type of diabetes. The body does not produce enough insulin or does not use insulin properly.

Once the autoimmune process begins, it usually cannot be reversed, and an individual needs injected insulin to survive. Type 1 diabetes accounts for about 5–10% of the diagnosed diabetes cases, whereas type 2 diabetes is more prevalent in the general population, making up 90–95% of diagnosed cases and can be inherited, especially among certain ethnic populations. Physiologically, individuals with type 2 diabetes can produce insulin, but their body is resistant to it and cannot use it effectively, depending on the progression of the disease. Type 1 diabetes is usually diagnosed in the youth or young adulthood; however, anyone at any age can be diagnosed with type 1 diabetes. Type 2 diabetes is usually diagnosed in adulthood, yet unhealthy youth can be diagnosed with type 2 diabetes. Lastly, the treatment for type 1 and type 2 diabetes is different. Type 1 diabetes requires injectable insulin to constantly replace what the body cannot make; type 2 diabetes requires a diet with a controlled amount of carbohydrates, exercise, oral medication, and potentially injectable insulin if the aforementioned methods cannot effectively control blood glucose (CDC, n.d.a). Refer to Table 19.2 for more details.

Regardless of the type of disease, individuals with diabetes are unable to produce insulin and/or effectively use it; therefore, daily monitoring of blood sugar levels and attention to one's diet is essential. Monitoring for current blood sugar levels can be accomplished with a **glucometer**, lancing device for pricking the finger to extract a drop of blood, and a testing strip. A **continuous glucose monitor (CGM)**; Figure 19.3) can also monitor real-time blood sugar levels. Wearing a CGM is particularly helpful to see how one's blood sugar is trending, especially if it is dropping or climbing at a fast rate, as the device shows blood sugar trends using up and down arrows on the display. Again, regardless of the type of diabetes, diet is particularly important to people with type 2 diabetes, but diet needs to be factored into the circumstances when planning exercise sessions for people witheither type of diabetes.

For those with diabetes, there are several healthcare professionals who become part of a team to help manage the disease. Quarterly checkups should occur with an endocrinologist, certified diabetes educator, and registered dietician to manage blood sugar control and lifestyle choices. Pharmacistsare also a key part of diabetes management because they can address

Glucometer A device used to measure blood glucose from a drop of blood.

Continuous glucose monitor (CGM) A wearable medical device that continuously measures blood sugar.

Table 19.2
Type 1 Versus Type 2 Diabetes

	Type 1 Diabetes	**Type 2 Diabetes**
Previous names	Juvenile diabetes	Adult-onset diabetes
Incidence	5–10% of the population with diabetes	90–95% of the population with diabetes
Diagnosis	Diagnosis most common during youth but can be diagnosed at any age	Diagnosis most common during adulthood but can be diagnosed earlier
Heredity	Family history uncommon but possible	Family history common but not necessary; prevalent in certain ethnicities
Disease specifics	Autoimmune disease; no cure; not reversible	Reversible to a point
	Body unable to produce insulin but can use outside source of insulin	Body able to produce insulin but cannot use it effectively
Treatment	Injected insulin required to live	Diet, exercise, oral medication; last resort injected insulin

Data from Centers for Disease Control and Prevention. (n.d.). Basics: Diabetes. Retrieved from https://www.cdc.gov/diabetes/basics/diabetes.html

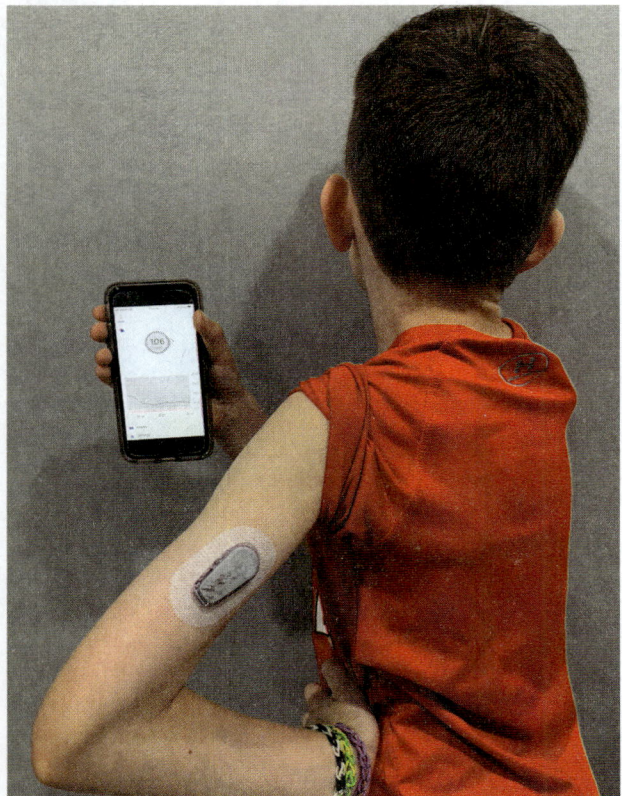

Figure 19.3 Continuous glucose monitor.
Courtesy of Cindy Trowbridge.

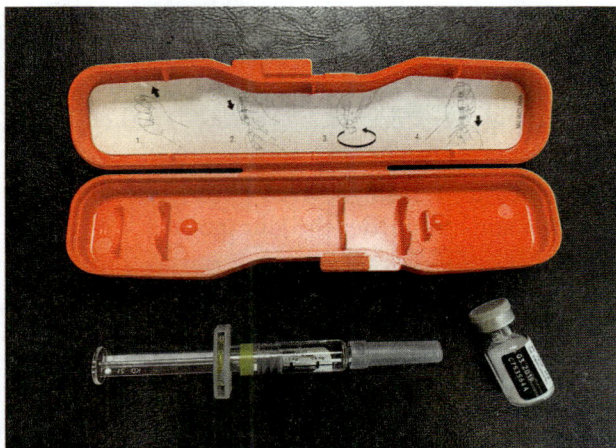

Figure 19.4 Glucagon kit.
Courtesy of Cindy Trowbridge.

concerns related to medications. The person with diabetes is also monitored for common complications via other medical professionals, such as dentists, eye doctors, mental health professionals, and primary care doctors (National Institute of Diabetes and Digestive and Kidney Diseases [NIDDKD], n.d.).

Blood Sugar 101

For an individual who does not have diabetes, normal fasting blood sugar level is 60–100 mg/dL (3.3–5.5 mmol/L), and 2 hours after eating a meal the blood sugar level is less than 140 mg/dL (7.8 mmol/L). The goal for a person with diabetes is to keep his or her blood sugar level within a normal range of 80–120 mg/dL (4.4–6.6 mmol/L) as much as possible. Under normal circumstances, doing this can be quite a challenge. The danger arises when the blood sugar level is below 70 mg/dL (3.9 mmol/L); this condition is referred to as **hypoglycemia**, or as a "low" in the community of people with diabetes. The following signs and symptoms can develop quickly because the blood sugar level can drop at a quick rate:

- Perspiration
- Extreme hunger
- Dizziness
- Tachycardia
- Loss of motor coordination
- Unusual behavior, such as aggression or confusion followed by loss of consciousness

If left untreated, this condition can be life threatening. If an individual with diabetes is unconscious, call 911. Then, locate the **glucagon kit** (Figure 19.4), and administer glucagon as per the kit's instructions. It would be wise for teammates, friends, coaches, or anyone else who would be close to an individual with diabetes to be educated about how to administer glucagon in the event of an emergency (ADA, n.d.b).

When individuals with diabetes experience signs and symptoms of hypoglycemia, they should do the following:

- Stop activity.
- Check their blood sugar level with the glucometer.
- Immediately administer at least 15 grams of fast-acting carbohydrate, such as a juice or sports drink, if their blood sugar level is below 70 mg/dL.

Hypoglycemia Low blood sugar level.

Glucagon kit A container holding a syringe of saline and a vial of dry glucagon to be mixed together and injected in the event of diabetic coma.

- Recheck their blood sugar level with the glucometer after 10–15 minutes; if it is still below 70 mg/dL (3.9 mmol/L), administer 15 grams of fast-acting carbohydrate. Repeat this cycle until their blood sugar level reaches the normal range.
- If they do not improve or go unconscious, call 911, and administer the glucagon.

People who have had diabetes for a long time can feel their "lows" and know when they need to consume fast-acting carbohydrate. In this case, they may consume carbohydrate before checking their blood sugar level. Conversely, people who have had diabetes for a long time may not feel their "lows", or people with diabetes may have episodes of low blood sugar that are associated with altered mental status and may need assistance to treat the low blood sugar, or may have an unexplained pattern of low blood sugar (less than 54 mg/dL or 3 mmol/L); this is called **hypoglycemic unawareness**. Such unawareness is cause for serious concern, and they should follow up with their endocrinologist. People with hypoglycemic unawareness can act abnormally or erratically and not be aware enough to test their blood sugar level. In this circumstance, others should make them aware that they need to test their blood sugar level, or they should do it for them and ask them to consume fast-acting carbohydrate. It is possible to regain awareness by having very controlled blood sugar or very limited low blood sugar for several weeks.

Hypoglycemic unawareness The inability to sense low blood sugar, likely from having low blood sugar too often.

Hyperglycemia Excessively high level of blood sugar.

Ketone A molecule produced by metabolizing fat that can be measured in the urine and blood.

Ketoacidosis Metabolic state with extremely high ketone concentration in the blood, often the result of not enough insulin and too high a blood glucose level.

Diabetic coma A life-threatening condition caused by complications of having high blood sugar for too long, resulting in an altered state or unconsciousness.

Diabetic ketoacidosis (DKA) A serious condition that usually results from extended periods of high blood sugar causing a high concentration of ketones in the blood, this creates an acidic environment in the body, which can lead to organ damage and other complications.

The opposite of low blood sugar is high blood sugar and is called **hyperglycemia**. Hyperglycemia occurs when the blood sugar level is greater than 200 mg/dL (11.1 mmol/L). The following signs and symptoms can develop slowly:

- Fruity odor on the breath
- Extreme thirst
- Frequent urination
- Nausea and/or vomiting
- Loss of consciousness

If this condition is left untreated after an extended period of time (hours or days), the body will metabolize fat for energy and, as a result, creates a substance called **ketones**, which will make the blood more acidic. If a person with diabetes is in this state long enough, he or she will be in **ketoacidosis** or, worse, a **diabetic coma**. This condition can be life threatening as well. Unfortunately, many individuals are diagnosed with diabetes after the initial signs and symptoms have been present for some time and they are in **diabetic ketoacidosis (DKA)**, or a highly acidic state.

When people with diabetes experience signs and symptoms of hyperglycemia, they should do the following (NIDDKD, n.d.):

- Stop activity.
- Hydrate with water (no carbohydrate).
- Check their blood sugar level with the glucometer.
- Check for ketones via urine dipstick or ketone blood meter.
- Give insulin if you know the dosage to correct the blood sugar and call their endocrinologist's emergency number for guidance on what medication and dosage to take to further lower the blood sugar level if needed, or whether to seek immediate medical attention.
- If they are unconscious from a high blood sugar level, call 911, monitor for vital signs, and treat for shock.

Blood Sugar and Exercise

A detailed explanation of the specific mechanisms for controlling blood sugar level is beyond the scope of this text; however, it is very important to know that blood sugar levels in individuals with diabetes may fluctuate greatly from low blood sugar to high blood sugar levels during exercise. The goal is to keep blood sugar levels near normal (100–180 mg/dL, or 5.5–10 mmol/L) while exercising. Exercise is beneficial for both types of diabetes; however, extra attention to exercise intensity, insulin dosage, and diet is critical for safe participation. Adjusting these factors to ensure safe exercise can be accomplished with the assistance of a **certified diabetes educator** and/or an **endocrinologist**. For more information about diabetes, refer to NATA's position statement (Jimenez et al., 2007) and the ADA's standards of medical care (ADA, 2021).

Pregame or Exercise Plan

About 2 hours before a game or exercise, individuals with diabetes should monitor their blood sugar levels and adjust their insulin and diet to meet the target goal for blood sugar levels for exercise commencement. The blood sugar target range will vary, depending on the type of exercise or activity. However, when blood sugar levels are too low before exercise, carbohydrate should be consumed and/or insulin levels lowered to raise blood sugar levels to the target range before exercise. Likewise, when blood sugar levels exceed 300 mg/dL (16.6 mmol/L) and ketones are present before exercise, the body is already in an acidic state, and exercise can create additional acidity. This combined situation of high blood sugar level and exercise can cause a dangerous acidic condition in the body. Therefore, when blood sugar levels are above 300 mg/dL (16.6 mmol/L) and/or ketones are present, exercise must be delayed until ketones are cleared and blood sugar level is lowered.

Generally, **aerobic exercise** of moderate intensity, sustained over a period of time, results in maintenance of or even a decrease in blood sugar levels. For this type of exercise (e.g., long-duration running and walking), the target blood sugar level at exercise commencement should be on the higher end, about 200 mg/dL (11.1 mmol/L). To achieve this level, it is recommended that people with diabetes decrease their dosage of insulin and/or increase their carbohydrate intake accordingly about 2 or more hours before exercise begins.

Commonly, **anaerobic exercise** involving high-intensity, short-duration activities (80% VO_2 max or greater, such as football, hockey, basketball and soccer) results in increases of blood sugar levels during exercise. For this type of exercise, target blood sugar level at exercise commencement should be about 100–150 mg/dL (5.5–8.3 mmol/L). To achieve this level, it is recommended that people with diabetes maintain their normal routine, assuming that keeps them in the normal blood sugar range, or increase their dosage of insulin and/or decrease their carbohydrate intake accordingly about 2 or more hours before exercise begins.

Many other factors to consider before exercise is the timing and location of insulin injection. It is common to delay exercise 1–4 hours after injection, depending on the type of insulin (e.g., fast acting or other) because the combination of exercise and insulin will most likely lower blood sugar levels faster than if the individuals did not exercise. Regarding the injection site, it is ideal to inject insulin into an area of the body that will not be actively used as much during exercise. Lastly, if individuals are receiving preactivity treatments, keep in mind that hot and cold local treatments over the injection site may cause absorption rate differences (ADA, 2021; Jimenez et al., 2007).

Individuals with diabetes should plan to bring the following items to the game or exercise session and notify a friend, family member, or teammate of their exercise plans or have an exercise buddy:

- Glucometer and its supplies (i.e., testing strips, lancing device, and lancets)
- Glucagon kit
- Fast-acting sugar (e.g., juice, sports drinks, glucose tablets, or gels)
- Water

Certified diabetes educator A healthcare professional who has special education in the management of diabetes.

Endocrinologist A physician who specializes in the endocrine system and hormones.

Aerobic exercise Exercise of long duration and usually at low to medium intensity that requires the body to use oxygen to meet the energy demands.

Anaerobic exercise Exercise of short duration and high intensity that does not require the body to use oxygen to meet energy demands.

- Medical information, ID, or emergency contact information
- Cell phone
- Money (dollar bills or quarters for vending machines)
- Insulin and associated supplies (i.e., needles and pump)
- Extra supplies of all of the above

During Game or Exercise Plan

Because of the effect of exercise on blood sugar levels, it is recommended to frequently monitor blood sugar levels during exercise to ensure levels are within an acceptable range and treat accordingly. Individuals with diabetes need to bring their supplies to the activity area for easy access. If they are exercising outdoors over great distances, their supplies need to be transported with them for easy access at all times.

Postgame or Exercise Plan

Similarly, it is recommended to monitor blood sugar levels immediately after exercise and perhaps consume 15 grams of fast-acting carbohydrate after aerobic exercise. It is also common for a low blood sugar level to occur 8–12 hours after aerobic exercise because the body continues to recover from exercise.

It is also recommended to check blood sugar level around this time. Be advised that 8–12 hours after exercise may occur in the middle of the night; therefore, an alarm should be set. It is also recommended to monitor blood sugar levels after anaerobic exercise and treat accordingly for low blood sugar, however, it is common to have high blood sugar levels after high intensity anaerobic exercise. As the body recovers from exercise, blood sugar levels will lower naturally; therefore, it is usually not recommended to give a full corrective dose of insulin immediately after high intensity aerobic activity. Refer to Table 19.3 for a quick review.

Blood Sugar and the Environment

Extreme ambient temperatures (below 32°F [5.7°C] and above 86°F [30°C]) may also affect insulin absorption. In addition to temperature, the level of hydration and other factors in the environment can also play a role in blood sugar levels. For example, even though cold weather can slow the absorption rate of insulin in a hydrated person with diabetes, the cold weather can cause low blood sugar levels because of the energy needed to maintain body temperature. Conversely, even though hot weather can increase the absorption rate of insulin, high blood sugar levels may result in a dehydrated person with diabetes. It is recommended to monitor blood sugar levels frequently in extreme environmental conditions.

Table 19.3
Blood Glucose Monitoring and Treatment Before, During, and After Exercise*

	Aerobic Exercise	Anaerobic Exercise
Blood sugar goal at start of game/exercise	200 mg/dL (11.1 mmol/L)	100–150 mg/dL (5.5–8.3 mmol/L)
Before activity (2 hours before)	Decrease insulin dosage and/or increase carbohydrate content of food.	Increase insulin dosage and/or decrease carbohydrate content of food.
During activity	Monitor blood sugar levels and treat accordingly.	Monitor blood sugar levels and treat accordingly.
Post activity	Monitor blood sugar levels, especially 8–12 hours after, and treat accordingly.	Monitor blood sugar levels and treat accordingly.

*This table represents only suggested blood sugar levels for optimal performance of activity. Each individual will need to find what works best for them given any unique circumstances. Note: If blood sugar is over 300 mg/dL (16.6 mmol/L) and/or ketones are present, delay aerobic or anaerobic exercise until blood sugar levels are lower and ketones are cleared.

Miscellaneous Issues

The information presented in this chapter generally describes what individuals with diabetes experience before, during, and after exercise regarding the factors they need to consider for safe participation. Keep in mind that not all people with diabetes respond to diet, exercise, insulin, or the environment exactly the same. It may take repeated trials and, hopefully, not too many serious errors to find a routine that results in good blood sugar control and performance. Also, practice routines may need to be different from game routines given the hormonal response to game situations. There are many successful athletes with diabetes, such as Gary Hall (Olympic gold medal swimmer with type 1 diabetes) and Kendall Simmons (former Pittsburgh Steelers professional football player with type 1 diabetes), who have found a way to successfully compete with diabetes with the help of medical professionals (e.g., certified diabetes educators, endocrinologists, registered dieticians, team physicians, and certified athletic trainers), coaches, parents, friends, and teammates. Encourage individuals with diabetes to find their way.

A management flow chart covering the major treatment approaches for diabetes-related emergencies is shown in Figure 19.5.

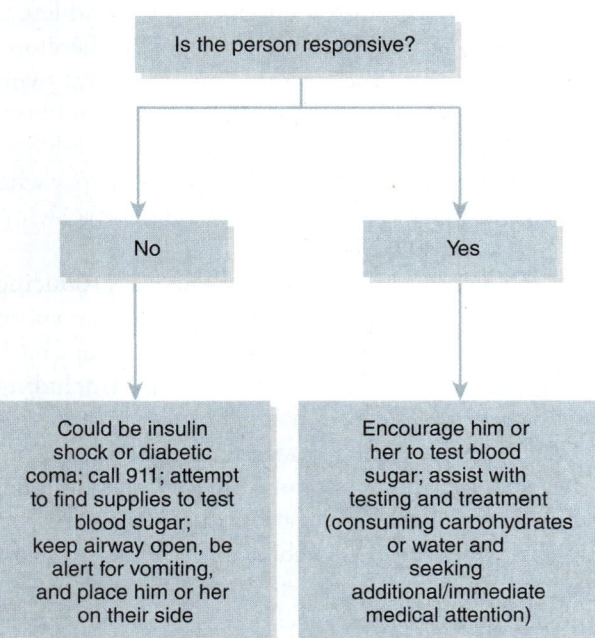

Figure 19.5 Management procedures for diabetes-related emergencies.

WHAT IF ❓

You are coaching high school softball. During practice one afternoon your right fielder comes to you complaining of extreme hunger and acting strangely. You notice during your conversation that she is perspiring heavily although it is a cool, cloudy afternoon. You know from her preseason physical evaluation that she has diabetes. What condition would these signs and symptoms indicate? What would be the appropriate first aid for this young athlete?

Epilepsy and Sports Participation

Epilepsy is a neurological disorder of the brain associated with a wide variety of symptoms. The most well-known symptom of epilepsy is a **seizure**, which is a sudden episodic change in behavior or appearance due to an abrupt imbalance of electrical activity in the brain (Epilepsy Foundation, n.d.e). Seizures take many forms and may involve motor systems, perceptions, and even the mood of the athlete. According to the Epilepsy Foundation (n.d.a), 1 out of 26 people in the United States will develop epilepsy in their lifetime. Seizures can happen at any age and affect both males and females; however, they tend to begin in young children or in older adults.

There are three forms of epileptic seizure the coach, educator, or care provider is likely to encounter among athletes (Epilepsy Foundation, n.d.d). The first type, a **generalized onset seizure**, affects both

---

Epilepsy A chronic neurological disorder characterized by sudden attacks of brain dysfunction, including altered consciousness, abnormal motor activity, sensory phenomena, and/or inappropriate behavior.

Seizure Sudden onset of uncoordinated muscular activity and changes in consciousness lasting an unpredictable time.

Generalized onset seizure A seizure that affects both sides of the brain; is dramatic and severe, often characterized by violent convulsions and loss of consciousness.

sides of the brain and includes **tonic–clonic seizures** (i.e., rigid muscles–rhythmical jerking movements; once known as grand mal seizures), atonic seizures (i.e., weak or limp muscles), and absence seizures (i.e., brief twitches in a specific part of the body or staring spells). Tonic–clonic seizures involve the most dramatic symptoms. This seizure is characterized by generalized convulsions involving a fall to the ground and uncontrolled shaking of the arms and legs plus body twitching. During the seizure, the person is unconscious, but the eyes may be open, thereby creating the illusion that the person is awake. The typical generalized tonic–clonic (i.e., grand mal) seizure lasts from 2–5 minutes. The second type is called a **focal onset seizure**; this type of seizure begins on one side of the brain. When these seizures happen, the person is awake and aware (**focal onset aware seizure**), and, immediately following the seizure, the person will recover and may not know one has occurred. Another type of focal onset seizure occurs when the person is confused (**focal onset impaired seizure**; Epilepsy Foundation, n.d.d). An athlete suffering this type of seizure will suddenly lose contact with surroundings and demonstrate any number of unusual behaviors, including mumbling; picking at or removing clothing; automatisms, or repeated movements, such as clapping; or walking around in an apparently random fashion. This type of seizure may last for up to 5 minutes, after which time the athlete will recover but will remain confused and disoriented, possibly for a considerable time. The athlete will have no memory of activity during the seizure. The third type of seizure is called an **unknown onset seizure**, meaning that it is not witnessed by anyone to know what type it is or the beginning of the seizure is not known. As the seizure is investigated, the seizure may be diagnosed as focal or general (Epilepsy Foundation, n.d.d).

Seizures may be triggered by common events, such as a specific time of day or night, illness, drug use, stress, or menstrual cycle, or when sleep deprived, not eating well, or seeing flashing lights. Additionally, increased thermal temperature and being physically tired from exercise are triggers.

From the coach's standpoint, two major concerns must be addressed regarding an athlete with epilepsy—safety in the chosen activity and proper first aid care should a seizure occur. Many questions have been raised within the lay and medical communities regarding what activities may pose a risk for the athlete with epilepsy. With the advent of anticonvulsant drugs, the vast majority of these athletes can control seizures. It has been reported that over half of people with epilepsy who take anti-seizure medication can remain free from seizures; however, approximately 36% do not respond to seizure medication (Epilepsy Foundation, n.d.b). The prevailing medical evidence suggests that high-risk activities for athletes afflicted with epilepsy include aquatic sports, sports in which falling is possible, and potentially contact and collision sports (Epilepsy Foundation, n.d.c).

Obviously, a seizure occurring while an athlete is in the water carries the risk of drowning; therefore, athletes who may suffer seizures should always swim with a buddy, alert pool personnel of their condition, and wear a life vest. However, it is generally advised that the benefits to a young athlete with epilepsy who is interested in water sports, such as competitive swimming, far outweigh the risks.

Athletes interested in sports capable of producing a dangerous fall, such as cycling, ice skating or speed skating, skydiving, mountain climbing, and horseback riding, should be evaluated thoroughly (including assessment of seizure control history on an individual basis) before participating (Epilepsy Foundation, n.d.c). In the case of mountain climbing, an additional risk is incurred due to elevations that reduce oxygen and involve atmospheric changes. Whether athletes participate in activities that are hazardous in the event of losing consciousness, such as water skiing, should be decided individually with their doctor. In such activities, the risks of injury related to a seizure exceed whatever benefits may be derived from participation.

Tonic–clonic seizures A seizure that involves stiffening, twitching, or jerking phases of muscle activity in addition to experiencing changes in sensation and mood leading up to the seizure; once called a grand mal seizure.

Focal onset seizure A partial seizure occurring in just one area of the brain.

Focal onset aware seizure A seizure that does not cause loss of awareness.

Focal onset impaired seizure A seizure that affects a larger part of the brain and likely causes unawareness.

Unknown onset seizure A seizure in which it is difficult to determine if it is of focal or generalized onset, perhaps because it was not witnessed by anyone.

A persistent myth has been that athletes with epilepsy should not be involved in contact and collision sports because the potential jarring of the brain may increase the likelihood of seizure. Research, however, does not support this premise; in fact, it appears that athletes with epilepsy have no more risk from participation in such sports than does anyone else. The personal physician, parents, and athlete should collaborate to make reasonable decisions about participation. Of course, athletes with epilepsy involved in contact sports should take the same safety precautions as other athletes by wearing helmets, facemasks, and mouth guards.

There is no reason that any youngster with epilepsy should be excluded from most school or community sports programs. In fact, such children can benefit a great deal from participation, particularly regarding their self-esteem and overall physical fitness.

It is important for coaching personnel to educate all participants about epilepsy in the event that an athlete suffers from a seizure. In this way, fear and anxiety on the part of teammates can be minimized (Carter & McGrew, 2021; Epilepsy Foundation, n.d.c).

First aid care for epileptic seizures is determined by the type of seizure and the immediate circumstances. Obviously, a generalized tonic–clonic seizure that takes place in the water will require first aid quite different from the first aid for a complex partial seizure that occurs in the wrestling arena. For the most part, first aid for any type of seizure involves protection of the athlete from self-injury, followed by psychological support. The appropriate first aid care for an athlete suffering an epileptic seizure is provided in **Time Out 19.2**.

TIME OUT 19.2

First Aid Care for Epileptic Seizure in an Athlete (Generalized Onset [Tonic–Clonic Seizure])

- Coaching staff should know who on their team has epilepsy, the specific type of the disorder, and any related medications the athlete is taking.
- Note the approximate time, to the minute, that the seizure began, because this is very important information to relay to the patient and any advanced medical care providers.
- If the seizure occurs in an aquatic setting, the priority must be to remove the victim from the water immediately and maintain the airway.
- Ask other athletes to move away from the victim and to resume their practice and/or game-related activities.
- *Do not* attempt to restrain the athlete during the seizure.
- *Do not* put anything in the person's mouth. Efforts to hold the tongue down can injure the teeth or jaw. Seizure victims will not swallow their tongue.
- Remove any clothing around the neck that might restrict breathing.
- Move potentially harmful objects away from the immediate area of the athlete.
- If the athlete is not wearing some type of helmet (e.g., football, lacrosse, and hockey), place something soft under the athlete's head.
- As the seizure passes, place the athlete onto his or her side, sometimes called the "recovery position."
- As the athlete regains consciousness, be sure to provide psychological support and treat for any injuries incurred or signs or symptoms of shock.
- Initiate the emergency plan, including contacting EMS if:
  - The seizure lasts more than 5 minutes.
  - The victim is having trouble breathing.
  - Another seizure occurs.
  - Injuries were sustained and need advanced treatment.
  - Victim remains unconscious after seizure has ended.

Review Questions

1. Define the acronyms *URI* and *LRI*.
2. What types of organisms are related to respiratory infections?
3. Define the term *gastroenteritis*.
4. Briefly describe the history of Lyme disease in the United States.
5. What is the mode of transmission for Lyme disease?
6. Describe the major signs and symptoms of Lyme disease.
7. True or false? Lyme disease is caused by a virus.
8. What is the causative agent of infectious mononucleosis?
9. What is the risk related to collision sports and mononucleosis?
10. Describe the common signs and symptoms of EIA.
11. What can a coach do to assist an athlete suffering from EIA?
12. Which ethnicities are likely to carry the sickle cell trait?
13. What conditions are likely to cause a sickle cell crisis?
14. Describe several ways you can prevent a sickling crisis in athletes with SCT.
15. Explain what rhabdomyolysis is and how to prevent it.
16. What are the recommended levels of blood glucose for the athlete with diabetes?
17. List the signs and symptoms of hyperglycemia.
18. List the signs and symptoms of hypoglycemia.
19. What is the difference between infield management for hyperglycemia and hypoglycemia?
20. Define *epilepsy*.
21. What are the management guidelines for an athlete suffering an epileptic seizure?

References

American Diabetes Association. (n.d.). Standards of medical care in diabetes 2021. Retrieved from https://diabetesjournals.org/care/issue/44/Supplement_1

Aronowitz, R. A. (1991). Lyme disease: The social construction of a new disease and its social consequences. *The Milbank Quarterly*, 79–112.

Bartlett, A., Williams, R., & Hilton, M. (2016). Splenic rupture in infectious mononucleosis: A systematic review of published case reports. *Injury, 47*(3), 531–538.

Campbell, J. P., & Turner, J. E. (2018). Debunking the myth of exercise-induced immune suppression: Redefining the impact of exercise on immunological health across the lifespan. *Frontiers in Immunology, 9*, 648.

Carter, J. M., & McGrew, C. (2021). Seizure disorders and exercise/sports participation. *Current Sports Medicine Reports, 20*(1), 26–30.

Caterisano, A., Decker, D., Snyder, B., Feigenbaum, M., Glass, R., House, P., Sharp, C. P., Waller, M., & Witherspoon, Z. (2019). CSCCa and NSCA joint consensus guidelines for transition periods: Safe return to training following inactivity. *Strength & Conditioning Journal, 41*(3), 1–23.

Centers for Disease Control and Prevention (CDC). (n.d.a). About diabetes. Retrieved from https://www.cdc.gov/diabetes/basics/diabetes.html

Centers for Disease Control and Prevention (CDC). (n.d.b). Allergies. Retrieved from https://www.cdc.gov/healthcommunication/toolstemplates/entertainmented/tips/allergies.html

Centers for Disease Control and Prevention (CDC). (n.d.c). Diabetes basics. Retrieved from https://www.cdc.gov/diabetes/basics/index.html

Centers for Disease Control and Prevention (CDC). (n.d.d). Hepatitis A questions and answers for health professionals. Retrieved from https://www.cdc.gov/hepatitis/hav/havfaq.htm

Centers for Disease Control and Prevention (CDC). (n.d.e). Hepatitis B questions and answers for health professionals. Retrieved from https://www.cdc.gov/hepatitis/hbv/hbvfaq.htm

Centers for Disease Control and Prevention (CDC). (n.d.f). Lyme disease. Retrieved from https://www.cdc.gov/lyme/

Centers for Disease Control and Prevention (CDC). (n.d.g). Lyme disease maps: Most recent year. Retrieved from https://www.cdc.gov/lyme/datasurveillance/maps-recent.html

Centers for Disease Control and Prevention (CDC). (n.d.h). Recent surveillance data. Retrieved from https://www.cdc.gov/lyme/datasurveillance/recent-surveillance-data.html

Centers for Disease Control and Prevention (CDC). (2017). Tickborne diseases of the United States: A reference manual for health care providers. Retrieved from https://www.cdc.gov/lyme/resources/TickborneDiseases.pdf

Centers for Disease Control and Prevention (CDC). (2018a). Lyme disease. Retrieved from https://www.cdc.gov/lyme/index.html

Clark, A., & Mach, N. (2016). Exercise-induced stress behavior, gut-microbiota-brain axis and diet: A systematic review for athletes. *Journal of the International Society of Sports Nutrition, 13*, 43.

Cleary, M., Ruiz, D., Eberman, L., Mitchell, I., & Binkley, H. (2007). Dehydration, cramping, and exertional rhabdomyolysis: A case report with suggestions for recovery. *Journal of Sports Rehabilitation, 16*(3), 244–259.

Epilepsy Foundation. (n.d.a). About epilepsy: The basics. Retrieved from https://www.epilepsy.com/learn/about-epilepsy-basics

Epilepsy Foundation. (n.d.b). If first medicine doesn't work. Retrieved from https://www.epilepsy.com/learn/treating-seizures-and-epilepsy/treatment-101-basics/if-first-medicine-doesnt-work

Epilepsy Foundation. (n.d.c). Learn. Retrieved from https://www.epilepsy.com/learn/professionals/hallway-conversations/epilepsy-and-exercise-hallway-conversation

Epilepsy Foundation. (n.d.d). Types of seizures. Retrieved from https://www.epilepsy.com/learn/types-seizures

Epilepsy Foundation. (n.d.e). What is a seizure? Retrieved from https://www.epilepsy.com/learn/about-epilepsy-basics/what-seizure

Harris, M. D. (2011). Infectious disease in athletes. *Current Sports Medicine Reports, 10*(2), 84–89.

Jimenez, C., Corcoran, M., Crawley, J., Hornsby Jr., W. G., Peer, K., Philbin, R., & Riddell, M. (2007). National Athletic Trainers' Association position statement: Management of the athlete with type 1 diabetes mellitus. *Journal of Athletic Training, 42*(4), 536–545.

Kim, J., Lee, J, Kim, S., Ryu, H. Y., Cha, H. S., & Sung, D. J. (2016). Exercise-induced rhabdomyolysis mechanisms and prevention: A literature review. *Journal of Sport and Health Science, 5*(3), 324–333.

Ko, J. S., & Chiampas, G. (2021). The collapsed athlete. In D. J. Engel & D. M. Phelan (Eds.), *Sports cardiology* (pp. 343–359). New York, NY: Springer, Cham.

Kramer, A. (2020). An overview of the beneficial effects of exercise on health and performance. In J. Xiao (Ed.), *Physical exercise for human health*. New York, NY: Springer, Cham.

Lalloo, U. G., Kalla, I. S., Abdool-Gaffar, S., Dheda, K., Koegelenberg, C. F. N., Greenblatt, M., Feldman, C., Wong, M. L., van Zyl-Smit, R. N., & Asthma Working Group of the South African Thoracic Society. (2021). Guidelines for the management of asthma in adults and adolescents: Position statement of the South African Thoracic Society–2021 update. *African Journal of Thoracic and Critical Care Medicine, 27*(4).

Leaver-Dunn, D., Robinson, J. B., & Laubenthal, J. (2000). Assessment of respiratory conditions in athletes. *Athletic Therapy Today, 5*(6), 14–19.

Liao, W. L., Chang, T. P., Chen, S. J., & Kao, C. H. (2015). Benign paroxysmal positional vertigo is associated with an increased risk of fracture: A population-based cohort study. *Journal of Orthopaedic & Sports Physical Therapy, 45*(5), 406–412.

Manspeaker, S., Henderson, K., & Riddle, D. (2016). Treatment of exertional rhabdomyolysis in athletes: A systematic review. *JBI Evidence Synthesis, 14*(6), 117–147.

MedlinePlus. (2021). Infectious mononucleosis. Retrieved from https://medlineplus.gov/infectiousmononucleosis.html

Mitchell, B. L. (2018). Sickle cell trait and sudden death. *Sports Medicine-Open, 4*(1), 1–6.

National Institute of Diabetes and Digestive and Kidney Diseases (NIDDKD). (n.d.). Managing diabetes. Retrieved from https://www.niddk.nih.gov/health-information/diabetes/overview/managing-diabetes

Nye, N. S., Kasper, K., Madsen, C. M., Szczepanik, M., Covey, C. J., Oh, R., Kane, S., Beutler, A., Leggit, J. C., Deuster, P. A., & O'Connor, F. G. (2021). Clinical practice guidelines for exertional rhabdomyolysis: A military medicine perspective. *Current Sports Medicine Reports, 20*(3), 169–178.

O'Connor, F. G., Franzos, M. A., Nye, N. S., Nelson, D. A., Shell, D., Voss, J. D., Anderson, S. A., Coleman, N. J., Thomson, A. A., Harmon, K. G., & Deuster, P. A. (2021). Summit on exercise collapse associated with sickle cell trait: Finding the "way ahead." *Current Sports Medicine Reports, 20*(1), 47–56.

Oh, R. C., Arter, J. L., Tiglao, S. M., & Larson, S. L. (2015). Exertional rhabdomyolysis: A case series of 30 hospitalized patients. *Military Medicine, 180*(2), 201–207.

Report of the Special Presidential Committee to Investigate the January 2011 Hospitalization of University of Iowa Football Players. (2011). Retrieved from https://www.healthy.arkansas.gov/images/uploads/resources/Rhabdomyolysis_-_University_of_Iowa_Board_of_Regents_Report.pdf

Rice, S. G. (2008). Medical conditions affecting sports participation. *Pediatrics, 121*(4), 841–848.

San Francisco Department of Public Health. (n.d.a). Hepatitis A. Retrieved from http://www.sfcdcp.org/hepatitisa.html

San Francisco Department of Public Health. (n.d.b) Hepatitis B. Retrieved from https://www.sfcdcp.org/infectious-diseases-a-to-z/hepatitis-b/

Simpson, R. J., Campbell, J. P., Gleeson, M., Krüger, K., Nieman, D. C., Pyne, D. B., Turner, J. E., & Walsh, N. P. (2020). Can exercise affect immune function to increase susceptibility to infection? *Exercise Immunology Review, 26*, 8–22.

Stack, M. A., & Hakemi, A. (2011). Diagnosis and treatment of exercise induced bronchospasm: A review. *Journal of the American Academy of Physician Assistants, 24*(6), 26–30.

U.S. Anti-Doping Agency. (2018). Wallet card 2018. Retrieved from https://usada.org/wp-content/uploads/wallet-card.pdf

Walsh, N. P., & Oliver, S. J. (2016). Exercise, immune function and respiratory infection: An update on the influence of training and environmental stress. *Immunology & Cell Biology, 94*(2), 132–139.

CHAPTER 20

Special Medical Concerns for the Adolescent Athlete

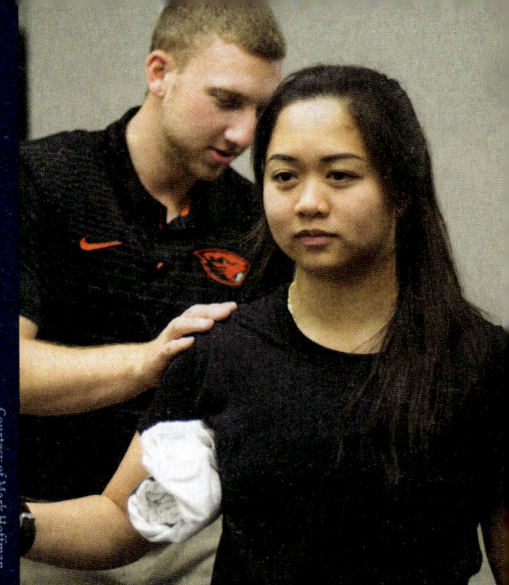

MAJOR CONCEPTS

Approximately 36 million youths between the ages of 5 and 18 years participate in a wide array of organized sports nationwide (Statistic Brain Research Institute, 2017), and roughly 30 million children ages 6 to 14 participated in one or more activities or sports in 2015 (Sports & Fitness Industry Association, 2016). By the age of 6 years, 66% of boys and 52% of girls are on sports teams (Statistic Brain Research Institute, 2017). An additional 7.8 million children are involved in secondary school–sponsored activities (National Federation of State High School Associations, n.d.). With that large number of participants has come rather startling injury data. Estimates are that approximately 2.6 million sports- and recreation-related injuries in children up to age 19 were treated in a hospital emergency department in 2009 (Centers for Disease Control and Prevention, n.d.). The number of injuries that occur is likely much higher than the estimated 2.6 million because many injuries receive care by a medical professional outside of an emergency department. Some of these injuries can be prevented.

Though young athletes suffer the greatest number of injuries of all sports participants, they often receive limited medical care. The availability and expertise of sports medicine providers, including physicians, Board of Certification–certified athletic trainers, and physical therapists, increases as athletes reach more elite levels of competition. Accordingly, the relatively small number of athletes competing at the Olympic and professional levels have unlimited access to specialty medical care. Collegiate athletes usually have the services of a full-time athletic trainer and one or more active team physicians, but the situation changes dramatically at the high school level. In 1994, only 37% of secondary schools employed a full-time athletic trainer, and, in 2005, approximately 42% of public secondary schools used athletic training services (Pryor et al., 2015). At the youth sports level, there is rarely any involvement by trained medical personnel. As a result, coaches and parents are often left to provide initial care for injured athletes.

Youth Sports in America

Organized youth sports have been a part of American culture for more than a century. As 19th-century America became increasingly industrialized and urbanized, local schools and churches formed youth sports organizations to help "build character" through physical activity. In the 1890s, the YMCA first began offering young men the opportunity to compete against each other. The founding of New York City's Public School Athletic League in 1903 ushered in the explosion of organized sports participation in the first half of the 20th century, which culminated with the birth of Little League Baseball in 1939. The 1970s then saw an influx of girls and young women entering the traditionally male-dominated youth sports culture as barriers were overcome both legally and socially ("The Living Law," n.d.). However, there were some backlashes against youth sports throughout the years; many educational leaders opposed competition, citing its potentially harmful psychological effects. Educators also observed a corresponding decrease in free play activities as children immersed themselves in organized sports. They feared "premature specialization" in certain sports would lead to injuries and interfere with the normal physical and mental development of childhood. Formal school budgets have been cut, causing physical education to be removed from the curriculum. Based on these examples, many formal school athletic programs were disbanded, beginning a shift in philosophy that has had repercussions in youth sports for many years. Physical educators and other teachers started to play a diminishing role in coaching school-sponsored sports for young participants, thereby allowing thousands of parents and other volunteers to take their places. Unfortunately, the majority of these well-meaning volunteers have had no formal training in coaching or in child developmental phases. As a result, concerns have continued to be raised about the potential for young athletes to suffer physical and emotional harm from sports competition. In response to such concerns, for example, many youth baseball and soccer leagues have stopped keeping score or recording wins and losses, Little League Baseball established pitch counts, and many athletes are encouraged not to specialize too early (LaParade et al., 2016). However, despite these oppositions, youth sports have never been more popular.

Factors in Youth Sports Participation

Why do children and adolescents play organized sports? There are a variety of answers. Not surprisingly, the primary motivating factor for many young athletes is having fun. Other often-cited rationales have been making friends through team involvement, developing skills, and improving physical fitness (Nationwide Children's Hospital, n.d.).

Unfortunately, the reasons for discontinuing participation are fear of injury, lack of playing time, overemphasis on competition, and dislike of the coach in high school students. Sadly, attrition among boys and girls results from an "absence of fun". Lately, free play among youth has shifted to parent- or coach-driven activities and formalized, competitive athletic leagues (e.g., club sports, Amateur Athletic Union), leading to sports specialization at younger ages. This is a highly concerning topic in the medical field because specialization at a young age has been found to lead to increased rates of injury, burnout, lowered motivation and withdrawal from sport, and psychological concerns (LaPrade et al., 2016). Additionally, this model of competitive youth sports has made it difficult for families without extensive financial means to participate in organized leagues, and has forced some to find other community-based options for activity (Pandya, 2021). With the expansion of youth sports, there is also concern that the lack of qualified healthcare providers, such as athletic trainers, at practices and events may contribute to injury rates and inappropriate care for acute injuries similar to those of schools located in lower socioeconomic areas that have less access to certified athletic trainers (Huggins et al., 2019; Post et al., 2019).

In 2019, the Youth Early Sport Specialization Summit sponsored by the American Medical Society for Sports Medicine concluded that there is great variation in participation guidelines, both within and between sports, and training aspects, as well as a lack of coordination between medical organizations, sport organizations, and governing bodies. They recommend incorporating more specific language in organizational communications, such as more quantified details and enforcement on training load per age or development stage, and providing appropriate training and timing for sports specialization (Tenforde et al., 2022).

Epidemic of Youth Sports Injury

Injuries can span the gamut from catastrophic to those that result in very little time loss from practice or competition. Catastrophic injuries are typically categorized as fatal (i.e., death), nonfatal (i.e., life-altering complications), and serious (i.e., significant time loss).

Fatal injuries are those resulting from asthma, brain injuries, cervical spine injuries, diabetes, exertional heatstroke, exertional hyponatremia, exertional sickling, lightning, and sudden cardiac arrest (Casa et al., 2012). Noncatastrophic injuries also occur commonly in high school athletes, and there seem to be timing (practice vs. competition) and team- and gender-specific factors that contribute to the different injury rates. Analysis from High School RIO™ from the 2006–2007 through 2018–2019 school years suggests that most injuries in high school sports are acute in nature, especially during competition, and of those acute injuries, the most common involved ligament structures and concussions. Football had the most acute and overuse injuries among all sports analyzed, and girls' soccer had the most acute and overuse injuries among the female sports analyzed (Ritzer et al., 2021). Acute injuries were not the only types of injuries suffered; overuse or repetitive trauma injuries represented approximately 50% of pediatric sports-related injuries (Valovich McLeod et al., 2011). Additionally, it has been found that approximately 10.5% of injuries from the 2005–2006 through 2015–2016 high school injury data in the High School RIO™ surveillance system were recurrent in nature and more often resulted in greater playing time loss and surgical management (Welton et al., 2018). These data can be used by healthcare providers, coaches, physical educators, and parents to safeguard young athletes during sports participation.

Two alliances have been established to educate the public about the rate and types of injuries that happen in youth sports. The overall purposes of these alliances are to increase knowledge about sports injury prevention, recognition, and treatment so sporting careers and even lives can be saved. Both the Youth Sports Safety Alliance and STOP Sports Injuries offer websites full of valuable information, which can be downloaded, about different sports and the role that coaches, parents, and athletes can play in guaranteeing safe participation. The Youth Sports Safety Alliance was started by the National Athletic Trainers' Association (NATA) and has brought together more than 100 other organizations that care about youth athletes. In particular, the Alliance commits to several calls to action, which are listed in **Time Out 20.1**. STOP Sports Injuries was initiated by the American Orthopaedic Society for Sports Medicine (AOSSM) in 2007 and has been joined by several other medical or athletic societies.

TIME OUT 20.1

Youth Sports Safety Alliance

GENERAL RECOMMENDED ACTIONS

- Ensure that youth athletes have access to qualified healthcare professionals—physician, athletic trainer, school nurse, or other healthcare professional—preferably in a designated space where physical exams and private conversations can occur.
- Educate the public about the signs and symptoms of sports injuries and conditions as well as the potential risks associated with sports and nutritional supplements and performance-enhancing substances.
- Assure preparticipation examinations, including specific screening for cardiac history and symptoms, eating disorders, depression, and female athlete triad, and appropriate baseline testing (i.e., concussion) be performed for all athletes.
- Ensure that sports equipment, uniforms, playing surfaces, facilities, and environmental conditions be checked for safety and best conditions to prevent injury and spread of communicable disease.
- Insist that research into youth sports injuries be supported and published.

(continues)

> **TIME OUT 20.1** *(continued)*
>
> **SPECIFIC RECOMMENDED ACTIONS FOR CARDIAC, NEUROLOGICAL, ENVIRONMENTAL, AND NUTRITIONAL CONDITIONS**
>
> - Support a national registry of sports-related catastrophic injuries and fatalities.
> - Request that appropriate emergency action plans and safety protocols and procedures be established and routinely rehearsed as well as protocols for injury and illness prevention and return to activity and school.
> - Eliminate the culture of "playing through pain" without assessment, and be educated on certain medical conditions that have consequences of "playing through pain" or environmental conditions.
> - Ensure that general and sports-specific safety education be a priority for every administrator, coach, parent, and player.
> - Educate regarding signs and symptoms of sudden cardiac arrest; traumatic brain injury; cervical spine injury; exertionally or environmentally induced distress; and psychosocial problems, such as depression, substance abuse, and disordered eating.
> - Require that automated external defibrillators (AEDs) be immediately accessible at all venues as well as a trained individual who can use the AED and properly assess serious injuries and conditions and follow guidelines for treating heat illness.
> - Require healthcare professionals, coaches, and officials be trained in cardiopulmonary resuscitation (CPR) and AED use.
> - Require medical clearance to return to activity for heat-related conditions, concussion and other brain injuries, and cardiac events.
> - Require proper referral of athletes to appropriate medical professionals when psychosocial or dietary problems are suspected.
>
> Modified from The Youth Sports Safety Alliance National Action Plan for Sports Safety. http://www.youthsportssafetyalliance.org/sites/default/files/docs/National-Action-Plan.pdf. Accessed: May 5, 2017. Used with permission.

In 2017, the NATA published recommendations for youth sports organizations similar to the general recommended actions and specific recommended actions for cardiac, neurological, environmental, and nutritional concerns of the Youth Safety Alliance (Time Out 20.1), but the NATA also has recommendations for potentially life-threatening medical conditions and lightning (Huggins et al., 2017). Among the most popular recommendations for potentially life-threatening medical conditions are asthma, anaphylaxis, sickle cell trait, diabetes, and epilepsy. The NATA recommends that these conditions be disclosed to coaches and medical personnel and these individuals educated about the conditions and how to prevent, recognize, and treat them. Lastly, the NATA encourages proper medications and devices (e.g., inhaler, epinephrine injector, glucometer, and insulin) be with athletes at all times as well as proper communications be carried out in emergency events.

The Growing Athlete

Prepubescence

Children grow slowly and steadily in height and weight from about 5–9 years old. It is typical for both boys and girls to grow in height 2–2.5 inches (5–7 cm) and add weight of 4–7 pounds (2–3 kg) per year during this time. Also, boys and girls will also tend to follow their same growth percentage on the growth charts over these years. During prepubescence, boys and girls will grow at the same rate, have the same strength comparatively, and show improvements in balance and coordination due to gradually increasing myelination.

The longitudinal growth of bones arises from the diaphysis and the physis (i.e., growth plate) located near the ends of long bones (Figure 20.1). Though a rather complex structure, the physis is basically an anatomic framework on which rows of a

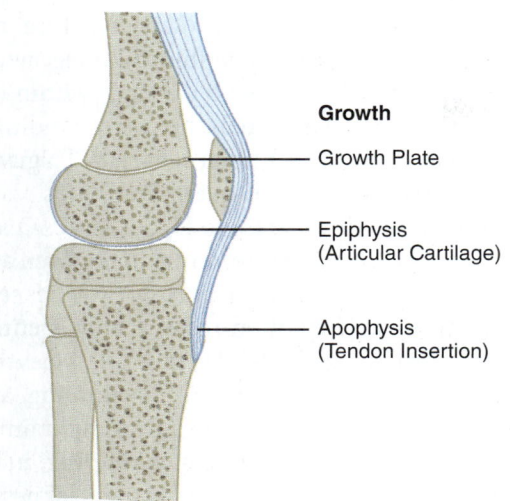

Figure 20.1 Long bone, showing physis, articular cartilage, and apophysis.

cartilaginous matrix are progressively laid down to allow for longitudinal growth. Each layer undergoes a series of physiological transformations, culminating in complete ossification (i.e., new bone formation). All bones continually lengthen beginning with embryonic development, but puberty signals a particularly rapid phase of bone growth. In contrast, skeletal muscle has no "growth center" corresponding to that found in long bones. In fact, muscles grow in length in a manner similar to how they grow in size—they respond to increasing forces. The progressive lengthening of the bone stimulates the muscles to correspondingly become longer. Lastly, during the growing years of prepuberty and puberty, not only are the bones and muscles growing, but nerve myelination is also occurring.

Puberty

Before proceeding with a discussion of common injury patterns, an understanding of the uniqueness of the growing athlete is required. It has often been said that children are not just "little adults." Nowhere does this saying apply more than in athletics. Emotionally and physically, children and adolescents respond far differently to the rigors of sports activity than do their adult counterparts.

Before reaching physical maturity, the young athlete's body is in a dynamic state. Change is constant as growth and development take place. Puberty is defined as the time when children develop secondary sexual characteristics, experience an increase in the rate of linear growth, and add muscle mass. Puberty happens at different ages for girls and boys and is highly influenced by genetics. At times, the **chronological age** of an individual does not match his or her **biological age**. For example, puberty usually begins at an average age of 10 years in girls and is signaled by the onset of breast development; at around the age of 12 years, boys will begin puberty, with an increase in testicular volume being the first physical sign. However, this development is not the case in every individual, as in a 12-year-old girl who has not started development yet (i.e., "late bloomer"), but others have.

There are three ways to assess what stage of maturation a young person is in. First, acquiring an X-ray of the left hand can assess **bone age**, meaning it can determine at what stage of bone ossification the body is in. Not everyone receives an X-ray during puberty, but an X-ray can be very helpful in assessing individuals who have started puberty too early or too late. Second, **Tanner stages** break down the development of secondary sexual characteristics into five stages, with stage 1 representing prepuberty and stage 5 representing full maturation of an adult. This method is much less costly and quicker than an X-ray, but it can be uncomfortable for the individual to share this information with health professionals and parents may not agree to disclosing such information. Third, taking measurements, such as weight, height, bone length, and peak height velocity, can provide **somatic information** to help determine stage of development. Usually, parents and youths are more comfortable sharing this type of information compared to that necessary to determine the Tanner stage of development. It is important to know how an individual is maturing because this can provide clues to injuries and will dictate how an individual trains for sport.

Chronological age Age since birth.

Biological age Age of individual based on stage of bone or biological development.

Bone age The age of a person as determined by the current stage of bone ossification.

Tanner stages Outlines five stages of physical maturation.

Somatic information In the context of growth and development, physical measurements such as peak height velocity, mass, leg length, etc., that assist in determining maturation.

Longitudinal growth accelerates during early puberty, with **peak height velocity** (i.e., "growth spurt") being attained at an average of age 12 years in girls and 14 years in boys. In young women, this time frame typically corresponds to just before the onset of menses. On average, menarche occurs 2 years after breast development begins. Most girls will see no more than 5 centimeters of height added after menarche, with their peak height velocity occurring 6–12 months before menarche. Boys attain peak height velocity later in puberty than do girls, corresponding to Tanner stage 3 or 4 of sexual maturity (i.e., near adult pubic hair distribution and genital development). Peak height velocity may result in linear growth rates of almost 10 centimeters per year. Growth during puberty may account for up to 20% of final adult height. Bone growth ends once the physis closes, signaling the attainment of skeletal maturity. The average age of full skeletal development is approximately 14 years for girls and 16 years for boys, but there may be much variation (Brown et al., 2017).

In terms of muscle, youths will increase muscle mass first before they are then able to withstand high forces. The average boy will see a doubling of his total muscle mass between the ages of 10 and 17 years, experience peak muscle mass between 18 and 25 years old, and achieve peak strength between 20 and 30 years old. Girls will achieve peak muscle mass between 16 and 20 years old and peak strength at 20 years old (Haff & Triplett, 2016). And, as stated earlier, nerve myelination will gradually develop and be completed at sexual maturity.

Injury Mechanisms

Macrotrauma and microtrauma events are the two basic injury categories seen in sports. **Macrotrauma** results from a single, high-force traumatic event. Examples include compound and comminuted fractures, joint dislocations, and tendon or ligament ruptures. Though young athletes may suffer these injuries, they are more likely to suffer trauma to the growth plate (i.e., physis) than to tear a ligament or fracture

Peak height velocity Known as the "growth spurt," or the maximum vertical height gained in the shortest period of time, usually during the development years.

Macrotrauma Injury from a single, high-force event.

Microtrauma Injury from overuse or repetitive stress.

the shaft of a long bone. As with any structure, the weakest point is the most susceptible to damage when subjected to a force. The growth cartilage within the physis offers less resistance than the correspondingly stronger bones and joints (Brown et al., 2017; Nguyen et al., 2017). **Microtrauma**, or overuse, injuries result from chronic, repetitive stress to local tissues. Overuse injuries are increasingly common in children and adolescents and represent the majority of injuries seen in young athletes. They often result from repetitive activities or chronic submaximal loading of tissues that occurs in activities such as throwing, swimming, and distance running. Multiple factors, including training errors, improper technique, excessive training, inadequate rest, early specialization, and muscle weaknesses and imbalances, can lead to these injuries (Valovich McLeod et al., 2011). Many of these factors are discussed in more detail throughout the chapter.

Ligament Injuries

Severe ligamentous injuries are less common in youth and adolescent athletes than in adults, but they still do occur. An increased laxity of the ligaments prior to skeletal maturity and the relative plasticity of the long bones contribute to ligamentous injuries. As previously discussed, the physis offers less resistance to force than do the ligaments and, in many instances, is the site of injury. The physis may act to absorb more of the forces. For example, if a young athlete suffers a lateral blow to the knee, the valgus force will more likely result in a distal femoral or proximal tibial physis fracture than in the medial collateral ligament sprain often seen in skeletally mature athletes (Figure 20.2).

However, before puberty, ligamentous injuries may occur more commonly than previously thought. Before the pubertal growth spurt, the physis and its attachment site to the underlying bone may actually be stronger than the ligaments. When evaluating potential ligament injuries in adolescents, the basic principle of comparing the injured joint with the contralateral joint must always be remembered. The examiner may initially suspect ligamentous disruption owing to the increased laxity of immature joints. Similar laxity in the contralateral joint confirms a normal finding.

Tendon and Bone Injuries

The physes, apophyses, and articular surfaces of long bones are three key anatomic structures susceptible to injury in the young athlete (Figure 20.1). These

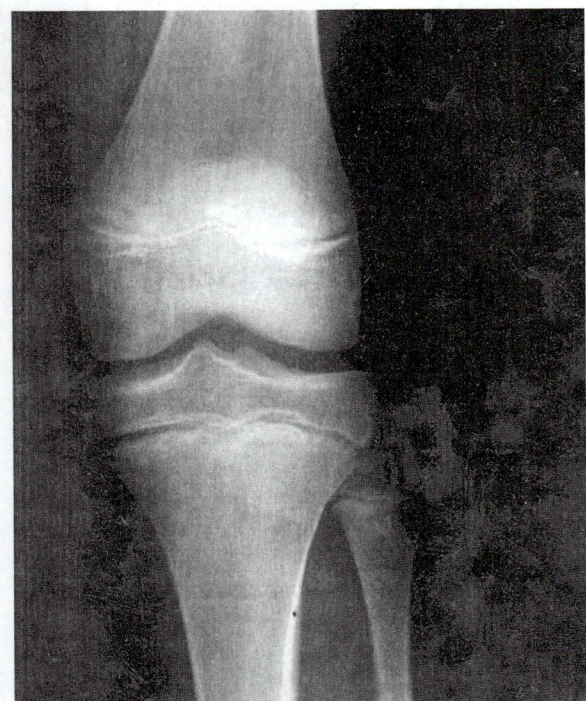

Figure 20.2 Stress X-ray of a fracture at the growth plate of a tibia in a skeletally immature athlete. Without the stress applied to the fracture by the radiology technologist to the medial aspect of the tibia, it would be difficult to visualize the fracture.

Courtesy of Ron Pfeiffer.

Table 20.1
Common Sites of Apophysitis

Anatomic Site	Condition
Tibial tubercle	Osgood–Schlatter disease
Inferior pole of patella	Sinding–Larsen–Johansson disease
Calcaneus	Sever's disease
Medial distal humerus	Little league elbow
Fifth metatarsal base	Iselin's disease
Iliac crest	Iliac apophysitis
Ischial tuberosity	Ischial apophysitis

three structures share the presence of growth cartilage. The apophysis represents the site at which large muscle–tendon units attach to bones. Similar in structure to the physis, these tendon sites typically mature and completely ossify before the closure of the physes. The articular cartilage may be more susceptible to stress injury in young athletes because the surface and underlying matrix have not yet achieved maturity. Therefore, it is likely unable to attenuate stress as well as the adult tissue can. During times of rapid growth (i.e., growth spurt), the bones grow first, and the muscles lag behind in length, setting up the potential for injury (Wik et al., 2020). For example, a force applied to a joint that is likely to affect a ligament in the adult will most likely cause injury to growth areas in youths and adolescents. And chronic lower loads of force as compared to a sudden applied force are more likely to injure the site where tendon and bone meet.

Chronic microtraumatic injuries to the immature apophysis and the resultant inflammation have long been recognized. In 1903, Osgood and Schlatter each described traction injury at the tibial tubercle and named the condition Osgood–Schlatter disease (Osgood, 1903). Other commonly involved sites include the calcaneus (i.e., Sever's disease) and medial humerus (i.e., little league elbow; Table 20.1). Apophyseal injuries provide excellent examples of the multiple factors that lead to injury in the growing athlete. As discussed, muscles lengthen in response to bone growth. Therefore, a susceptible period exists when the muscle is shorter than necessary for optimal function in relation to the bone. The result is constant tension on the apophysis, which is exacerbated by repetitive activity. With repeated traction placed on the apophysis, there may be some weakening within the growth cartilage matrix, culminating in inflammation, pain, and loss of function (Brown et al., 2017; Nguyen et al., 2017).

Young athletes are more susceptible to **apophysitis** during times of rapid bone growth, but overtraining, poor technique, and chronic misuse may all inflict damaging forces across joints and contribute to injury (Valovich McLeod et al., 2011). Infrequently, macrotraumatic injuries can also occur at the apophysis. High-force injuries may result in the complete disunion of the apophyseal growth cartilage, the adolescent equivalent of a complete tendon avulsion. Initial treatment of apophyseal injuries is similar to the treatment of other musculoskeletal injuries and includes ice, anti-inflammatory medications, modification of activity levels (complete or relative rest),

Apophysitis Inflammation or stress injury where a tendon attaches near or around growth plates of bones resulting in pain and/or excessive pulling of the bone causing structural changes.

bracing, and stretching of various muscle groups. Calcaneal apophysitis (i.e., Sever's disease) is often particularly amenable to the placement of a heel lift in the shoe of the involved foot. The heel lift acts to functionally shorten the pull of the gastrocnemius and soleus muscles, thus lessening the tension at the calcaneal apophysis. Typically, some of the symptoms associated with apophysitis linger for quite some time until bone growth slows.

Growth Plate Injuries

Injuries to the physis may result from microtrauma and macrotrauma. In the 1960s, Salter and Harris (1963) classified five injury patterns seen after trauma to the physis. The Salter–Harris type I fracture is by far the most common physis injury and represents a "separation" of the cartilaginous zone from the bone (Figure 20.2). The diagnosis is most often made based on physical exam findings because radiographs are typically normal. Such an injury should always be suspected when the athlete presents with a joint injury but with tenderness predominantly over the distal or proximal portion of the bone and a normal joint examination. Injuries to the distal fibula and distal radius are most often seen. Treatment consists of casting for 4–6 weeks, and complications are rare.

Injuries in the Salter–Harris classification system become progressively more serious as the corresponding type number increases. Types III and IV involve fractures of the bone's articular surface and usually require surgical repair. Type V injuries represent a compression of the growth plate and carry the highest incidence of premature closure and growth arrest. Over the years, another type of growth plate injury has been recognized. Chronic, repetitive axial loading of a physis may lead to microvascular injury and resultant growth arrest. This injury is most commonly seen in gymnasts who present with radial deviation of their hands secondary to overgrowth of the ulna as compared with the shortened radius.

Over the past several decades, a number of physeal injury classification systems have arisen. While the Salter–Harris system has stood the test of time and remains the most commonly used system, it does not adequately describe all possible fracture variants. Therefore, two additional physeal injuries deserve special mention. Ogden (1981) described an injury that may occur at the perichondral region of the physis (Figure 20.3). In the early 1990s, Peterson (1994)

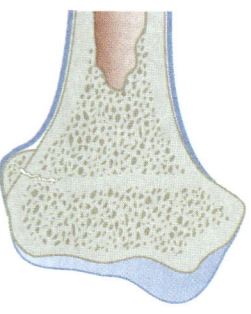

Figure 20.3 Rang–Ogden type IV injury.

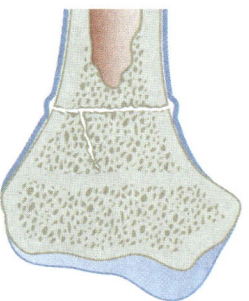

Figure 20.4 Peterson type I injury.

WHAT IF ?

A 15-year-old tackle football player, a linebacker, severely limps toward the sideline after having been involved in a tackle during a scrimmage. He reports having felt his knee twist severely and that he experienced a popping, or "letting go" feeling, when the injury occurred. He notes tenderness along the top of the tibia bone along his knee joint line. This pain was made worse by asking him to simply stand on the injured leg. Based on the information presented in this chapter, what would you conclude are possible injuries given this athlete's injury history, signs, and symptoms?

proposed a classification system with many similarities to the Salter–Harris scheme. His main addition was that of the Peterson type I fracture—a transverse fracture of the metaphysis with a longitudinal extension into the physis, often seen in the distal radius (Figure 20.4).

Growth Cartilage

The articular surfaces of all bones are covered with cartilage. Immature growth cartilage differs biomechanically and biologically from that found in adults.

Athletic Trainers SPEAK OUT

Why is it so important to have athletic trainers in the secondary school setting?

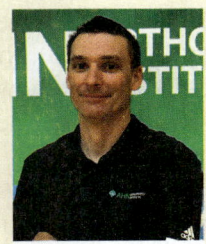

Courtesy of Matthew Dady.

The single most important reason for an athletic trainer (AT) in the secondary school setting is making sure that the student-athletes are being properly cared for and their safety is ensured. The addition of an AT to a secondary school is a decision made with the medical care of the student-athlete in mind. Deciding to include an AT will add value to the secondary school and the athletic programs. When examining the six domains of athletic training—prevention, clinical evaluation, immediate care, treatment and rehabilitation, organization and administration, and professional responsibilities—the AT should be proficient in all of these areas, leading to successful outcomes. Having an athletic trainer at the secondary school setting will also remove the healthcare decision-making by coaches and administrators for injured athletes.

In many instances, the ATs in these settings often are responsible for all decisions regarding athletic injuries and other medical or health-related concerns. It is vital that we use our skills to properly evaluate and treat each athlete within our scope of practice. Often, this may require further evaluation by physicians or through emergency care. ATs at the secondary school will likely make decisions about budgeting, emergency action plans, rehabilitation protocols, equipment, and environmental safety issues. Making and managing these decisions is where ATs show their importance in the secondary school setting. One of the most crucial aspects of being an AT in the secondary school setting is the continuum of care and communication between athletes, coaches, and parents or guardians. In many cases, this will be the athlete's and their parents' or guardians' first exposure to an injury and the steps necessary for full recovery. As an AT in the secondary setting, you will be involved in that athlete's injury from the point of the acute injury through rehabilitation and, finally, returning to play. Safe return to play is an especially important role for the AT as parents or guardians will likely be looking for guidance.

—**Matthew Dady, MS, ATC, LAT**

Matthew Dady is a Staff Athletic Trainer contracted through the Allegheny Health Network to Chartiers-Houston Jr/Sr High Schools in Houston, Pennsylvania.

In addition to providing a low-friction articulating surface, cartilage acts to absorb and disperse forces in weight-bearing joints. Growth cartilage may be somewhat softer than its adult equivalent and subjects the underlying tissues to damage. Though less common than the two injury patterns mentioned earlier, injuries do occur. The primary example is osteochondritis of the radial head capitellum, found in little league elbow. Such injuries may impart long-term damage to the articular cartilage.

There are also cartilaginous areas in the body that develop into boney tissue as one matures. For example, there is cartilage between the boney sections of the patella in youths, and, as they enter puberty, the cartilage slowly decreases and bone formation increases. If muscle forces during activity are too great, this cartilage is at risk of injury (Brown et al., 2017; Nguyen et al., 2017).

Contributors to Injury

Sports medicine specialists nationwide are in agreement that sports-related injuries among adolescents and children have risen dramatically since the 1990s. Multiple factors are responsible for the rise and are most easily categorized as intrinsic and extrinsic contributors to injury. Intrinsic characteristics are individual biological and psychosocial attributes associated with internal aspects, such as chronological age, bone or biological age, ability, strength, and flexibility, whereas extrinsic characteristics are associated with external aspects, such as the playing field condition or the environment (Mandorino et al., 2022; Windt & Gabbett, 2017). Though multiple factors exist, this discussion focuses on those believed to be the most important and amenable to change. It must also be remembered that many injuries are the result of a combination of factors rather than a single entity.

Intrinsic Factors

The most important intrinsic factor involved in youth sports injuries is the growing body itself. The susceptibility to injury of growth cartilage, bone, and the muscle–tendon unit represents factors that are under only limited control. During the pubescent growth spurt, when the peak height velocity is occurring, the bone is temporarily more porous and prone to injury, such as epiphyseal fractures (Windt & Gabbett, 2017). In addition, during peak height velocity, there is a change in the center of mass, potential muscle imbalances, and muscle–tendon tightness.

However, several other intrinsic factors have been identified as predisposing pediatric athletes to overuse injuries. In particular, previous injury and associated laxity or instability to joints and overall experience with sport techniques play very important roles. Previous injury may result in tissue changes, including fibrosis, which may cause limited range of motion and function (Mandorino et al., 2022). Also, young males with taller stature, thinner body structure, less strength, decreased muscle flexibility, and high degrees of ligamentous laxity are particularly prone to overuse injuries, especially when paired in repeated contests with larger male athletes of the same age, because of the constant wear and tear applied to weaker joints and muscles. Additionally, the "late bloomers" may suffer injuries from trying to keep up with the stronger and faster athletes who have already developed (Windt & Gabbett, 2017). From a biomechanical perspective, young females with taller and thinner body structures are also prone to overuse injuries, and their decreased muscle flexibility will often contribute to genu valgum (i.e., knock-knee) or overpronation of the feet (Valovich McLeod et al., 2011). For example, biomechanical malalignment at the knees and feet may lead to increased incidence of medial tibial stress syndrome (i.e., shin splints) and stress fractures (Valovich McLeod et al., 2011) as well as areas of weakness elsewhere.

Extrinsic Factors

Cultural Deconditioning

Despite record numbers of youngsters involved in organized sports, obesity among youths continues to rise. In a 2015–2016 analysis by the National Health and Nutrition Examination Survey (NHANES), the obesity prevalence was 18.5% in youths, which shows an increased trend since the previous report (Hales et al., 2017).

The degree of obesity in children and adolescents has been correlated to decreased activity and increased caloric intake over the years, but other factors, such as socioeconomics of family, community, and national policies and genetic or biological factors, also play a role in the rise of obesity in youths (Lee & Yoon, 2018). Specifically, increased screen time on electronic devices has only contributed to decreased activity over the years. Concomitantly, free play, the spontaneous physical activity of childhood, has continued to decline. Along with the decrease in free play, simple activities such as walking to school or bicycling from one destination to another have also declined. Youths ages 6–17 years are recommended to complete 60 minutes or more of moderate- to vigorous-intensity aerobic exercise a day, and at least 3 days a week as part of the 60 minutes a day should include age-appropriate muscle and bone strengthening according to the 2018 Physical Activity Guidelines for Americans. Types of muscle-strengthening exercise include tug-of-war, playing on playground equipment, and resistance exercises. Types of bone-strengthening exercises include hopping, skipping, jumping, and running (U.S. Department of Health and Human Services, 2018). However, only 21% of youths aged 19 years in the United States complete 60 minutes or more of activity a day, and only roughly 27% of high school students complete the 60 minutes or more of activity a day (Kann et al., 2016; National Physical Activity Plan Alliance, 2016).

At the time of its origin, organized youth activity was intended to be an adjunct to free play. Currently, organized sports have become the basis of physical activity for most children. Therefore, we now see young athletes enter into sports with no underlying base of physical fitness or skill in sports, leaving them prone to acute and chronic injury. Many of them drop out of organized sports because of the lack of fun, time, or playing time; issues with coaches; or too much pressure. And some of those who do participate in youth sports may be consuming too many calories and unhealthy food and beverages.

Obesity in youths is an important health issue for various reasons. First, if youths do not achieve normal body weight before puberty, they are more prone to staying obese as an adult and have an increased risk of cardiovascular and metabolic disease, such as type 2 diabetes, and cancer in adulthood. And those conditions can lead to premature death (Weihrauch-Blüher et al., 2018). Second, as these obese youths participate in physical activity or childlike activities, such as free play during recess and school hours, they are more at risk for macrotrauma and major bone injuries due to more forces applied to the body when they exercise or fall. For example, obese youths may suffer more complicated fractures and be more at risk for postoperative complications and failures than are nonobese youths. Other orthopedic conditions obese youths are prone to are slipped capital femoral epiphysis (Fedorak et al., 2018) and Blount disease (Confroy et al., 2021).

Training Errors or Improper Technique

An important figure in the life of any young athlete is his or her coach. Unfortunately, there is a nationwide shortage of qualified individuals to fulfill these vital roles; and as a result, many young athletes are never taught proper preseason conditioning methods, nor do they learn the basic fundamentals vital to their sport. In addition, athletes and coaches alike fall prey to the "more is better" philosophy of training, attempting to accomplish too much, too soon in an attempt to improve but setting the stage for injury instead.

Formally trained or not, many coaches simply do not have the requisite knowledge base for instructing young athletes on the principles of sport techniques and conditioning. Volunteers without formal training often base their coaching style and teaching of fundamentals on personal experiences. Even trained coaches will likely have learned many of the technical aspects of their job by observing and listening to other coaches. Both of these styles of acquiring knowledge are prone to misinformation, with improper theory being perpetuated for years. Weight training (discussed in further detail later in the chapter) is a particularly important area where improper training can lead to serious injury.

Excessive Training, Inadequate Rest, and Early Specialization

A recent position statement on overuse injuries in pediatric athletes developed by the National Athletic Trainers' Association (Valovich McLeod et al., 2011) identifies several recommendations regarding excessive training, inadequate rest, and early specialization. These are merely recommendations, and the authors noted that more research is needed to clarify their validity; however, they are a place to start in an effort to prevent overuse injuries in young athletes. Valovich McLeod and colleagues (2011) recommended the following:

- Pediatric athletes should have at least 1–2 days off per week from competitive practices, competitions, and sport-specific training.
- Progression of training intensity, load, time, and distance should increase by only 10% each week to allow for adequate adaptation.
- Pediatric athletes should participate on only one team of the same sport per season and practice or play no more than 5 days per week.
- Pediatric athletes should take time off between sport seasons and up to 2–3 nonconsecutive months away from one specific sport.
- If pediatric athletes do participate in simultaneous or consecutive seasons, then it is important to follow guidelines on the cumulative amount of specific activities (e.g., pitch counts, miles run, or meters swimming).

In addition to these recommendations, the AOSSM published a consensus statement in 2016 that defined early single-sport specialization to be participating in intense training or competition in organized sports for over 8 months per year, participating in one sport, and in children less than roughly 12 years old. The AOSSM reiterated the consensus statement of the American Medical Society for Sports Medicine, which suggests that a variety of physical (i.e., injury) and mental health (e.g., burnout and depression) concerns are attributed to early sports specialization (DiFiori et al., 2014). The incidence of overuse injuries, insufficient sleep, overtraining, psychological burnout, and eating disorders may be reduced if children can avoid excessive scheduling and sport-time commitments and can focus on fun, skill development, and lifelong physical activity skills, especially during the prepubescent years. Although the perceived need for large volumes of sport-specific practice stem from past research over 20 years ago, current research has not supported this notion. In fact, the early specialization focus is likely more from the push for athletic college scholarships. Interestingly, researchers have found that early specialization has not benefited high-caliber national- or professional-level performance. For those who are involved with early sport specialization, the AOSSM recommends that children be monitored for burnout and overuse injury if their participation hours are more than their age per week or they have more than 16 hours of intense training per week. AOSSM also recommends that periodized strength and conditioning training for children be planned to help with diverse skill development and reduce injury risk. Periodization becomes particularly important when the athlete is going through his or her growth spurt, or peak height velocity. During this time of rapid growth, activity programs should be modified for less intensity and volume and address muscle imbalances and flexibility (LaPrade, 2016).

Ultimately, many factors may have contributed to the youth sport specialization problem. However, a recent review of sport organization guidelines (Tenfrode et al., 2022) demonstrated a lack of consensus over how youth athletes should train relative to psychological approaches, physical loads, facilities and resources, and timing and monitoring of training. Therefore, youth sport organizations should consider using frameworks to develop youth sport participation guidelines.

Equipment

Although less important than the factors previously discussed, athletic equipment can play a role in injury. Football helmets must be up to current standards and fit properly. Shoulder pads also must be of the correct size and fit. Proper footwear can play a significant role in lower extremity injuries among young distance runners. Footwear should be inspected for the quality of the impact absorption material; good fit; and ability to compensate for alignment changes, particularly during heel strike. All other equipment not mentioned should fit properly, and manufacturers' guidelines should be adhered to. Unfortunately, budget constraints may restrict the purchase of new or upgraded equipment; however, at all times, equipment must meet manufacturers' guidelines for the safety of the individuals who wear it.

Playing Surfaces

The condition of athletic fields at the high school and youth sports levels may range from near professional quality to abysmal. All playing surfaces should be inspected before events to search for potential hazards, such as sprinkler heads, holes, and other hazardous objects. Any issues need to be addressed before allowing play.

Injury Imitators

Any discussion of adolescent musculoskeletal injuries must include a review of pathological conditions that may initially present with similar physical findings to common injuries. An old medical axiom is that "common illnesses happen commonly." However, we must always consider common presentations of uncommon conditions. This section briefly reviews some of the serious medical conditions that may be initially confused with musculoskeletal trauma. When evaluating injured adolescents, one must bear in mind three principles regarding such conditions:

1. **Physical findings inconsistent with injury history.** In general, the extent of the physical findings should be comparable to the severity of the injury described by the athlete or witnessed by others. Finding a complete rupture of the anterior talofibular ligament following an ankle inversion is consistent. Severe tenderness, edema, and erythema of the entire foot 2–3 days after a similar injury does not make sense. Additionally, absence of any trauma history coupled with physical examination findings consistent with injury (e.g., swelling, erythema and tenderness) should especially raise concerns for a more serious underlying pathological process.

2. **Unusual local symptoms.** Exquisite tenderness, erythema, or pain out of proportion to the injury mechanism should raise suspicion for other pathology. Severe night pain and pain on awakening in the morning are also unusual aspects of typical musculoskeletal injuries that should be further investigated.

3. **Systemic symptoms.** A young athlete with musculoskeletal complaints coupled with any

combination of fever, weight loss, night sweats, nausea, or vomiting requires urgent medical attention and a thorough evaluation.

> ### WHAT IF ❓
>
> A 14-year-old female cross-country runner has been complaining to you for the past week about hip pain. She reports that these symptoms started shortly after the team began running high-intensity practices that included extremely explosive sprints with emphasis placed on driving the knees as high as possible. When asked to point to where the pain is most severe, she points to the area of the anterior superior iliac spine on her right hip. In addition, she reports that simply raising up her right leg, as if to bring her knee to her face, causes considerable pain at that same site. Based on the information presented in this chapter, what would you conclude are possible injuries given this athlete's injury history, signs, and symptoms?

Oncological Considerations

Adolescence is the peak age for occurrence of long bone tumors. Such tumors are rare. When they do occur, their onset is typically insidious, and the symptoms may be mistaken for a traumatic etiology early on in the course of illness. Unfortunately, delay in treatment can decrease chances for survival. Bone tumors often result in local pain and tenderness, edema, and night pain. Other complaints may include fever and weight loss. Osteosarcomas most commonly arise in the metaphyses of the femur, tibia, and humerus. Ewing's sarcoma is typically found in the midshaft of long bones but may also arise in the pelvis. Diagnosis is made by plain radiographs and confirmed by biopsy. Treatment for both types of tumors consists of tumor excision and intensive chemotherapy. Five-year survival rates are near 80%.

Rheumatological Considerations

When an athlete presents with complaints of pain or swelling in more than one joint, particularly in the absence of trauma, a diagnosis of juvenile rheumatoid arthritis (JRA) must be considered. Pauciarticular JRA presents with involvement of only a few joints, typically of the lower limbs, but the sacroiliac joint may also be inflamed. Affected individuals initially complain of pain and stiffness on awakening in the morning, with symptoms improving with increased activity. Symptoms are progressive. JRA may result in severe low back and lower extremity pain, disability, and additional systemic symptoms (e.g., fever or rash). Diagnosis is made by clinical history and blood testing.

Infectious Considerations

Variations in the blood supply to the joints and physes make young athletes more susceptible to bone and joint infections than their adult counterparts. Bone infections (i.e., **osteomyelitis**) may present similarly to bone tumors, with fevers being more common in infection. Plain radiographs are normal early in the course, with diagnosis typically made by bone scan or magnetic resonance imaging (MRI). Infections are treated with 4–6 weeks of antibiotics, usually intravenously. Adolescents are also at risk for localized muscle infections. **Pyomyositis** results from bacterial invasion of the muscle tissue. Symptoms include fever, pain, and local tenderness. Diagnosis may be made by MRI. Treatment typically requires surgical drainage and 4–6 weeks of intravenous antibiotics (Lovejoy et al., 2017). Lyme disease, a bacterial infection, may also present with joint involvement and other systemic symptoms. Methicillin-resistant *Staphylococcus aureus* (MRSA) can also present with systemic symptoms, but a skin lesion characterizes its presence.

Neurovascular Considerations

Reflex neuropathic dystrophy (RND) merits discussion because early intervention and treatment greatly aid in the resolution of symptoms. Though the exact pathogenesis is unknown, there is usually some degree of psychogenic overlay. Most common in girls between the ages of 9 and 16 years, RND is preceded by minor injury about half of the time and usually involves the lower extremities. Severe pain and dysfunction are the predominant presenting complaints. Physical findings

---

Osteomyelitis Infection of bone or bone marrow with associated inflammation.

Pyomyositis Bacterial infection of muscles resulting in pus-filled abscesses.

include marked tenderness (i.e., **hyperesthesia**) and signs of local autonomic dysfunction, which may include cyanosis, coolness, diffuse edema, or increased perspiration. Laboratory tests are usually inconclusive. Once the diagnosis is made, patients are placed in an aggressive physical therapy program to regain function of the affected extremity. Treatment may also include individual or family counseling.

Psychological Considerations

All members of the sports medicine team are familiar with athletes who malinger or seek secondary gain from their injuries. However, coaches and athletic trainers must also watch for the subtle signs of depression and other mental health concerns. Athletes presenting with a continuum of seemingly minor yet troublesome injuries should be further questioned about sleep habits, activities, and mood. An athlete's endorsement of symptoms such as poor sleep, early awakening, abandonment of pleasurable activities (i.e., **anhedonia**), and feelings of worthlessness indicates potential depression, and referral to a physician, psychologist, or school counselor is mandatory.

Strength Training

Adolescent strength training has become increasingly popular in recent years. Long thought of as being unnecessary, or even harmful, weight training for adolescents and preadolescents has come under a new focus with concentration on benefits, safety, and the appropriate age at which to begin participation (Faigenbaum, 2017, 2018; Stricker et al., 2020). Studies examining the incidence and types of injuries incurred while weight training have shown varying results. High injury rates are typically attributed to improper supervision in combination with the nature of the lifting technique—Olympic lifts, single lifts with maximum weight, or bad form.

A concern in adolescent weight training is that skeletal immaturity may allow for growth plate injuries to occur or adverse effects on linear growth. Although there have been reports of growth plate injury caused by weight training, many of these injuries were felt to be caused primarily by unsupervised training programs and the need to lift maximal weights. Other research reports little to no risk of injury during resistance training at young stages of development (Faigenbaum, 2017; Stricker et al., 2020).

Therefore, because of this potential risk, the American Academy of Pediatrics (AAP) issued guidelines for adolescent weight training (Stricker et al., 2020). In its statement, it suggests that youth strength training has been shown to increase strength and improve cardiovascular health, body composition, bone density, mental health, and blood lipids when proper supervision and form are instilled. Before puberty, many of the gains achieved through strength training are attributable to neuromuscular adaptations. These adaptations may allow the young athlete to achieve greater and faster hypertrophy in the postpubertal stages because of the learning that occurred in the prepubertal stages. Specifically, preadolescents increase strength by increasing the number of motor neurons, not necessarily by hypertrophy, during strength training. While it has been found that strength training during youth and through puberty improves markers of health and strength, youths who do not participate in physical activity tend to become adults who are at risk for adverse health outcomes (Faigenbaum, 2018; Stricker et al., 2020). Having stated that, caution should be applied and medical clearance obtained before starting strength training or physical activity when children have pre-existing hypertension, cardiomyopathy, pulmonary hypertension, Marfan's syndrome, cancer treatment history, and seizure disorders or are taking certain drugs for chemotherapy.

The AAP guidelines called for close supervision by knowledgeable coaches and medical professionals to ensure proper exercise form, progression, and periodization for children and adolescents who strength train. Resistance training should be individualized to accommodate varying physical development stages, training and technical competencies, and psychosocial aspects. Ideally, children should learn about the body and health; acquire a lifelong desire for physical activity; be informed of proper form and etiquette; and, above all, have fun. Strength training should not be viewed as a competition because of the various stages of development. For example, when a young athlete is

Hyperesthesia Nonpainful touch stimuli becomes painful.

Anhedonia No longer experiencing pleasure from activities that once were enjoyable.

experiencing his or her growth spurt, high volume and intensity are likely to contribute to injury. Rather, the individual should focus on flexibility and correcting muscle imbalances.

Additionally, the AAP, in conjunction with the NSCA and the 2014 International Consensus position statement on youth resistance training, advised beginning a body-weight strengthening program (e.g., frog jumps, bear crawls, crab walks) when children begin sports participation, perhaps as young as 5 years old. If children have the desire to begin a strength training program, they must be receptive to coaching and able to follow instructions. If a child is not coachable or loses interest in strength training, the program should be discontinued. Additional recommendations are found in Table 20.2.

Can strength training prevent injury? As mentioned earlier, strength training increases neuromuscular coordination and muscle mass and strength. Assuming all other variables are equal, these neuromuscular adaptations may allow young athletes to perform better at their chosen sports. Also, these adaptations may make the young athlete less susceptible to the microtrauma of overuse injuries. Strength training should not be expected to prevent all serious acute injuries that are inherent in sports, but it may lessen the athlete's risk for injury (Stricker et al., 2020).

Safety

Safety should be the focus of all adolescent weight-training programs. The main way to avoid injury is to provide young athletes with proper supervision and guidelines. Other possible strategies may include eliminating use of single-repetition maximum lifts, limiting the use of Olympic and powerlifting techniques, and offering safer alternative techniques for lifting.

One area of concern with the adolescent population and strength training is the measurement of strength. The predominant way to measure strength is through the use of the one-repetition maximum lift (1-RM). This technique is commonly used in squatting, the bench press, and other Olympic or powerlifting lifts. The 1-RM consists of a one-time maximal

Table 20.2
AAP Recommendations for Youth Strength Training

1. Receive medical clearance to begin youth strength training.
2. Incorporate aerobic and resistance training as well as skill training into physical activities.
3. Follow proper form and techniques as well as progressions and periodizations as instructed by a qualified supervisor (adequate ratio of supervisor to youths).
4. Avoid powerlifting; body building; maximal lifts; and rapid, explosive movements until physical and skeletal maturity.
5. Educate about the risks of performance-enhancing drugs and substances.
6. Begin with no or low resistance until form is perfected; then, add body weight or other forms of resistance. Begin with 1–2 sets of 8–12 repetitions at low resistance intensity (e.g., ≤60% 1-RM) and progress to 2–4 sets of 6–12 repetitions of increased resistance intensity (e.g., ≤80% 1-RM) while correctly performing exercises; an increase in 5–10% weight or resistance can be applied.
7. Include exercises for all muscle groups through a full range of motion, working large muscle groups and multijoints, then progressing to smaller muscle groups and single joints; core exercises should be included. Sport-specific exercises can be included subsequently.
8. Include dynamic warm-up and cooldown exercises before and after 20–30-minute workouts twice a week for at least 8 weeks to acquire benefits.
9. Include aerobic conditioning if general health benefits are the goal.
10. Ensure adequate hydration during workouts and nutrition in general.
11. Any injury or illness from strength training should be evaluated before resuming strength training.

Modified from Stricker, P. R., Faigenbaum, A. D., McCambridge, T. M., & Council on Sports Medicine and Fitness. (2020). Resistance training for children and adolescents. *Pediatrics, 145*(6), e20201011.

exertion of force used to move the weight. This one-time effort requires near perfect execution of form and puts an inordinate amount of stress on the body. In skeletally mature populations, this may be a valid and accurate way to assess strength, but it has not been recommended for youth and adolescents in the past (Faigenbaum, 2017); however, if properly administered by qualified professionals, the AAP recommends the 1-RM or alternative methods (e.g., grip strength, vertical jump) to evaluate strength and fitness (Stricker et al., 2020).

One such alternative technique is to use a 1-RM equivalent. This technique allows the athlete to assess maximum strength without the increased chance of injury. It can be calculated as follows:

$$(\text{weight lifted} \times \text{number of repetitions} \times 0.03) + \text{weight lifted} = 1\text{-RM}$$

Although this technique is not precise enough for Olympic or powerlifting standards, it does provide a safer alternative for assessing strength in adolescent populations.

Another way to limit injury is to avoid placing the body in positions that may put the joints and limbs at a mechanical disadvantage, which increases the risk for injury. Following are four examples of common lifting mistakes with a description of the proper and safe lifting techniques to avoid them.

Lat Pulldown

Problem

When the weight is pulled down behind the neck, the neck is placed in excessive flexion, and the shoulder joints are loaded at the extreme of external rotation. Also, the line of pull in relation to the bar and the latissimus dorsi muscle is such that this position does not oppose the latissimus dorsi and, thus, does not provide quality resistance.

Solution

A safer way to perform this exercise is to sit down with the bar directly overhead. Grabbing the bar with the hands approximately shoulder width apart, the athlete should lean back slightly so the bar passes just in front of the head, pulling the bar straight down in front of the head to chin level. This movement will allow for a more optimal line of pull on the latissimus dorsi and decrease stress on the shoulder joint. The torso should not rock back and forth while performing this exercise, to avoid low back injury.

Bench Press

Problem

Hyperextension of the shoulders (i.e., dropping the bar to the chest or the elbows behind the plane of the body) puts the pectoralis major at a mechanical disadvantage, contributes to shoulder instability, and puts excessive stress on the acromioclavicular joint.

Solution

A safer way to perform this exercise is to keep the elbows even with the plane of the body (i.e., do not drop elbows beyond the level of the chest wall). This will decrease stress on the shoulder joint and allow for a better mechanical advantage, thus providing better resistance for the muscle. To ensure proper depth of the elbows, the use of a partner to watch elbow depth is beneficial. Once proper depth has been achieved, a towel placed on the chest may be used as a reminder. As the bar touches the towel, the push phase of the movement begins. When performing the chest press, as with any exercise, control of the weight must be maintained. The bar should never be bounced off the chest.

Military Press

Problem

Extreme shoulder external rotation and abduction during a behind-the-neck military press puts stress on the shoulder capsule, contributing to shoulder instability.

Solution

A safer way to perform this exercise and eliminate these stresses is to do the military press in front of the head. Also, by not allowing the shoulder to drop below 60° abduction, the deltoid muscle moves the weight through the range of motion without putting undue stress on the rotator cuff.

Squats

Problem

When performing a squat in which the thighs are parallel to or lowered to the floor, there is an excessive amount of shear force on the knee in a position where the articular cartilage is thinnest.

Solution

When weight training, the individual should avoid deep squats and maintain lumbar spine stability. Alternative lifts to the squat may include the leg press and the box squat. When employing the box squat, the box must be used only as a guide for appropriate depth of movement. The box itself should never be used to drop down to and rest on or bounce off of to gain momentum. When performing the leg press, the depth of the movement should entail not allowing the knees to be bent at greater than a 90° angle.

Adolescent weight training, like any activity, has the potential to result in musculoskeletal injury. However, the rate of injury does not seem to be any higher than that of other activities adolescents participate in on a daily basis. Through proper teaching, close supervision, and adherence to suggested guidelines, the rate of injuries can be further reduced. Strength training is a safe and beneficial means of exercise for adolescent populations.

Prevention of Injury

Though all sports activities carry an inherent risk of injury, certain principles can be applied that will help decrease the number of injuries sustained. Strength and conditioning techniques have already been covered, and multiple studies show the benefits of such training for athletes of all ages. Following are other important areas of intervention.

Preparticipation Physical Examination

All athletes should have a complete evaluation before their entry into organized sports. The preparticipation physical examination (PPE) is not intended to be a comprehensive medical examination but rather focused on sports participation. Particular attention should be paid to previous musculoskeletal injuries because there is a high rate of recurrence if they have not been properly rehabilitated. Ideally, a physician with training and specific knowledge in the adolescent athlete population should conduct the examination.

Treatment and Rehabilitation of Injuries

The relative lack of medical care for young athletes has resulted in injuries going undiagnosed and in diagnosed injuries not being properly rehabilitated. In 2009, only 42% of secondary schools had access to athletic trainers (Pryor, 2015). Fortunately, as of 2013, approximately 60% of secondary schools now have access to athletic trainers; however, this rate is still too low when it comes to protecting the young athletic population. First, injuries that are undiagnosed can lead to serious health complications. Second, when an athlete is injured, he or she is highly susceptible to reinjury of that limb or joint over the next several years. Improperly treated first-time injuries or reinjury might eventually limit participation in physical activity later in life, thereby leading to other health complications (Valovich McLeod et al., 2011). Many of these "old injuries" can be assessed during the PPE, but coaches and athletic trainers must ensure that all injuries receive proper initial and follow-up care.

Stretching Programs

To improve overall flexibility and mobility, specific exercises should be a routine part of all conditioning programs before and during the sports season. Major muscle groups and joints benefit from a dynamic warm up before activity, which increases tissue temperature and blood flow and has other positive physiological effects (Behm et al., 2016; Opplert & Babault, 2018). Prior to activity, dynamic stretching lasting greater than 2 minutes with a fast frequency of movement may increase performance and help to increase range of motion. Although static stretching and proprioceptive neuromuscular facilitation have been shown to decrease acute injury with running, sprinting, and other repetitive activities, these techniques have not been shown to decrease all causes of injury or overuse conditions. It is unclear if any stretch technique will decrease exercise-induced muscle soreness, yet after exercise, any stretch technique seems to temporarily increase range of motion. Therefore, stretching of any kind is of benefit depending upon the context in which it is used (Behm et al., 2016).

Coaching Techniques

Coaches can play a valuable role in the prevention of acute and chronic injuries among their young athletes. However, they must be knowledgeable in the fundamental techniques of their sport and know the proper principles of strength and conditioning. A basic understanding of the anatomic variations of young athletes is also helpful.

The overall training load and progression toward more intense training early in the course of a sports season are major determinants in the development of overuse injuries, along with other factors previously discussed. In addition to placing increased stress on the muscles and joints, the body is more likely to fatigue, thus compromising form and technique, which increases the risk of injury even more. As discussed earlier, an increase in total training volume or intensity of no more than 10% per week has been suggested to provide coaches with a model of how to limit injury risk (Stricker et al., 2020). For example, a young distance runner who begins the week running 3 miles per day would increase that distance to no more than 3.3 miles the next week. The same principle can be applied to young pitchers, swimmers, or gymnasts regarding the overall length of their training sessions.

Female Athletes

At the time of the PPE or, if appropriate, for a specific injury or complaint, a detailed menstrual history should be obtained from all female athletes. Any history of primary amenorrhea (i.e., absence of menses by age 16) or secondary amenorrhea (i.e., absence of menses for more than three consecutive cycles after regular monthly cycles have become established) should be further explored. Many female athletes believe that menstrual irregularities (i.e., absent menses or scant flow) during their competitive season are normal and will not perceive them as a problem unless specifically questioned. Such irregularity is typically indicative of poor nutritional intake, which is often the result of burning more calories than are being consumed. This energy (i.e., calorie) deficit may be unintentional (i.e., poor eating habits) or intentional (i.e., disordered eating).

Female athletes with a history of primary or secondary amenorrhea should be evaluated by a physician. Nutrition education or referral to a nutritionist may also be appropriate. Any history of previous stress fractures should also prompt a thorough training history (e.g., overload, poor technique, or "too much, too soon") and a review of menstrual history and nutritional intake because such injuries should raise suspicion for the presence of the female athlete triad (i.e., eating disorder, amenorrhea, and osteoporosis).

Prescription Stimulant Medications

The increasing use of stimulant medications for the treatment of attention deficit hyperactivity disorder (ADHD) is an emerging area of uncertainty and discussion in the sports medicine field. The majority of ADHD medications (i.e., methylphenidate [Ritalin], dextroamphetamine [Dexedrine], and amphetamine plus dextroamphetamine [Adderall]) are stimulants and have been well documented as having improved the quality of life and academic success of individuals using them. In addition to the benefits seen in the classroom, when given appropriate medication, young athletes with ADHD also show increased ability to concentrate on tasks during athletic practices. Currently, athletes with ADHD should continue to take their medications as prescribed, regardless of athletic activity, and parents/guardians, athletes, and medical providers should be aware that taking these medications increases the risk of heat illness, and that they can potentially interfere with concussion diagnosis and recovery. Additionally, many sports organizations (e.g., NCAA, IOC) have banned stimulant use and may have specific policies to adhere to in order to continue taking the medication while participating in athletics. Future research should further define the ergogenic potency of these medications within the ADHD population (Stewman et al., 2018).

Review Questions

1. Where are the common areas for apophysitis?
2. What does research indicate is the primary motivating factor for children to engage in organized sports?
3. What is the most common cause reported for withdrawing from sports among high school students?
4. On average, boys will see how much of an increase in muscle mass between the ages of 10 and 17 years?
5. What is the anatomic term for the point on a long bone where large muscle–tendon units attach?
6. True or false? Changes in bone length occur more slowly than length changes in muscle–tendon structures.

7. What is the technical term for a growth plate?

8. Where can you find reliable and valid information regarding adolescents and injury?

9. True or false? Severe ligament injuries are more common in children than in adults.

10. What specific anatomical structure and injury does the term *Salter–Harris classification* refer to?

11. According to the text, what is the most important intrinsic factor related to youth sports injuries?

12. Describe the factors that contribute to youth sports injury.

13. What are the recommended steps to help reduce overtraining, inadequate rest, and early specialization?

14. True or false? Most youth sports coaches have no formal training.

15. Define the terms *osteomyelitis* and *pyomyositis*.

16. Briefly explain the guidelines on adolescent strength training in children.

17. Using the 1-RM equivalent equation presented in the text, calculate the 1-RM equivalent for 120 pounds lifted for 10 repetitions on the bench press.

References

Behm, D. G., Blazevich, A. J., Kay, A. D., & McHugh, M. (2016). Acute effects of muscle stretching on physical performance, range of motion, and injury incidence in healthy active individuals: A systematic review. *Applied Physiology, Nutrition, and Metabolism, 41*(1), 1–11.

Brown, K. A., Patel, D. R., & Darmawan, D. (2017). Participation in sports in relation to adolescent growth and development. *Translational Pediatrics, 6*(3), 150.

Casa, D. J., Guskiewicz, K. M., Anderson, S. A., Courson, R. W., Heck, J. F., Jimenez, C. C., . . . Walsh, K. M. (2012). National Athletic Trainers' Association position statement: Preventing sudden death in sports. *Journal of Athletic Training, 47*(1), 96–118.

Centers for Disease Control and Prevention (CDC). (n.d.). A national action plan for child injury prevention: Protecting our nation's future. Retrieved from https://www.cdc.gov/safechild/pdf/nap_overview_v12.pdf

Confroy, K., Miles, C., Kaplan, S., & Skelton, J. A. (2021). Pediatric obesity and sports medicine: A narrative review and clinical recommendations. *Clinical Journal of Sport Medicine, 31*(6), e484–e498.

DiFiori, J. P., Benjamin, H. J., Brenner, J., Gregory, A., Jayanthi, N., Landry, G., & Luke, A. (2014). Overuse injuries and burnout in youth sports: A position statement from the American Medical Society of Sports Medicine. *Clinical Journal of Sport Medicine, 24*(1), 3–20.

Faigenbaum, A., & Micheli, L. (2017). Youth strength training. Retrieved from https://www.acsm.org/docs/default-source/files-for-resource-library/smb-youth-strength-training.pdf?sfvrsn=85a44429_2

Faigenbaum, A. D. (2018). Youth resistance training: The good, the bad, and the ugly—the year was 2017. *Pediatric Exercise Science, 30*, 19–24.

Fedorak, G. T., Brough, A. K., Miyamoto, R. H., & Raney, E. M. (2018). The epidemiology of slipped capital femoral epiphysis in American Samoa. *Hawai'i Journal of Medicine & Public Health, 77*(9), 215–219.

Haff, G. G., & Triplett, N. T. (2016). *Essentials of strength training and conditioning*. (4th ed.). Champaign, IL: Human Kinetics.

Hales, C. M., Carroll, M. D., Fryar, C. D., & Ogden, C. L. (2017). Prevalence of obesity among adults and youth: United States, 2015–2016. Retrieved from https://www.cdc.gov/nchs/data/databriefs/db288.pdf

Hickey, G., & Fricker, P. (1999). Attention deficit hyperactivity disorder, CNS stimulants and sport. *Sports Medicine, 27*(1), 11–21.

Huggins, R. A., Coleman, K. A., Attanasio, S. M., Cooper, G. L., Endres, B. D., Harper, R. C., Huemme, K. L., Morris, R. F., Pike Lacey, A. M., Peterson, B. C., Pryor, R. R., & Casa, D. J. (2019). Athletic trainer services in the secondary school setting: The athletic training locations and services project. *Journal of Athletic Training, 54*(11), 1129–1139.

Huggins, R. A., Scarneo, S. E., Casa, D. J., Belval, L. N., Carr, K. S., Chiampas, G., . . . Weston, T. (2017). The inter-association task force document on emergency health and safety: Best-practice recommendations for youth sports leagues. *Journal of Athletic Training, 52*(4), 384–400.

Jamtvedt, G., Herbert, R. D., Flottorp, S., Odgaard-Jensen, J., Håvelsrud, K., Barratt, A., . . . Oxman, D. (2010). A pragmatic randomised trial of stretching before and after physical activity to prevent injury and soreness. *British Journal of Sports Medicine, 44*(14), 1002–1009.

Kann, L., McManus, T., Harris, W. A., Shanklin, S. L., Flint, K. H., Hawkins, J., . . . Zaza, S. (2016). Youth Risk Behavior Surveillance—United States, 2015. *MMWR, 65*(6), 1–174.

LaPrade, R. F., Agel, J., Baker, J., Brenner, J. S., Cordasco, F. A., Côté, J., Engebretsen, L., Feeley, B. T., Gould, D., Hainline, B., Hewett, T., Jayanthi, N., Kocher, M. S., Myer, G. D., Nissen, C. W., Philippon, M. J., & Provencher, M. T. (2016). AOSSM early sport specialization consensus statement. *Orthopaedic Journal of Sports Medicine, 4*(4), 1–8.

Lee, E. Y., & Yoon, K. H. (2018). Epidemic obesity in children and adolescents: Risk factors and prevention. *Frontiers of Medicine, 12*(6), 658–666.

The Living Law. (n.d.). Retrieved from http://www.titleix.info/History/The-Living-Law.aspx

Lloyd, R. S., Faigenbaum, A. D., Stone, M. H., Oliver, J. L., Jeffreys, I., Moody, J. A., ... & Myer, G. D. (2014). Position statement on youth resistance training: The 2014 International Consensus. *British Journal of Sports Medicine, 48*(7), 498–505.

Lovejoy III, J. F., Alexander, K., Dinan, D., Drehner, D., Khan-Assad, N., & Lacerda, I. R. (2017). Team approach: Pyomyositis. *JBJS Reviews, 5*(6), e4.

Mandorino, M., Figueiredo, A. J., Gjaka, M., & Tessitore, A. (2022). Injury incidence and risk factors in youth soccer players: A systematic literature review. Part II: Intrinsic and extrinsic risk factors. *Biology of Sport, 40*(1), 27–49.

McCambridge, T. M., & Stricker, P. R. (2008). Strength training by children and adolescents. *Pediatrics, 121*(4), 835–840.

National Federation of State High School Associations (NFHS). (n.d.) School athletics participation survey. Retrieved from http://www.nfhs.org/ParticipationStatics/PDF/2014-15_Participation_Survey_Results.pdf

National Physical Activity Plan Alliance. (2016). 2016 United States report card on physical activity for children and youth. Retrieved from http://www.physicalactivityplan.org/reportcard/2016FINAL_USReportCard.pdf

Nationwide Children's Hospital. (n.d.). Allowing youth sports to be child's play. Retrieved from https://www.nationwidechildrens.org/specialties/sports-medicine/sports-medicine-articles/allowing-youth-sports-to-be-childs-play

Nguyen, J. C., Sheehan, S. E., Davis, K. W., & Gill, K. G. (2017). Sports and the growing musculoskeletal system: Sports imaging series. *Radiology, 284*(1), 25–42.

Ogden, J. A. (1981). Injury to the growth mechanism of the immature skeleton. *Skeletal Radiology, 6*(4), 237–253.

Opplert, J., & Babault, N. (2018). Acute effects of dynamic stretching on muscle flexibility and performance: An analysis of the current literature. *Sports Medicine, 48*(2), 299–325.

Osgood, R. B. (1903). Lesions of the tibial tubercle occurring during adolescence. *Boston Medical and Surgical Journal, 148*, 114–117.

Pandya, N. K. (2021). Disparities in youth sports and barriers to participation. *Current Reviews in Musculoskeletal Medicine, 14*, 441–446.

Peterson, H. A. (1994). Physeal fractures: Part 3: Classification. *Journal of Pediatric Orthopaedics, 14*(4), 439.

Post, E., Winterstein, A. P., Hetzel, S. J., Lutes, B., & McGuine, T. A. (2019). School and community socioeconomic status and access to athletic trainer services in Wisconsin secondary schools. *Journal of Athletic Training, 54*(2), 177–181.

Pryor, R. R., Casa, D. J., Vandermark, L. W., Stearns, R. L., Attanasio, S. M., Fontaine, G. J., & Wafer, A. M. (2015). Athletic training services in public secondary schools: A benchmark study. *Journal of Athletic Training, 50*(2), 156–162.

Ritzer, E. E., Yang, J., Kistamgari, S., Collins, C. L., & Smith, G. A. (2021). An epidemiologic comparison of acute and overuse injuries in high school sports. *Injury Epidemiology, 8*(1), 1–11.

Salter, R. B., & Harris, W. R. (1963). Injuries involving the epiphyseal plate. *Journal of Bone & Joint Surgery, 45*(3), 587–622.

Sports & Fitness Industry Association. (2016). 2016 Sports, fitness, and leisure activities topline participation report. Retrieved from https://www.sfia.org/reports/411_2016-Sports%2C-Fitness%2C-and-Leisure-Activities-Topline-Participation-Report

Statistic Brain Research Institute. (2017). Youth sports program statistics. Retrieved from http://www.statisticbrain.com/youth-sports-statistics/

Stewman, C. G., Liebman, C., Fink, L., & Sandella, B. (2018). Attention deficit hyperactivity disorder: Unique considerations in athletes. *Sports Health, 10*(1), 40–46.

Stricker, P. R., Faigenbaum, A. D., McCambridge, T. M., & Council on Sports Medicine and Fitness. (2020). Resistance training for children and adolescents. *Pediatrics, 145*(6), e20201011.

Tenforde, A. S., Montalvo, A. M., Nelson, V. R., Myer, G. D., Brenner, J. S., ... & Herman, D. C. (2022). Current sport organization guidelines from the AMSSM 2019 Youth Early Sport Specialization research summit. *Sports Health, 14*(1), 135–141.

U.S. Department of Health and Human Services. (2018). Physical activity guidelines for Americans. Retrieved from https://health.gov/paguidelines/second-edition/pdf/Physical_Activity_Guidelines_2nd_edition.pdf

Valovich McLeod, T., Decoster, L., Loud, K., Micheli, L., Parker, J., Sandrey, M., & White, C. (2011). National Athletic Trainers' Association position statement: Prevention of pediatric overuse injuries. *Journal of Athletic Training, 46*(2), 206–220.

Weihrauch-Blüher, S., Schwarz, P., & Klusmann, J. H. (2018). Childhood obesity: Increased risk for cardiometabolic disease and cancer in adulthood. *Metabolism, 92*, 147–152.

Welton, K. L., Kraeutler, M. J., Pierpoint, L. A., Bartley, J. H., McCarty, E. C., & Comstock, R. D. (2018). Injury recurrence among high school athletes in the United States: A decade of patterns and trends, 2005–2006 through 2015–2016. *Orthopaedic Journal of Sports Medicine, 6*(1), 2325967117745788.

Wik, E. H., Martínez-Silván, D., Farooq, A., Cardinale, M., Johnson, A., & Bahr, R. (2020). Skeletal maturation and growth rates are related to bone and growth plate injuries in adolescent athletics. *Scandinavian Journal of Medicine & Science in Sports, 30*(5), 894–903.

Windt, J., & Gabbett, T. J. (2017). How do training and competition workloads relate to injury? The workload–injury aetiology model. *British Journal of Sports Medicine, 51*(5), 428–435.

Youth Sports Safety Alliance. (n.d.). National action plan for sports safety. Retrieved from http://www.youthsportssafetyalliance.org/sites/default/files/docs/National-Action-Plan.pdf

Glossary of Terms

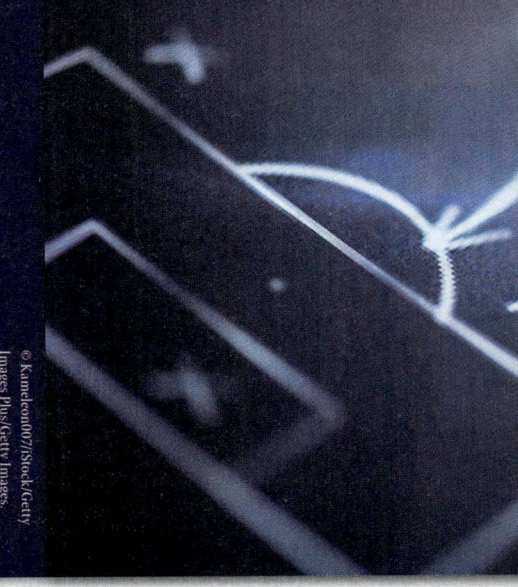

A

Abrasions—Rubbing or scraping off of skin.

Acclimatization—The process in which physiology is adapted to suit a new or change in environment (i.e., temperature, altitude, light, etc.).

Achilles tendon rupture—Complete tear of the Achilles tendon.

Achilles tendonitis—Inflammation of the Achilles tendon.

Acne mechanica—Sports acne that results from pressure, heat, or friction.

Acromioclavicular (AC) joint—Articulation (arthrodial) formed by the distal end of the clavicle and the acromion process.

Acute appendicitis—Severe inflammation of the appendix caused by trapped feces or an occurrence of a virus, bacteria, or parasite and accompanied by increasing symptoms (i.e., pain, fever, nausea) within 24 to 48 hours; is considered a medical emergency.

Acute injury—Injury characterized by rapid onset, resulting from a traumatic event.

Acute mountain sickness—Symptoms such as headache, nausea, vomiting, dizziness, and shortness of breath that come on within 24 hours of ascending into altitude; also called altitude sickness.

Adenosine triphosphate (ATP)—The molecule that is the body's direct source of energy.

Adequate Intake (AI)—The daily intake level based on observed or experimentally determined estimates of nutrient intake by a group(s) of apparently healthy people.

Adjustment disorder—An emotional or behavioral reaction in response to specific events. It is considered unhealthy if the reaction lasts longer than 3 months.

Aerobic exercise—Exercise of long duration and usually at low to medium intensity that requires the body to use oxygen to meet the energy demands.

Aerobic fitness—The amount of work that can be accomplished using the oxidative system of converting nutrients into energy. Also called aerobic power.

Aerobic system—An energy system that makes ATP with the use of oxygen.

Agonist muscles—Muscles that are considered the prime movers of a joint.

Allergy—An overreaction of the immune system to any substance that initiates an inflammatory response.

Altitude sickness—Symptoms such as headache, nausea, vomiting, dizziness, and shortness of breath that come on within 24 hours of ascending into altitude; also called acute mountain sickness.

Amenorrhea—Absence or suppression of menstruation.

Amino acids—Building blocks of proteins.

Anaerobic exercise—Exercise of short duration and high intensity that does not require the body to use oxygen to meet energy demands.

Anaerobic fitness—The amount of work that can be accomplished using nonoxidative pathways to produce energy.

Anaerobic system—An energy system that makes ATP and lactic acid without oxygen.

Analgesic—Agent that relieves pain without causing a complete loss of sensation.

Anaphylaxis—A serious, sudden, and life-threatening allergic reaction that usually presents with throat or tongue swelling, shortness of breath, and other grave symptoms.

Anatomic—Pertaining to anatomy.

Angiogenesis—Formation of capillaries that interconnect, resulting in the formation of new vessels.

Anhedonia—No longer experiencing pleasure from activities that once were enjoyable.

Anisocoria—Unequal size pupils that may be related to an acute condition such as head injury or occur naturally. It is important to perform a thorough clinical evaluation to determine the appropriate management.

Ankle sprain—Injury to any of the ligaments of the ankle.

Anorexia nervosa—A disorder characterized by a pattern of self-starvation with a concomitant obsession with being thin and an overwhelming fear of being fat.

Antagonist muscles—Muscles that counteract the action of the agonist muscles.

Anterior—Located before or in front of.

Anterograde amnesia—Inability to recall events that have occurred after an amnesia-inducing injury.

Antibiotic resistance—When bacteria adapt and become resistant to antibiotic medication.

Anti-inflammatory drug—Drug designed to prevent swelling. Two basic categories are currently in use: steroidal and nonsteroidal.

Antioxidants—Protective compounds that fight against free radicals or highly reactive molecules.

Antipyretic—Agent that relieves or reduces fever.

Anxiety—Feelings of apprehensiveness, powerlessness, and impending danger along with physical symptoms of increased heart rate and breathing rate, sweating, and trembling to the point where it interferes with one's ability to perform daily functions.

Apophysis—Bony outgrowth to which muscles attach.

Apophysitis—Inflammation or stress injury where a tendon attaches near or around growth plates of bones resulting in pain and/or excessive pulling of the bone causing structural changes.

Apoptosis—Process of programmed cell death. Biochemical events can lead to changes in cell characteristics, thereby causing cell death.

Arachidonic acid—Chemical released when cells are damaged that serves as a precursor to the formation of other inflammatory chemicals, including leukotrienes and prostaglandins.

Athletic energy deficit—Occurs when an athlete does not consume enough calories to properly sustain body function and his or her caloric needs for exercise. Also known as relative energy deficiency in sport (RED-S).

Athletic training student aides—Students who observe and experience the field of athletic training under the direct supervision of a certified or licensed athletic trainer.

Attention deficit hyperactivity disorder (ADHD)—A disorder characterized by an abnormal level of inattentiveness, hyperactivity, and/or impulsiveness that interferes with social and academic function.

Automated external defibrillator (AED)—A lightweight, portable device that delivers an electric shock through the chest to the heart. The shock can potentially reset an irregular heartbeat and allow a normal rhythm to resume following sudden cardiac arrest.

Avascular necrosis—Tissue death due to lack of blood supply.

Avulsion fracture—Piece of bone is pulled off by tendons or ligaments likely due to strong forces.

Avulsions—Forcible tearing away or separation.

B

Bacteria (sing. bacterium)—Microorganisms that are usually single-celled and found in most environments on Earth. They are very versatile, can survive in extreme conditions, and can be both harmful and helpful. It is estimated that the human body contains more bacterial cells than human cells.

Ballistic stretching—Stretching technique that uses quick, sudden, and repetitive bouncing motions.

Bandage—Material used to hold a dressing in place.

Basal metabolic rate (BMR)—The amount of energy needed to sustain functioning at rest (calculated after 12–18 hours of no exercise).

Bed bugs—Small insects in mattresses and other furniture that come out at night to feed on blood.

Bennett's fracture—Fracture and/or dislocation of the base of the first metacarpal bone (thumb) and trapezium (wrist).

Biological age—Age of individual based on stage of bone or biological development.

Biomechanics—Branch of study that applies the laws of mechanics, internal or external, to the living body.

Bipolar disorder—A manic-depressive illness that involves cycling mood swings from major depression to mania, during which individuals feel full of energy.

Blister—Excessive friction causing a buildup of fluid between the tissues of the skin.

Blood glucose—The amount of sugar in the blood, measured in milligrams per deciliter (mg/dL) or millimol per liter (mmol/L).

Blood-borne pathogen—Infectious organism in human blood that can lead to disease and is spread through direct contact with an infected person's blood.

Body composition—The makeup of the body divided into lean body weight, or fat free mass, and fat.

Body mass index (BMI)—A value derived from a person's height and weight that indicates nutritional status.

Bone age—The age of a person as determined by the current stage of bone ossification.

Bonking—Extreme fatigue that occurs from depleting carbohydrate stores.

Boundary layer—Thin layer of warm air around the skin.

Boutonnière deformity—Buttonhole deformity whereby the proximal interphalangeal joint of the finger is forced through the central band of the tendon of the extensor digitorum muscle.

Boxer's fracture—Fracture of the proximal or neck section of the fourth and/or fifth metacarpal bones.

Bradykinin—Inflammatory chemical released when tissues are damaged; it causes increased pain in the area and may play a role in the production of other inflammatory chemicals, such as prostaglandins.

Branched chain amino acids (BCAAs)—Essential amino acids.

Bronchitis—Inflammation of the bronchial tree.

Bulimia nervosa—A disorder characterized by repeated bouts of binge eating followed by some form of purging, such as vomiting, use of laxatives, fasting, and vigorous and excessive exercise.

Bunion—Inflammation and joint deformity of the first metatarsal phalangeal joint usually accompanied by pain and dysfunction.

Bursa—Small, fluid-filled sac, typically located over bony prominences, that assists in cushioning and reducing friction.

Bursitis—Inflammation of a bursa.

C

Callus—Rough, raised, and thickened area of skin due to friction.

Calorie—Kilocalorie; unit of energy equal to 1,000 calories.

Carbohydrate loading—A nutritional technique used to maximize the volume of stored carbohydrate in the muscle and liver to improve performance.

Carbohydrate—A macronutrient consisting of carbon, hydrogen, and oxygen atoms that provides energy for high-intensity exercise.

Carbuncle—Group of bacterial infected hair follicles with pus. They are larger and deeper than furuncles.

Cardiopulmonary resuscitation (CPR)—A technique involving repeated compression of a patient's chest and rescue breathing to restore the blood circulation of a person who has suffered cardiac arrest.

Carpal tunnel syndrome—A complex set of symptoms resulting from pressure on the median nerve as it passes through the carpal tunnel of the wrist, causing soreness and numbness.

Carpal tunnel—Anatomic region of the wrist where the median nerve and the majority of the tendons of the anterior forearm pass into the hand.

Catastrophic injury—Injury involving damage to the brain and/or spinal cord that presents a potentially life-threatening situation or the possibility of permanent disability.

Cauliflower ear—Blood and fluid accumulates in the pinna (auricle) of the ear due to friction or pressure and disrupts normal blood flow, resulting in excessive scarring and deformity; common in wrestlers.

Cellulitis—A potentially serious bacterial skin infection. The skin appears red, swollen, and warm and painful to the touch.

Cerebral contusion—Bruising of the brain tissue.

Certified diabetes educator—A healthcare professional who has special education in the management of diabetes.

Certified Strength and Conditioning Specialist (CSCS)—Professional who trains athletes in order to improve athletic performance by using scientific knowledge of many disciplines such as exercise physiology to design testing and workout sessions, strength training and coordination programs, and provide nutrition and injury prevention guidance.

Chilblain—An exaggerated inflammatory response to cold exposure for 1–5 hours due to prolonged vasoconstriction of skin blood vessels.

Cholesterol—A sterol or fat-like substance found in cell membranes that helps produce vitamin D, steroid hormones, and bile.

Chondromalacia—Abnormal softening of cartilage between the patella and the femur.

Chronic injury—Injury characterized by a slow, insidious onset, implying a gradual development of structural damage.

Chronic traumatic encephalopathy (CTE)—Condition that can be identified only after death with a brain autopsy. It is a degenerative disease characterized by a distinct collection of tau proteins in several areas of the brain that affect function.

Chronological age—Age since birth.

Central nervous system (CNS)—Consists of the brain and spinal cord and is the processing center for bodily functions.

Cold urticaria—Condition in which the skin reacts to exposure to cold with localized edema associated with severe itching.

Colic—Intra-abdominal pain.

Colitis—Inflammation of the colon.

Collagen—The major protein of connective tissue.

Colles' fracture—Transverse fracture of the distal radius.

Commission—A legal liability arising when individuals perform acts that are not legally theirs to perform.

Common cold—A viral infectious disease of the upper respiratory tract that primarily affects the nose. The throat, sinuses, and larynx may also be affected.

Commotio cordis—A rare, lethal disruption of heart rhythm as a result of abrupt, blunt, nonpenetrating trauma to the chest/heart area.

Compartment syndrome—Inflammation of one of the lower leg compartments leading to increased pressure within the compartment and diminished sensation, blood flow, and function of the foot and ankle.

Complement system—Refers to the part of the immune system that involves the complement proteins which assist host defense and inflammation.

Complete protein—A protein that contains all 9 essential amino acids (e.g., meat, dairy, eggs, and soy).

Complex carbohydrates—Polysaccharides that contain more nutrients and fiber compared to simple carbohydrate.

Concentric contraction—Occurs when a muscle shortens and contracts resulting in joint movement.

Conduction—Heating through direct contact with a medium.

Connective tissue—The most common tissue in the body; includes ligaments, bones, retinaculum, joint capsules, cartilage, fascia, and tendons.

Contact dermatitis—Inflammation or an allergic reaction of the skin caused by direct contact with an irritating substance.

Continuous glucose monitor (CGM)—A wearable medical device that continuously measures blood sugar.

Contrecoup—Brain contusion injury to the opposite side of the site of impact.

Contusion—Bruise or injury to soft tissue that does not break the skin.

Convection—Heating through another medium, such as air or liquid.

Core body temperature—Internal body temperature usually measured orally or rectally.

Corn—Thickened skin similar to a callus that develops in response to friction or pressure.

Costochondral separation—Injury to the ribs at the attachment of the cartilage.

Coup—Brain contusion injury to the same side as the site of the impact.

Crepitation—Crackling, grating, or grinding sound heard during the movement of a broken bone or joint.

Critical force—The force at which the tissue's ability to withstand stress and strain is exceeded.

Cryotherapy—Therapeutic use of cold.

Cerebrospinal fluid (CSF)—Clear fluid that surrounds the spinal cord and brain.

D

de Quervain's disease—Inflammation of sheaths surrounding the extensor tendons of the thumb.

Dehydration—Process of losing body water through sweating, diarrhea, respiration, and vomiting.

Depressed skull fracture—A fracture of the skull where it is sunken in from a trauma; can occur with or without a cut in the scalp.

Detached retina—The retina in the back of the eye pulls away from the blood vessels and is deprived of oxygen and nutrients; this is a medical emergency.

Diabetic coma—A life-threatening condition caused by complications of having high blood sugar for too long, resulting in an altered state or unconsciousness.

Diabetic ketoacidosis (DKA)—A serious condition that usually results from extended periods of high blood sugar causing a high concentration of ketones in the blood, this creates an acidic environment in the body, which can lead to organ damage and other complications.

Dietary Reference Intakes (DRI)—This value includes the Recommended Dietary Allowance (RDA) and average daily level of intake sufficient to meet the nutrient requirements of nearly all (97–98%) healthy people.

Diplopia—Double vision.

Disaccharide—Two monosaccharide molecules combined; include lactose (milk sugar), sucrose, and maltose.

Dislocation of the tibiofemoral joint—Complete separation of the tibia and femur joint ("knee joint"), which is usually visually obvious and a medical emergency.

Dislocation—The displacement of contiguous surfaces of bones comprising a joint.

Distal interphalangeal (DIP) joint—The joint formed by the articulation between the middle and distal phalanges of the digits (hinge type of joint).

Dorsiflexion—Bending the foot toward the dorsum, or shin; the opposite of plantar flexion.

Dressing—Covering, either protective or supportive, that is applied to an injury or wound.

Dynamic stretching—A voluntary stretching technique that uses full-range, sport-like motions to warm up.

Dyspnea—Difficult or painful breathing.

Dysthymia—Characterized by nondisabling depressive symptoms that are chronic but do not cause changes in usual functioning.

E

Eccentric exercises—Exercises that concentrate or focus on the eccentric contraction of the movement (the muscle lengthens while it contracts); sometimes referred to as the negative muscle contraction.

Ecchymosis—Black-and-blue discoloration of the skin caused by hemorrhage.

Edema—Abnormal accumulation of fluid in the interstitial tissue; disruption of homeostatic fluid balance in the tissues.

Endocrinologist—A physician who specializes in the endocrine system and hormones.

Environmental—The aggregate of surrounding things, conditions, or influences related to one's surroundings.

Epicondylitis—Inflammatory response of the soft tissue that attaches to the epicondyle.

Epidemiology—The study of the distribution of disease or injury within a population and its environment.

Epidural (extradural) hematoma—Bleeding between the dura and the cranial bones.

Epilepsy—A chronic neurological disorder characterized by sudden attacks of brain dysfunction, including altered consciousness, abnormal motor activity, sensory phenomena, and/or inappropriate behavior.

Epiphyseal plate—A hyaline cartilage plate at the end of each long bone where the growth center of the bone resides.

Epiphysis—Cartilaginous growth region of a bone.

Epistaxis—Nosebleed.

Ergogenic aid—Anything, however, usually supplements and pharmacological sources, that has the potential to increase the work output of the person consuming or using it.

Erythema—Red discoloration of the skin.

Essential amino acids—Nine amino acids (histidine, isoleucine, leucine, lysine, methionine, phenylalanine, threonine, tryptophan, and valine) that the body cannot make and therefore must obtain from the diet.

Etiology—Science dealing with causes of disease or injury.

Euhydration—The state of being optimally hydrated so body systems can function normally.

Evaporation—The process of turning liquid into vapor, and the means by which the body cools itself via sweating.

Eversion (medial) ankle sprain—Injury to the medial ligaments due to excessive eversion.

Eversion—Movement that entails turning the sole of the foot outward.

Exercise mode—Refers to the specific activity being performed (e.g., running, swimming, or cycling).

Exercise order—Specific order in which exercises should be performed within a session.

Exercise progression—Involves gradually increasing the frequency, intensity, and/or duration of training to achieve set goals.

Exercise selection—Choosing a training exercise based on the movement and the muscular requirements of the sport.

Exercise-associated hyponatremia (EAH)—A life-threatening medical condition created when there is a low concentration of sodium in the blood (<135 mEq/L) due to overconsumption of fluids and not enough sodium intake or extreme sodium loss.

Exercise-associated muscle cramp (EAMC)—Involuntary, extremely painful muscle spasm associated with exercise, usually involves the gastrocnemius and hamstrings.

Exercise-induced asthma (EIA)—A constriction of the airway resulting from participation in exercise. Also known as exercise-induced bronchoconstriction (EIB), the term preferred by the American College of Allergy, Asthma, and Immunology.

Exercise-related transient abdominal pain (ETAP)—Commonly called a "stitch in the side," pain that is benign and self-limiting but may be stabbing or sharp when severe or achier and cramping when less intense. It can be recurrent and tends to be resistant to treatment.

Exertional heat exhaustion (EHE)—Involves generalized fatigue, hypotension, and cardiovascular insufficiency that occurs during exercise when heavy sweating, hypohydration, and elevated core body temperature occur.

Exertional heat illnesses (EHIs)—A general term given to physical conditions that can occur when exercising in the heat.

Exertional heatstroke (EHS)—Excessive heat buildup, with core temperatures exceeding 104°F (40°C) in the body, resulting in the body's inability to cool itself quickly, which may cause organs to malfunction. This is a medical emergency (cool first then transport).

Exertional rhabdomyolysis (ER)—Skeletal muscle breaks down, and its contents, such as creatine kinase, myoglobin, and electrolytes, enter the bloodstream; myoglobin may also be present in the urine.

Exertional sickling—A life-threatening condition resulting from many factors that cause lack of blood flow and cell death (e.g., too intense conditioning, heat, hypohydration, high altitude, illness).

Exophthalmos—A bulging of the eye anteriorly out of the orbit.

Exostosis—Bony outgrowths that protrude from the surface of a bone where there is not typical bony formation.

Extracellular fluid—Fluid outside of cells; also called interstitial fluid.

Extrinsic injury risk factors—Anything outside the body that can affect an individual, such as environmental temperature.

F

Fascia—Connective tissue that covers, supports, and connects, yet separates muscles, organs, vessels, nerves, and other structures.

Fat—A macronutrient consisting of carbon, hydrogen, and oxygen atoms that provides energy for low-intensity, long-duration exercise.

Fat-soluble vitamins—Vitamins A, D, E, and K, which are stored in the fat tissue; can be toxic to the body if they are in excess.

Female athlete triad—Condition when a female athlete has disordered eating (energy deficit), menstrual irregularities, and osteoporosis/osteopenia.

Femoral fracture—Fracture of the femur, which can be in several different areas of the bone.

Femoral neck stress fracture—A rare stress injury to the bony matrix in the femoral neck of the femur usually due to repetitive stress or overload.

Femoroacetabular impingement (FAI)—Pinching of tissues around the hip joint due to the femoral head not being congruent with the acetabulum.

Fiber—Nondigestible carbohydrate.

Fibroblast—Immature, fiber-producing cell of connective tissue that can mature into one of several cell types.

Fibroblastic phase—The second of the healing phases in which the body is beginning to build the infrastructure necessary for the injured site to recover.

Flail chest—A portion of the rib cage is separated from the rest of the chest wall, usually due to trauma, making breathing very difficult.

Flexibility—The range of motion in a given joint or combination of joints.

Focal onset aware seizure—A seizure that does not cause loss of awareness.

Focal onset impaired seizure—A seizure that affects a larger part of the brain and likely causes unawareness.

Focal onset seizure—A partial seizure occurring in just one area of the brain.

Folliculitis—Inflammation and bacterial infection of a hair follicle.

Fracture—A break or crack in a bone.

Fracture-dislocation—An injury resulting in both the fracture of a bone and dislocation at the joint.

Friction—Heat producing.

Frostbite—Freezing of tissues from excessive exposure to cold.

Frostnip—Less severe form of frostbite.

Functional knee brace—Braces used after a rehabilitation program while the athlete returns to sport.

Fungus (pl. fungi)—A eukaryotic organism such as yeasts, molds, and mushrooms.

Furuncle—Bacterial infection of a hair follicle that goes into the deeper layers of the skin. A small pocket of pus forms called a boil.

G

Gamekeeper's thumb—Sprain of the ulnar collateral ligament of the metacarpophalangeal joint of the thumb.

Ganglion—Herniation of the synovium surrounding a tendon and subsequent filling of the area with synovial fluid, resulting in a visible bump seen through the skin.

Gastritis—Inflammation of the stomach lining.

Gastroenteritis—Inflammation of the stomach and intestines.

Gastrointestinal (GI) system—The organ system that takes in food, digests it to extract and absorb energy and nutrients, and expels the remaining waste as feces. The mouth, esophagus, stomach, and intestines are part of this organ system.

Generalized onset seizure—A seizure that affects both sides of the brain; is dramatic and severe, often characterized by violent convulsions and loss of consciousness.

Glenohumeral (GH) joint—Articulation (spheroid) formed by the head of the humerus and the glenoid fossa of the scapula.

Glenohumeral internal rotation deficit (GIRD)—An adaptive process in which the throwing shoulder experiences a loss of internal rotation, usually caused by posterior capsular and rotator cuff tightness, owing to the repetitive cocking that occurs with the overhead throwing motion.

Glucagon kit—A container holding a syringe of saline and a vial of dry glucagon to be mixed together and injected in the event of diabetic coma.

Glucometer—A device used to measure blood glucose from a drop of blood.

Glycemic index (GI)—A rating based on how quickly carbohydrates are digested and absorbed into the bloodstream. The quicker the blood glucose rises, the higher the rating.

Golfer's elbow—Medial humeral epicondylitis related to incorrect golf technique.

Gradual onset injury—A condition that manifests itself over time where there is no single identifiable event and the distress or disability progressively increases.

H

Hamstrings—Group of three muscles on the posterior thigh that perform knee flexion (i.e., semimembranosis, semitendinosis, and biceps femoris).

Harris-Benedict equation—Equation used to calculate resting energy expenditure.

Heat syncope—Orthostatic dizziness or fainting due to heat exposure, hypohydration, and lack of blood flow to the brain; usually occurs during sudden change of position after not moving for a while.

Heel spur—Bony formation on calcaneus as a result of plantar fasciitis.

Hematoma—A localized collection of extravasated blood, usually clotted, that is confined within an organ, tissue, or space.

Hematuria—Blood, which can appear red or brown, in the urine.

Hemopneumothorax—Blood and air collect in the pleural cavity (space between the lungs and chest wall).

Hemorrhage—A profuse escape of blood from a ruptured blood vessel.

Hemostasis—Platelets and clotting factors in the bloodstream move to the site of injury to prevent excessive blood pooling; the mechanism that leads to the end of bleeding. This step helps attract other chemicals and cells to fully begin the inflammation phase.

Hemothorax—Blood collects in the pleural cavity (space between the lungs and chest wall).

Hepatitis B virus (HBV)—A liver infection that can lead to cirrhosis or liver cancer.

Hepatitis C virus (HCV)—A short-term or chronic liver infection.

Hernia—Protrusion of a part of an organ or tissue through an abnormal opening.

Herniated disk—Rupture or protrusion of the nucleus pulposus through the annulus fibrosus of an intervertebral disk.

Herpes gladiatorum—A common skin condition caused by herpes simplex virus type 1 (HSV-1).

Herpes simplex virus (herpes)—Categorized into two types: herpes type 1 (HSV-1, or oral herpes) and herpes type 2 (HSV-2, or genital herpes).

Herpes simplex virus type 1 (HSV-1)—Causes the common cold sore, or fever blister.

High altitude cerebral edema (HACE)—Fluid and swelling accumulation in the brain due to high altitude exposure.

High altitude pulmonary edema (HAPE)—Fluid and swelling accumulation in the lung due to high altitude exposure.

High-density lipoprotein (HDL)—A substance that transports lipids in the blood and lymph. Also referred to as "good cholesterol" because it is considered protective against cardiovascular disease. Levels should be >60 mg/dL.

Hip adductors—Group of three main muscles on the medial thigh that perform hip adduction (i.e., adductor magnus, adductor longus, adductor brevis).

Hip dislocation—Head of the femur fully displaces from the acetabulum.

Hip pointer—Contusion and associated hematoma to the superior/anterior portion of the iliac crest.

Histamine—Powerful inflammatory chemical that causes an increase in vascular permeability and vasodilation.

Hormones—Various internally secreted compounds formed in endocrine glands that affect the functions of specifically receptive organs or tissues.

Human immunodeficiency virus (HIV)—A virus that destroys important immune function, making it hard to fight disease and infection.

Human papillomavirus (HPV)—Over 120 distinct types of these viruses have been identified, at least two of which are related to plantar warts.

Humeroradial joint—Articulation (arthrodial) formed by the proximal end of the radius and the distal end of the humerus, specifically the capitellum.

Humeroulnar joint—Articulation (ginglymus) formed by the proximal end of the ulna, specifically the trochlear notch, with the distal end of the humerus, specifically the trochlea.

Hydrogenation—A process where hydrogen atoms are added to unsaturated fat to make unsaturated oils more conducive to baking and cooking.

Hyperesthesia—Nonpainful touch stimuli becomes painful.

Hyperextension—Extreme stretching of a body part. Joint range of motion beyond normal extension of the vertebral joints where there is compression on posterior bony structures.

Hyperglycemia—Excessively high level of blood sugar.

Hyperhydration—An excess of body water that causes enlarged intracellular and extracellular fluid volume.

Hyperosmolality—Increased concentration of a solution.

Hyperthermia—A body temperature above 104°F (40°C).

Hypertrophic cardiomyopathy (HCM)—The heart muscle becomes abnormally thick (i.e., hypertrophied), which makes it hard for the heart to pump blood.

Hypertrophy—Enlargement of a body part caused by an increase in the size of its cells.

Hyphema—Accumulated blood in the anterior chamber of the eye from torn blood vessels within anterior eye structures.

Hypoglycemia—Low blood sugar level.

Hypoglycemic unawareness—The inability to sense low blood sugar, likely from having low blood sugar too often.

Hypohydration—The provision of less than the normal amount of water to the body to meet its metabolic demands, creating a shortage of body water (mild, moderate, severe).

Hyponatremia—Low blood sodium levels due to too much water consumption and/or sodium deficiency.

Hypothermia—A body temperature below 95°F (35°C).

Hypovolemic shock—Inability of the cardiovascular system to maintain adequate circulation to all parts of the body.

I

Idiopathic—Cause of the condition is unknown.

Immediate energy system—The energy system that produces ATP at the fastest rate. Also known as the phosphagen system.

Impetigo—Skin infection caused by both streptococci and staphylococci bacteria.

Incision—Wound created when a sharp-edged object cuts through skin.

Incomplete protein—A protein that lacks one or more of the essential amino acids. This does not imply that they are inadequate or not needed in the diet.

Incubation period—Time between an exposure to an infectious agent and the appearance of symptoms of that infection.

Infectious mononucleosis—Viral infection characterized by general fatigue and enlargement of organs, such as the spleen.

Inflammation phase—The first of the healing phases in which the body is responding to the threat of infection while trying to assess and contain the original injury.

Ingrown toenail—Partial toenail growth laterally into the skin around the nail causing pain and inflammation.

Inhaler—A pressurized canister in which a prescribed medication for asthma is housed. When used properly, the medication is propelled into the lungs.

Injury—Physical harm or damage to the body.

Insidious—Slow onset or signs and symptoms occur with no obvious mechanism.

Insulin—A hormone that transports glucose from the blood into the cells of the body.

Intracellular fluid—Fluid contained inside the cell.

Intracerebral hematoma—Bleeding within the brain tissues.

Intracranial injury—Head injury characterized by disruption of blood vessels, either veins or arteries, resulting in the development of a hematoma or swelling within the confines of the cranium.

Intrinsic injury risk factors—Anything inherent to the body that cannot be changed, such as age or bony characteristics, or that is changeable, such as fitness level, both of which can affect the individual.

Inversion (lateral) ankle sprain—Injury to the lateral ligaments due to excessive inversion.

Inversion—Movement that entails turning the sole of the foot inward; inner border of the foot lifts.

Iontophoresis—Using an electrical current to drive a chemical/medication directly through the skin.

J

Jersey finger—Torn flexor tendon of finger typically due to the finger being caught in a jersey and pulled forcefully into extension.

Joint capsule—Saclike structure that encloses the ends of bones in a diarthrodial joint.

Jumper's knee—Irritation anywhere within the patellar tendon complex.

K

Kehr's sign—Pain radiating into the left shoulder that is normally associated with an injury to the spleen.

Ketoacidosis—Metabolic state with extremely high ketone concentration in the blood, often the result of not enough insulin and too high a blood glucose level.

Ketone—A molecule produced by metabolizing fat that can be measured in the urine and blood.

Kyphosis—Exaggeration of the normal curve of the thoracic spine.

L

Labral tear—Tear in cartilage surrounding hip or shoulder joint.

Lacerations—Cuts and gashes.

Lean body weight (LBW)—The amount of weight that is from lean body tissues; also called fat free mass.

Leukocyte—White blood cell.

Lice—Infestation of small insects in hair (head or pubic area) that causes intense itching.

Lipids—Fat molecules classified as triglycerides, phospholipids, and sterols.

Little league elbow—Condition related to excessive throwing that results in swelling of the growth plate at the medial epicondyle of the elbow (i.e., medial humeral epicondylitis).

Little league shoulder—Condition related to excessive throwing that results in pain and swelling in the growth plate in the upper humerus bone (i.e., proximal humeral epiphysitis).

Load volume—The total amount of weight lifted in a given workout session.

Locus of control—People's belief, or lack thereof, of being in control of events occurring in their lives.

Lordosis—Abnormal curvature of the lumbar vertebrae.

Low-density lipoprotein (LDL)—A substance that transports lipids in the blood and lymph. Also referred to as the "bad cholesterol" because it is considered to increase risk of cardiovascular disease. Levels should be <100 mg/dL.

Lower respiratory infection (LRI)—Infection that involves the lungs, bronchi, and larynx.

Luxation—Complete dislocation of a joint.

Lyme disease—Bites from infected blacklegged ticks that transfer bacteria to humans, resulting in a skin rash and other symptoms.

Lysosome—Cellular organelle that contains enzymes that break down waste materials and cellular debris.

M

Macrocycle—The largest unit of time (i.e., 1 year) when planning exercise to achieve a particular goal.

Macronutrients—Carbohydrates, proteins, and fats that provide calories for our energy needs.

Macrotrauma—Injury from a single, high-force event.

Major depression—Characterized by a combination of five or more symptoms and noticeable changes in usual functioning, such as sleep, eating, work, or school.

Major minerals—Minerals needed in quantities greater than 100 mg daily (i.e., calcium, phosphorus, magnesium, sodium, chloride, potassium, and sulfur).

Malaise—Discomfort and uneasiness caused by an illness.

Malfeasance—An act of commission in which wholly unlawful conduct is performed.

Mallet finger—Deformity of the distal interphalangeal joint of the finger caused by an avulsion of the tendon of the extensor digitorum muscle from the distal phalanx.

Marfan syndrome—Inherited disorder affecting connective tissue in the heart, blood vessels, eyes, and bones. Vision problems and defects in the large blood vessels leaving the heart are two primary conditions associated with this genetic disorder.

Maturation and remodeling phase—The third of the healing phases in which the body is completing the process of recovery and tissue is beginning to be formed according to how it will be used.

Menisci—Fibrocartilaginous structures within the knee joint for protection of the condyles.

Mesocycle—Smaller units of time in a macrocycle (i.e., weeks to months).

Metaphysis—The portion of growing bone located between the shaft and the epiphysis.

Methicillin-resistant *Staphylococcus aureus* (MRSA)—A type of staph bacteria that is resistant to several antibiotics.

Microcycle—Smallest units of time in a macrocycle (i.e., 2–4 weeks).

Micronutrients—Essential vitamins and minerals required in very small amounts for our body functions but that do not have caloric value or provide direct energy.

Microtrauma—Injury from overuse or repetitive stress.

Minerals—Micronutrients that lack carbon, are made of a variety of elements, and must be consumed regularly for proper body function.

Minor, or trace, minerals—Minerals needed in quantities of less than 100 mg daily (i.e., iron, zinc, chromium, fluoride, copper, manganese, iodine, molybdenum, and selenium).

Misfeasance—An act of commission in which lawful conduct is improperly performed.

Modality—Therapeutic agent or technique that helps create an optimal healing environment.

Molluscum contagiosum—Caused by the poxvirus, which manifests as a skin infection.

Mononucleosis—Viral illness that creates a variety of symptoms, including fever, muscle aches, and fatigue.

Monosaccharide—Simplest form of sugar and the basic unit of carbohydrate. Includes fructose, glucose, and galactose.

Monounsaturated fat—A fatty acid molecule with one double or triple bond per molecule that prevents hydrogen from bonding.

Morton's foot—Shortened first metatarsal or elongated second metatarsal bone that causes most of the weight bearing to be on the second metatarsal.

Morton's neuroma—Abnormal growth on nerves between the metatarsal heads.

Muscle endurance—The ability to sustain repeated contractions against a submaximal load.

Muscle power—The ability to generate force as quickly as possible, or a rate of work.

Muscle strength—The maximal amount of force that can be generated by muscles.

Myalgia—General muscle pain.

Myelin—A structure, composed of fats and proteins, that insulates the axon of a nerve.

Myocarditis—Infection of the heart with inflammation and damage to the heart muscle.

Myositis ossificans traumatica—Inflammation of muscle as a result of repeated traumatic blows, which causes bleeding and then bony deposits to collect within muscle.

Myositis ossificans—The abnormal calcification or ossification of bone within muscle tissue after an injury.

N

Negligence—The failure to do what a reasonably careful and prudent person would have done under the same or similar circumstances or doing something that a reasonably careful and prudent person would not have done under the same or similar circumstances.

Neurapraxia—A temporary loss of motor and sensory function owing to blockage of nerve conduction.

Neurocognitive insufficiency—Slower reaction time and cognitive processing of movement patterns.

Neuromechanical—The interaction of the nervous system with mechanical activity that creates movement.

Neuromuscular—Having characteristics of both nervous and muscular tissue.

Nonsteroidal anti-inflammatory drugs (NSAIDs)—Class of agents that block specific reactions in the inflammatory process.

Nystagmus—Vision condition where the eyes make repetitive, uncontrolled movements when tracking.

O

Occupational Safety and Health Administration (OSHA)—Agency of the U.S. Department of Labor that is responsible for establishing and enforcing safety and health standards in the workplace.

Omission—A legal liability arising when a person does not perform a necessary action.

Orbital hematoma—Bruising and bleeding associated with a blow to the eye and eye orbit; commonly referred to as a black eye.

Orthopedic surgeon—Physician who assesses and attempts to correct deformities and dysfunction of the musculoskeletal system.

Osgood-Schlatter disease—Epiphyseal inflammation of the tibial tubercle or apophysitis of the tibial tubercle.

Osteitis pubis—Inflammation of the pubis symphysis joint, causing pain, possible dysfunction, and degeneration.

Osteoblast—Bone cell that synthesizes bone.

Osteochondritis dissecans (OCD)—Condition in which a fragment of cartilage and underlying bone are detached from the articular surface; also called "joint mice."

Osteochondrosis—Self-limiting derangement of normal bone growth in developing bone at the growth plate.

Osteoclast—Bone cell that breaks down bone tissue for the purposes of maintaining, repairing, and remodeling bony tissue.

Osteomyelitis—Infection of bone or bone marrow with associated inflammation.

Osteoporosis—When the body loses too much bone, makes too little bone, or both, then the bones become porous and weak, making them more likely to fracture.

Otitis externa—External auditory canal infection.

Otitis media—Inner ear infection.

P

Palpation—The act of feeling with the hands for the purpose of determining the structural integrity of the tissue beneath.

Parasite—Microscopic organism that lives on or in a host and may cause disease or skin lesions, some of which are contagious.

Patellar fracture—Fracture of the patella, which can be in several areas of the bone.

Patellar subluxation/dislocation—Patella moves partially (subluxation) or completely (dislocation) out of its groove with the femur.

Patellofemoral joint—Articulation of the patella and femur, specifically the posterior surface of the patella and the anterior surface of the femoral condyles.

Pathogenic—Causing disease.

Peak height velocity—Known as the "growth spurt," or the maximum vertical height gained in the shortest period of time, usually during the development years.

Periodization—The organization of training into a cyclical structure to attain the optimal development of an athlete's performance capacities.

Permethrin—Broad-spectrum insecticide that can be infused in clothes to prevent insects from approaching and biting.

Pes cavus—Abnormally high longitudinal arch which may lead to compensation patterns.

Pes planus—Abnormally flat foot or loss of the longitudinal arch which may lead to compensation patterns.

Phagocytosis—The uptake of large particles from the extracellular matrix into the cell for the purpose of cleaning up debris and assisting with immune system function.

Phalanges—Anatomic name for the bones of the fingers and toes.

Pharyngitis—Inflammation of the pharynx or throat.

Phonophoresis—The use of ultrasound to assist with the topical or transdermal delivery of drugs or possibly other substances into the tissues of the body.

Phospholipids—Lipids that are both fat and water soluble; located in the cell membranes of the body.

Physical exam—The process of evaluating an individual for signs and symptoms associated with injury or illness.

Plaintiff—The individual who was injured and brings the lawsuit.

Plantar fasciitis—Inflammation of the plantar tissues of the foot.

Plantar flexion—Moving the top of the foot away from the shin, as in pointing the foot and ankle in dance.

Pneumonia—Inflammation of the lungs.

Pneumothorax—Air collects in the pleural cavity (space between the lungs and chest wall) causing the lung to collapse.

Peripheral nervous system (PNS)—Consists of nerves that reside outside of the spinal cord and brain that relay information from brain to body.

Point tenderness—Pain produced when an injury site is palpated.

Poison ivy, oak, sumac—Plant sap that contacts the skin and causes an itchy, irregular rash.

Polysaccharide—Many, up to thousands, of monosaccharides linked together; examples include glycogen, starch, and cellulose (fiber).

Polyunsaturated fat—A fatty acid molecule with many double or triple bonds that prevents at least two hydrogen atoms from bonding.

Preparticipation physical examination (PPE)—A clinical examination performed by a physician on physically active individuals to assess their physical and mental health before participation in sports or physical activities to determine their physical readiness.

Prophylactic knee brace—Braces used to prevent collateral ligament injuries or stabilize the knee, usually for linemen in football.

Proprioceptive neuromuscular facilitation (PNF)—Stretching techniques that involve combinations of alternating contractions and stretches.

Prostaglandins—Perhaps some of the most powerful chemicals produced in the body; related to the inflammatory process, they cause a variety of effects, including vasodilation, increased vascular permeability, pain, fever, and clotting.

Protein—In terms of the diet, a macronutrient consisting of carbon, hydrogen, oxygen, and nitrogen; mainly found in connective and muscle tissue, there are 20 different types of amino acids which can be combined to form a protein.

Proximal interphalangeal (PIP) joint—The joint formed by the articulation between the proximal and middle phalanges of the digits (hinge type of joint).

Pubic aponeurosis—Complex fascial layer formed by a confluence of fibers from the rectus abdominus, adductor longus, gracilis, transversus abdominus and internal oblique (conjoint tendon), and external oblique.

Pulmonary contusion—A direct blow to the thorax that results in lung trauma.

Puncture—Wound created when an object punctures the skin and creates a hole.

Purulent—Consisting of, or forming, pus.

Pyoderma—Pus-producing infection of the skin.

Pyomyositis—Bacterial infection of muscles resulting in pus-filled abscesses.

Q

Q angle—Angle made by a line from the anterior superior iliac spine and the center of the patella and a line from the center of the patella to the center of the tibia.

Quadriceps—Group of four muscles (vastus medialis, vastus intermedius, vastus lateralis, and rectus femoris) of the anterior thigh that perform knee extension.

R

Radiation—Emission and diffusion of rays of heat.

Radiocarpal joint—Articulation (ellipsoidal) formed by the distal end of the radius and three bones of the wrist: navicular, lunate, and triquetral.

Radioulnar joints—Two articulations (pivot) formed by the proximal and distal radius and ulna, known commonly as the proximal and distal radioulnar joints.

Recommended Dietary Allowance (RDA)—Average daily intake sufficient enough to meet daily nutrient requirements.

Rectal core body temperature—The temperature of the core as measured in the rectal cavity.

Regeneration—Damaged tissue is replaced by cells of the same type along with scar tissue, but the tissue retains most of its original structure.

Relative humidity—The moisture content in the air that is expressed as a percentage. The percentage is the percent of moisture in the air that can be retained at a given temperature and pressure.

Repair—Original tissue is replaced by scar tissue or repaired tissue.

Repetition volume—The number of repetitions a weight is lifted.

Resolution—Complete healing whereby dead cells and cellular debris are removed, and the tissue is left functionally the same.

Rest periods—Usually specific to the amount of time allowed between sets in a given training session; can be used in a broader sense to describe the recovery between training days.

Resting energy expenditure (REE)—Energy used to maintain basic physiologic function, which accounts for approximately 60–75% of energy expenditure.

Resting metabolic rate (RMR)—The minimal amount of energy needed to meet the body's demands at rest (calculated hours after a meal or exercise and is usually slightly higher than BMR).

Retrograde amnesia—Inability to recall events that occurred just before an injury.

Rhabdomyolysis—As a result of overexertion or traumatic injury, muscle fibers are damaged and die, which, in turn, causes a release of their contents into the bloodstream; this condition can lead to serious complications, such as renal (i.e., kidney) failure.

Rhinitis—Irritation and inflammation of the mucous membrane inside the nose. Common symptoms are a stuffy nose, runny nose, sneezing, and postnasal drip.

Risk factor—Causative agent in a sports injury.

Rotator cuff—Group of four muscles crossing the glenohumeral joint: subscapularis, supraspinatus, infraspinatus, and teres minor.

S

Salter-Harris fracture—A category of fractures that involves the growth plate.

Saturated fat—A fatty acid molecule in which hydrogen atoms occupy all the available bonding sites; solid at room temperature.

Scabies—Infestation of small mites in the skin that causes intense itching.

Scapular dyskinesis—Abnormal mobility or function of the scapula both statically and dynamically.

Scoliosis—Lateral and/or rotary curvature of the spine.

Second impact syndrome—Significant brain swelling that can occur rapidly if a person suffers a second concussion before symptoms from an earlier concussion have subsided.

Secondary enzymatic injury—Indirect result of tissue trauma. Healthy tissues surrounding primary injury die as a result of aggressive eating of healthy tissue within the area of the original injury. Waste products also damage cell membranes of healthy cells, causing cell death.

Secondary metabolic injury—Indirect result of tissue trauma. Healthy tissues surrounding primary injury die from lack of blood flow and metabolic supplies. The energy needed exceeds that of the energy available.

Seizure—Sudden onset of uncoordinated muscular activity and changes in consciousness lasting an unpredictable time.

Self-concept—The image of the self that is constructed from the beliefs one holds about oneself.

Sensitizer—A chemical that initiates an allergic reaction.

Shin splints—Exercise-induced tibia pain; also called medial tibial stress syndrome, tibial stress injury, or chronic exertional compartment syndrome.

Shivering—A body response to cold temperatures characterized by fast muscle contractions in an effort to increase body heat.

Shoulder pointer—Contusion and subsequent hematoma in the region of the acromioclavicular joint.

SICK scapula—A combination of scapular malposition, inferior medial border prominence, coracoid process tenderness, and dyskinesis of scapular movement.

Sickle cell trait—A condition in which red blood cells are shaped like a "sickle," which causes decreased blood flow and eventually leads to breakdown of muscle tissue (i.e., fulminant rhabdomyolysis).

Sign—Objective evidence of an abnormal situation within the body.

Simple carbohydrates—Monosaccharides.

Sinusitis—Acute inflammation of one or more of the paranasal sinuses.

Slipped capital femoral epiphysis—Head of femur displaces relative to neck of femur.

Snapping hip syndrome—A lateral hip pain with only certain motions caused when soft tissue "snaps" over the greater trochanter of the femur.

Soft tissue—Includes muscles, fascia, tendons, joint capsules, ligaments, blood vessels, and nerves.

Somatic information—In the context of growth and development, physical measurements such as peak height velocity, mass, leg length, etc., that assist in determining maturation.

Spear tackler's spine—Diagnosed via X-ray, the cervical spine shows changes, including a narrowing of the spine at the neck or loss of the normal curvature of the spine, and/or changes resulting from trauma to the spine; a strict contraindication for further participation in tackle sports.

Spearing—A practice in tackle football whereby a player performs either a tackle or a block using the head as the initial point of contact.

Spondylolisthesis—Forward slippage of vertebra, usually between the fifth lumbar and the sacrum.

Spondylolysis—Defect in the neural arch (i.e., pars interarticularis) of the vertebrae.

Sports medicine—Branch of medicine concerned with the medical aspects of sports participation.

Sprain—Injury to a joint and the surrounding structures, primarily ligaments and/or joint capsules.

Sputum—Bronchial secretions.

Standard precautions—Protective measures that have been recommended by the Centers for Disease Control and Prevention (CDC) for use in dealing with blood and body fluids or other potentially hazardous materials.

Static stretching—Passively stretching a muscle by placing it in a maximal lengthened position and holding it there for extended periods of time (anywhere from 10 to 60 seconds or longer).

Sternoclavicular (SC) joint—Articulation (arthrodial) formed by the union of the proximal clavicle and the manubrium of the sternum.

Sterols—Lipids primarily made of carbon and hydrogen.

Strain—Injury involving muscles and tendons or the junction between the two, commonly known as the musculotendinous junction.

Stress fracture—Small crack or break in a bone related to excessive, repeated overloads; also known as overuse fracture or march fracture.

Stressor—Anything that affects the body's physiological or psychological condition and upsets the homeostatic balance.

Subdural hematoma—Bleeding below the dura mater.

Subluxation—Partial or incomplete dislocation of an articulation.

Subtalar joint—Articulation (arthrodial) formed by the inferior surface of the talus and the superior surface of the calcaneus.

Subungual hematoma—Blood formation under a nail.

Sudden onset injury—A condition resulting from a specific identifiable episode resulting in a rapid onset of experienced distress or disability.

Sun protection factor (SPF)—Rating of a sunscreen is determined by the sunscreen's ability to absorb harmful ultraviolet light over time.

Sunburn—Reaction to too much UV exposure whereby the skin turns red and may blister.

Swan neck deformity—A rupture to the volar plate of the PIP joint causing a deformity that resembles a swan's neck with the head (bent DIP) and long neck (hyperextended PIP).

Sweat loss—The amount of sweat lost during physical activity calculated by body weight before and after activity.

Sweat rate—The amount of sweat produced per hour for a given activity.

Symptom—Subjective evidence of an abnormal situation within the body.

Syndrome—Group of typical symptoms or conditions that characterize a deficiency or disease.

T

Tâche noir—Trauma-related black spots on the palm.

Tackler's exostosis—Formation of a benign growth projecting from the humerus that is caused by repeated blows to the upper arm region; common in tackle football.

Talocrural (ankle) joint—Articulation formed by the distal tibia and fibula with the superior surface (dome) of the talus.

Talon noir—Trauma-related black spots on the heel.

Tanner stages—Outlines five stages of physical maturation.

Team physician—A medical doctor who agrees to provide at least limited medical coverage to a particular sports program or institution and ideally has additional training in sports medicine.

Tendinitis—Inflammation of a tendon.

Tenosynovitis—Inflammation of the sheath of a tendon.

Testicular contusion—Bruise to the testicles from direct trauma.

Testicular torsion—Twisting of the testicles from traumatic or nontraumatic events.

Thermal effect of activity (TEA)—The energy used for nonrest activities.

Thermal effect of food (TEF)—The energy used to process food.

Thermal gradient—The temperature difference and distance between two points, or the change in temperature over a given distance (e.g., difference in temperature between core and extremities).

Thermogenesis—The creation of heat by various methods.

Thermoregulation—The processes involved in order to maintain an optimal physiological range of core body temperature.

Thermotherapy—Therapeutic use of heat.

Thoracic cage—Thoracic vertebrae, their corresponding ribs, and the sternum.

Thoracic outlet syndrome (TOS)—A group of disorders that occur when nerves or blood vessels in the space between the collarbone (clavicle) and the first rib are compressed, causing pain in the shoulders and neck and possibly numbness in the fingers.

Thrombosis—Local coagulation or clotting of the blood.

Tibiofemoral joint—Articulation of the tibia and femur, or "knee" joint, specifically the articulation between both femoral condyles and both tibial condyles.

Tibiofibular syndesmosis sprain—Injury to the distal tibiofibular ligament, also known as a high ankle sprain.

Tinea versicolor—Fungus infection resulting in the formation of circular skin lesions that appear either lighter or darker than adjacent skin.

Tinea—Group of fungi-related skin infections, commonly called ringworm, which can affect various parts of the body—groin area (i.e., tinea cruris), feet and toes (i.e., tinea pedis), and scalp (i.e., tinea capitis).

Temporomandibular joint (TMJ)—The joint created by the temporal and mandibular bones; it allows our jaw to open and close.

Tonic-clonic seizures—A seizure that involves stiffening, twitching, or jerking phases of muscle activity in addition to experiencing changes in sensation and mood leading up to the seizure; once called a grand mal seizure.

Tort—A private wrong or injury, suffered by an individual as a result of another person's conduct.

Total daily energy expenditure (TDEE)—An estimation of calories burned per day when exercise is taken into account.

Total glenohumeral rotation range of motion (TRM)—The entire measurement arc of passive range of motion of the shoulder, including external and internal rotation.

Training duration—The length of time of the training session.

Training frequency—The number of training sessions per week or day.

Training intensity—The effort expended during an exercise session.

Training volume—The amount of work performed during a training session or period of time (i.e., number of repetitions multiplied by the amount of weight used, number of miles).

Trait anxiety—A general disposition or tendency to perceive certain situations as threatening and to react with an anxiety response.

Trans fat—The result of hydrogenation; has a negative association with cardiovascular health.

Transition phase—2–4 weeks of adjusted exercise to bring an athlete to peak performance or the next phase of the plan.

Trauma—Wound or injury.

Triglycerides—Simple lipids made of a glycerol molecule and three fatty acids that are stored in muscles and the liver; protect organs and insulate the body as well as carry substances through the blood.

Trochanteric bursitis—Bursitis of the trochanter bursa due to tight lateral soft tissue of the hip.

Tunnel of Guyon—Anatomic region formed by the hook of the hamate bone and the pisiform bone, whereby the ulnar nerve passes into the hand.

Turf toe—Hyperextension of the first metatarsal phalangeal joint causing a sprain to the ligaments and inflammation.

Type 1 diabetes—Insulin-dependent type of diabetes mellitus usually diagnosed in children and adolescents, but anyone can be diagnosed at any age. In this autoimmune disease, the body does not produce insulin.

Type 2 diabetes—Non-insulin-dependent type of diabetes. The body does not produce enough insulin or does not use insulin properly.

U

Universal and standard precautions—The practice of avoiding contact with a person's bodily fluids, by means of the wearing of nonporous articles, such as medical gloves, goggles, and face shields. The practice was expanded and is now known as standard precautions.

Unknown onset seizure—A seizure in which it is difficult to determine if it is of focal or generalized onset, perhaps because it was not witnessed by anyone.

Unsaturated fat—A fatty acid molecule in which the available bonding sites are not occupied by hydrogen; liquid at room temperature.

Upper respiratory infection (URI)—Infection involving the nose, throat, ears and sinuses, tonsils, and associated lymph glands.

Urticaria—Hives that occur from a change in body temperature during exercise.

V

Valgus—Outward force on a bone segment distal to a joint causing an opening on the medial (inside) of the joint.

Varus—Inward force on a bone segment distal to a joint causing an opening on the lateral (outside) of the joint.

Vasoconstriction—Decrease in the diameter of a blood vessel resulting in decreased blood flow.

Vasodilation—Increase in the diameter of a blood vessel resulting in increased blood flow.

Ventricular fibrillation—The heart beats with rapid, erratic electrical impulses. The ventricles quiver, diminishing the effectiveness of expelling blood from the heart.

Vertigo—Type of dizziness that causes a perception of motion and includes a loss of balance.

Very low-density lipoprotein (VLDL)—A substance that transports lipids in the blood and lymph. Currently there is no recommended level.

Virus—Infectious agent that lacks cell structure and causes contagious conditions.

Vitamins—Thirteen micronutrients that must be consumed regularly because they are essential to health and performance but have no caloric value nor provide direct energy.

Volkmann's contracture—Contracture of muscles of the forearm related to a loss of blood supply caused by a fracture and/or dislocation of either of the bones in the forearm or the humerus.

W

Wart—Circular raised area of skin caused by HPV.

Water-soluble vitamins—Vitamins B and C, which are easily transported through the blood but are not stored in the body and are excreted through the kidneys and urine.

Wet bulb globe temperature (WBGT)—Measure of temperature, humidity, wind speed, and solar radiation to determine heat stress.

Wind chill factor—The outdoor temperature after taking wind into account; this is usually lower than the air temperature.

Index

Note: Page numbers followed by *f* or *t* indicate material in figures or tables, respectively.

A

AAFP. *See* American Academy of Family Physicians
AAOS. *See* American Academy of Orthopaedic Surgeons
AAP. *See* American Academy of Pediatrics
AAS. *See* anabolic androgenic steroids
abdominal region. *See also* thorax and abdomen injuries
    anatomy, 321–322, 322*f*
    muscle strains, 326
    pain in, 334–335
abdominal rigidity, 163
abnormal patellofemoral configuration, 366
abrasions, 240, 410
Academy of Nutrition and Dietetics (2009), 135
acclimatization, 434, 434*t*, 441*t*, 446–447
acetabulum, 339, 340*f*
acetylsalicylic acid, 184
Achilles tendinitis, 390
Achilles tendon, 6, 6*f*, 381, 389–391
    complex, 394
    rupture, 390
ACL. *See* anterior cruciate ligament
ACL Research Retreat of 2012, 369
acne mechanica, 416
acromioclavicular (AC) joint, 14, 262, 262*f*, 266, 269–271, 270*f*
acromion process, 269
active assisted exercise, 186
active exercise, 186
Act of God, 56
acute appendicitis, 335
acute fracture symptoms, 10
acute injuries, 5, 5*f*, 489
    pain and, 178–180
acute mountain sickness, 455
ADA. *See* American Diabetes Association
Adderall (amphetamine and dextroamphetamine), 147, 504
adductor muscles, 342
adenosine triphosphate (ATP), 113
adequate intake (AI), 121
ADHD. *See* attention deficit hyperactivity disorder
adhesive strapping techniques, 396
adjustment disorders, 104
adolescent fractures, hip/pelvis, 343–346
adolescent medical concerns, 487
    American youth sports, 488
    coaching techniques, 503–504
    cultural deconditioning, 496–497
    epidemic of youth sports injury, 489–490
    equipment, 498
    extrinsic factors, 496–498
    female athletes, 504
    growing athlete, 490–492
    growth cartilage, 494–495
    growth plate injuries, 494
    infectious imitators, 499
    injury contributors, 495–498
    injury imitators, 498–500
    injury mechanisms, 492–495
    injury prevention, 503–504
    intrinsic factors, 496
    ligament injuries, 492
    neurovascular imitators, 499–500
    oncological imitators, 499
    playing surfaces, 498
    preparticipation physical examination, 503
    prepubescence, 490–491
    prescription stimulant medications, 504
    psychological imitators, 500
    puberty, 491–492

adolescent medical concerns (*continued*)
  rehabilitation of previous injuries, 503
  rheumatological imitators, 499
  safety, 501–502
  sports participation factors, 488
  strength training, 500–503
  stretching programs, 503
  tendon and bone injuries, 492–494
  training errors, 497
AEDs. *See* automated external defibrillators
aerobic dance, 17
aerobic exercise, 479
aerobic fitness/aerobic power, 75–76
aerobic system, 113
aerosol coolants, 180
afterdrop, 452
AHCT. *See* athletic health care team
airway assessment, 160–161
airway obstructions, 43, 158, 325
albuterol, 471
alcohol detoxification, 333
alertness assessment, 160
allergic reactions, 414, 425
allergies, 469
altitude-related conditions, 454–456, 456*f*
altitude sickness, 455
amenorrhea, 102, 504
American Academy of Family Physicians (AAFP), 60, 70, 72
American Academy of Orthopaedic Surgeons (AAOS)
  continuing education courses, 40
  initial check, 159
American Academy of Pediatrics (AAP), 15, 70
  adolescent weight training, 500
  PPE guidelines, 60
American College of Sports Medicine (ACSM), 127*t*
American Diabetes Association (ADA), 475
American Heart Association, 155
  BOC certification courses, 40
  CPR and AED courses, 59
American Medical Association (AMA), 8
American Medical Society for Sports Medicine, 60, 70
American Orthopaedic Society for Sports Medicine, 60
American Osteopathic Academy of Sports Medicine, 60, 70
American Red Cross, 43, 59
American Society for Testing and Materials (ASTM), 237
amino acids, 116, 139, 143*t*, 146
ammonia capsules, 209
amphetamine (Adderall), 147, 504
anabolic androgenic steroids (AAS), 331
anabolic steroids, 147
anaerobic exercise, 479
anaerobic fitness, 76–77
anaerobic system, 113

analgesics, 180
anaphylaxis, 469
anatomic rationale, 370
anatomic snuffbox, palpation in, 302, 303*f*
anatomy
  abdominal region, 321–322
  arm/wrist/hand injuries, 285–286, 286*f*
  hip/pelvis injuries, 339–343
  internal organs, 322–323, 323*f*, 324*f*
  lower leg/ankle/foot, 378–383
  lumbar spine, 253–254, 253*f*–254*f*, 254*t*
  shoulder, 261–267, 262*f*–264*f*, 265*t*–266*t*, 266*f*, 267*f*
  thigh/knee/leg injuries, 353–357
  thoracic spine, 247–248, 248*f*
  thorax, 321–322, 322*f*
anconeus, 286
androstenedione (andro), 144*t*, 148
angiogenesis, 177, 182
anhedonia, 97, 500
anisocoria, 210
ankle joint, 379
  ligaments, 381*f*
ankles
  anatomy, 378–383
  fractures, 383–384
  injuries, 384–389. *See also* lower leg, ankle, and foot injuries
  skeletal injuries, 383–384
  soft-tissue injuries, 384–394
  taping/bracing, 388
  tendon-related injuries, 389–391
ankle sprains, 385, 387–389, 401
ankle taping, 388
  preventive, 400–404
  procedure, 404*f*
annular ligament of elbow, 286, 286*f*
annulus, 256
anorexia nervosa, 100–101
anterior, 23
anterior compartment, muscles of, 381
anterior cruciate ligament (ACL), 367, 369–373
  injuries, 74
  osteoarthritis in knee and, 20–21
  soccer, 26
anterior dislocation of GH joint, 271, 271*f*, 272*f*
anterior longitudinal ligaments, 253*f*
anterior muscles, 354
anterior shoulder pain, 23
anterior talofibular, 381, 385
  ligaments, 381, 385
anterograde amnesia, 199
antibiotic resistance, 418
anticonvulsant drugs, 482
antihistamines, 454

anti-inflammatory drugs, 180
antioxidants, 121
antipyretic effects, 184
anxiety, 94, 98, 98t
apophyseal injuries, 493
apophysis, 22, 491f, 493, 494
apophysitis, 294, 296, 493
apoptosis, 175, 176
appendix, rupture, 335
Appropriate Medical Care for the Secondary School-Aged Athlete (NATA), 60
aquatic sports and epilepsy, 482
arachidonic acid, 175, 184
arachnoid membrane, 192, 193f
arch problems, 395–397
arch taping procedure, 395
arm injuries
    anatomy, 285–286, 286f
    biceps brachii injuries, 289–291
    elbow fractures, 295–296, 296f
    myositis ossificans traumatica, 288–289
    osteochondritis dissecans of elbow, 299–300
    triceps brachii injuries, 291
    upper arm fractures, 291–293
    upper arm soft tissue injuries, 286–291
arnica, 143t
arteries of arm, 266f
articular cartilage, 177, 491f, 493
articular surfaces of long bones, 492
articulation between vertebrae, 257
artificial turf, 411
aspirin, 184
assessment of injuries, 158–165
    airway, 158, 160–161, 325
    alertness, 160
    breathing, 161
    circulation, 161–162
    head injuries, 207t, 208–209
    hemorrhage, 159–160
    medical history, 163–164
    palpation, 164–165
    physical exam, 162–165
    responsiveness, 160
    scene safety, 158
    shock, 165
Association for Applied Sport Psychology, 97
assumption of risk, 56
asthma, 469–472
ASTM. *See* American Society for Testing and Materials
athletes
    diabetes, 475–481
    dietary guidelines for
        during competition, 138
        daily maintenance, 136–138
        for post exercise, 138–139
        precompetition diets, 138
    diets, 109
    ergogenic substances used by, 143t–144t
    growing
        bone growth, 490–491
        puberty, 491–492
    injured, 139
    nutritional knowledge of, 135–136
    oral/injectable steroids, 147
    SCT, 472–473
    tape/braces for, 401
Athletes Targeting Healthy Exercise and Nutrition Alternatives (ATHENA), 103, 136
athletic energy deficit, 132
athletic health care team (AHCT), 37–49
    athletic training settings, 43–46
    clinics and hospitals, 46
    colleges and universities, 44–45
    key team members, 39–43
    AT salaries, 46, 47t
    secondary school level, 47–49
    secondary school setting, 45–46
    sports medicine, defined, 38–39
    youth athletes, 46–47
Athletic Medicine Unit. *See also* athletic health care team (AHCT)
athletic trainers. *See also* Board of Certification (BOC)-certified athletic trainers
    certification subjects, 41
    clinics and hospitals, 46
    colleges and universities, 44–45
    exertional heat illness, 444
    job settings, 43
    professional sports, 43
    AT salaries, 46, 47t
    secondary school setting, 45–46
athletic training settings, 43–46
atlantoaxial joint, 195
ATP. *See* adenosine triphosphate
attention deficit hyperactivity disorder (ADHD), 103–104, 104t, 504
    stimulants, 147
auricula, 239
auricular hematoma, 238
automated external defibrillators (AEDs), 328f
    BOC certification training, 43
    coach training/certification in, 39, 59
    commotio cordis, 328
    and CPR, 327
    emergency care training, 155, 156f
    emergency plans and, 152, 157
avascular necrosis, 358
AVPU scale, 160

avulsion, 9, 383, 410
    tooth, 232
avulsion fractures, 296, 346
    hip/pelvis, 346
    tendon-bone strain, 9
axial loading of cervical spine, 219–220

B

bacteria, defined, 410
bacterial infections, 499
    skin, 418–422
badminton, GH joint-related impingement syndrome, 277
balanced diet, 137
ball-and-socket joint, 339, 340f
ballistic stretching, 80, 81
bandage, 412, 413, 415
bands of extensor tendons, 313, 313f
barrier devices, 43
basal metabolic rate (BMR), 110
baseball
    contusions, 10
    head/face injuries, 20
    injury data, 2
    Little League elbow, 22
    protective chest equipment, 330
    sports participation growth, 2
baseball finger. *See* mallet finger
baseline concussion screening, 205–208, 207t
bases, types of, 68
basketball, 20–23
    commotio cordis, 328
    contusions, 10
    GH joint–related impingement syndrome, 277
    injury rates by gender, 20
    knee ligament sprains, 21
    lower-extremity injuries, 20, 21f
    protective chest equipment, lack of, 331
batting cages, 68
BCAAs. *See* branched chain amino acids
bed bugs, 425
bench press, 502
Bennett's fracture, 308, 308f
beta-2 agonists, 471
beta-alanine, 145
beta-hydroxy beta-methylbutyrate (HMB), 146
biceps brachii, 23, 286
    injuries, 289–291
    muscle tendon, 279, 279f
biceps femoris muscle, 342, 354
biceps tendon, 279
biomechanical deficiencies, 393
biomechanical rationale, 370
biomechanics of sport, 98

bipolar disorder, 95
black eye, 236
bladder injuries, 334
blisters and calluses, 397–398
blood
    blood glucose levels, 114, 475
    exposure to, 238
    transfusions and HBV, 473
    in urine, 334
blood-borne pathogens, 159, 411
blood sugar, 477
    and environment, 480
    and exercise, 478–479
Board of Certification (BOC)-certified athletic trainers, 109
    as AHCT members, 39
    ankle taping procedure, 396
    CAATE accreditation, 41
    injury recognition, 14
    rehabilitative exercise and, 186
    secondary school level, 47–49
    secondary schools, 45–46
    youth athletes, 46–47
BOC Exam Candidate Handbook, 41
body composition, 81, 140, 141
body image, 101
body weight management, nutrition and, 140–141
boils, 420
bone infections, 499
bone injuries, 492–494
bone scans, 12
bones of hand and wrist, 308f
bonking, 129
boundary layer, 450
boutonnière deformity, 313–314, 313f
boxer's fracture, 308, 309
boxing, bleeding wounds, 411
brachialis, 286
brachial plexus, 221–222, 221f, 266, 267f
bradykinin, 172
brain contusions, 10
brain stem, 194
branched chain amino acids (BCAAs), 117
breach of duty, 55
breast injuries, 326–327
breathing assessment, 161, 208–209
bronchitis, 464
buddy taping, 309
budgetary constraints, 69
bulimia nervosa, 100–101
bunions, 397, 397f
burners, 221
bursa, 300
bursitis, 276

C

caffeine, 146
calcaneal apophysitis, 494
calcaneofibular ligaments, 381
calcium, 124–125
calf muscles, 381
calluses (fracture healing), 12, 177, 177f, 398, 413–414
    blisters and, 397–398
calories, 110
Canadian Standards Association (CSA), 237
capsular ligaments, 262f, 271
carbohydrate loading, 116
carbohydrates (CHO), 113–116, 139
carbuncles, 419–421
cardiac arrest, 158
cardiac contusion, 327, 332
cardiac issues
    cardiac arrest, 208
    pathology, 329
    sudden death, 328
cardiac medical history, 71
cardiopulmonary resuscitation (CPR), 327
    after circulation assessment, 162, 209
    athletic trainers and, 43
    coach's training in, 22, 39
    emergency care training, 155–158, 155f
    emergency plans and, 152, 154
    sudden cardiac arrest, 328
CARE. See Concussion Assessment, Research and Education
carpal tunnel, 303, 304, 305f
    syndrome, 304
carrdiac issues
    cardiogenic shock, 165
cartilage, 356, 358
catastrophic injuries, 197, 218, 219t, 489
cauda equina, 339
cauliflower ear, 24, 238
causative factors in injury, 66–67
caution, 97
CECS. See chronic exertional compartment syndrome
cellulitis, 419
cellulose, 114
Centers for Disease Control and Prevention, 410
central nervous system (CNS), 160, 194, 438
cerebellum, 194
cerebral contusion, 202
cerebral edema, 200
cerebral meninges, 192–194, 193f
cerebrospinal fluid (CSF), 192, 193
cerebrum, 194
Certificate of Added Qualifications in Sports Medicine (CAQ), 39

certified athletic trainers (ATs), 136
certified diabetes educator, 479
cervical protrusions, 210
cervical spine injuries, 218–224
    brachial plexus injuries, 221–222, 221f
    fractures and dislocations, 222–224
    guidelines for appropriate care of, 227–228
    ice hockey, 222
    mechanisms of injury, 219–221
    sprains, 222
    strains, 222
cervical vertebrae, 195
CEUs. See continuing education programs
CGM. See continuous glucose monitor
checklist, symptom-scale, 212
cheerleading, 27–28, 197
chemical cold-packs, 180
chemotactic factors, 174
chemotaxis, 174
chest protector, 330, 331f
chickenpox, 454
CHO. See carbohydrates
Cholesterol, 119, 120t
chondromalacia, 366
chronic Achilles tendinitis, treatment for, 390
chronic exertional compartment syndrome (CECS), 393
chronic GH joint subluxation, 279
chronic injuries, 5, 6f
chronic obstructive pulmonary disease, 335
chronic traumatic encephalopathy (CTE), 200
circulation assessment, 161–162, 208–209
classifications of injury, 8–14
clavicle, 262, 267–268, 268f
CNS. See central nervous system
coaches
    advice for, 103
    AHCT responsibilities, 39
    education, 135–136
    first contact with injured student, 51, 52f
    legal protections, 58–59
    liability insurance coverage, 58
    negligent actions, 57–58
    nutritional knowledge of, 135–136
    and student team leaders, 136
coaching techniques, 503–504
coccygeal plexus, 340
coccyx, 254, 258, 339
cold-related conditions, 449–454
cold treatment for inflammation, 180
cold urticaria, 454
colic, 464
colitis, 464
collagen, 177, 186

collateral ligaments, 310, 311, 368
    injuries, 368
Colles' fracture, 300, 301, 301f
comminuted fractures, 11f
commission, 55
    act of, 55
Commission on Accreditation of Athletic Training Education (CAATE), 41, 42
Committee on the Medical Aspects of Sports, 8
common cold, 462
common integument, 409
common sites of, 493t
commotio cordis, 328
community-acquired methicillin-resistant *Staphylococcus aureus* (CA-MRSA), 420
comparative negligence, 56
compartment syndrome, 391–392
competition, environment, 67
competitive stress, 89–91
complement system, 174
complete proteins, 117
complex carbohydrates, 114
complex partial seizure, 483
compound fractures, 10
compression, 169, 170f, 180, 181
computerized neurocognitive assessment, 208
concentric contraction, 275
concussion (mild traumatic brain injury), 26, 198–199
    baseline screening, 205–208, 207t
    consensus statements, 204–206
    rehabilitation, 213–215
Concussion Assessment, Research and Education (CARE), 205
concussion education, 216–218
conduction, 432, 450
condyloid joint, 310
connective tissue, 169, 170
conoid ligaments, 269
consensus statements, 204–206
Consumer Product Safety Commission (CPSC), 27
contact ACL injuries, 369
contact/collision sports and epilepsy, 483
contact dermatitis, 414
contact lens problems, 237
continuing education programs (CEUs), 43
continuous glucose monitor (CGM), 476, 477f
contrecoup injury, 198
contributory negligence, 56
contusions, 10
    cardiac, 327
    cerebral, 202
    defined, 10
    of elbow, 300

    pulmonary, 332
    shoulder, 275
    testicular/scrotal, 348
convection, 432, 450
coracoacromial arch, 277, 277f
coracoclavicular ligament, 262f, 269
coracohumeral ligament, 262f, 271
coracoid process, 279
core body temperatures, 431
core exercises, 79
corns, 413–414
coronal plane MRI of a torn ACL, 368f
corporate athletic trainers, 43
cortisone, 184
costochondral joint, 322
costochondral separation, 325
costoclavicular ligaments, 274
coup injury, 198
CPR. *See* cardiopulmonary resuscitation
crabs, 425
cranial injury, 203
cranium, 192, 192f
creatine, 143t, 145
crepitation, 11
crepitus, 164
critical force, 5, 170
cruciate ligaments, 356, 367, 369
    injuries, 368–373
cryotherapy, 180–184
CSA. *See* Canadian Standards Association
CSF. *See* cerebrospinal fluid
CTE. *See* chronic traumatic encephalopathy
cultural deconditioning, 496–497
cup protector, 348, 351
cycling, clavicle fractures, 267–268, 268f
cystic fibrosis, 335

D

daily fiber intake, 114
date rape drug, 148
deformity
    as acute fracture symptom, 10
    as dislocation symptom, 14
degenerative enzymes, 174
degradation effect, 174
dehydration, symptoms and treatment, 432
dehydroepiandrosterone (DHEA), 144t, 148
deltoid muscle, 264f
dental injuries, 232–234
Department of Defense (DOD), 205
depressed skull fractures, 203
depression, 95–97, 500
de Quervain's disease, 306

dermis, 409, 420
detached retina, 235, 237
dexamethasone, 184
dexedrine, 147, 504
dextroamphetamine, 147
DHEA. *See* dehydroepiandrosterone
diabetes, 475–481, 481*f*
diabetic coma, 478
diabetic ketoacidosis (DKA), 478
diaphragm, 322
diathermy, 180
   machines, 69
dietary carbohydrates, 114
dietary fiber, 114
dietary guidelines for athletes
   during competition, 138
   daily maintenance, 136–138
   for post exercise, 138–139
   precompetition diets, 138
dietary nitrate, 143*t*
dietary protein, 118
dietary reference intake (DRI), 121, 122*t*–123*t*
Dietary Supplement Health and Education Act (DSHEA), 142
diets
   post exercise, 138–139
   precompetition, 138
DIP joint. *See* distal interphalangeal joint
diplopia, 236, 239
disaccharides, 113
disk protrusion/herniation at lumbar vertebrae, 256*f*
dislocated hip, 345
dislocations, 13–14
   cervical, 222, 223
   defined, 13–14
   of elbow, 294, 295*f*
   fracture, 308
   of hand, 310–314
   of jaw, 239
   manubrium, 325
   wrist, 303–304, 303*f*, 304*f*
disordered eating. *See* eating disorders
displaced fractures, 325
distal forearm fractures, 300–302
distal interphalangeal (DIP) joint, 311, 312
diving, 239
DKA. *See* diabetic ketoacidosis
doctrine of sovereign immunit, 57
documentation of injuries, 60
DOD. *See* Department of Defense
dorsalis pedis, pulse of, 391
dorsal radiocarpal ligament, 303, 303*f*, 304*f*
dorsiflexion, 223, 379, 380, 389, 390

doughnut-shaped pads, 395
dressing for wounds, 412
DRI. *See* dietary reference intake
drills, 80
dugout locations, 68
duodenal ulcer, 334
dura mater, 192
dynamic flexibility, 79
dynamic stretching, 79, 80
dyspnea, 251
dysthymia, 95

E

EAPs. *See* emergency action plans
eardrum, 238
ear injuries, 238–239
eating disorders, 98–100, 497
   anorexia nervosa and bulimia nervosa, 100–101
   prevention of, 102–103
   research, 100
   sport specificity and, 101–102
   treatment of, 103
ECC. *See* emergency cardiac care
eccentric contractions, 7, 170, 276
ecchymosis, 10
echinacea, 143*t*
echocardiogram/echocardiography, 329
ECM. *See* erythema chronicum migrans
edema, 175, 178, 454
EIA. *See* exercise-induced asthma
EIB. *See* exercise-induced bronchospasm
elbow dislocation, 294, 295*f*
elbow injuries, 293–300
   contusions, 300
   epicondylitis, 296–299, 297*f*
   fractures, 295–296, 296*f*
   ODC, 299–300
   splinting of, 293*f*, 295
   sprains and dislocations, 294–295, 295*f*
elbow joint, 286, 286*f*
   epicondylitis of, 296–299, 297*f*
elbow sprains, 294–295, 295*f*
electrolyte imbalances, 102
electrotherapies, 180
elevation of injury, 181
emergency action plans (EAPs), 84, 152, 328
   airway assessment, 160–161
   breathing assessment, 161
   circulation assessment, 161–162
   circulatory system, 161–162
   elements, 152
   emergency care training, 155
   hemorrhage assessment, 159–160

emergency action plans (EAPs) (*continued*)
    initial assessment of injuries, 158–165
      medical history, 163–164
      palpation, 164–165
      physical exam, 162–165
      practices for athletics, 154–155
      removal from field/court, 165
      respiratory system, 160
      responsiveness of athlete, 160
      return to play condition, 165–166
      shock, 165
emergency cardiac care (ECC), 43
Emergency Care and Safety Institute, 155
emergency care training
    AED, 155, 156f
    CPR, 155, 155f
    initial responders' limitations, 157–158
    injury evaluation procedures, 156–157
emergency medical services (EMS), 151, 231, 470
    access routes, 68
    availability, 223
emergency plans, 59, 151
emotional responses, 94t
empty calorie foods, 114
EMS. *See* emergency medical services
encephalon, 192
endocrinologist, 479
endurance, 462
    sports, nutrition and, 129–130
energy
    athletic energy deficit, 129
    expenditure, 110–111
enlarged spleen, 334
environmental bases, 369
environmental injuries, 431–457
    altitude-related conditions, 454–456
    altitude sickness, 455
    chilblain, 453–454
    cold-related conditions, 449–454
    cold urticaria, 454
    exertional heat illnesses, 434–441
    frostbite/frostnip, 452–453
    heat-related conditions, 431–449
    high altitude cerebral edema, 455–456
    high altitude pulmonary edema, 455
    hypothermia, 451–452
    immersion (trench) foot, 454
    lightning, 456–457
    prevention, heat illness, 441–449, 446t–449t
ephedra, 143t, 146, 147
epicondylitis, 294
    of elbow joint, 296–299, 297f
epidemiology, 14
    of sports injuries, 14–15

epidermis, 409, 424
epidural (extradural) hematoma, 202
epigastric pain, 334
epilepsy, 164, 481–483
epiphyseal plate, 280
epiphysis, 12, 13
epistaxis, 237
epithelial tissue, 170
epoxy resins, 414
Epstein-Barr virus, 466, 467
equilibrium and inner ear, 238
equipment fitting, injury prevention and, 498
equipment inspections, 61
erector spinae muscles, 255, 255f
ergogenic aids, 143t–144t, 504
    nutritional, 145–146
    stimulants and anabolic-androgenic substances, 146–148
ergonomics, 43
erythema, 172
erythema chronicum migrans (ECM), 465
erythropoietin (EPO), 147
esophageal problems, 334
essential amino acids, 117
estrogen inhibitors, 144t
ETAP. *See* exercise-related transient abdominal pain
ethics of sports-injury care, 52–54
ethyl chloride, 180, 182
etiology of spondylolisthesis, 257
euhydration, 433
evaluation process in injury assessment, 156–157
evaporation, 432, 438
eversion of foot, 380
Ewing's sarcoma, 499
exercise, 114, 115
    aerobic, 479
    anaerobic, 479
    and blood sugar, 478–479
    and immune response, 461–469
    post exercise diet, 138–139
exercise-associated hyponatremia, 439–440, 440f
exercise-associated muscle cramps, 435–436
exercise-induced asthma (EIA), 164, 470–472
exercise-induced bronchospasm (EIB), 472
exercise mode, 76
exercise order, 79
exercise progression, 76
exercise rehabilitation, 186–187
exercise-related transient abdominal pain (ETAP), 335
exercise selection, 79
exertional heat exhaustion, 436–437, 437f
exertional heat illnesses (EHIs), 15, 434–441, 442t–443t
    exercise-associated hyponatremia, 439–440, 440f
    exercise-associated muscle cramps, 435–436
    exertional heat exhaustion, 436–437, 437f

exertional heatstroke, 437-439, 439t
heat syncope, 435
hypohydration, 434-435, 434t
exertional rhabdomyolysis, 473-475
exertional sickling, 436
exophthalmos, 203
exostosis, 288
explosive power training, 78
extensor/supinator forearm muscles, 286, 288f
extensor tendons, bands of, 313, 313f
external acoustic meatus, 238
external ear, 238
external locus of control, 91
external oblique muscles, 323f
extracellular fluid, 126
extrinsic factors, 66-69
extrinsic overuse injuries, 6
eyes
    anatomy, 234f
    injuries, 234-237, 235t, 236f
    protection, 21-22

F

face
    anatomy, 195
    fractures, 239, 240f
    wounds, 239-240
facemask removal, 225, 226f, 230, 231f
facilities, 68-69
    inspections, 61
FAI. *See* femoroacetabular impingement
false ribs, 321, 322f
Family Educational Rights and Privacy Act (FERPA), 73
fascia, 7
fatalities
    from cardiac problems, 328
    cheerleading, 197
    in soccer, 27
fats, 118-121, 120t
fat-soluble vitamins, 121
fatty acid, 119
FDP muscle. *See* flexor digitorum profundus muscle
Federation Internationale de Football, 27
female athletes, 128, 504
    contact ACL injuries, 369
    knee injuries in basketball, 20
    noncontact ACL injury, 369
female athlete triad, 129, 504
femoral fractures, 357-358
    of right leg, 357f
femoral hernias, 348
femoral neck stress fracture, 343
femoroacetabular impingement (FAI), 347
FERPA. *See* Family Educational Rights and Privacy Act

fiber, 114
fibrin, 130
fibroblastic repair phase, 171, 176-178
fibroblasts, 177
fibula, fracture of, 384f
fibular (lateral) collateral ligament, 356
finger-sweep method, 161, 161f
first aid care
    of Achilles tendon, 390
    AC joint sprains, 270-271
    asthma victims, 472, 472f
    of avulsion fractures, 346
    biceps brachii muscle, 290-291
    biceps tendon problems, 280
    boutonnière deformity, 314
    of brachial plexus injury, 222
    cardiac/pulmonary contusion, 333
    certification, 59
    cervical fractures, 223
    cervical spine strains, 222
    clavicle fracture, 268
    of compartment syndrome, 392
    costochondral separation, 325
    de Quervain's disease, 306
    dislocated hip, 345
    distal forearm fractures, 302
    elbow
        fractures, 296
        sprains and dislocations, 294-295
    epicondylitis/apophysitis, 299
    epileptic seizures, 483
    femoral fracture, 358
    gamekeeper's thumb, 311
    ganglion, 307
    GH joint dislocation, 273
    hand fractures, 309
    herniated disk, 256
    of hip pointer, 344
    humeral fractures, 291-292, 293f
    inflamed bursa, 363
    jersey finger, 313
    jumper's knee, 366
    knee ligaments injury, 371
    of lateral ankle sprain, 386
    lower leg/foot fracture, 384
    lumbar sprains/strains, 256
    mallet finger, 312
    of muscle strains, 361
    muscular contusion, 359
    nerve injuries to wrist, 305-306
    OCD, 363
    ODC, 299-300
    olecranon bursitis, 300
    Osgood-Schlatter disease, 365

first aid care (*continued*)
  of pelvis fracture, 343
  rib fractures, 249–251
  rotator cuff injuries, 276
  SC joint injuries, 274
  shin splints, 393
  shoulder contusions, 275
  SLAP, 273–274
  of sprains, 222
  sternum/rib fracture, 325
  subluxation/dislocation of patella, 364
  suspected torn meniscus, 367
  swan neck deformity, 314
  testicular/scrotal contusions, 348
  of tib/fib syndesmosis sprain, 387
  training, 39
  triceps muscle, 291
  upper arm contusions, 289
  vertebral fractures, 249
  wrist
    fractures, 303
    sprains and dislocations, 304
first-degree sprains/strains, 9
fitness components, 74
flail chest, 325
flexibility, 79–81
flexor carpi ulnaris, 305
flexor digitorum profundus (FDP) muscle, 312
flexor/pronator forearm muscles, 286, 289f
floating ribs, 321
"Fluid Replacement for the Physically Active," 440
focal onset aware seizure, 482
focal onset impaired seizure, 482
focal onset seizure, 482
folliculitis, 420–421
football
  bleeding wounds, 411
  brain/spinal cord injuries, 19
  commotio cordis, 328
  contusions, 10
  liver injury, 333
  myositis ossificans traumatica, 288
  pelvis fractures, 343
  spearing, 19
  spondylolisthesis, 257
  thoracic strains, 251
foot disorders, 394–400
foot injuries. *See* lower leg, ankle, and foot injuries
forearm injuries
  axial loading of, 299
  wrist injuries and, 300–302, 301f
    fractures, 302–303, 302f, 303f
    nerve injuries, 304–306, 305f
    sprains and dislocations, 303–304, 303f, 304f
    tendon problems, 306–307, 306f, 307f
forearm muscles, 286, 288f, 289f
foreseeability, 55
formaldehyde resin allergies, 414
fracture-dislocation, 308
fractures, 10, 325–326, 383–384
  elbow, 295–296, 296f
  hand, 308–309, 308f–310f
  scaphoid bone, 302, 302f
  sternal, 325
  stress X-ray of, 493f
  types, 10, 11f. *See also* specific bones and sports
  upper arm, 291–293
  wrist, 302–303, 302f, 303f
free play decline, 496
friction blisters, 413
friction burns, 24
frostbite/frostnip, 452–453
fructose, 114
functional activities, 187
functional knee braces, 375
functional loss and return to play, 165
fungus, defined, 410
fungus infections, 417–418
furuncles, 419–421
furuncles, carbuncles, and folliculitis, 419–421

G

galea aponeurotica, 192
gamekeeper's thumb, 310–311, 310f
gamma-hydroxybutyrate (GHB), 144t, 148
ganglion of wrist, 307, 307f
gastritis, 464
gastrocnemius, 381
gastroenteritis, 464
gastrointestinal infections (GI), 464
gemelli muscles, 341
general conditioning programs, 74
generalized onset seizure, 481
GHB. *See* gamma-hydroxybutyrate
GH joint. *See* glenohumeral joint
GI. *See* gastrointestinal infections; glycemic index
ginseng, 143t
GIRD. *See* glenohumeral internal rotation deficit
glenohumeral internal rotation deficit (GIRD), 278
glenohumeral (GH) joint, 14, 75, 261–262, 271–274, 271f, 272f
glenohumeral joint–related impingement syndrome, 277–279, 277f, 278f
glenoid fossa, 262, 271, 272f, 275, 285
glenoid labrum, 23, 262
glucagon kit, 477, 477f

glucocorticoids, 184
glucometer, 476
gluteus minimus muscle, 340
glycemic index (GI), 114–115, 115t
glycerol, 119
glycogen, 115–116, 138
   loading, 115–116
golfer's elbow, 298
Good Samaritan law, 56, 58
gracilis muscle, 342, 343
gradual onset injury, 6
grand mal seizure, 482
greater multangular (trapezium) bone, 308
greenstick fractures, 11f, 268, 325
groin injuries, 359
groin pulls, 359
groin strains, prevention of, 350
growth cartilage, 494–495
growth in adolescents, 492
growth plates, 494
guarana, 143t, 146, 147
gymnastics, 27, 141, 233
   GH joint impingement syndrome, 277
   kyphosis, 249
   microvascular injury, 494
   spondylolisthesis, 257

H

HACE. *See* high altitude cerebral edema
Hageman factor (XIIa), 174
Hamilton, Breanna, 179
hamstring muscles, 342, 354, 359
hand fractures, 308–309, 308f–310f
hand injuries, 307, 308f
   fractures, 308–309, 308f–310f
   sprains and dislocations, 310–314
HAPE. *See* high altitude pulmonary edema
Harris–Benedict equation, 111
HAV. *See* hepatitis A virus
HBV. *See* hepatitis B virus
HCM. *See* hypertrophic cardiomyopathy
head, neck, and face injuries
   anatomy, 192–194
   background information for head injuries, 195–197
   brachial plexus injuries, 221–222, 221f
   breathing assessment, 208–209
   central nervous system, 194
   cervical spine injuries, 218–224
   circulation assessment, 208–209
   concussion, 198–199
   contact lens problems, 237
   cranial injury, 203
   dislocations, 222–224
   ear injuries, 238–239
   eye injuries, 234–237, 235t, 236f
   face, 195, 239, 240f
   football emergency procedures for treatment, 226–231
   fractures, 222–224
   initial check, 208
   intracranial injury, 201–203
   maxillofacial region injuries, 231–240
      dental injuries, 232–234
      eye injuries, 234–237, 235t, 236f
      face injury, 239, 240f
      nose injuries, 237–238
   mechanism of, 197–198
   meninges, 192–194, 193f
   neck (cervical spine), 195, 224
   nose, 237–238
   nose injuries, 237–238
   peripheral nervous system, 194–195
   physical exam, 209–218, 212t, 216t, 217t
   post-concussive syndrome, 200
   second impact syndrome, 200–201, 201f
   sideline assessment, 211–213, 212t
   skull, 192, 192f, 193f
   sprains, 222
   strains, 222
   treatment guidelines, 203–218, 224–226
head-tilt/chin-lift technique, 161, 161f
healing process, acute phase of, 390
Health Insurance Portability and Accountability Act (HIPPA), 60, 73
heart
   injuries, 327–331
   murmurs/arrhythmias, 335
heat cramps, 436
Heat index, 432, 433f
heat-related conditions
   exertional heat illnesses, 434–441
   prevention, heat illness, 441–449
heat syncope, 435
heat treatment for inflammation, 180
heel spurs, 394–395
helmets, 226f
   baseball, 21–22
   removal dangers, 161, 209, 229f
hematoma formation, 10, 172–173
   contusion with, 392f
   intracerebral, 202
hematuria, 258, 334
hemopneumothorax, 333
hemorrhage, 9
   assessment, 159–160
   sprains and, 9
hemostasis, 173

hemothorax, 250, 325
hepatitis A virus (HAV), 467–468
hepatitis B virus (HBV), 411, 467–468
hepatitis infection, 467–468
herbal supplements, 143t–144t, 146
hernias, 348–349
herniated disk, 256
herpes
	herpes gladiatorum, 422–423, 422f, 427t
	HSV-1, 423
	wrestling and, 24
herpes simplex virus type 1 (HSV-1), 423
high altitude cerebral edema (HACE), 455–456
high altitude pulmonary edema (HAPE), 455
"high ankle sprain", 387
high-density lipoprotein (HDL), 119
high-force injuries, 493
hip adductors, 354
hip extensors, 342f
hip flexors, 342f
HIPPA, Health Insurance Portability and Accountability Act. See Health Insurance Portability and Accountability Act
hip/pelvis injuries
	anatomy, 339–343
	avulsion fractures, 346
	hernias, 348–349
	hip dislocation, 345
	hip pointer, 344
	male genitalia injuries, 348
	nerve problems, 350
	osteitis pubis, 344–345
	other hip problems, 346–348
	pelvis fractures, 343
	prevention of, 350–351
	sacroiliac joint injury, 345
	skeletal injuries, 343–345
	slipped capital femoral epiphysis, 343–344
	soft-tissue injuries, 346–350
	sports-related injuries, 343–350
histamine, 172
history of injury, 11, 163, 163f
HIV. See human immunodeficiency virus
hockey
	commotio cordis, 328
	pelvis fractures, 343
hormones, 370
	effect of sex, 370
horseshoe-shaped pad, 386, 386f
horseshoe stirrups, 402f
HPV. See human papillomavirus
HSV-1. See herpes simplex virus type 1
human immunodeficiency virus (HIV), 411

human papillomavirus (HPV), 424
humeral head, 275
humeroradial joint, 285, 286
humeroulnar joint, 285
hydration stations, 437f
hydration techniques, 109
hydrocollator packs, 180
hydrocortisone, 184
hydrogenation, 119
hydrogen peroxide, 412
hydroxymethylbutyrate, 144t
hyoid, 195
hyperesthesia, 500
hyperextension, 257
	of cervical spine, 222
hyperflexion of cervical spine, 219, 221
hyperglycemia, 475t, 478
hyperhydration, 439
hyperosmolality, 138
hypersomnia, 97
hyperthermia, 431
hypertrophic cardiomyopathy (HCM), 327, 329, 329f, 335
hypertrophy/endurance phase (periodization), 82
hyphema, 236
hypoglycemia, 477
hypoglycemic unawareness, 478
hypohydration, 434–435, 434t, 435
hypothalamus, 432, 451
hypothenar eminence, 305
hypothermia, 451–452
hypovolemic shock, 160, 162, 165

I

ICE. See ice, compression, and elevation
ice, compression, and elevation (ICE), 300
ice hockey, thoracic strains, 251
idiopathic nature, 366
IFS. See interferential stimulation
iliac artery/vein, 340
iliacus muscle, 341
iliocostalis muscles, 322
iliopsoas group, 341
IM. See infectious mononucleosis
immediate energy system, 113
immediate-onset injury, 399
immune response, 461–469
immune serum globulin (ISG), 467, 463
impetigo, 419–420, 419f, 427t
impingement syndrome, 277–279, 277f, 278f
incisions, 410
incomplete proteins, 117
incubation period, 424
industrial/corporate athletic trainers, 44

infections, skin, 416-426
infectious imitators, 499
infectious mononucleosis (IM), 466-467
inferior nasal concha bones, 195
inflamed bursae, 363-364
inflammatory process, 172, 173f
inflammatory response phase, 172-176
infraspinatus muscles, 263, 264f, 267
ingrown toenail, 399f
inguinal hernias, 348
inhaler, 470
initial assessment of injuries, 158-165
initial check, injury
    dental injuries, 232-233
    eye, 236-237, 236f
    head, 208
injuries, 5
    acute/chronic, 5, 6f
    contributors, 495-498
    data, 3
    evaluation procedures, 156-157
    imitators, 498-500
    mechanisms, 492-495
    recognition, 14
    recurrent, 28-29
injury prevention, 82-85, 503-504
injury process, 169-187
    cryotherapy, 180-184
    exercise rehabilitation, 186-187
    fibroblastic repair phase, 176-178
    inflammatory process, 172, 173f
    inflammatory response phase, 172-176
    intervention procedures, 180-185
    mechanical forces, 170, 170f
    nonsteroidal anti-inflammatory drugs, 184-185, 185t
    pain and acute injury, 178-180
    pharmacologic agents, 184-185
    physics of injury, 169-171
    physiology of injury, 171-178
    prevention, 180
    remodeling phase, 178
    steroidal anti-inflammatory drugs, 184
    thermotherapy, 180-184
injury-specific exercise, 187
inner ear and equilibrium, 238
innominate bones, 339
insidious, 237
institution-based athletics, 154
insulin, 114, 475-476
intercarpal joints, 303
interclavicular ligaments, 274
intercostal muscles, 251, 322
interferential stimulation (IFS), 180

internal hemorrhaging, 160
internal injuries, thorax/abdomen, 327-335, 328f, 329f, 330t, 331f-333f
internal locus of control, 91
internal oblique muscles, 322, 323f
internal organs, 322-323, 323f, 324f
    injury with fracture, 258
International Olympic Committee (IOC), 471, 504
interstitial spaces, 172
intervention procedures, 180-185
intervention strategies
    extrinsic factors, 67-69
    intrinsic factors, 69-82
intervertebral joints, 321
intra-articular cartilaginous disk, 269
intracellular fluid, 126
intracerebral hematoma, 202
intracranial injury, 201-203
intracranial pressure, 199
intrinsic factors, 66, 67t, 69-82
intrinsic overuse injuries, 6
inversion ankle sprains, 401
inversion of foot, 380
invertebral disk injuries, 253
IOC. *See* International Olympic Committee
iontophoresis, 184
iron, 126
ischium, 339
ISG. *See* immune serum globulin

J

jaw-thrust technique, 161, 161f
jersey finger, 312-313, 312f
jock itch, 417
joint capsules, 7, 9
joint dysfunction, as dislocation symptom, 14
joint mice. *See* osteochondritis dissecans (OCD)
JRA. *See* juvenile rheumatoid arthritis
jumper's knee, 364-366
juvenile rheumatoid arthritis (JRA), 499

K

Kehr's sign, 334
keratolysis, 424
ketoacidosis, 478
ketones, 478
kidneys
    contusions, 10
    heat susceptibility, 334
    injuries, 334
kinesiology, 275
knee bracing, 374-376

knee injuries
    participation of athletes with, 372t–373t
    preventing, 371
knee joint, 353
    ligaments of, 356f
Koch, Steven, 326
kyphosis, 249

L

labyrinth, 238
lacerated spleen, 334
lacerations, 410
lacrimal bones, 195
lacrosse, commotio cordis, 328
lactose, 113
laser surgery, 423
lateral ankle sprain, 385, 387
lateral flexion of cervical spine, 222
latex allergy, 415
latex gloves, 233
latissimus dorsi muscle, 263, 263f, 264f, 265t, 322, 323t
lat pull down, 502
Laudner, Kevin, 281
law and sports injury, 51–63
    actions when sued, 61–62
    coach's liability, 56–58
    coach's protections, 58–59
    ethics of sports-injury care, 52–54
    Good Samaritan law, 56, 58
    state regulation of athletic training, 62
    torts, 54–56
lean body weight (LBW), 141
leukocytes, 174, 175
leukotrienes, 175
levator scapulae muscle, 263, 264f, 265t
liability insurance coverage, 58
lice, 425
ligaments, 286
    of ankle joint, 381f
    damage categories, 269
    injuries, 492
    knee joint, 356f
lightning, 69, 456–457
    safety, 457
    treatment, 457
lipids, 118
liquid nitrogen, 423, 424
litigation. *See also* law and sports injury
    coach liability, 14
Little League Baseball in 1939, 488
Little League elbow, 22, 296, 297, 493
Little League shoulder, 280
liver injuries, 333

load volume, 77
local symptoms, unusual, 498
locus of control, 91
long bone tumors, 499
long-distance running, hypothermia, 451
longissimus muscle, 322
long-term treatment with adhesive tape, 394
lordosis, 253
low back pain, 334
low-cost alternative method, 395
low-density lipoprotein (LDL), 119
lower extremity biomechanics, 370
lower-extremity injuries, 18, 21
lower leg, ankle, and foot injuries
    anatomy, 378–383
    ankle taping, preventive, 400–404
    sports injuries
        ankle injuries, 384–389
        arch problems, 395–397
        blisters and calluses, 397–398
        bunions, 397
        compartment syndrome, 391–392
        foot disorders, 394–400
        fractures, 383–384
        heel spurs, 394–395
        Morton's foot, 395
        plantar fasciitis, 394
        shin splints, 392–394
        skeletal injuries, 383–384
        soft-tissue injuries, 384–394
        tendon-related injuries, 389–391
        toe injuries, 398–400
lower respiratory infections (LRI), 463–464
low glycemic index carbohydrates, 114
LRI. *See* lower respiratory infections
lumbar disk injuries, 256
lumbar plexus, 340
lumbar vertebrae, 253
lung injuries, 332–333, 332f, 333f
luxation, 13
lyme disease, 416, 425, 426f, 465–466, 499
lysosomes, 174

M

macrocycle, 81
macronutrients, 109, 110
macrophages, 175, 176, 181
macrotrauma, 492
magnetic resonance imaging (MRI), 12, 499
major depression, 95
major minerals, 123
malaise, 463, 464
male genitalia injuries, 348

malfeasance, 55
mallet (baseball) finger, 311–312, 311f, 312f
malocclusion, 239
maltose, 113
mandible, 195, 232
mandibular condyle, 239
mandibular fossa, 239
manubrium of sternum, 274
Marfan syndrome, 331
maturation phase, 171, 178
maxilla, 195, 232
maxillofacial region injuries, 231–240
    dental injuries, 232–234
    eye injuries, 234–237, 235t, 236f
    face injury, 239, 240f
    nose injuries, 237–238
mechanical dysfunction, 366
mechanical forces of injury, 170, 170f
mechanisms of injury
    cervical spine, 219–221
    head, 197–198
medial, ankle sprain, 385
medial epicondylitis, 298
medial tibial stress syndrome (MTTS), 392
mediastinum, 322
medical history of injury assessment, 163–164
melanomas, 415
meninges, 192–194, 193f
menisci injuries, 366–367
menstruation, 504
mental health
    anorexia nervosa and bulimia nervosa, 100–101
    anxiety disorders, 98, 98t
    behavioral disorders, 98–100
    mood disorders, 95–98
    neurodevelopmental disorders, 103–104
    prevention, 102–103
    research of eating habits, 101
    role of care provider, 104–105
    specificity and eating disorders, 101–102
    treatment, 103
mesocycles, 81
metabolic emergencies, 164
metacarpal bones, 308, 309
metacarpophalangeal (MP) joint, 310f
metaphysis, 12, 13
methicillin-resistant *staphylococcus aureus* (MRSA), 24, 417, 421–422
methylphenidate (Ritalin), 147
microcycle, 81
micronutrients, 110, 121
microtrauma, 383, 492, 494
microvascular injury, 494
middle ear, 238

mid-shaft humeral fractures, 291, 292f
mild hypothermia, 452
mild traumatic brain injury, 195
military press, 502
minerals, 123–126, 124t
minimal competitive weight, 141
minor, or trace, minerals, 124, 124t
misfeasance, 55
missing organs, 73
modalities for pain, 180, 180t
moderate hypothermia, 452
molluscum contagiosum, 423–424, 423f
monocytes, 174, 176
mononucleosis, 334, 454
monosaccharides, 113, 114
monounsaturated fats, 119
Morton's foot, 395
Morton's neuroma, 395
mosaic wart, 424
mouth guards, 21–22, 233
movable soccer goals, 27
MRI. *See* magnetic resonance imaging
MRSA. *See* methicillin-resistant *staphylococcus aureus*
MTTS. *See* medial tibial stress syndrome
multivitamin supplement, 126
muscle endurance, 77–79
muscle power, 77–79
muscle protein, 139
muscles, 291, 294
    activity/innervation, 322, 323t
    of arm, 286, 287f
    strains, 326
muscle strength, 77–79
muscular tissue, 170
musculotendinous junction (MTJ), 9, 170
myalgia, 462, 464
myelin, 194
myocarditis, 462
myositis ossificans, 10, 358–359
myositis ossificans traumatica, 288–289

N

nasal bones, 195
NATA. *See* National Athletic Trainers' Association
National Association of Anorexia Nervosa and Associated Disorders (ANAD), 100
National Athletic Trainers' Association (NATA), 29, 112, 127t, 140, 229, 471, 489
    AHCT description, 41–41
    BOC certification, 41–42
    heat-related illness, 436
    MRSA, 422
    recognition/treatment, 328

National Collegiate Athletic Association (NCAA), 136, 197, 233, 237
   banned drugs, 504
   contact ACL injuries, 369
   deaths in athlete population, 327
   football injury survey, 18
   guideline (medical evaluations, immunizations, and records), 71
   noncontact ACL injury, 369
   soccer goal construction, 25
   wrestling/skin infection guidelines, 426
National Collegiate Athletic Association (NCAA) Injury Surveillance Program (ISP), 20
National Federation of State High School Associations (NFHS), 18, 25, 71, 132
National Football League (NFL), 220, 369
National Safety Council
   CPR and AED training, 59
   fracture symptoms, 10
   wound treatment guidelines, 412
National Strength and Conditioning Association (NSCA), 75, 77, 147
NCAA. *See* National Collegiate Athletic Association
neck (cervical spine), 195
   injuries
      football emergency procedures for treatment, 226–231
      treatment guidelines for, 224–226
negative body image, 102
negative pressure, 332f
negligence, 52–56
nerves, 339
   CNS, 438
   injuries to wrist, 304–306, 305f
   problems, 350
nervous tissue, 170
neural arch, 257, 257f
neurapraxia, 220
neurodevelopmental disorders, 103–104
neurogenic shock, 165
neuroma, 395
neuromuscular activity, 370
neuromuscular electrical stimulation (NMES), 180
neuropsychological testing, 60
neurovascular imitators, 499–500
neutrophils, 174
New York City Public School Athletic League, 488
NFL. *See* National Football League
nipple irritation, 327
nitric oxide (NO), 146
NMES. *See* neuromuscular electrical stimulation
nonathlete's diet, 136
noncatastrophic injuries, 489

noncontact ACL injury, 369
nonsteroidal anti-inflammatory drugs (NSAIDs), 184–185, 185t
nose injuries, 237–238
NSAIDs. *See* nonsteroidal anti-inflammatory drugs
NSCA. *See* National Strength and Conditioning Association
nucleus pulposus, 256
nutrients overview
   carbohydrate, 113–116
   energy expenditure, 110–111
   energy systems, 113
   fat, 118–121
   minerals, 123–126
   protein, 116–118
   vitamins, 121–123, 121f, 122t–123t
   water, 126–128
   weight loss, 111–113
nutrition
   body composition, 81
   body weight management, 140–141
   dietary guidelines for athletes
      during competition, 138
      daily maintenance, 136–138
      for post exercise, 138–139
      precompetition diets, 138
   endurance athletes, 129–130
   endurance sports, 129–130
   female athletes, 129
   and injury recovery, 139–140
   nutritional knowledge, 135–136
   strength/power athletes, 130–131
   supplements, 145–146
   team sport athletes, 131–132
   wrestling, 132, 134

O

obesity in children and adolescents, 496
oblique fractures, 11f
oblique muscles, 322
observation of injury, 162, 164–165
Occupational Safety and Health Administration (OSHA), 411
OCD. *See* osteochondritis dissecans
omega-3 fatty acids, 140
omega-6 fatty acids, 140
omission, 55
oncologic imitators, 499
one-repetition maximum lift (1 RM), 502
orbital hematoma, 236
orthopedic surgeons, 38, 357
Osgood-Schlatter disease, 364–366, 493
OSHA. *See* Occupational Safety and Health Administration

ossification, 491
osteitis pubis, 344–345
   prevention of, 350
osteoarthritis, 21
osteoblasts, 177
osteochondritis dissecans (OCD), 299–300, 362–363
osteochondrosis, 280
osteoclasts, 177
osteomyelitis, 499
osteoporosis, 102, 504
osteosarcomas, 499
otitis externa, 463
otitis media, 463
oval window rupture, 239
over the counter (OTC) sale, 146
overuse injuries, 6, 280–281, 467, 492, 496
   definition, 83
   drawbacks, 82, 83f
   emergency action plan, 84
   guidelines, 83–84
   return-to-play criteria, 84
oxidative energy conversion, 75

P

pain, 10
   and acute injury, 178–180
palatine bones, 195
palmar radiocarpal ligament, 303, 303f, 304f
palpation
   in anatomic snuffbox, 302, 303f
   injury assessment, 164–165, 164f
   thoracic strains, 251
parasites, defined, 410
parasites infections, 424–426
parasitic skin infections, 426
paratroopers, braces in, 388
parental consent forms, 60
pars interarticularis, 257
passive exercise, 186
passive stretching, 80
patella
   dislocation/subluxation, 364
      fractures, 358
      patellar tendon, 6, 7f
      patellar tracking, 366
patellofemoral conditions, 366
patellofemoral joint, 354
   injuries, 362–366
pathogenic eating behaviors, 99
PCS. *See* post-concussive syndrome
pectineus muscle, 342
pectoralis major/minor muscles, 263, 263f, 265t, 322

pectoral muscles, strains in, 326
pelvis, 254
   fractures, 343
penetrating eye injuries, 235
periodization, 75, 81–82
periosteum of cranial bone, 192
peripheral mechanical stabilization, 373
peripheral nervous system (PNS), 194–195
permethrin, 466
peroneus brevis, 381, 391
personal hydration needs calculations, 445t
personality traits, 91–92
personality variables, 91
pes anserinus group, 342, 343
pes cavus, 395
pes planus, 395
Peterson type I injury, 494, 494f
phagocytosis, 175
phalangeal dislocations, 314, 314f
phalanges, 307
   fractures of, 309
pharmacologic agents, 180, 184–185
pharyngitis, 463
phase 1
   stress model, 93
phase 2
   stress model, 93
phase 3
   stress model, 93
phonophoresis, 184
phospholipids, 119, 175
physes, 493
physical exam during injury assessment, 162–165, 209–218, 212t, 216t, 217t
   concussion education, 216–218
   home instructions, 213–215
   postconcussion care, 213–215
   return to learn, 215, 217t
   return to play, 215, 216t
   sideline assessment, 211–213, 212t
physical findings inconsistent with injury history, 498
physics of sports injury, 169–171
physiology of sports injury, 171–178
pia mater, 193–194, 193f
PIP joint. *See* proximal interphalangeal joint
piriformis muscle, 340
plaintiff, 54, 55
plantar fasciitis, 394
plantar flexion, 379, 380
plantar warts, 424
plasma proteins, 175
platelets, 175
playing surfaces, 69, 498

pleural sac, 322, 332
pneumonia, 464
pneumothorax, 250, 250f, 325, 332, 332f, 333
PNF. *See* proprioceptive neuromuscular facilitation
PNS. *See* peripheral nervous system
point tenderness, 163
poison (plants) allergy, 414
pole-vaulting, pelvis fractures, 343
polycarbonate, 237
polymorphs, 176
polysaccharides, 113
polyunsaturated fats, 119
popliteus muscle, 381
postconcussion care, 213–215
post-concussive syndrome (PCS), 200
posterior cruciate ligament, 356, 367
posterior longitudinal ligaments, 255
posterior rib fracture, 250
posterior SC dislocation, 274
posterior talofibular ligaments, 381
posterior tibial artery, 381
postexercise rehydration, 446
postgame, 480, 480t
postgraduate classes, 60–61
post-traumatic amnesia (PTA), 199
postural problems, 72
postural stability testing, 60
power phase (periodization), 82
PPE. *See* preparticipation physical examination/evaluation
practice/competition environment, 68
precompetition diets, 138
prednisolone, 184
prednisone, 184
pregame, 479–480
"Pre-hospital Care of the Spine-Injured Athlete," 226, 229
premature specialization, 488
preparticipation physical examination/evaluation (PPE), 60, 70–74
    components, 73, 74t
    by coordinated medical team, 72
    females' menstrual history, 503
    as requirement, 60
prepatellar bursitis, 364f
prescription stimulant medication, 504
preseason conditioning, 74, 497
preventive ankle taping, 400–404
    advantages and disadvantages of, 400
prewrap, application of, 401
PRICE. *See* protection, rest, ice, compression, and elevation
primary amenorrhea, 504
professional sports settings, 43–46
pronator forearm muscles, 286, 289f

prophylactic adhesive-taping procedure, 388
prophylactic knee brace, 373, 374t
proprioception training exercises, 388
proprioceptive neuromuscular facilitation (PNF), 80
prostaglandins, 172, 174, 184
protection, rest, ice, compression, and elevation (PRICE), 181
protective cup, 348, 351
protective equipment, 69, 69t
    heart/lung injury, 330
    padding, 69
protective eyewear, 237
proteins, 116–118, 139
    consumption after exercise, 139
protein supplementation, 117–118
protein supplements, 117–118
proteoglycans, 177
proximal humeral epiphysiolysis, 280
proximal interphalangeal (PIP) joint, 313, 314
proximal musculotendinous junction (MTJ), 170
proximate cause, 55
psoas muscles, 341
psychogenic shock, 165
psychologic imitators, 500
psychology of competition
    personality variables, 91
    stress and athlete, 89–91
psychology of injury
    eating disorders, 98–100
    mental health
        anorexia nervosa and bulimia nervosa, 100–101
        anxiety disorders, 98, 98t
        behavioral disorders, 98–100
        mood disorders, 95–98
        neurodevelopmental disorders, 103–104
        prevention, 102–103
        research of eating habits, 101
        role of care provider, 104–105
        specificity and eating disorders, 101–102
        treatment, 103
    personality traits, 91–92
    psychological stress, 92–93, 93f
    psychology of competition, 89–91
    psychosocial variables, 92, 92t
    recommendations, 95
psychometric tests, 92
psychosocial variables of injury, 92, 92t
PTA. *See* post-traumatic amnesia
puberty, 491–492
pubic bones, 339
pubic lice, 425
pubis, 339

pulmonary contusion, 332–333
punctures, 410
purulent lesions, 419
pyoderma, 419
pyomyositis, 499

Q

Q angle, 366, 366f
quadriceps, 354, 366
quadriceps muscles, 341, 354, 354f, 366

R

radiation, 432, 449
radiocarpal joint, 286
radioulnar joints, 285, 286
range of motion (ROM), 79
    factors determining, 79
    rehabilitative exercise for, 186
Rang-Ogden type IV injury, 494, 494f
RDA. See recommended dietary allowance
recommended dietary allowance (RDA), 121
recovery (rest) periods, 77
rectal core body temperature, 438
rectus abdominis muscles, 322
rectus femoris muscle, 341, 347, 354, 360
REE. See resting energy expenditure
referred pain, 334
reflex neuropathic dystrophy (RND), 499
refractometer, 141
regeneration, 171
rehabilitation
    of previous injuries, 503
    programs, 394
rehabilitative exercises, 178, 186–187
rehydration, 445–446
relative humidity, 432
remodeling phase, 171, 178
removal from activity area, 165
renal failure, 334
repair, 171
repetition maximum (RM), 77
repetition volume, 77
repolarization phase of contracting heart, 328
rescue breathing, 158
research, athlete, 100
resistance training, 76–77
resistive exercise, 186
resolution, 171
respiratory infections
    LRI, 463–464
    URI, 462–463

respiratory system, 160
    injury assessment, 160
    respiratory arrest, 208
responsiveness of athlete, 160
rest, ice, compression, and elevation (RICE), 250
resting energy expenditure (REE), 111
resting metabolic rate (RMR), 110
rest periods, 78
retinaculum, 300
retrograde amnesia, 199
return to learn condition, 215, 217t
return to play condition, 165–166, 215, 216t
return-to-play criteria, 84
rhabdomyolysis, 158
rheumatologic imitators, 499
rhinitis, 462
rhodiola, 143t
rhomboid muscle, 263, 264f, 322
rib fractures, 249–251, 325
rib joints, 321
RICE. See rest, ice, compression, and elevation
rigid ankle brace, 389f
ringworm, 24, 417, 417f
risk factors, 14
    identification of, 14
Ritalin (methylphenidate), 147, 504
1-RM equivalent, 502
RMR. See resting metabolic rate
RND. See reflex neuropathic dystrophy
ROM. See range of motion
room dimensions, 69
rotational deformity, 309
rotation of cervical spine, 222
rotator cuff, 6, 7f, 267, 275–276, 276f
running
    chronic injuries, 5, 6f
    snapping hip syndrome, 347
ruptured eardrum, 239
ruptured rectus femoris muscle, 360
    case study of, 360

S

sacral, 258
sacral plexus, 340, 340f
sacroiliac (SI) joints, 255, 339, 345
sacrum, 254, 339
SAD. See seasonal affective disorder
safety fences, 68
safe weight loss and management, 140
sagittal plane MRI of a torn ACL, 368
salmeterol, 471

Salter-Harris fractures, 12–13, 13f, 494
sanitation facility location, 68
sartorius muscle, 341
saturated fats, 119
scabies, 424–425
scalp, 193f
scaphoid bone, fracture of, 302, 302f
scapula, 263, 268
scapular dyskinesis, 278
scar tissue, 171, 178
Scheuermann's disease, 249
sciatic nerve, 340, 350
SC joint. See sternoclavicular joint
scoliosis, 249
scrotal contusions, 348
seasonal affective disorder (SAD), 97–98
secondary amenorrhea, 504
secondary enzymatic injury, 175, 181
secondary metabolic injury, 175, 181
secondary school setting, 45–46
secondary sexual characteristics, 490, 491
second-degree sprains/strains, 9
second impact syndrome (SIS), 199, 200–201, 201f
second-user CPR, 43
seizure, 481
self-concept as risk factor, 91
self-help strategies, 97
semicircular fibrocartilaginous disks, 356
semimembranosus muscle, 342
semirigid orthoses, 394
sensitizers, 414
septal hematoma, 238
septal injuries, 238
serratus anterior muscle, 263, 264f
serum hepatitis (HBV), 411
severe hypothermia, 452
Sever's disease, 494
shear forces, 170, 170f
shin splints, 12, 392–394
shivering, 449
shock in injury assessment, 165
shoes, 350
shoulders
    acromioclavicular joint injuries, 269–271, 270f
    anatomy, 261–267, 262f–264f, 265t–266t, 266f, 267f
    biceps tendon, 279–280, 279f
    contusions, 275
    fractured clavicle, 267–268, 268f
    fractured scapula, 268
    girdle muscles, 75, 263, 263f, 264f, 265t
        actions, and innervations of, 265f–266f
    glenohumeral (GH) joint, 271–274, 271f, 272f
    joint, 262
    Little League, 280
    muscles, 262, 263, 263f, 264f, 265t
    overuse injuries, 280–281
    pointer, 275
    rotator cuff, 275–276, 276f
    skeletal injuries, 267–268, 268f, 269f
    soft-tissue injuries, 269–281
    sternoclavicular joint injuries, 274–275
    strains, 275–281, 276f–279f
    subluxation, 163
    tip pain, 334
sickle cell trait, 436, 472–473
SICK scapula, 277–278
side aches, 335
sideline assessment, head injuries, 211–213, 212t
sign, defined, 162
signs and symptoms
    Achilles tendon, 390
    AC joint sprains, 270
    asthma, 469–472
    avulsion fractures, 346
    biceps tendon problems, 279–280
    boutonnière deformity, 313
    brachial plexus injury, 221
    cervical spine sprains, 222
    cervical spine strains, 222
    clavicle fracture, 268
    coccyx fracture, 258
    compartment syndrome, 391
    concussion (mild head injury), 198
    dehydration, 432
    dental injuries, 232
    de Quervain's disease, 306
    of dislocated hip, 345
    distal forearm fractures, 300–301
    ear injuries, 238–239
    EIA, 471
    elbow fractures, 296
    elbow sprains and dislocations, 294, 295f
    epicondylitis/apophysitis, 298–299
    exertional heat exhaustion, 436–437
    exertional heatstroke, 438
    eye injuries, 235
    femur fracture, 358
    frostbite (deep freezing), 452
    frostnip (superficial freezing), 452
    gamekeeper's thumb, 311
    ganglion, 307
    GH joint injuries, 272
    hand fractures, 309
    herniated disk, 256
    herpes gladiatorum, 422–423
    humeral fractures, 291

hypohydration, 435
hypothermia, 452
impetigo and cellulitis, 419–420
impingement syndrome, 278
inflamed bursa, 363
injuries to biceps brachii muscle, 290
injuries to triceps brachii muscle, 291
jersey finger, 312–313
jumper's knee, 365
knee ligaments injury, 371
lateral ankle sprain, 386
lower leg/foot fracture, 384
lumbar sprains/strains, 255
mallet finger, 312
muscle strains, 361
muscular contusion, 359
nerve injuries to wrist, 305
OCD, 363
ODC, 299
olecranon bursitis, 300
Osgood-Schlatter disease, 365
plantar warts, 424
rotator cuff injuries, 276
SC joint injuries, 274
shin splints, 393
shoulder contusions, 275
sickle cell trait, 473
SLAP, 273
subluxation/dislocation of patella, 364
suspected torn meniscus, 367
swan neck deformity, 314
testicular contusions, 348
of tib/fib syndesmosis sprain, 387
tinea infection, 418
tinea versicolor, 418
upper arm contusions, 288–289
vertebral fractures, 249
wrist fractures, 302–303
wrist sprains and dislocations, 303–304
zygomatic bone fracture, 239
SI joint. See sacroiliac joints
silver fork deformity, 301, 301f
simple carbohydrates, 114
simple fats, 119
sinusitis, 462
SIS. See second impact syndrome
skeletal injuries, 249–251, 357–358, 383–384
    hip/pelvis, 343–345
    shoulder, 267–268, 268f, 269f
skin, 410f, 427t–428t
    allergic reactions, 414, 425
    bacterial infections, 418–422
    care provider role, 426–428
    exacerbation skin conditions, 416
    infections, 23, 416–426
    inflammatory conditions, 414–416
    MRSA, 24, 421–422
    plantar warts, 424
    ringworm, 417–418
    tinea versicolor, 418
    ultraviolet light and, 415–416
    viral infections, 422–424
    wounds, 410–413
    wrestling and skin infections, 426
skull anatomy, 192, 192f, 193f
slipped capital femoral epiphysis, 343–344
snapping hip syndrome, 347
soccer, 25
    data, 25
    injury rates, 2, 3, 25
    jumping and pelvic avulsion, 346
    osteitis pubis, 345
social physique anxiety, 100
social support, psychological recovery and, 95
softball
    anterior shoulder pain, 23
    game vs. practice injury rates, 21
    injury data, 2, 3, 21
    protective chest equipment, 330, 331f
soft orthotics, 395f
soft tissue, defined, 7
soft tissue injuries, 384–394
    avulsion fractures, 346
    hernias, 348–349
    male genitalia injuries, 348
    nerve problems, 350
    shoulder, 269–281
    to thigh, 358–362
    to upper arm, 286–291
soleus muscles, 381, 390
sovereign immunity, 56, 57
spearing, 19, 220
spear tackler's spine, 223
SPF. See sun protection factor
spheroidal articulation, 271
spinal curvature, 249
spinalis muscle, 322
spinal nerves, 194
spine
    lumbar disk injuries, 256
    lumbar spine
        anatomy, 253–254, 253f–254f, 254t
        sprains, 255–256, 255f
        strains, 255–256, 255f
    rib fractures, 249–250
    skeletal injuries, 249–251

spine (continued)
　spinal curvature, 249
　spondylolisthesis, 257, 257f
　spondylolysis, 257, 257f
　strains, thoracic spine, 251
　thoracic cage, 248, 248f
　thoracic spine anatomy, 247, 248f
　traumatic fractures, 257–258
　vertebral fractures, 249
spine boards, 225f
spleen injuries, 334
splinting
　of elbow injury, 293f, 295
　techniques, 314, 315f
spondylolisthesis, 257, 257f
spondylolysis, 257, 257f
spontaneous pneumothorax, 332
sport environment, 100
sports bras, 326
sports classifications, 15–17, 16t–17t
sports hernias, 349, 349f
sports injury, concept of, 1–31, 152
　ankle injuries, 384–389
　baseball/softball, 21–23
　basketball, 20–21
　cheerleading, 27–28
　classifications of injury, 8–14
　contusions, 10
　dislocations, 13–14
　epidemiology, 14–15
　fractures, 10–13
　gymnastics, 27
　injury recognition, 14
　knee joint, 356f
　lower leg
　　arch problems, 395–397
　　blisters and calluses, 397–398
　　bunions, 397
　　compartment syndrome, 391–392
　　foot disorders, 394–400
　　fractures, 383–384
　　heel spurs, 394–395
　　Morton's foot, 395
　　plantar fasciitis, 394
　　shin splints, 392–394
　　skeletal injuries, 383–384
　　soft-tissue injuries, 384–394
　　tendon-related injuries, 389–391
　　toe injuries, 398–400
　lumbar disk, 256
　menisci, 366–367
　patellofemoral conditions, 366
　patellofemoral joint, 362–366
　physics of, 169–171
　physiology of, 171–178
　recurrent injuries, 28–29
　Salter-Harris fractures, 12–13, 13f
　skeletal, 267–268, 268f, 269f, 357–358, 383–384
　soccer, 25–27
　soft-tissue, 269–281
　　to thigh, 358–362
　spondylolisthesis, 257, 257f
　spondylolysis, 257, 257f
　sports classifications, 15–17, 16t–17t
　sprains, 9, 255–256, 255f
　strains, 9–10, 255–256, 255f
　stress fractures, 11–12
　tackle football, 18–20
　traumatic fractures, 257–258
　volleyball, 24–25
　wrestling, 23–24
　youth sports and fitness participation, 1–3
　youth sport specialization, 29–31, 31t
sports injury prevention
　aerobic fitness, 75–76
　body composition, 81
　causative factors, 66–67
　extrinsic factors, 67–69
　flexibility, 79–81
　heat illness, 441–449
　intervention strategies, 67–82
　intrinsic factors, 69–82
　muscle strength, power, and endurance, 77–79
　nutrition, 81
　overuse injuries, 82–84
　periodization, 81–82
　prevention and conditioning, 74–75
sports medicine, 38–39
　clinic, 43
　defined, 38–39
　fellowships, 39
　specialists involved in, 38
sports nutrition programs, 136
sport specificity and eating disorders, 101–102
sport task, 100
sprains, 9, 384
　cervical spine, 222
　defined, 9
　dislocations as, 13–14
　elbow, 294–295, 295f
　of hand, 310–314
　lumbar spine, 251, 255–256, 255f
　softball, 21
　wrist, 303–304, 303f, 304f
sprinting and pelvic avulsion fracture, 346
sputum, 464

squash, 277
squats, 502–503
"squeeze" test, 387
stabilization of head and neck, 203, 204f
standard ankle-taping procedure, 388
Standard Nomenclature of Athletic Injuries (SNAI), 8, 9
standard precautions, 159
standing toe touch, 80
Staphylococcus aureus, 418, 419
starch, 114
state regulation of athletic training, 62
static flexibility, 79
static stretching, 80
sternal fracture, 325
sternoclavicular (SC) joint, 262, 263f, 266, 274–275, 322
sternocostal joints, 322
steroidal anti-inflammatory drugs, 184
steroids, 147, 333, 412
sterols, 119
stingers, 221
stirrups, 401, 402f
    horseshoe, 402f
stitch in the side, 335
STOP Sports Injuries, 489
strains, 9–10
    abdominal muscle, 326
    cervical spine, 222
    defined, 9
    injuries, prevention of, 359
    lumbar spine, 255–256, 255f
    muscle, 326
    thoracic spine, 251
strength phase (periodization), 81
strength/power athletes, 130–131
strength training, 500–503
Streptococcus, 418, 419
stress fractures, 11–12, 383
stressful life events, 92
stress-injury model, 92
stressor, 93
stress X-ray of fracture, 493f
stretching exercises, 80, 503
subacromial space, 277
subclavian artery, 266
subclavius muscle, 263, 265t
subcutaneous fat, 140
subdural hematoma, 202
subluxations, 13, 279, 325
subscapularis muscles, 263, 264f, 267
subsequent ankle sprains, control of, 387
subsyndromal SAD, 97
subtalar joint, 379, 380
subungual hematoma, 398

sucrose, 113, 114
sudden death, 328
sudden onset injury, 6
sugars, 113, 114
Suicide, 96, 97t
sunburn protection, 416
sun protection factor (SPF), 415
superior dislocation of SC joint, 274
supinator forearm muscles, 286
Supplement 411, 145
supplementation, protein, 117–118
supracondylar fractures, 295
supraglenoid tubercle, 279
supraorbital regions, 195
supraspinatus muscle tendon, 6, 263, 264f, 267, 277
surgically implanted fixation, 308
suture joints, 192
suturing, 240
swan neck deformity, 314, 315f
sweat evaporation process, 127
sweat loss, 435
sweat rate, 444
swelling as acute fracture symptom, 10
swimming, GH joint-related impingement syndrome, 277
sympathetic eye movement, 236
symphysis pubis joint, 339, 344
symptomatic SAD, 97
symptoms, defined, 162
syndesmosis sprain, 387
syndrome, 277
synovial fluid, 307
synoviated articulation, 274
synthetic rubber additive allergies, 414
syphilis, 454
systemic symptoms, 498–499

T

table tennis, GH joint impingement syndrome, 277
tâche noir, 414
tackler's exostosis, 288
TACO. *See* tarp-assisted cooling oscillation
talocrural joint, 381, 402
talon noir, 414
Tanner stages of sexual maturity, 491
taping
    ankles, 395
    wrist and thumb, 314–315, 315f–317f
tarp-assisted cooling oscillation (TACO), 439
TDEE. *See* total daily energy expenditure
TEA. *See* thermal effect of activity
teacher as athletic trainer, 45
team dynamics, 104
team physicians, 39–40

team sport athletes, 131–132
TEF. *See* thermal effect of food
temporomandibular joint (TMJ), 239, 240*f*
tenderness, complaints of, 10
tendinitis, 276, 279, 304
tendons, 379, 389–391
    finger, 311*f*
    injuries, 389–391, 492–494
    muscles, 357
    problems of wrist, 306–307, 306*f*, 307*f*
    thumb, 306*f*
tennis
    GH joint impingement syndrome, 277
    and pelvic avulsion fracture, 346
tennis elbow, 298
tenosynovitis, 306
TENS. *See* transcutaneous electrical nerve stimulation
tensile forces, 170, 170*f*
tensor fasciae latae muscle, 341
terbutaline sulfate, 471
teres major/minor muscles, 263, 264*f*, 267
terrible-triad injury, 371
testicle injuries, 348
testicular contusion, 348
testicular/scrotal contusions, 348
testosterone precursors, 148
therapeutic exercise, 186–187
therapeutic heat, 180
thermal effect of activity (TEA), 110
thermal effect of food (TEF), 110
thermal gradient, 449
thermal injuries, indoor activities and, 68
thermogenesis, 449
thermoregulation, 126, 432
thermotherapy, 180–184
thigh, knee, and leg injuries
    anatomy, 353–357
    knee ligament, 367–373
    menisci injuries, 366–367
    patellofemoral conditions, 366
    patellofemoral joint, 362–366
    prevention, 373–376
    skeletal, 357–358
    soft-tissue injuries to thigh, 358–362
third-degree sprains/strains, 9
thoracic cage, 248, 248*f*
thoracic outlet syndrome (TOS), 251–252, 251*f*
thorax and abdomen injuries, 321–335
    abdominal pain, 334–335
    anatomy, 321–322
    bladder injuries, 334
    breast injuries, 326–327
    external injuries, 325–327
    fractures, 325–326
    heart injuries, 327–331
    internal injuries, 327–335, 328*f*, 329*f*, 330*t*, 331*f*–333*f*
    internal organs, 322–323, 323*f*, 324*f*
    kidney injuries, 334
    liver injuries, 333
    lung injuries, 332–333, 332*f*, 333*f*
    spleen injuries, 334
thumb taping, wrist and, 314–315, 315*f*–317*f*
tib/fib syndesmosis sprain, 386, 387
tibia, fracture of, 384*f*
tibial (medial) collateral ligament, 367
tibial stress injury (TSI), 393
tibiofemoral joint, 354
    dislocation of, 358
tibiofibular syndesmosis sprain, 386
tick removal, guidelines for, 466
ticks, 425
time lost as injury definition, 5
Tinactin, 418
tinea, 417–418, 417*f*, 427*t*
tinea versicolor (TV), 418
tissue, types of, 170
TMJ. *See* temporomandibular joint
toe injuries, 398–400
Tomczyk, Christopher P., 224
tonic-clonic seizure, 482, 483
tooth avulsion, 232
tooth enamel erosion, 102
topical analgesic allergies, 414
torn meniscus, 367
tort, 54–56
TOS. *See* thoracic outlet syndrome
total daily energy expenditure (TDEE), 110
total glenohumeral rotation range of motion (TRM), 278
track and field, GH joint impingement syndrome, 277
training duration, 76
training error, 497
training frequency, 76
training intensity, 76
training volume, 77
trait anxiety, 91
trait theory, 91
trait variables, 91
transcutaneous electrical nerve stimulation (TENS), 180
trans fat, 119
transition phase in training cycle, 82
transport device, 165
transverse carpal ligaments, 300
transverse fractures, 11*f*
transverse humeral ligament, 279
trapezium bone, 308
trapezius muscle, 263, 264*f*, 265*t*, 322

trapezoid ligaments, 269
trauma, 171
traumatic fractures, 257–258
traumatic injuries, 383
treatment guidelines
    dental injuries, 232–233
    exercise-induced asthma, 471
    exertional heat exhaustion, 437
    exertional heatstroke, 439
    eye injuries, 236–237
    head injury, 203–218
    hypothermia, 452
    for neck injuries, 224–226
    nose injury, 237–238
    plantar warts, 424
    tinea infection, 418
triamcinolone, 184
triceps brachii injuries, 291
triglycerides, 119
TRM. *See* total glenohumeral rotation range of motion
trochanteric bursitis, 347
true ribs, 321
TSI. *See* tibial stress injury
tunnel of Guyon, 304–305, 305*f*
turf burn, 296
turf toe, 399
    taping, 399
TV. *See* tinea versicolor
tympanic membrane, 238
type 1 (insulin dependent) diabetes, 475, 476*t*
type 2 (non-insulin dependent) diabetes, 475, 476*t*
typical physical exams, 70

U

ulnar collateral ligaments, 310
ulnar nerve, 294, 304–305
ultrasound diathermy, 180
ultrasound therapies, 69
ultraviolet A (UVA) light rays, 415–416
ultraviolet B (UVB) light rays, 415–416
uncus of temporal lobes, 200–201
unilateral spondylolysis, 257
universal and standard precautions, 411
University of North Carolina, 4
unknown onset seizure, 482
unresponsive to any stimulus assessment, 160
unsafe weight management practices, 140
unsaturated fats, 119
upper arm. *See* arm injuries
upper extremities, 66–67
upper respiratory infections (URI), 462–463
urine dipstick method, 141
urticaria, 416

U.S. Anti-Doping Agency (USADA), 144
U.S. Food and Drug Administration (FDA), 117, 144–145
U.S. National Registry of Sudden Death in Young Athletes, 327
U.S. society, 70
UVA light rays. *See* ultraviolet A light rays

V

valgus forces, 294
varicella, 454
varus forces, 294
vascular engorgement of brain tissue, 201
vasoactive substances, 174
vasoconstriction, 172, 173, 175
vasodilation, 172, 173, 452
ventricular fibrillation, 327
vertebral fractures, 249
vertebral joints, 321
vertigo, 462, 463
very low-density lipoprotein (VLDL), 120
vestibulocochlear nerve, 238
violent force injures, 367
violent trauma, 383
viral infections, 422–424
viruses, defined, 410
vitamins, 121–123, 121*f*, 122*t*–123*t*
Volkmann's contracture, 295, 296*f*
volleyball
    data, 25
    GH joint impingement syndrome, 277
vomer, 195

W

WADA. *See* World Anti-Doping Agency
waist, 302
Walls, Robert, 252
warm-up exercises, 80
warts, 424
water
    body weight, 140
    as nutrient, 126–128
water-soluble vitamins, 121
weight chart, 445
weight cutting, 132
weight gain, in injured athletes, 139
weight lifting, spondylolisthesis, 257
weight loss, 111–113
weight management, nutrition and, 140–141
weight-training exercises, 77
wet bulb globe temperature (WBGT), 432
whiplash injuries, 198, 222
whirlpool bath safety risks, 69

wind chill chart, 451
wind chill factor, 450, 450f
Wolfe, Beth, 292–293
World Anti-Doping Agency (WADA), 144
wounds, skin, 410–413
wrestling, 23–24, 132, 134
    AC joint injuries, 267
    bleeding wounds, 411
    GH joint injuries, 267
    herpes gladiatorum, 422
    nutrition and, 132, 134
    skin problems, 426
    takedowns/escapes, 23, 23f
    thoracic strains, 251
Wrestling Minimum Weight Project (WMWP), 132
wrist dislocations, 303–304, 303f, 304f
wrist fractures, 302–303, 302f, 303f
wrist injuries
    and forearm, 300–302, 301f
        fractures, 302–303, 302f, 303f
        nerve injuries, 304–306, 305f
        sprains and dislocations, 303–304, 303f, 304f
        tendon problems, 306–307, 306f, 307f
    nerve injuries to, 304–306, 305f
    sprains, 303–304, 303f, 304f
    tendon problems of, 306–307, 306f, 307f
    and thumb taping, 314–315, 315f–317f
written contracts, 59

X

X-ray diagnoses of stress fractures, 12, 12f

Y

YMCA, 488
youth sports
    in America, 488
    injury, epidemic of, 489–490
    participation, factors in, 488
youth sports–based athletics, 154–155
Youth Sports Safety Alliance, 489–490

Z

zingiberis rhizoma, 143t
zygomatic bones, 195
    fracture, 239